Suicide Gene Therapy

METHODS IN MOLECULAR MEDICINE™

John M. Walker, SERIES EDITOR

96. **Hepatitis B and D Protocols:** *Volume 2, Immunology, Model Systems, and Clinical Studies,* edited by *Robert K. Hamatake and Johnson Y. N. Lau, 2004*

95. **Hepatitis B and D Protocols:** *Volume 1, Detection, Genotypes, and Characterization,* edited by *Robert K. Hamatake and Johnson Y. N. Lau, 2004*

94. **Molecular Diagnosis of Infectious Diseases,** *Second Edition,* edited by *Jochen Decker and Udo Reischl, 2004*

93. **Anticoagulants, Antiplatelets, and Thrombolytics,** edited by *Shaker A. Mousa, 2004*

92. **Molecular Diagnosis of Genetic Diseases,** *Second Edition,* edited by *Rob Elles and Roger Mountford, 2003*

91. **Pediatric Hematology:** *Methods and Protocols,* edited by *Nicholas J. Goulden and Colin G. Steward, 2003*

90. **Suicide Gene Therapy:** *Methods and Reviews,* edited by *Caroline J. Springer, 2003*

89. **The Blood–Brain Barrier:** *Biology and Research Protocols,* edited by *Sukriti Nag, 2003*

88. **Cancer Cell Culture:** *Methods and Protocols,* edited by *Simon P. Langdon, 2003*

87. **Vaccine Protocols,** *Second Edition,* edited by *Andrew Robinson, Michael J. Hudson, and Martin P. Cranage, 2003*

86. **Renal Disease:** *Techniques and Protocols,* edited by *Michael S. Goligorsky, 2003*

85. **Novel Anticancer Drug Protocols,** edited by *John K. Buolamwini and Alex A. Adjei, 2003*

84. **Opioid Research:** *Methods and Protocols,* edited by *Zhizhong Z. Pan, 2003*

83. **Diabetes Mellitus:** *Methods and Protocols,* edited by *Sabire Özcan, 2003*

82. **Hemoglobin Disorders:** *Molecular Methods and Protocols,* edited by *Ronald L. Nagel, 2003*

81. **Prostate Cancer Methods and Protocols,** edited by *Pamela J. Russell, Paul Jackson, and Elizabeth A. Kingsley, 2003*

80. **Bone Research Protocols,** edited by *Miep H. Helfrich and Stuart H. Ralston, 2003*

79. **Drugs of Abuse:** *Neurological Reviews and Protocols,* edited by *John Q. Wang, 2003*

78. **Wound Healing:** *Methods and Protocols,* edited by *Luisa A. DiPietro and Aime L. Burns, 2003*

77. **Psychiatric Genetics:** *Methods and Reviews,* edited by *Marion Leboyer and Frank Bellivier, 2003*

76. **Viral Vectors for Gene Therapy:** *Methods and Protocols,* edited by *Curtis A. Machida, 2003*

75. **Lung Cancer:** *Volume 2, Diagnostic and Therapeutic Methods and Reviews,* edited by *Barbara Driscoll, 2003*

74. **Lung Cancer:** *Volume 1, Molecular Pathology Methods and Reviews,* edited by *Barbara Driscoll, 2003*

73. **E. coli:** *Shiga Toxin Methods and Protocols,* edited by *Dana Philpott and Frank Ebel, 2003*

72. **Malaria Methods and Protocols,** edited by *Denise L. Doolan, 2002*

71. **Haemophilus influenzae Protocols,** edited by *Mark A. Herbert, Derek Hood, and E. Richard Moxon, 2002*

70. **Cystic Fibrosis Methods and Protocols,** edited by *William R. Skach, 2002*

69. **Gene Therapy Protocols,** *Second Edition,* edited by *Jeffrey R. Morgan, 2002*

68. **Molecular Analysis of Cancer,** edited by *Jacqueline Boultwood and Carrie Fidler, 2002*

67. **Meningococcal Disease:** *Methods and Protocols,* edited by *Andrew J. Pollard and Martin C. J. Maiden, 2001*

66. **Meningococcal Vaccines:** *Methods and Protocols,* edited by *Andrew J. Pollard and Martin C. J. Maiden, 2001*

METHODS IN MOLECULAR MEDICINE™

Suicide Gene Therapy

Methods and Reviews

Edited by

Caroline J. Springer

*Cancer Research UK Centre for Cancer Therapeutics
at the Institute of Cancer Research, Sutton, Surrey, UK*

HUMANA PRESS ✴ TOTOWA, NEW JERSEY

ISSN: 1543-1894

Printed in the United States of America. 10 9 8 7 6 5 4 3 2 1

Library of Congress Cataloging-in-Publication Data
Suicide gene therapy : methods and reviews / edited by Caroline J. Springer.
      p. ; cm. -- (Methods in molecular medicine, ISSN 1543-1894)
  Includes bibliographical references and index.
  ISBN 978-1-61737-283-4   e-ISBN 978-1-59259-429-0
  1. Cancer--Gene therapy. [DNLM: 1. Neoplasms--therapy. 2. Gene Therapy--methods. QZ 266 S948 2004] I. Springer, Caroline J. II. Series.
  RC271.G45S85 2004
  616.99'4042--dc21

                                              2003014330

Preface

Gene therapy has expanded rapidly over the last decade. The number of clinical trials reported by 2001 included 532 protocols and 3436 patients. Phase I trials predominate with 359 trials of 1774 patients versus Phase II (57 trials with 507 patients) and Phase III (3 trials of 251 patients). The disease overwhelmingly targeted by gene therapy is cancer: involving 331 trials with 2361 patients. Despite the somewhat disappointing results of clinical trials to date, gene therapy offers tremendous promise for the future of cancer therapy.

The area of gene therapy is vast, and both malignant and nonmalignant cells can be targeted. *Suicide Gene Therapy: Methods and Reviews* covers gene therapy that targets malignant cells in a treatment that has become known as "suicide gene therapy." Basically, this approach uses the transduction of cancer cells with a gene for a foreign enzyme that, when expressed, is able to activate a nontoxic prodrug into a highly cytotoxic drug able to kill the cancer cell population. This is a major area in cancer gene therapy—in 2001 this technique was represented by 52 clinical protocols with a total of 567 patients. Additional trials used multiple gene therapy protocols that also involved suicide gene therapy (83 with 497 patients), indicating that the interest in this area is considerable.

Suicide Gene Therapy: Methods and Reviews aims to cover comprehensively, both in theoretical and practical terms, the rapidly evolving area of suicide gene therapy for cancer. A multidisciplinary approach to this topic is presented here, focusing always on the state-of-the-art—from basic research to clinical practice. *Suicide Gene Therapy: Methods and Reviews* is the first book on this topic to integrate theory and practice. The reader will find an extensive review of the theoretical background of suicide gene therapy, covering all major aspects, including the design and use of vectors for gene transduction, various enzyme and prodrug systems, the mechanistic analysis of the bystander effect, the design and synthesis of prodrugs, immunological implications, and the clinical impact. The reader will find also the basic methodology used to explore, study, and expand this area.

Finally, I'd like to emphasize that in my opinion suicide gene therapy represents an area where outstanding progress has been made and that provides new hope for the treatment of cancer, especially cancer of solid tumors.

Caroline J. Springer

Acknowledgments

My sincere thanks to the authors: you were all a pleasure to work with. Also thanks to Ms. Regan Barfoot, who worked tirelessly to bring the book to fruition. This book would not have been possible without grants from Cancer Research UK (SP2330/0201 and SP2330/0102).

Contents

Preface v

Contributors xi

1 Introduction to the Background, Principles,
  and State of the Art in Suicide Gene Therapy
  Ion Niculescu-Duvaz and Caroline J. Springer *1*

2 Introduction to Vectors for Suicide Gene Therapy
  Caroline J. Springer *29*

3 Construction of VNP20009: *A Novel, Genetically Stable
  Antibiotic-Sensitive Strain of Tumor-Targeting* Salmonella
  for Parenteral Administration in Humans
  **Kenneth Brooks Low, Martina Ittensohn, Xiang Luo, Li-Mou Zheng,
  Ivan King, John M. Pawelek, and David Bermudes** *47*

4 Nonreplicating DNA Viral Vectors for Suicide Gene Therapy:
  The Adenoviral Vectors
  Masato Yamamoto and David T. Curiel *61*

5 Replication-Selective Oncolytic Adenoviruses
  **Gunnel Halldén, Stephen H. Thorne, Jingping Yang,
  and David H. Kirn** *71*

6 Retroviral Vectors for Suicide Gene Therapy
  Colin Porter *91*

7 Nonviral Liposomes
  Andrew D. Miller *107*

8 Peptide- and Polymer-Based Gene Delivery Vehicles
  Richard Brokx and Jean Gariépy *139*

9 Design of Prodrugs for Suicide Gene Therapy
  **Dan Niculescu-Duvaz, Ion Niculescu-Duvaz,
  and Caroline J. Springer** *161*

10 Cytochrome P450-Based Gene Therapies for Cancer
  E. Antonio Chiocca and David J. Waxman *203*

11 Tumor Sensitization to Purine Analogs by *E. coli* PNP
  Kimberly V. Curlee, William B. Parker, and Eric J. Sorscher *223*

12 Enzyme–Prodrug Systems: *Carboxylesterase/CPT-11*
  Mary K. Danks and Philip M. Potter *247*

13 Enzyme–Prodrug Systems:
    Thymidine Phosphorylase/5'-Deoxy-5-Fluorouridine
    Alexandre Evrard, Joseph Ciccolini, Pierre Cuq,
    and Jean-Paul Cano 263

14 Methods to Improve Efficacy in Suicide Gene Therapy Approaches:
    Targeting Prodrug-Activating Enzymes Carboxypeptidase G2
    and Nitroreductase to Different Subcellular Compartments
    Silke Schepelmann, Robert Spooner, Frank Friedlos,
    and Richard Marais 279

15 Extracellular β-Glucuronidase for Gene-Directed
    Enzyme–Prodrug Therapy
    Sabine Brüsselbach 303

16 Enhancement of Suicide Gene Prodrug Activation
    by Random Mutagenesis
    Jean-Emmanuel Kurtz and Margaret E. Black 331

17 Combination Suicide Gene Therapy
    Wolfgang Uckert, Brian Salmons, Christian Beltinger,
    Walter H. Günzburg, and Thomas Kammertöns 345

18 Immune Response to Suicide Gene Therapy
    Shigeki Kuriyama, Hirohisa Tsujinoue, and Hitoshi Yoshiji 353

19 Targeting Cancer With Gene Therapy Using Hypoxia as a Stimulus
    Gabi U. Dachs, Olga Greco, and Gillian M. Tozer 371

20 Radiation-Activated Antitumor Vectors
    Simon D. Scott and Brian Marples 389

21 In Vitro and In Vivo Models for the Evaluation of GDEPT:
    Quantifying Bystander Killing in Cell Cultures and Tumors
    William R. Wilson, Susan M. Pullen, Alison Hogg,
    Stephen M. Hobbs, Frederik B. Pruijn, and Kevin O. Hicks 403

22 Suicide Gene Therapy in Liver Tumors
    Long R. Jiao, Roman Havlik, Joanna Nicholls,
    Steen Lindkaer Jensen, and Nagy A. Habib 433

23 Clinical Trials With GDEPT:
    Cytosine Deaminase and 5-Fluorocytosine
    Nicola L. Brown and Nicholas R. Lemoine 451

24 The Nitroreductase/CB1954 Enzyme–Prodrug System
    Nicola K. Green, David J. Kerr, Vivien Mautner,
    Peter A. Harris, and Peter F. Searle 459

25 Side Effects of Suicide Gene Therapy
Marjolijn M. van der Eb, Bertie de Leeuw, Alex J. van der Eb,
and Rob C. Hoeben 479

26 Antibody-Directed Enzyme–Prodrug Therapy
R. Barbara Pedley, Surinder K. Sharma, Robert E. Hawkins,
and Kerry A. Chester 491

27 Bioreductive Prodrugs for Cancer Therapy
Beatrice Seddon, Lloyd R. Kelland, and Paul Workman 515

Index 543

Contributors

CHRISTIAN BELTINGER • *University Children's Hospital, Ulm, Germany,*

DAVID BERMUDES • *Vion Pharmaceuticals, New Haven, CT*

MARGARET E. BLACK • *Department of Pharmaceutical Sciences, Washington State University, Pullman, WA*

RICHARD BROKX • *Department of Medical Biophysics, University of Toronto, Toronto, Ontario, Canada*

NICOLA L. BROWN • *Cancer Research UK Molecular Oncology Unit, Imperial College of Science, Technology and Medicine; Hammersmith Hospital, London, United Kingdom*

SABINE BRÜSSELBACH • *Institute of Molecular Biology and Tumour Research (IMT), Philipps-University Marburg, Marburg, Germany*

JEAN-PAUL CANO • *Department of Toxicology, Faculty of Pharmacy, University of Montpellier, Montpellier, France*

KERRY A. CHESTER • *Cancer Research UK Targeting and Imaging Group, Department of Oncology, Royal Free and University College Medical School, London, United Kingdom*

E. ANTONIO CHIOCCA • *Molecular Neuro-Oncology Laboratory, Neurosurgery Service, Massachusetts General Hospital; Harvard Medical School, Boston, MA*

JOSEPH CICCOLINI • *Department of Pharmacokinetics and Toxicokinetics, Faculty of Pharmacy, University of Aix-Marseille, Marseille, France*

PIERRE CUQ • *Department of Toxicology, Faculty of Pharmacy, University of Montpellier, Montpellier, France*

DAVID T. CURIEL • *Division of Human Gene Therapy, Departments of Medicine, Pathology and Surgery, and the Gene Therapy Center, University of Alabama at Birmingham, Birmingham, AL*

KIMBERLY V. CURLEE • *Department of Human Genetics, University of Alabama at Birmingham, Birmingham, UK*

GABI U. DACHS • *Tumour Microcirculation Group, Gray Laboratory Cancer Research Trust, Mount Vernon Hospital, Northwood, UK*

MARY K. DANKS • *Department of Molecular Pharmacology, St. Jude Children's Research Hospital, Memphis, TN*

ALEX J. VAN DER EB • *Departments of Molecular Cell Biology and of Radiation Genetics, Leiden University Medical Center, Leiden, The Netherlands*

MARJOLIJN M. VAN DER EB • *Departments of Molecular Cell Biology and of Surgery, Leiden University Medical Center, Leiden, The Netherlands,*

ALEXANDRE EVRARD • *Department of Toxicology, Faculty of Pharmacy, University of Montpellier, Montpellier, France*

FRANK FRIEDLOS • *The Cancer Research UK Centre for Cancer Therapeutics, The Institute of Cancer Research, London, United Kingdom*

JEAN GARIÉPY • *Department of Medical Biophysics, University of Toronto, Toronto, Ontario, Canada*

OLGA GRECO • *Tumour Microcirculation Group, Gray Laboratory Cancer Research Trust, Mount Vernon Hospital, Northwood, UK*

NICOLA K. GREEN • *Hybrid Systems Ltd., Littlemore Park, Oxford, United Kingdom*

WALTER H. GÜNZBURG • *Institute of Virology, University of Veterinary Sciences, Vienna, Austria*

NAGY A. HABIB • *Liver Surgery Section, Division of Surgery, Anaesthetics, and Intensive Care, Faculty of Medicine, Imperial College of Science Technology and Medicine, London, United Kingdom*

GUNNEL HALLDÉN • *Viral and Genetic Therapy Programme, Cancer Research UK and Imperial College School of Medicine, Hammersmith Hospital, London, United Kingdom*

PETER A. HARRIS • *Kudos Pharmaceuticals Ltd., Cambridge, United Kingdom*

ROMAN HAVLIK • *Liver Surgery Section, Division of Surgery, Anaesthetics, and Intensive Care, Faculty of Medicine, Imperial College of Science Technology and Medicine, London, United Kingdom*

ROBERT E. HAWKINS • *Cancer Research UK Department of Medical Oncology, Christie CRUK Research Centre, Christie Hospital NHS Trust, Manchester, United Kingdom*

KEVIN O. HICKS • *Auckland Cancer Society Research Centre, The University of Auckland, Auckland, New Zealand*

STEPHEN M. HOBBS • *Institute of Cancer Research, Sutton, Surrey, United Kingdom*

ROB C. HOEBEN • *Department of Molecular Cell Biology, Leiden University Medical Center, Leiden, The Netherlands*

ALISON HOGG • *Auckland Cancer Society Research Centre, The University of Auckland, Auckland, New Zealand*

MARTINA ITTENSOHN • *Vion Pharmaceuticals, New Haven, CT*

STEEN LINDKAER JENSEN • *Liver Surgery Section, Division of Surgery, Anaesthetics, and Intensive Care, Faculty of Medicine, Imperial College of Science, Technology, and Medicine, London, United Kingdom*

LONG R. JIAO • *Liver Surgery Section, Division of Surgery, Anaesthetics, and Intensive Care, Faculty of Medicine, Imperial College of Science, Technology, and Medicine, London, United Kingdom*

THOMAS KAMMERTÖNS • *Max-Delbrück-Center for Molecular Medicine, Berlin, Germany*

LLOYD R. KELLAND • *Cancer Research UK Centre for Cancer Therapeutics, Institute of Cancer Research, Sutton, Surrey, United Kingdom*

DAVID J. KERR • *Department of Clinical Pharmacology, University of Oxford, Oxford, United Kingdom*

IVAN KING • *Vion Pharmaceuticals, New Haven, CT*

DAVID H. KIRN • *Department of Pharmacology, Oxford University Medical School, Oxford, United Kingdom*

SHIGEKI KURIYAMA • *Third Department of Internal Medicine, Kagawa Medical University, Kagawa, Japan*

JEAN-EMMANUEL KURTZ • *Department of Pharmaceutical Sciences, Washington State University, Pullman, WA*

BERTIE DE LEEUW • *Department of Molecular Cell Biology, Leiden University Medical Center, Leiden; Department of Neuro-Oncology, Erasmus University, Rotterdam, The Netherlands*

NICHOLAS R. LEMOINE • *Cancer Research UK Molecular Oncology Unit, Imperial College of Science, Technology, and Medicine; Hammersmith Hospital, London, United Kingdom*

KENNETH BROOKS LOW • *Department of Therapeutic Radiology, Yale University School of Medicine, New Haven, CT*

XIANG LUO • *Vion Pharmaceuticals, New Haven, CT*

RICHARD MARAIS • *Cancer Research UK Centre for Cell and Molecular Biology, The Institute of Cancer Research, London, United Kingdom*

BRIAN MARPLES • *Radiation Oncology Department, Karmanos Cancer Institute, Detroit, MI*

VIVIEN MAUTNER • *Cancer Research UK Institute for Cancer Studies, University of Birmingham, Birmingham, United Kingdom*

ANDREW D. MILLER • *Imperial College Genetic Therapies Centre, Department of Chemistry, Imperial College London, London, United Kingdom*

JOANNA NICHOLLS • *Liver Surgery Section, Division of Surgery, Anaesthetics, and Intensive Care, Faculty of Medicine, Imperial College of Science, Technology, and Medicine, London, United Kingdom*

DAN NICULESCU-DUVAZ • *Cancer Research UK Centre for Cancer Therapeutics at the Institute of Cancer Research, Sutton, Surrey, UK*

ION NICULESCU-DUVAZ • *Cancer Research UK Centre for Cancer Therapeutics at the Institute of Cancer Research, Sutton, Surrey, UK*

WILLIAM B. PARKER • *Southern Research Institute, Birmingham, AL*

JOHN M. PAWELEK • *Department of Therapeutic Radiology, Yale University School of Medicine, New Haven, CT*

R. BARBARA PEDLEY • *Cancer Research UK Targeting and Imaging Group, Department of Oncology, Royal Free and University College Medical School, London, United Kingdom*

COLIN PORTER • *Section of Cell and Molecular Biology at the Institute of Cancer Research, London, United Kingdom*

PHILIP M. POTTER • *Department of Molecular Pharmacology, St. Jude Children's Research Hospital, Memphis, TN*

FREDERIK B. PRUIJN • *Auckland Cancer Society Research Centre, The University of Auckland, Auckland, New Zealand*

SUSAN M. PULLEN • *Auckland Cancer Society Research Centre, The University of Auckland, Auckland, New Zealand*

BRIAN SALMONS • *Austrian Nordic Biotherapeutics AG, Vienna, Austria*

SILKE SCHEPELMANN • *The Cancer Research UK Centre for Cancer Therapeutics, The Institute of Cancer Research, London, United Kingdom*

SIMON D. SCOTT • *Department of Radiation Oncology, Karmanos Cancer Institute, Detroit, MI*

PETER F. SEARLE • *Cancer Research UK Institute for Cancer Studies, University of Birmingham, Birmingham, United Kingdom*

BEATRICE SEDDON • *Cancer Research UK Centre for Cancer Therapeutics, Institute of Cancer Research, Sutton, Surrey, United Kingdom*

SURINDER K. SHARMA • *Cancer Research UK Targeting and Imaging Group, Department of Oncology, Royal Free and University College Medical School, London United Kingdom*

ERIC J. SORSCHER • *Departments of Medicine and of Physiology and Biophysics, University of Alabama at Birmingham, Birmingham, AL*

ROBERT SPOONER • *Section of Cell and Molecular Biology at the Cancer Research UK Centre for Cancer Therapeutics, The Institute of Cancer Research, London, United Kingdom*

CAROLINE J. SPRINGER • *Cancer Research UK Centre for Cancer Therapeutics at the Institute of Cancer Research, Sutton, Surrey, UK*

STEPHEN H. THORNE • *Palo Alto Veterans Administration Medical Center and Stanford University Medical Center, Palo Alto, CA*

GILLIAN M. TOZER • *Tumour Microcirculation Group, Gray Laboratory Cancer Research Trust, Mount Vernon Hospital, Northwood, UK*

HIROHISA TSUJINOUE • *Third Department of Internal Medicine, Nara Medical University, Nara, Japan*

WOLFGANG UCKERT • *Max-Delbrück-Center for Molecular Medicine, Berlin, Germany*

DAVID J. WAXMAN • *Division of Cell and Molecular Biology, Department of Biology, Boston University, Boston, MA*

WILLIAM R. WILSON • *Auckland Cancer Society Research Centre, The University of Auckland, Auckland, New Zealand*

PAUL WORKMAN • *Cancer Research UK Centre for Cancer Therapeutics, Institute of Cancer Research, Sutton, Surrey, United Kingdom*

MASATO YAMAMOTO • *Division of Human Gene Therapy, Departments of Medicine, Pathology, and Surgery, and the Gene Therapy Center, University of Alabama at Birmingham, AL*

JINGPING YANG • *Genetic Therapy Inc./A Novartis Company, Gaithersburg, MD*

HITOSHI YOSHIJI • *Third Department of Internal Medicine, Nara Medical University, Nara, Japan*

LI-MOU ZHENG • *Vion Pharmaceuticals, New Haven, CT*

1

Introduction to the Background, Principles, and State of the Art in Suicide Gene Therapy

Ion Niculescu-Duvaz and Caroline J. Springer

1. Introduction to the Background and Principles of Suicide Gene Therapy

Chemotherapy is widely used with surgery and radiotherapy for the treatment of malignant disease. Selectivity of most drugs for malignant cells remains elusive. Unfortunately, an insufficient therapeutic index, a lack of specificity, and the emergence of drug-resistant cell subpopulations often hamper the efficacy of drug therapies. Despite the significant progress achieved by chemotherapy in the treatment of disseminated malignancies, the prognosis for solid tumors remains poor. A number of specific difficulties are associated with the treatment of solid tumors, where the access of drugs to cancer cells is often limited by poor, unequal vascularization and areas of necrosis. The histological heterogeneity of the cell population within the tumor is another major drawback. Attempts to target therapies to tumors have been addressed by using prodrugs activated in tumors by elevated selective enzymes and are described in Chapter 27. An alternative strategy that use antibodies to target tumors with foreign enzymes that subsequently activate prodrugs is described in Chapter 26.

One approach aimed at enhancing the selectivity of cancer chemotherapy for solid tumors relies on the application of gene therapy technologies. Gene therapies are techniques for modifying the cellular genome for therapeutic benefit. In cancer gene therapy, both malignant and nonmalignant cells may be suitable targets. The possibility of rendering cancer cells more sensitive to drugs or toxins by introducing "suicide genes" has two alternatives: toxin gene therapy, in which the genes for toxic products are transduced directly into tumor cells, and enzyme-activating prodrug therapy, in which the transgenes encode enzymes that activate specific prodrugs to create toxic metabolites. The latter approach, known as suicide gene therapy, gene-directed enzyme prodrug therapy (GDEPT) *(1,2)*, virus-directed enzyme prodrug therapy

From: *Methods in Molecular Medicine, Vol. 90, Suicide Gene Therapy: Methods and Reviews*
Edited by: C. J. Springer © Humana Press Inc., Totowa, NJ

(VDEPT) *(3)*, or gene prodrug activation therapy (GPAT) *(4)* may be used, in isolation or combined with other strategies, to make a significant impact on cancer treatment. In this chapter, the terms GDEPT and suicide gene therapy are used.

The terms suicide gene therapy and GDEPT can be used interchangeably to describe a two-step treatment designed to treat solid tumors. In the first step, the gene for a foreign enzyme is delivered and targeted in a variety of ways to the tumor where it is to be expressed. In the second step, a prodrug is administered that is activated to the corresponding drug by the foreign enzyme expressed in the tumor. Ideally, the gene for the enzyme should be expressed exclusively in the tumor cells compared to normal tissues and blood. The enzyme must reach a concentration sufficient to activate the prodrug for clinical benefit. The catalytic activity of the expressed protein must be adequate to activate the prodrug under physiological conditions. Because expression of the foreign enzymes will not occur in all cells of a targeted tumor in vivo, a bystander effect (BE) is required, whereby the prodrug is cleaved to an active drug that kills not only the tumor cells in which it is formed but also neighboring tumor cells that do not express the foreign enzyme *(5)*.

The main advantages of optimised suicide gene therapy systems are as follows:

1. Increased selectivity for cancer cells, reducing side effects.
2. Higher concentrations of active drug at the tumor, compared to the concentrations accessible by classical chemotherapy.
3. Bystander effects generated.
4. Tumor cell enzyme transduction and kill may induce immune responses that enhance the overall therapeutic response.
5. Prodrugs are not required to exhibit intrinsic specificity for cancer cells; they are designed to be activated by the foreign enzymes, which is technically easier to achieve.

A number of hurdles are still to be overcome. The most important are the following:

1. The vectors for gene transduction that target the tumor and achieve efficient infection of cancer cells.
2. Ideally, the vectors should be also nonimmunogenic and nontoxic.
3. The control of gene expression at the tumor.

These issues will be addressed in this chapter and in Chapters 2–8 on vectors and should be read in conjunction with reviews on the background and principles of GDEPT *(6–8)*, viral vectors *(9–15)*, and nonviral vectors *(16,17)*, the kinetics of activation *(18)*, enzymes for GDEPT *(19)*, the BE *(20)*, and prodrugs designed for GDEPT *(21–23)*.

Herein we summarize the state of the art of suicide gene therapy highlighting recent progress and the areas that to date have hampered the development of suicide gene therapy.

2. Enzymes and Prodrugs Used in Suicide Gene Therapy Systems

There are specific requirements of the enzymes used in GDEPT. They should have high catalytic activity (preferably without the need for cofactors), should be different from any circulating endogenous enzymes, and should be expressed in sufficient concentration for therapeutic efficacy. The enzymes proposed for suicide gene therapy can be characterized into two major classes. The first class comprise enzymes of nonmammalian origin with or without human counterparts. Examples include viral thymidine kinase (TK), bacterial cytosine deaminase (CD), bacterial carboxypeptidase G2 (CPG2), purine nucleotide phosphorylase (PNP), thymidine phosphorylase (TP), nitroreductase (NR), D-amino-acid oxidase (DAAO), xanthine–guanine phosphoribosyl transferase (XGPRT), penicillin-G amidase (PGA), β-lactamase (β-L), multiple-drug activation enzyme (MDAE), β-galactosidase (β-Gal), horseradish peroxidase (HRP), and deoxyribonucleotide kinase (DRNK). Those enzymes that do have human homologs have different structural requirements with respect to their substrates in comparison to the human counterparts. Their main drawback is that they are likely to be immunogenic. The second class of enzymes for suicide gene therapy comprises enzymes of human origin that are absent from or are expressed only at low concentrations in tumor cells. Examples include deoxycytidine kinase (dCK), carboxypeptidase A (CPA), β-glucuronidase (β-Glu), and cytochrome P450 (CYP). The advantages of such systems resides in the reduction of the potential for inducing an immune response. However, their presence in normal tissues is likely to preclude specific activation of the prodrugs only in tumors unless the transfected enzymes are modified for different substrate requirements.

The genes can be engineered to express their product either intracellularly or extracellularly in the recipient cells *(1)*. The extracellularly expressed variants are either tethered to the outer cell membrane *(1,24)* (*see also* Chapter 14) or secreted from cells (*see* Chapter 15). There are potential advantages to each approach. Where the enzyme is intracellularly expressed, the prodrug must enter the cells for activation and, subsequently, the active drug must diffuse through the interstitium across the cell membrane to elicit a BE. Cells in which the enzyme is expressed tethered to the outer surface or secreted are able to activate the prodrug extracellularly. A more substantial BE should therefore be generated in the latter system, but spread of the active drug into the general circulation is a possible disadvantage *(1,24)*.

The design of prodrugs tailored for GDEPT is described in depth in Chapter 9. The basic prodrug and drug requirements of a suicide gene therapy system are briefly described herein.

Good pharmacological properties, good pharmacokinetic properties of prodrugs, low cytoxicity of prodrugs with high cytotoxicity of the activated drugs, and effective activation of prodrugs by the expressed enzyme are all important features. Prodrugs should be chemically stable under physiological conditions and be highly diffusible in the tumor interstitium. The released drugs should be as potent as possible, highly diffusible, ideally active in both proliferative and quiescent cells, and induce BEs.

The activation of the prodrugs is a key step in suicide gene therapy. It is an advantage if the expressed enzyme can activate the prodrug directly to the drug, without the need for additional steps requiring further catalysis, because it is possible for the host endogenous enzymes needed for the latter steps to become defective or deficient in cancer cells.

Two basic types of prodrug have been used in GDEPT: the directly linked and the self-immolative prodrugs. The directly linked prodrugs can be defined as a pharmacological inactive derivative of a drug, which requires chemical transformation to release the active drug. In terms of anticancer activity, the conversion of the prodrug to an active drug results in a sharp increase in its cytotoxicity. In a directly linked prodrug, the active drug is released directly following the activation process (*see* Chapter 9).

A self-immolative prodrug can be defined as a compound generating an unstable intermediate which, following the activation process, will extrude the active drug in a number of subsequent steps. The most important feature is that the site of activation is normally separated from the site of extrusion. The activation process remains an enzymatic one. However, the extrusion of the active drug relies on a supplementary spontaneous fragmentation. Potential advantages of self-immolative prodrugs are the possibility of altering the lipophilicity of the prodrugs with minimal effect on the activation kinetics and the possibility to improve unfavorable kinetics of activation as a result of unsuitable electronic or steric features of the active drug. The range of drugs that can be converted to prodrugs is greatly extended and is unrestricted only by the structural substrate requirements for a given enzyme.

A large number of enzyme–prodrug systems have been developed for GDEPT in the recent years and are summarized in **Table 1**.

2.1. Quantitative Data

In order to compare different GDEPT systems in terms of therapeutic efficiency, each system should be characterized by relevant quantitative parameters. Some parameters refer to the activation process that can be described by kinetic parameters (K_M, V_{max}, and k_{cat}) (*see* **Table 2**). The concentration of the drug and the rate at which it is released at the activation site depends on the kinetic parameters of the enzyme–prodrug system. Often, published V_{max} and K_M values are not compared under equivalent conditions, whilst measuring the maximum velocity of the activation reaction and the concentration of substrate needed to reach half of this maximum velocity. Thus, there are insufficient data on enzyme–prodrug systems to allow GDEPT systems to be compared. As a rule, however, a low K_M and high V_{max} (or k_{cat}) would be expected to favor the systems. The comparison of the yeast CD with bacterial CD bears out this prediction. The yeast enzyme, which proved to be more effective than its bacterial counterpart in GDEPT experiments, exhibits lower K_M and higher V_{max} than the bacterial homolog (*see* **Table 2**). Unfortunately, comparable values for the V_{max} of these enzymes cannot be obtained because the V_{max} has been determined under very different experimental conditions for the various systems and is expressed in different ways, making direct comparisons impossible. Despite these caveats, it appears from the data in **Table 2** that prodrugs such as CMDA (a substrate of CPG2), GCV (a substrate of HSV-TK), and CPT-11 (a substrate of CA) are superior to 5-FC (a substrate of CD) or 5'-FDUR (a substrate of TP) because the latter have high K_M and low V_{max}. The turnover number, k_{cat}, provides additional information about the reaction rate, but the implications of this measure for tumor cell killing is unclear, because it is not yet known if sudden release of the active drug is more effective than a slow, constant release or if quiescent and proliferating cells differ in their sensitivity to drugs released at different rates.

Two biological parameters can be use to compare the different GDEPT systems. These are the potential of activation of a given system and its degree of activation. The first parameter is defined as the ratio of the IC_{50} of the prodrug to the IC_{50} of the released drug in a control nontransfected cell system. It represents the maximum possible efficiency of a given enzyme–prodrug system towards a cell line. The degree of activation is defined as the ratio of the IC_{50} of the prodrug in the nontransfected cell line to the IC_{50} of the prodrug in the transfected or infected cell line and demonstrates the efficiency of the system in a cell line *(18)*. These parameters allow a fair comparison between suicide gene therapy systems in vitro and should also be helpful in designing new systems.

2.2. New Systems

Most of the GDEPT systems summarized in **Table 2** are described comprehensively in this volume (*see* Chapters 9–15). However, a number of new systems have been reported in the last three years and will be briefly reviewed here.

The horseradish peroxidase (HRP) enzyme/indole-3-acetic acid (IAA) prodrug system is described with the potential for hypoxia-regulated gene therapy *(41)*. At physiological pH, IAA is activated by HRP to a long-lived species (radical) that is able to cross cell membranes, and has significantly increased cytotoxicity than the prodrug. This system is claimed to be active against T24 bladder carcinoma cells in vitro *(41)*. Another recently developed system is CYP1A2/acetaminophen *(37)*. Acetaminophen is converted to the chemically reactive metabolite *N*-acetyl-benzoquinoneimine (NABQI). Incubation of H1A2MZ cells with acetaminophen (4–20 m*M*) causes extensive cytotoxicity. When 5% of cells expressing CYP1A2 were treated with acetaminophen, complete cell killing resulted in 24 h. A potent BE was reported. Similar activity was described against the HCT116 colon carcinoma cells and SKOV-3 ovarian cancer cells but not with MDA MB 361 cells, where a 50% transfection is required to achieve total cell kill *(37)*.

Tyrosinase has been investigated as a potential prodrug-activating enzyme for GDEPT. However, its use was hampered by the low expression of tyrosinase transgenes in nonmelanotic cells and by the low activity of the enzyme. Recently, mutants of tyrosinase, which accumulate in various cellular compartments (the wild-type enzyme is present only in melanosomes), overcome these difficulties. A GDEPT system, mutated tyrosinase/*N*-acetyl-4S-cysteaminyl phenol (NAcSCAP) or 4-hydroxyphenyl propanol (HPP), was recently developed. Expression of the mutated enzyme was induced by transfection of human tumor cells (9L gliosarcoma, MCF-7 breast adenocarcinoma, and HT-1080 fibrosarcoma). Further administration of NAcSCAP or HPP stopped cell proliferation and induced cell death in a dose-dependent manner *(42)*.

Escherichia coli uracil phosphoribosyl transferase (UPRT) (E.C. 2.4.2.9) (the homologs in human cells are orotate phosphoribosyl transferase [E.C. 2.4.2.10] or uridine-5'-monophosphate synthase) catalyzes the conversion of uracil to uridine-5'-monophosphate. This enzyme is also able to mediate the conversion of 5-FU into 5-

Table 1
Enzyme–Prodrug Systems

System no.	Names and codes	Origin	Prodrugs	Released (pro)drugs	K_M (μM)	V_{max} (nM/mg/min)	k_{cat} (min^{-1})
1	Carboxyl esterase (CE)	Human, rabbit	Irinotecan 7-ethyl-10-[4-(1-piperidino)-1-piperidino]-carbonyloxy-(20S)-camptothecin	SN-38 7-ethyl-10-hydroxy-(20S)-camptothecin	23–52.9	1.43×10^{-3}	—
2	Carboxypeptidase A (CPA)	Human	MTX-α-peptides	MTX	8.2.–96	—	12,250±1135
3	Carboxypeptidase G2 (CPG2)(E.C.3.4.22.12)	Pseudomonas R16	CMDA ZD-2767P Self-immolative prodrugs	CMBA, Phenol-bis-iodo nitrogen mustard. Alkylating agents, anthracycline antibiotics	3.4 2.0	— —	34,980 1,770

No.	Enzyme	Species	Substrate	Product			
4	Cytochrome P450 human CYP2B1, 2B6,2C8, 2C9, 2C18 and 3A	Human, rat, rabbit	Oxazaphosphorines: cyclophosphamide (CP) ifosfamide (IF);	Alkylating agents	300	39.1	—
	Rat: CYP2B1		Ipomeanol, 2-aminoanthracene (2-AA);	Toxic metabolites	480	17.8	—
	Rabbit: CYP 4B1 (with or without P450 reductases)		Acetaminophen	N-acetyl benzoquinone imine (NABQI)			
5	Cytosine deaminase (CD) E.C. 3.5.4.1 (with or without uracilphosphoribosyl transferase, UPRT)	E. coli, yeast	5-Fluorocytosine (5-FC)	5-Fuorouracil (5-FU)	17,900 800	11.7 68	—
6	D-Amino-acid oxidase (DAAO)	Rohdotorula gracilis, (yeast)	D-Alanine	Hydrogen peroxide	—	—	—
7	Deoxycytidine kinase, (dCK), E.C.2.7.1.21	Human	Cytosine arabinoside	Cytosine arabinoside monophosphate	25.6	—	—

Table 1 (*continued*)
Enzyme–Prodrug Systems

System no.	Names and codes	Origin	Prodrugs	Released (pro)drugs	K_M (μM)	V_{max} (nM/mg/min)	k_{cat} (min^{-1})
8	Deoxyribonucleotide kinase (DmNK)	Drosophila melanogaster	Analogs of pyrimidine and purine 2-deoxynucleosides	Analogs of pyrimidine and purine 2'-deoxynucleotide monophosphates	—	—	—
9	DT-Diaphorase (DT-D)	Human, rat	Bioreductive agents: E09, etc.	Reduced forms	—	—	—
10	β–Galatosidase (β–Gal) E.C. 3.2.1.23	*E. coli*	Self-immolative prodrugs from anthracycline antibiotics	Anthracycline antibiotics	—	—	—
11	β-Glucuronidase (β-Glu)	Human	Self-immolative HM-1826	Doxorubicin	10.2	39.4	—
12	Horseradish peroxidase (HPP)	Plant	Indole-3-acetic acid (IAA)	?	—	—	—
13	β–Lactamase (β-L)	Bacterial	Self-immolative cephem prodrugs	Alkylating agents, *Vinca* alkaloids, anthracycline antibiotics	160	—	3,300–72,000
14	Methionine-α,γ–liase (MET)	*Pseudomonas putida*	Selenomethionine	Methylselenol	—	—	—

Table 1(*continued*)
Enzyme–Prodrug Systems

System no.	Names and codes	Origin	Prodrugs	Released (pro)drugs	K_M (μM)	V_{max} (nM/mg/min)	k_{cat} (min^{-1})
15	Multiple drug activating enzyme (MDAE)	Tomato	Acetylated 6-TG, MTX, and other purines	6-TG, MTX, cytotoxic purines	—	—	—
16	Nitroreductase (NR)	E. coli	CB-1954 and analogs; Self-immolative prodrugs	Alkylating agents; Alkylating agents pyrazolidines, enediynes	900	—	180
17	Penicillin G amidase (PGA)	E. coli	—		—	—	—
18	Purine nucleotide phosphorylase, (PNP), E.C. 2.4.2.1	E. coli	Purine nucleosides	6-methylpurine, 2-fluoroadenine	14–23	422–638[a]	—
19	Thymidine kinase (TK) E.C. 2.7.1.21	Herpes simplex virus	Modified pyrimidine nucleosides: GCV, ACV, valacyclovir, etc.	Monophosphate nucleotide analogs	11–15.8(47) 305–375	$1.3–22 \times 10^{-3}$ $3–4 \times 10^{-4}$	
20	Thymidine kinase, (TK)	Varicella-zoster virus	FIAU, purine nucleosides araM		56	680[b]	—

9

Table 1 (*continued*)
Enzyme–Prodrug Systems

System no.	Names and codes	Origin	Prodrugs	Released (pro)drugs	K_M (µM)	V_{max} (nM/mg/min)	k_{cat} (min^{-1})
21	Thymidine phosphorylase (TP), E.C. 2.4.2.4	Human	Pyrimidine analogs, 5-DFUR	5-Fluorodeoxyuridine monophosphate 5-FdRMP	325	0.17–2.28	—
22	Xanthine-guanine phosphoribbosyl transferase (XGPT)	E. coli	6-Thiopurines	6-Thiopurine nucleoside	—	—	—

ACV, acyclovir; ara-M, 6-methoxypurine arabinoside; CB1954, 5-aziridinyl-2,4-dinitrobenzamide; CMBA, N,N-2(-chloroethyl)(2-mesyloxyethyl)aminobenzoic acid; CMDA, N,N-(2-chloroethyl)(2-mesyloxyethyl)aminobenzoyl-L-glutamic acid; 5'-DFUR, 5'-deoxy-5-fluorouridine; EO9,3-hydroxy-5-aziridinyl-1-methyl-(1H-indole-4,7-dione)-propenol;FIAU, 1-(2'-deoxy-2-fluoro-b-D-arabinofuranosyl)-5-iodouracil; GCV, ganciclovir; HM-1826, N-(4-b-glucuronyl-3 nitro-benzyloxy-carbonyl)-doxorubicin; MTX, methotrexate; 6-TG, 6-thioguanine; ZD2767, 4-[bis(2-iodoethyl)aminophenyl]-oxycarbonyl-L-glutamic acid

[a] µM/min/n.
[b] Relative maximal velocity.

FU-monophosphate. The system UPRT/5-FU was suggested for GDEPT based on this conversion *(43)*. The transfection of the UPRT gene into Colon 26 murine colon carcinoma cells followed by 5-FU treatment in syngeneic immunocompetent mice bearing these tumors led to tumor regressions. However, the UPRT/5-FU system was less efficient in the rare tumors in nude mice suggesting that $\alpha\beta$-T-cells are required for the antitumor effect. The BE was marginal *(43)*. An attempt to increase the sensitivity to 5-FU of MCF-7 cells mammary tumors by transfecting the gene for pyrimidine nucleosides phosphorylase (PyNP) failed *(44)*.

2.3. Improved Strategies

A number of strategies involving the components of suicide gene therapy, including the efficacy of the enzymes, the activation processes, the prodrugs, and the administration schedules, were recently developed in order to enhance the efficacy of the systems.

2.3.1. Mutation of the Enzymes

Techniques able to increase the efficacy of enzymes to activate prodrugs within GDEPT systems have been reviewed *(19)*. A number of enzymes such as CPG2 *(24)*, CPA *(39)*, and β-glucuronidase *(38,45)* have been engineered to be expressed extracellularly (secreted or tethered to the outer cell membrane) (*see also* Chapter 14). It was also demonstrated that the intracellular location of the enzyme (distributed between the nuclear compartment and the cytoplasm or targeted to the mitochondrion) might be important for the efficacy of the NR/GDEPT system *(35)*.

A different strategy builds on crystallographic descriptions of the active site of the enzyme, which should permit the molecular modeling and, eventually, the rational synthesis, of substrates that are well suited for suicide gene therapy system. One approach consists of modifying the active site of the enzyme by site-directed mutagenesis, in order to increase its catalytic efficiency towards an existing substrate *(46,47)* (*see also* Chapter 16). This technique was applied to obtain mutants of HSV-TK showing improved kinetics of activation for GCV and ACV *(47)*. Briefly, restricted set of random sequences aimed at modifying the active site of the TK enzyme was introduced into the HSV-TK-1 gene. The mutants, thus obtained, conferred increased sensitivity to both GCV and ACV in the transfected cells. The mutated HSV-TK1 gene transfected into C6 glioma cells provided a 33- to 294-fold and 3- to 182-fold increase in GCV and ACV cytotoxicities, respectively.

The HSV-TK-75 mutant of the same enzyme (containing a four-amino-acid alteration) performed significantly better (in vitro and in vivo) compared to the wild type, as a radiosensitizer following ACV administration in RT2 glioma cells. The superiority of ACV over GCV for the treatment of brain tumors is advocated because it penetrates the blood–brain barrier better.

Site-directed mutagenesis of carboxypeptidase A was also achieved in order to improve the efficacy of this enzyme toward specifically modified substrates that are less prone to interfere with its human homolog or other human peptidases *(39)*. Recently, tyrosinase mutants were reported, which make the tyrosinase–prodrug GDEPT system workable *(42)* (*see also* **Subheading 2.2.**).

Table 2
Bystander Effect

No.	GDEPT system	Bystander effect in vitro	Bystander effect in vivo	Refs.
1	HSV-TK/GCV	>10% (need cell-to-cell contact) at 50% transfection in prostate cancer cells: best effect in DU-145 cells; low in LNCaP, none in PC-3.	—	25
2	HSV-TK/GCV	In MC-26 murine colon carcinoma cells: 30 % of transduced cells completely inhibit proliferation; at 5% there is 90% inhibition at 4.58 μL/mL GCV dose.	In female BALB/c mice: 50% of transfected cells (+ 50% GM-CSF transfected cells) produce complete tumor regression in >80% of animals.	26
3	HSV-TK/GCV	In MNNG and MLM osteosarcoma cells a significant inhibition of proliferation is obtained with more than 5% transfected cells.	98% of mice which contain as little as 5% gene modified cells demonstrated complete and lasting regressions.	27
4	HSV-TK/GCV	Percentage of TK-positive cells to achieve 50% cell survival is 10–24 and 30–88 for the human pancreatic cell lines Pan89 and PanTuI, respectively.	No quantitative data.	28
5	HSV-TK/GCV	10% and 30% BT4C glioma cells TK-transfected are able to kill 78% and 86% of the cell population.	After 14 d of GCV treatment tumors containing more than 10% BT4C-TK cells show significant reduction in tumor size and prolonged survival times.	29
6	HSV-TK/GCV	In high-density cultures of 9L glioma cells, as little as 2% 9L-TK cells produce 50% cell kill. In low-density cultures 10% of transfected cells are needed to achieve the same effect.	No quantitative data.	30

		In vivo	In vitro	Ref
7	HSV-TK/GCV	In Lobund Wistar rats carrying MLL (subline of Dunning prostate cancer cells) tumors, 25% TK-transfected cells achieve 77.6% reduction in tumor size after GCV administration.	—	4
8	HSV-TK/ GCV (BVDU)	—	Only 2% surviving 9L glioma cells survived when a mixture containing 34% TK-transfected cells was treated with a mixture of the two prodrugs.	31
9	HSV-TK/GCV, BVDU; VZV-TK/BVDU; BVaraU	Strong tumor inibition is observed in 50% TK-transfected cells (HSV-TK/GCV) After 54 d the tumors of the treated animals are 8% compared to nontreated controls.	In MDA-MB-435 all systems produced a very low BE, except HSV-TK/GCV, which at 50% transfection kill 87% of the cell population. In 9L glioblastoma all systems at roughly 50% transfection killed 90% of cell population, except HSV-TK/GCV, which at 10% transfection killed 86% of the cell population.	27
10	CD/5-FC	No quantitative data.	In SW480, SK-BR-3, and Pancl cancer cells, transfection of CD gene in 10–20% of the cells is enough to kill the cell population. In the same cells, transfection of bicistronic CD+UPRT gene in approx 1% of cells produces a near complete cell kill.	33
11	CD/5-FC	—	Transfection 20% DHD/K12 colorectal cancer cells is sufficient to induce a cytotoxic effect in 79% (at 1 mM 5-FC) and 92% (at 2 mM 5-FC) of the cell population.	34

Table 2 *(continued)*
Bystander Effect

No.	GDEPT system	Bystander effect in vitro	Bystander effect in vivo	Refs.
12	NR/CB1954	In MDA-MB-361 cells 90% cell kill is achieved with 34% of cells transfected with NRwt or 40% cells transfected with NRmt.	—	35
13	NR/CB1954	In B-cell line, transfection of less than 5% cells with NR gene following CB1954 administration achieves approx 90% killing	Tumors containing either 30% or 100% transfected cells were growth inhibited but not cured.	36
14	CYP1A2/ acetaminophen	Exposure to 4 mM acetaminophen of a mixture of H12M7 cells containing 5% CYP1A2-transfected cells results in complete kill in 24 h. The same result was obtained with SK-OV-3 and HCT116 but not with MDA-MB-361 cells.	—	37
15	h-β-Glu/HMR1826	In JEG-3 human choriocarcinoma cells at 2% transfection of the *h-β-glu* gene followed by HMR1826 produces a dramatic BE (no quantitative data).	At 50% transfection strong antitumoral effect is shown in JEG-3 tumor-bearing animals and a weaker one in A549 lung tumor-bearing animals.	38
16	CPA/MTX-α-peptides	A culture of SCCVII cells expressing the CPA gene exhibits a SF < 0.001 (99.9% killing). At 5% transfection the SF is <0.1 (90% killing).	—	39
17	CPG2/CMDA	—	In animal bearing MDA-MB-361 tumor xenografts 10% stCPG2(Q)3 cells produce tumor regression and 6% cures. At 50% enzyme-expressing cells the number of cures is 50%.	40

BVDU, (E)-5-(2-bromovinyl)-2'-deoxyguanine; BVaraU, (E)-5-(2-bromovinyl)-1-β-D-arabinofuranosyl uracil; UPRT, uracil phosphoribosyltransferase; *see also* Table 1.

2.3.2. Multiple-Gene Transfection

A different strategy to develop more efficient suicide gene therapy systems uses transgenes with greater than one gene. Several different approaches have been reported.

Some prodrugs are activated by a metabolic cascade involving the sequential action of several enzymes. For example, in the activation of GCV to GCV triphosphate (GCVTP), three different kinases (HSV-TK, guanylate kinase, and nucleoside diphosphate kinase) are involved, acting in series. The multigene approach requires the cotransfection of genes for each of these enzymes and is expected to increase the overall yield of the desired final metabolite, the active drug. In the case of GCV, it has been claimed that the simultaneous transfection of these three genes allowed cells to convert >90% of the prodrug to GCVTP *(48)*. Likewise, the cotransfection of the genes for cyt-P450 and the P450-reductase significantly increased the conversion of CP to it toxic metabolites and, therefore, improved the overall efficiency of the cyt-P450/CP GDEPT system *(49)*.

The same strategy was applied to the CD/5-FC system, which showed poor results in cancer cell lines (such as breast and pancreatic carcinoma cell lines) resistant to 5-FU, because of defects in the downstream metabolism of 5-FU. Transduction of a bicistronic fusion gene encoding CD and uracil phosphotransferase was superior to the CD system alone both in vitro and in vivo *(33)*.

A different approach consisted of the transduction of two (or more) copies of the same gene in the target cells. It was demonstrated that the UMSCC29 and T98G human cancer cell lines containing two copies of the TK gene led to more effective metabolism of GCV and, therefore, exhibited enhanced sensitivity to the prodrug *(50)*.

An alternative approach consisted of transfecting target cells with two different suicide genes. These express enzymes able to activate two distinct types of prodrug, releasing anticancer drugs with different mechanisms of action and therefore making the system more effective. Examples were reported in which cells were infected with CYP+CD or TK+CD genes. In each case, the "double suicide gene" systems proved to be more effective both in vitro and in vivo compared to each single system *(51,52)*. Systems combining a suicide gene with an immunity enhancing gene were also reported *(53)*.

2.3.3. New Prodrugs for Old Systems

A different way of improving GDEPT systems is to design prodrugs with lower cytotoxicity. Also, complementary strategies of increasing the cytotoxicity of the released drugs or improving the activation process may be helpful. Some highly cytotoxic compounds (with IC_{50} in the nanomolar range) such as enediyines, cyclopropylindolines, and taxoids are now available, but, generally, their structures are complicated and efficient ways are needed to convert them to less toxic prodrugs. Designing self-immolative analogs of these prodrugs is one method, as are modifications that improve the uptake of the prodrug or alter the lipophilicity of the prodrug. New efforts were put into tailoring the prodrugs for use with an extracellular or intracellular activating enzyme (*see also* Chapter 9)

The most investigated enzyme used in a GDEPT system is HSV-TK. The prodrugs for activation by HSV-TK are GCV and ACV and similar analogs, which are not ideal because their kinetics are rather poor (high K_M and low V_{max}) and because they do not achieve the best compromise between potency and propensity to cross the blood–brain barrier. Despite the fact that GCV is, on average, 10-fold more potent then ACV, the latter is better able to cross the blood–brain barrier. These data prompted the assessment of new prodrugs: (*E*)-5-(2-bromovinyl)-2'-deoxyuridine (BVDU) and (*E*)-5-(2-bromovinyl)-1-β-D-arabinofuranosyl uracil (BVaraU) for the HSV- or VZV-TK systems *(31,32,54)*. Both compounds exhibited IC_{50} in the range 0.06–0.4 µ*M* in cells transfected with VZV-TK, whereas GCV was inactive. BVDU, elicited the same IC_{50} as GCV in HSV-TK transfected cells in contrast with BvaraU, which proved to be inactive. In vivo results confirm the effectiveness of BVDU in both HSV- and VZV-TK systems. However, in 9L gliosarcoma, BVDU was also inactive *(32)*. Experimental data showed that when BVDU and GCV were administered simultaneously, both the cell direct killing and the BE were enhanced. These facts led to the suggestion that suicide gene therapy using two different prodrugs metabolized by the same enzyme could be much more effective compared to the same system utilizing just one of them *(31)*.

In order to replace GCV with a less genotoxic alternative, penciclovir (PCV) (a GCV analog) was investigated. It was found that GCV was incorporated into the genomic DNA much more effectively than PCV, which is less genotoxic. For both prodrugs, apoptosis is the major route of cytotoxicity. However, because PCV induces apoptosis very effectively without major genotoxicity, it was recommended as a safer alternative to GCV *(55)*.

In order to avoid the bone marrow cytotoxicity associated with the HSV-TK/GCV system, the novel guanosine analog (1'*S*, 2'*R*)-9-{[1', 2'-bis(hydroxymethyl)cycloprop-1'-yl]methyl}guanine was designed. The compound had a similar potency to GCV when assayed in TK transfected cells in vitro but was devoid of an inhibitory effect against bone marrow progenitor cells and colony formation *(56)*.

2.3.4. Potentiation and Synergistic Effects

An alternative strategy to increase the efficiency of GDEPT systems was developed from a better understanding of the mechanisms of action of the released drugs based on synergistic or additive effects of compounds. This approach was applied to improve the HSV-TK/GCV and CD/5-FC systems. Combinations of these two GDEPT systems are assessed in Chapter 17.

Ponicidin (a diterpenoid isolated from *Rabdosia ternifolia*) was found preferentially to activate the HSV-1-TK kinase but not the cellular enzymes. The compound showed a synergistic antiviral effect with both GCV and ACV. When ponicidin was combined with GCV or ACV at a concentration devoid of antiviral activity (0.2 µ*M*/L), the cytotoxicities of both prodrugs in TK transfected cells were increased by 3- to 87-fold and 5- to 52-fold, respectively, as compared with prodrug alone *(57)*.

Four compounds with apoptosis inducing properties (butyrate, camptothecin, taxol, and 7-hydroxystaurosporine) were assayed in conjunction with the HSV-TK/GCV system. It was found that GCV+butyrate and GCV+7-hydroxystaurosporine combinations resulted in increased Bak and decreased Bcl-X_L protein levels, whereas the GCV+camptothecin and GCV+taxol combinations increased the level of both proteins. These results may be useful in increasing cell apoptosis in colon cancers using HSV-TK/GCV *(58)*.

Finally, hydroxyurea (HU) was suggested as a possible combination with GCV in the HSV-TK/GCV system, because HU is able to reduce the level of dGTP, which is the endogenous competitor of GCV-TP for DNA incorporation *(59)*. Isobologram analysis demonstrated that the combination GCV+HU is additive in HSV-TK transfected cell cultures and synergistic in HSV-TK bystander mixtures *(60)*.

A similar rationale was applied to enhance the capabilities of the CYP2B1/CP system. A strategy aimed at minimizing the hepatic toxicity without diminishing its antitumoral potency was devised by using a CP–methimazole combination. Methimazole (MMI) is an antithyroid drug, which reduces hepatic P450-reductase gene expression and, therefore, reduces the NADPH-dependent P450-reductase activity in the liver but does not affect the activity of P450-reductase in 9L glioma cells growing in vivo. The combination CP+MMI was shown to increase the therapeutic index of CP in CYP2B1/ CP models in vivo *(61)* (Chapter 10).

A bioreductive drug, tirapazamine, is also able to increase the efficacy of CYP2B6/ CP under hypoxic conditions (1% O_2) after transfection of 9L glioma cells *(62)*.

The optimization of administration schedules as a means of improving the efficacy of suicide gene therapy is another approach. It was reported that repeated transfections of HVJ liposomes combined with repeated injections of 5-FC elicited much better results in vivo than single transfections *(63)*. A CYP2B1/P450-reductase/CP system showed that daily (for 6 d) moderate-dose (140 mg/kg) administrations significantly improved the efficacy of the system *(64)*.

2.3.5. Radiosensitization

Radiotherapy is a valuable alternative to chemotherapy with or without surgery, in the complex strategy of cancer treatment. Therefore, its combination with suicide gene therapy has been proposed as an advantage. HSV-TK gene transfection was used to increase the radiosensitivity of various cell lines. Specific incorporation of halogenated pyrimidine radiosensitizers such as 5-bromo-2'-deoxycytidine (BrdC) as 5-bromo-2'-deoxyuridine (BrdU) was demonstrated in transfected cells, increasing their sensitization ratio 1.4–2.3 times, compared with β-Gal transfected cells *(65)*. The effect was confirmed in vivo using RT2 glioma cells in Fisher 344 rats and it was proposed that HSV-TK transfection followed by BrdC administration and radiation may be a useful clinical treatment for glioma *(65)*.

A similar strategy of radiosensitization was proposed with the HSV-TK/ACV system. Using a mutant of the wild-type enzyme (HSV-TK-75, which is more effective in metabolising ACV), an enhanced sensitizing effect was shown in RT2 glioma cells. The cells become more sensitive to low doses of radiation (2–4 Gy), suggesting that this combination could improve glioma treatment *(66,67)*.

Radiation-inducible promoters have been proposed to control the expression of transgenes in cancer cells *(68)*, in *Clostridium* bacteria *(69,70)*, and in other vectors *(see* Chapter 20).

Finally, improving the bystander effect is another option (*see* **Subheading 4.2.**).

3. Imaging

One of the major problems in suicide gene therapy is the lack of good visualization techniques to monitor the delivery and the distribution of therapeutic transgenes in vivo. For gene transfer analysis in vitro, enhanced green fluorescent protein (EGFP) has proved useful. This technique has recently been applied to the HSV-TK and CYP4B1/ipomeanol systems *(71)*.

One possible approach to the imaging of gene expression in animals utilizes positron-emission tomography (PET) with reporter genes (PRGs) and PET reporter probes (PRPs). This technology was used for imaging of the HSV-TK/GCV system *(72–74)*. Recently, ^{125}I-FIAU was proposed as an effective PRP for imaging of the HSV-TK expression in vivo *(75)*.

Magnetic resonance spectroscopy (MRS) is another method of tackling the imaging problem. A large number of studies has demonstrated a correlation between different cancer treatments in patients and modification of the MRS of the corresponding tumors. Recently, it was reported that the efficacy of the treatment with HSV-TK/ GCV system can be monitored in vivo using ^{31}P-MRS *(4)*.

4. The Bystander Effect

The BE in a suicide therapy system can be defined as the cytotoxic effect on nongenetically modified cells following prodrug administration when only a fraction of the tumor mass is genetically modified to express an activating enzyme *(76)*. The successes described in GDEPT would surely not be possible without the existence of such an effect. However, although the BE is difficult to quantitate, especially in vivo, models have been devised to examine the BE (*see* Chapter 21). Other phenomena (e.g., the immune response) can contribute strongly to the overall effect and are examined in Chapter 18. Data on the BE generated by various GDEPT systems in vitro and in vivo are summarized in **Table 2**.

4.1. Mechanisms of the Bystander Effect

The prodrugs activated in GDEPT systems can release active drugs that are either diffusible or nondiffusible across cell membranes. Diffusible toxic metabolites formed following prodrug activation and released from dead and dying genetically modified cells will spread, according to diffusion laws, within the tumor cell population. This mechanism is postulated for the majority of GDEPT systems, such as 5-FU formed from 5-FC; for the metabolites of CP or IP, aldophosphamide, phosphoramidic mustards or acrolein, for benzoic acid mustard released from CMDA, and for 6-MeP, formed from the corresponding deoxynucleoside. The most relevant feature of such a mechanism is that cell-to-cell contact is not required for the killing of untransfected cells either in vitro or in vivo. The BE relies only on the diffusibility of the active drugs in the tumor interstitium and across the tumor cell membranes and on their cytotoxic potential. A number of examples support this assumption (*see* **Table 2**).

For purine or pyrimidine nucleoside prodrugs, the mechanism of the BE is different, the toxic metabolites are generally phosphorylated and are, therefore, not diffusible across cell membranes. The HSV-TK/GCV system requires cell-to-cell contact to display a BE. The transfer of toxic metabolites from cell to cell mainly requires the existence of gap-junctional intercellular communications (GJICs), but other mechanisms could also be involved. The GJICs vary with the cell line and are measured using dye (e.g., Lucifer yellow) diffusion through gap junctions. It was demonstrated that the level of GJIC is predictive of the extent of the BE in vitro, whatever the origin of the cancer cell lines. Consistent with this model, a number of reports showed that tumor cells resistant to BE did not show dye transfer from cell to cell, whereas BE-sensitive tumor cells did *(20)*. However, there are some exceptions that suggest that the BE is not completely mediated by gap junctions, even if cell-to-cell contact is necessary *(77)*. BE has been observed in vivo and generally there is a relationship between in vitro and in vivo behavior. The BE in vivo can be enhanced by collateral immune effects.

Another effect called the "Good Samaritan effect" has also been described. This effect refers to the observation that transfected cells can be protected from the active drug, presumably by lowering the concentration of the cytotoxic metabolites through GJIC *(78,79)*. This can be considered as beneficial because the transgenes will last longer, producing more toxic metabolites, thus enhancing the BE. On the other hand, it can be regarded as detrimental, making the eradication of the whole cell population more difficult.

4.2. Improving the Bystander Effect

In the GDEPT systems involving diffusible metabolites, it is difficult to pinpoint methods to enhance the local transfer of the active drug. One possibility is to express the enzyme extracellularly on the surface of tumor cells (*see* Chapters 14 and 15). Another way is to release drugs that can cross the cell membrane by active transport.

There are a number of options for the improvement of the BE based on the GJIC hypothesis for the GDEPT systems releasing nondiffusible toxic metabolites. It was noted that the GJIC can be controlled pharmacologically by using dieldrin, a drug that decreases cell-to-cell communications. The dye transfer diminished and dieldrin also inhibited the BE. Cyclic-AMP, foskolin, corticoids, carotenoids, and flavanoids (such as flavanone, apigenin, and tangeretin) are able to induce GJIC in vitro. This effect may be cell-specific or connexin-specific. The BE was also induced in vivo with c-AMP and retinoids *(20)*. Apigenin and lovastatin, an inhibitor of HMG-CoA reductase, both upregulate gap-junction function and dye transfer in tumors expressing gap junctions *(80,81)*.

In one report studying human lung tumor cell lines of different origins, significant cell killing occurred when only 10% of cells expressed HSV-TK. In this system, GJICs were not apparent from measuring the rapid intercellular transport of Lucifer yellow, which detects "rapid-transfer" gap-junctional communications, although it could be seen by the slow transfer of a different dye, calcein-AM, which measures the "slow-transfer" gap junctions. However, neither an inhibitor (1-octanol) nor an enhancer (all-*trans* retinoic acid) of gap junctions affected the extent of the BE, suggesting either that low levels of gap junctions can produce a maximal BE or that bystander cell killing occurs by other means *(77)*.

The GJICs are heavily dependent on the activity of connexins. The type of connexin expressed does not appear to be crucial for the BE because similar results were obtained with cells expressing different types of connexin. It was, however, demonstrated that the transfection of connexin genes into a number of different tumor cells (i.e., PC12 adrenal pheochromocytoma, HT-116 colon carcinoma, N2A neuroblastoma, C6 glioma) significantly increased the BE for the HSV-TK/GCV system. In a recent example, it was demonstrated that transfection of the *Cx43* gene in MDA MB 435 breast cancer cell line restores GJIC and that high expression of Cx43 enhanced the BE of the HSV-TK/GCV system. On the other hand, the noncommunicating MDA MB 435 breast cancer cell line triggered a significant BE both in vitro and in vivo with the HSV-TK/GCV system, suggesting that mechanisms other than GJIC may be involved in the BE *(82)*.

Another explanation may be that the TK enzyme or the toxic metabolites can be transported by apoptotic vesicles in nontransfected cells. However, the fact that the BE can be induced in the absence of apoptotic death in hepatocarinoma cells and that the transfer of GCV-TP occurs before apoptotic degeneration is in opposition to this assumption *(82,83)*. Phagocytosis of material from dying TK-positive cells (e.g., hydrolases or other lytic enzymes) to bystander cells has also been suggested as a mechanism for the BE. Apoptosis was detected in bystander cells and it was found that this event could be inhibited by *Bcl2* expression. However, during the apoptosis-induction period, in bystander cells cocultured with HSV-TK expressing cells, no phagocytosis was observed. It has also been suggested that killing of tumor cells by apoptosis could heighten the immune response to wild-type tumor cells by a priming effect.

5. Immune Effect in Suicide Gene Therapy Systems

It is generally accepted that the immune response improves the efficacy of GDEPT systems in vivo. Several lines of evidence strengthen this view. The first is that although the BE has been observed in immunocompromised animals, data suggest that the BE in vivo is mediated largely through the release of cytokines *(84)* and, therefore, GDEPT systems are more efficient in immunocompetent animals.

The second is the existence of the "distant bystander effect." A distant BE has been reported in a number of situations when tumors anatomically separated and with no possible metabolic cooperation were inhibited after suicide gene therapy was administered only to one tumor *(4,85)*. An immune-related response has been proposed to explain this effect. However, there are conflicting opinions because previous reports described the occurrence of the distant BE in immunodeficient animals. A new model was devised recently by implanting colorectal tumors cell in two different lobes of the liver, followed by HSV-TK/GCV therapy to only one tumor. After GCV administration, the distant tumors regressed partially or totally, the distant BE being observed in

92% of animals. This study clearly demonstrated that the distant BE was the result of an immune response *(85)*.

The third line of evidence is given by the cotransfection of both suicide genes and immune enhancing genes. The transgenes containing both a suicide gene and granulocyte macrophage colony stimulating factor *(GM-CSF)* or interleukin *(IL)* gene proved to be more effective when compared to the suicide gene therapy alone. An HSV-TK suicide gene therapy system in conjunction with *GM-CSF* gene was administered in BaLB/c mice bearing M-26 colon carcinoma, followed by GCV administration. Although there were no differences in the size of tumors as compared with HSV-TK/GCV alone, tumors regrew only in mice receiving the TK gene alone. Such combined systems are also able to induce complete or partial resistance to a tumor rechallenge *(26)*. Great efficacy as well as antimetastatic activity was shown by the same HSV-TK+GM-CSF/GCV system in a model of metastatic breast cancer *(86)*. Similar observations were reported for the CD/5-FC system. It was found that intraperitoneal administration of adenoviral vector AdSCF/AdGM-SCF in mice bearing CT26 colon adenocarcinoma followed by treatment with AdCF/5-FC could suppress tumor growth and prolong the survival period *(87)*.

It has been suggested that some drugs released during suicide gene therapy in vivo could produce tumor necrosis and an inflammatory response, which may break down the immunological isolation and elicit an immune response *(88)*. Such drugs may have a definite advantage in comparison with those inducing apoptosis. It was believed that for the CYP2B1/IF system, the phosphoramide mustard resulting after activation causes DNA cross links inducing cell death by apoptosis. However, a recent study demonstrated a necrotic mechanism of cell death. This may have important implications for the activation of the immune system *(89)*.

6. Clinical Evaluation

There have been a number of clinical trials with different suicide gene therapies. An important consideration are the side effects of the different components. These may be elicited by the vectors, the enzyme, and/or the prodrugs and are reviewed in Chapter 25. Clinical studies with HSV-TK/GCV, CD/5-FC, and NR/CB1954 are reviewed in Chapters 22, 23, and 24, respectively.

7. Conclusions

Some hurdles must be overcome before GDEPT will become a clinically efficient treatment of cancers.

The simultaneous release of active drugs that can act by different mechanisms, leading to a synergistic effect on tumor cells and the design of more effective new types of prodrug, is another way to progress. Modalities to enhance and to control the BE, particularly if cell-permeable and cell-impermeable active metabolites can be released together may be useful to improve the therapies. Also, the occurrence of resistant populations is less likely for drugs with different mechanisms of action.

GDEPT systems have already shown efficacy in vivo. Future developments in this technology should use mutagenesis to obtain more efficient activation of a given prodrug or to adapt the active site so that it binds better to prodrugs that are not substrates for endogenous enzymes. The prodrugs, too, could be redesigned to create better substrates for the enzymes, to maximize drug release or the BE, to take advantage of self-immolative strategies of activation, or to allow the active drug to accumulate more readily in tumor cells. Finally, it will also be useful to investigate the ways in which different prodrug systems synergize with each other or with other cancer treatments. The combination of GDEPT with radiotherapy or immunotherapy has previously been investigated. Such approaches may involve either a sequential treatment schedule (GDEPT/radiation therapy or GDEPT/immunotherapy) or the transfection of suicide gene(s) together with genes able to increase the sensitivity of the tumors to radiation or enhance the potential of the host immune system with cytokine genes.

Improvements are needed in vector design area to enhance targeting and delivery of suicide genes. Multiple options are available, including nonviral vectors, more complex systems involving coexpression of suicide genes with immunological or tumor suppressor genes, and selectively replicating viruses (*see* Chapters 2–8).

References

1. Marais, R., Spooner, R. A., Light, Y., Martin, J., and Springer, C. J. (1996) Gene-directed enzyme prodrug therapy with a mustard prodrug/carboxypeptidase G2 combination. *Cancer Res.* **56**, 4735–4742.
2. Bridgewater, G., Springer, C. J., Knox, R., Minton, N., Michael, P., and Collins, M. (1995) Expression of the bacterial nitroreductase enzyme in mammalian cells renders them selectively sensitive to killing by the prodrug CB1954. *Eur. J. Cancer* **31A**, 2362–2370.
3. Huber, B. E., Richards, C. A., and Austin, E. A. (1995) VDEPT; an enzyme/prodrug gene therapy approach for the treatment of metastatic colorectal cancer. *Adv. Drug Delivery Rev.* **17**, 279–292.
4. Eaton, J. L., Perry, M. J. A., Todryk, S. M., et al. (2001) Genetic prodrug activation therapy (GPAT) in two rat prostate models generates an immune bystander effect and can be monitored by magnetic resonance techniques. *Gene Ther.* **8**, 557–567.
5. Hermiston, T. (2000) Gene-delivery from replication-selective viruses: arming guided missiles in the war against cancer. *J. Clin. Invest.* **105**, 1169–1172.
6. Roth, J. A. and Cristiano, R. G. (1997) Gene therapy for cancer: what have we done and where are we going? *J. Natl. Cancer Inst.* **89**, 21–30.
7. Niculescu-Duvaz, I., Spooner, R., Marais, R., and Springer, C. J. (1998) Gene-directed enzyme prodrug therapy. *Bioconj. Chem.* **9**, 4–22.
8. Springer, C. J. and Niculescu-Duvaz, I. (1999) Patent property of prodrug involving gene therapy (1996–1999). *Exp. Opin. Ther. Patents* **9**, 1381–1388.
9. Bilbao, G., Contreras, J. L., Gómez-Navarro, J., and Curiel, D. T. (1998) Improving adenoviral vectors for cancer gene therapy. *Tumor Target.* **3**, 59–79.
10. Nguyen, J. T., Wu, P., Clouse, M. E., Hlatky, L., and Terwilliger, E. F. (1998) Adeno-associated virus-mediated delivery of antiangiogenic factors as an antitumor stratergy. *Cancer Res.* **58**, 5673–5677.
11. Robbins, P. D. and Ghivizzani, S. C. (1998) Viral vectors for gene therapy. *Pharm. Ther.* **80**, 35–47.
12. Zhang, W. W. (1999) Development and application of adenoviral vectors for gene therapy of cancer. *Cancer Gene Ther.* **7**, 113–138.

13. Curiel, D. T., Gerritsen, W. R. and Krul, M. R. (2000) Progress in cancer gene therapy. *Cancer Gene Ther.* 7, 1197–1199.

14. Roth, M. G. and Curiel, D. T. (2000) Toward the optimal vector for prostate cancer gene therapy; a CaPCURE meeting report. *Cancer Gene Ther.* 7, 1507–1510.

15. Kirn, D. (2001) Clinical research results with dI 1520 (ONYX-015), a replication selective adenovirus for the treatment of cancer: what have we learned? *Gene Ther.* 8, 89–98.

16. Miller, A. D. (1998) Cationic liposomes for gene therapy. *Angew. Chem. Int. Ed.* 37, 1768–1785.

17. Schatzlein, A. G. (2001) Non-viral vectors in cancer gene therapy: principles and progress. *Anti-Cancer Drug Des.* 12, 275–304.

18. Springer, C. J. and Niculescu-Duvaz, I. (2000) Prodrug-activating systems in suicide gene therapy. *J. Clin. Investig.* 105, 1161–1167.

19. Encell, L. P., Landis, D. M. and Loeb, L. A. (1999) Improving enzymes for gene therapy. *Nature Biotechnol.* 17, 143–147.

20. Mesnil, M. and Yamasachi, H. (2000) Bystander effect in herpes simplex virus–thymidine kinase/ganciclovir cancer gene therapy: role of gap-junctional intercellular communications. *Cancer Res.* 60, 3989–3999.

21. Denny, W. A. and Wilson, W. R. (1998) The design of selectively-activated anti-cancer prodrugs for use in antibody-directed and gene-directed enzyme prodrugs therapies. *J. Pharm. Pharmacol.* 50, 387–394.

22. Niculescu-Duvaz, I., Friedlos, F., Niculescu-Duvaz, D., Davies, L., and Springer, C. J. (1999) Prodrugs for antibody- and gene-directed enzyme prodrug therapies (ADEPT and GDEPT). *Anticancer Drug Des.* 14, 517–538.

23. Springer, C. J. and Niculescu-Duvaz, I. (2002) Gene-directed enzyme prodrug therapy, in Anticancer Drug Development (Baguley, B., ed.), Academic, New York, pp. 137–135.

24. Marais, R., Spooner, R. A., Stribbling, S. M., Light, Y., Martin, J., and Springer, C. J. (1997) A cell surface tethered enzyme improves efficiency in gene-directed enzyme prodrug therapy. *Nature Biotechnol.* 15, 1373–1377.

25. Loimas, S., Toppinen, M.-R., Visakorpi, T., Janne, J., and Wahlfors, D. (2001) Human prostate carcinoma cells as target for herpes simplex virus thymidine kinase-mediated suicide gene therapy. *Cancer Gene Ther.* 8, 137–144.

26. Jones, R. K., Pope, I. M., Kinsella, A. R., Watson, A. J. M., and Christmas, S. E. (2000) Combined suicide and granulocyte–macrophage colony-stimulating factor gene therapy induces complete tumor regression and generates antitumor immunity. *Cancer Gene Ther.* 7, 1519–1528.

27. Walling, H. W., Swarthout, G. T., and Culver, K. W. (2000) Bystander-mediated regression of osteosarcoma via retroviral transfer of the herpes simplex virus thymidine kinase and human interleukin-2 genes. *Cancer Gene Ther.* 7, 187–196.

28. Howard, B. D., Boenicke, L., Schniewind, B., Henne-Bruns, D., and Kalthoff, H. (2000) Transduction of human pancreatic tumor cells with vesicular stomatitis virus G-pseudotyped retroviral vectors containing a herpes simplex virus thymidine kinase mutant gene enhances bystander effects and sensitivity to ganciclovir. *Cancer Gene Ther.* 7, 927–938.

29. Sandmair, A.-M., Turunen, M., Tyynela, K., et al. (2000) Herpes simplex virus thymidine kinase gene therapy in experimental rat BT4C glioma model: effect of the percentage of thymidine kinase-positive glioma cells on treatment effect, survival time, and tissue reactions. *Cancer Gene Ther.* 7, 413–421.

30. Kruse, C. A., Lamb, C., Hogan, S., Russell Smiley, W., Kleinschmidt-DeMasters, B., and Burrows, F. G. (2000) Purified herpes simplex thymidine kinase retroviral particles. II.

Influence of clinical parameters and bystander killing mechanisms. *Cancer Gene Ther.* **7,** 118–127.

31. Hamel, W., Zirkel, D., Mehdorn, H. M., Westphal, M., and Israel, M. A. (2001) E-5-(2-bromovinyl)-2'-deoxyuridine potentiates ganciclovir-mediated cytotoxicity on herpes simplex virus-thymidine kinase-expressing cells. *Cancer Gene Ther.* **8,** 388–396.

32. Grignet-Debrus, C., Cool, V., Baudson, N., et al. (2000) Comparative in vitro and in vivo cytotoxic activity of (E)-5-(2-bromovinyl)-2'-deoxyuridine (BVDU) and its arabinosyl derivative, (E)-5-(2-bromovinyl)-1-β-D-arabinofuranosyluracil (BVaraU), against tumor cells expressing either the Varicella zoster or the Herpes simplex virus thymidine kinase. *Cancer Gene Ther.* **7,** 215–223.

33. Erbs, P., Regulier, E., Kintz, J., et al. (2000) In vivo cancer gene therapy by adenovirus-mediated transfer of a bifunctional yeast cytosine deaminase/uracil phosphoribosyltransferase fusion gene. *Cancer Res.* **60,** 3813–3822.

34. Bentires-Alj, M., Helin, A.-C., Lechanteur, C., et al. (2000) Cytosine deaminase suicide gene therapy for peritoneal carcinomatosis. *Cancer Gene Ther.* **7,** 20–26.

35. Spooner, R. A., Maycroft, K. A., Paterson, H., Friedlos, F., Springer, C. J., and Marais, R. (2001) Appropriate subcellular location of prodrug-activating enzymes has important consequences for suicide gene therapy. *Int. J. Cancer* **93,** 123–130.

36. Westphal, E.-M., Ge, J., Catchpole, J. R., Ford, M., and Kennedy, S. C. (2000) The nitroreductase/CB1954 combination in Eptein–Barr virus-positive B cell lines: induction of bystander killing in vitro and in vivo. *Cancer Gene Ther.* **7,** 97–106.

37. Tatcher, N. J., Edwards, R. J., Lemoine, N. R., Doehmer, J., and Davies, D. S. (2000) The potential of acetaminophen as a prodrug in gene-directed enzyme therapy. *Cancer Gene Ther.* **7,** 521–525.

38. Heine, D., Muller, R., and Brusselbach, S. (2001) Cell surface display of a lysosomal enzyme for extra-cellular gene-directed enzyme prodrug therapy. *Gene Ther.* **8,** 1005–1010.

39. Hamstra, D. A., Page, M., Maybaum, J., and Rehemtulla, A. (2000) Expression of endogenously activated secreted or cell surface carboxypeptidase A sensitizes tumor cells to methotrexate-α-peptide prodrugs. *Cancer Res.* **60,** 657–665.

40. Stribbling, S. M., Friedlos, F., Martin, J., et al. (2000) Regressions of established breast cancer xenografts by carboxypeptidase G2 suicide gene therapy and the prodrug CMDA are due to a bystander effect. *Human Gene Ther.* **11,** 285–292.

41. Greco, O., Folkes, L. K., Wardman, P., Tozer, G. M., and Dachs, G. U. (2000) Development of a novel enzyme/prodrug combination for gene therapy of cancer: horseradish peroxidase/indole-3-acetic acid. *Cancer Gene Ther.* **7,** 1414–1420.

42. Simonova, M., Wall, A., Weissleder, R., and Bogdanov, A. (2000). Tyrosinase mutants are capable of prodrug activation in transfected non-melanotic cells. *Cancer Res.* **60,** 6656–6662.

43. Kawamura, K., Tasaki, K., Hamada, H., Takenaga, K., Sakiyama, S., and Tagawa, M. (2000) Expression of *Escherichia coli* uracil phosphoribosyltransferase gene in murine colon carcinoma cells augments the antitumoral effect of 5-fluorouracil and induces protective immunity. *Cancer Gene Ther.* **7,** 637–643.

44. Cuq, P., Rouquet, C., Evrard, A., Ciccolini, J., Vian, L., and Cano, J.-P. (2001) Fluoropyrimidine sensitivity of human MCF-7 breast cancer cells stably transfected with human uridine phosphorylase. *Br. J. Cancer* **84,** 1677–1680.

45. Weyel, D., Sedlacek, H. H., Muller, R., and Brusselbach, S. (2000) Secreted human β-glucuronidase: a novel tool for gene-directed enzyme prodrug therapy. *Gene Ther.* **7,** 224–231.
46. Black, M. E., Newcomb, T. G., Wilson, H. M., and Loeb, L. A. (1996) Creation of drug-specific herpes simplex virus type 1 thymidine kinase mutants for gene therapy. *Proc. Natl. Acad. Sci. USA* **93,** 3525–3529.
47. Black, M., Kokoris, M. S., and Sabo, P. (2001) Herpes simplex virus-1 thymidine kinase mutants created by semi-random sequence mutagenesis improve prodrug-mediated tumor cell killing. *Cancer Res.* **61,** 3022–3026.
48. Blanche, F., Cameron, B., Couder, M., and Crouzet, J. (1997). *Enzymes Combinations for Destroying Proliferative Cells,* US Patent W09735024, Rhone-Poulenc Roerer, p. 1–61.
49. Chen, L., Yu, L. J., and Waxman, D. J. (1997) Potentiation of cytochrome P450/cyclo-phosphamide-based cancer gene therapy by coexpression of the *P450 reductase* gene. *Cancer Res.* **57,** 4830–4837.
50. Kim, Y. G., Bi, W., Feliciano, E. S., Drake, R. R., and Stambrook, P. J. (2000) Ganciclovir-mediated cell killing and bystander effect is enhanced in cells with two copies of the herpes simplex virus thymidine kinase. *Cancer Gene Ther.* **7,** 240–246.
51. Kammertoens, T., Gelbmann, W., Karle, P., et al. (2000) Combined chemotherapy of murine mammary tumors by local activationof the prodrug ifosfamide and 5-fluorocytosine. *Cancer Gene Ther.* **7,** 629–636.
52. Rogulski, K. R., Wing, M. S., Paielli, D. L., Gilbert, J. D., Kim J. H., and Freytag, S. O. (2000) Double suicide gene therapy augments the antitumor activity of a replication-competent lytic adenovirus through enhanced cytotoxicity and radiosensitization. *Human Gene Ther.* **11,** 67–76.
53. Toda, M., Martuza, R. L., and Rabkin, S. D. (2001) Combination suicide/cytokine gene therapy as adjuvants to a defective herpes simplex virus-based cancer vaccine. *Gene Ther.* **8,** 332–339.
54. Candotti, F., Agbaria, R., Mullen, C. A., et al. (2000) Use of a herpes thymidine kinase/neomycin phosphotransferase chimeric gene for metabolic suicide gene therapy. *Cancer Gene Ther.* **7,** 574–580.
55. Thust, R., Tomicic, M., Klocking, R., Voutilainen, N., Wutzler, P., and Kaina, B. (2000) Comparison of the genotoxic and apoptosis-inducing properties of ganciclovir and penciclovir in chinese hamster ovary cells transfected with the thymidine kinase gene of herpes simplex virus-1: implication for gene therapeutic approaches. *Cancer Gene Ther.* **7,** 107–117.
56. Hasegawa, Y., Nishiyama, Y., Imaizumi, K., et al. (2000) Avoidance of bone marrow suppression using A-5021 as a nucleoside analog for retrovirus-mediated herpes simplex virus type I thymidine kinase gene therapy. *Cancer Gene Ther.* **7,** 557–562.
57. Hayashi, K., Hayashi, T., Sun, H.-D., and Takeda, I. (2000) Potentiation of ganciclovir toxicity in the herpes simplex virus thymidine kinase/ganciclovir administration system by ponicidin. *Cancer Gene Ther.* **7,** 45–42.
58. McMasters, R. A., Wilbert, T. N., Jones, K. E., et al. (2000) Two-drug combinations that increase apoptosis and modulate Bak and Bcl-X$_L$ expression in human colon tumor cell lines transduced with herpes simplex virus thymidine kinase. *Cancer Gene Ther.* **7,** 563–573.
59. Rubsam, L. Z., Davidson, L., and Shewach, D. S. (1998) Superior cytotoxicity with gancyclovir compared with acyclovir and 1-β-D-arabinofuranosylthymine in herpes simplex virus-thymidine kinase-expressing-cells: a novel paradigm for cell killing. *Cancer Res.* **58,** 3873–3882.

60. Boucher, P. D., Ostruszka, L. J., and Shewach, D. S. (2000) Synergistic enhancement of herpes simplex virus thymidine kinase/ganciclovir mediated cytotoxicity by hydroxyurea. *Cancer Res.* **60,** 1631–1636.
61. Huang, Z., Raychowdhury, K., and Waxman, D. J. (2000) Impact of liver P450 reductase suppression on cyclophosphamide activation, pharmacokinetics and antitumoral activity in a cytochrom P450-based cancer gene therapy model. *Cancer Gene Ther.* **7,** 1034–1042.
62. Jounaidi, Y. and Waxman, D. J. (2000) Combination of the bioreductive drug tirapazamine with the chemotherapeutic prodrug cyclophosphamide for P450/P450-reductase-based cancer gene therapy. *Cancer Res.* **60,** 3761–3769.
63. Kanyama, H., Tomita, N., Yamano, T., et al. (2001) Usefulness of repeated intratumoral gene transfer using hemagglutinating virus of Japan-liposome method for cytosine deaminase suicide gene therapy. *Cancer Res.* **61,** 14–18.
64. Jounaidi, Y. and Waxman, D. J. (2001) Frequent, moderate dose cyclophosphamide administration improves the efficacy of cytochrome P-450/cytochrome P-450 reductase based cancer gene therapy. *Cancer Res.* **61,** 4437–4444.
65. Brust, D., Feden, J., Farnsworth, J., Amir, C., Broaddus, W. C., and Valerie, K. (2000) Radiosensitization of rat glioma with bromodeoxycytidine and adenovirus expressing herpes simplex virus-thymidine kinase delivered by slow, rate-controlled positive pressure infusion. *Cancer Gene Ther.* **7,** 778–788.
66. Valerie, K., Brust, D., Farnsworth, J., et al. (2000) Improved radiosensitization of rat glioma cells with adenovirus-expressed mutant herpes simplex virus-thymidine kinase in combination with acyclovir. *Cancer Gene Ther.* **7,** 879–884.
67. Valerie, K., Hawkins, W., Farnsworth, J., et al. (2001) Substantially improved in vivo radiosensitization of rat glioma with mutant HSV-TK and acyclovir. *Cancer Gene Ther.* **8,** 3–8.
68. Kawashita, Y., Ohtsuru, A., Kaneda, Y., et al. (1999) Regression of hepatocelluar carcinoma in vitro and in vivo by radiosensitising suicide gene therapy under the inducible and spatial control of radiation. *Hum. Gene Ther.* **10,** 1509–1519.
69. Nuyts, S., Theys, J., Landuyt, W., Van Mellaert, L., Lambin, P., and Anne, J. (2001) Increasing specificity of anti-tumour therapy: cytotoxic proteins delivery by non-pathogenic Clostridia under regulation of radio-induced promoter. *Anticancer Res.* **21,** 857–862.
70. Nuyts, S., Van Mellaert, L., Theys, J., Landuyt, W., Lambin, P., and Anne, J. (2001) The use of radiation-induced bacterial promoters in anaerobic-conditions: a means to control gene expression in Clostridium-mediated gene therapy. *Radiat. Res.* **155,** 716–723.
71. Steffens, S., Frank, S., Fisher, U., et al. (2000) Enhanced green fluorescent proteinfusion proteins of herpes simplex virus type 1 thymidine kinase and cytochrome P450 4B1: applications for prodrug-activating gene therapy. *Cancer Gene Ther.* **7,** 806–812.
72. Tjuvajev, J.G., Finn, R., Watanabe, K., et al. (1996) Noninvasive imaging of herpes simplex virus thymidine kinase gene transfer and expression: a potential method for monitoring clinical gene therapy. *Cancer Res.* **56,** 4087–4095.
73. Tjuvajev, J.G., Avril, N., Oku, T., et al. (1998) Imaging herpes virus thymidine kinase gene transfer and expression by positron emission tomography. *Cancer Res.* **58,** 4333–4341.
74. Yagoubi, S. S., Wu, L., Liang, Q., et al. (2001) Direct correlation between positron emission tomographic images of two reporter genes delivered by two distinct adenoviral vectors. *Gene Ther.* **8,** 1072–1080.
75. Brust, P., Haubner, R., Friedrich, A., et al. (2001) Comparison of [^{18}F]FHPG and [$^{124/125}$I]FIAU for imaging herpes simplex virus type 1 thymidine kinase gene expression. *Eur. J. Nucl. Med* **28,** 721–729.

76. Huber, B. E., Austin, E. A., Richards, C. A., Davis, S. T., and Good, S. S. (1994) Metabolism of 5-fluorocytidine to 5-fluorouracil in human colorectal tumor cells transduced with the cytosine deaminase gene: significant antitumor effects when only a small percentage of tumor cells express cytosine deaminase. *Proc. Natl. Acad. Sci. USA* **91,** 8302–8306.

77. Imaizumi, K., Hasegawa, Y., Kawabe, T., Emi, N., Saito, H., Naruse, K., and Shimokata, K. (1998) Bystander tumoricidal effect and gap junctional communication in lung cancer cells. *Am. J. Respir. Cell Mol. Biol.* **18,** 205–212.

78. Wygoda, M. R., Wilson, M. R., Davis, M. A., Trosko, J. E., Rehemtulla, A., and Lawrence, T. S. (1997) Protection of herpes simplex virus thymidine kinase-transduced cells from ganciclovir-mediated cytotoxicityby bystander cells: the good Samaritan effect. *Cancer Res.* **57,** 1699–1703.

79. Andrade-Rosental, A. F., Rosental, R., Hopperstad, M. D., Wu, J. K., Vrionis, F. D., and Spray, D. C. (2000) Gap junctions: the "kiss of death" and the "kiss of life." *Brain Res. Rev.* **32,** 308–315.

80. Touraine, R. L., Vahanian, N., Ramsey, W. J., and Blaese, R. M. (1998) Enhancement of the herpes simplex virus thymidine kinase/ganciclovir bystander effect and its antitumor efficacy in vivo by pharmacologic manipulation of gap junctions. *Hum. Gene Ther.* **9,** 2385–2391.

81. Touraine, R. L., Ishii-Morita, H., Ramsey, W. J., and Blaese, R. M. (1998) The bystander effect in the HSVtk/ganciclovir system and its relation to gap junctional communication. *Gene Ther.* **5,** 1705–1711.

82. Grignet-Debrus, C., Cool, V., Baudson, N., Velu, T., and Calberg-Bacq, C.-M. (2000) The role of cellular- and prodrug-associated factors in the bystander effect induced by the *Varicella zoster* and *Herpes simplex* viral thymidine kinases in suicide gene therapy. *Cancer Gene Ther.* **7,** 1456–1468.

83. Kaneko, Y. and Tsukamoto, A. (1995) Gene therapy of hepatoma: bystander effect s and non-apoptotic cell death induced by thymidine kinase and ganciclovir. *Cancer Lett.* **96,** 105–110.

84. Ramesh, R., Marrogi, A. J., Munshi, A., Abboud, C. N., and Freeman, S. M. (1996) In vivo analysis of the "bystander effect": a cytokine cascade. *Exp. Hematol.* **24,** 829–838.

85. Agard, C., Ligeza, C., Dupas, B., et al. (2001) Immune-dependent distant bystander effect after adenovirus-mediated suicide gene transfer in a rat model of liver colorectal metastasis. *Cancer Gene Ther.* **8,** 128–136.

86. Majumdar, A., Zolotorev, A., Samuel, S., et al. (2000) Efficacy of herpes simplex virus thymidine kinase in combination with cytokine gene therapy in an experimental metastatic breast cancer model. *Cancer Gene Ther.* **7,** 1086–1099.

87. Cao, X., Huang, X., Ju, D.W., Zhang, W.P., Hamada, H., and Wang, J. (2000) Enhanced antitumoral effect of adenovirus-mediated cytosine deaminase gene therapy by induction of antigen-presenting cells through stem cell factor/granulocyte macrophage colony-stimulating factor gene transfer. *Cancer Gene Ther.* **7,** 177–186.

88. Rivas, C., Chandler, P., Melo, J. V., Simpson, E., and Apperley, J. F. (2000) Absence of in vitro or in vivo bystander effects in a thymidine kinase-transduced murine T-lymphoma. *Cancer Gene Ther.* **7,** 954–962.

89. Karle, P., Renner, M., Salmons, B., and Gunzburg, W. H. (2001) Necrotic, rather than apoptotic death caused by cytochrome P450-activated ifosfamide. *Cancer Gene Ther.* **8,** 220–230.

2

Introduction to Vectors for Suicide Gene Therapy

Caroline J. Springer

1. Introduction

Suicide gene therapy requires vectors or vehicles capable of efficient and selective gene delivery of the therapeutic genes to tumor cells. A number of vector systems has been proposed for gene therapy. These include: the viral vectors, adenoviruses (*see* Chapters 4 and 5), adeno-associated viruses (AAV), herpes simplex virus *(1)*, parvoviruses, lentiviruses, retroviruses *(2,3)* (*see* Chapter 6), naked DNA (with or without electroporation) *(4)*, bacteria (*see* Chapter 3)—and nonviral vectors—cationic lipids, liposomes, polyethyleneimine (PEI), polyamino acids, peptides, and dendrimers (*see* Chapters 7 and 8).

Three issues are of major importance: the targeting of the cancer cells, the efficiency of transduction, and the safety of administration in humans. Transduction efficiencies (in vitro and in vivo) for a number of systems are shown in **Table 1**.

2. Vectors in Suicide Gene Therapy

Adenoviruses have achieved better transduction rates (10–50%) in vivo than retroviruses (0.9–14.6%). Nonviral vectors (with electroporation) have achieved up to 8% transfection in vivo. Unusually high values (up to 59%) have been reported for nonviral vector transfection in vivo. However, the highest values (>80%) were reported for a combination of viral and nonviral vectors (adenovirus complexed with PEI or DEAE-dextran) (*see* **Table 1**).

For applications such as ex vivo infections, direct administration of the vector to target tissues in vivo, or locoregional delivery, the ability to target specific cells may not be necessary. Of 333 protocols that were ongoing in cancer gene therapy in February 2001, >38% used intratumoral or locoregional delivery. However, if systemic delivery is required, targeting will be of major importance.

From: *Methods in Molecular Medicine, Vol. 90, Suicide Gene Therapy: Methods and Reviews*
Edited by: C. J. Springer © Humana Press Inc., Totowa, NJ

Table 1
In Vitro and In Vivo Transduction Efficiencies

No.	Delivery vector	Gene delivered	Type of cells infected	In vitro (%)	In vivo (%)	Ref.
1	Nonviral (folate-containing cationic liposomes)	p53 (Squamous carcinoma head and neck tumor cells)	JSQ-3	10–70	40–50	5
2	Nonviral: DC-6 141 commercially available liposomes			1.0 0.23–0.62	—	6
3	Nonviral (HVJ liposomes + plasmids)	HSV-TK (herpes simplex virus-thymidine kinase)	HuH7 (Human hepatocellular carcinoma in male SCID mice)	—	19.7±6.0	7
4	Nonviral (DOTAP + plasmids)	CD (cytosine deaminase)	HCT116 MDA MB 435 9L glioma OVCAR-3	0.7 0.7 3.0 10.5	—	8
5	Nonviral (lipofectin + integrin targeted peptides + plasmids)	HRP	T24 human bladder carcinoma cells: pRK34-HRP pCI-EGFP	20–26 60–70	—	9

Table 1 *(continued)*
In Vitro and In Vivo Transduction Efficiencies

No.	Delivery vector	Gene delivered	Type of cells infected	In vitro (%)	In vivo (%)	Ref.
6	Nonviral (cationic liposome, PAAD + EBV-based plasmids)	HSV-TK (β-Gal)	HCC: HLE, PLC/PRF/5, and HuH7 pSES-TK (EBV) pS-TK	35 3	—	*10*
7	Nonviral HVJ-AVE liposomes)	*LacZ*	Purkinje cells of cerebral vermis and upper cervical cord	—	29.0–59.4	*11*
8	Adenovirus (adenovirus complexed with PEI, DEAE-dextran, lipofectamine, etc.)	β-Gal	Human adenocarcinoma cell line Mz-ChA-2 Ad-5 β-Gal + cationic lipids + lipofectamine + PEI + DEAE-dextran	1 36–12 85–10 >99 >99	>80 >80	*12*
9	Adenovirus (conjugated with polylysine)	HSV-TK	Human bladder cancer cells UM-UC-3 UM-UC-14	66^a 63^a	—	*13*

31

Table 1 *(continued)*
In Vitro and In Vivo Transduction Efficiencies

No.	Delivery vector	Gene delivered	Type of cells infected	In vitro (%)	In vivo (%)	Ref.
10	Adenovirus (replicative defective lacking E1 and E3 regions)	HSV-TK+GM-CSF+IL-2	Metastatic breast cancer cells 4T1	>50	15–22	*14*
11	Adenovirus (replication defective, replication conditional)	*LacZ*	Human glioblastoma cells U87DEGFR replicative defective virus replicative conditional virus	—	10[a] 40[a]	*15*
12	Adenovirus	Rabbit carboxyl esterase	Neuroblastoma cell lines: NB-1643 and 1691, SJNB-1, IMR-32 (MOI 50) PBMNC (MOI 500)	100 0	—	*16*
13	Adenovirus (containing a Myc-Max element)	HSV–TK	SCLC	90–100	—	*17*
14	Adenovirus [using the L-plastin promoter: Ad-Lp-lacZ(I) compared to Ad-CMV-LacZ (II)]	*LacZ*, CD	In explant cultures of: Ascites Primary tumor Metastatic tumor Normal peritoneum	(I) (II) 10–35 50–80 15–60 50–90 15–45 45–85 1–4 60–80	—	*18*
15	Adenovirus	*LacZ*	Human bladder cancer cell lines: KU-7 (MOI 50) and UMUC-2 (MOI100)	90	—	*19*

Table 1 (*continued*)
In Vitro and In Vivo Transduction Efficiencies

No.	Delivery vector	Gene delivered	Type of cells infected	In vitro (%)	In vivo (%)	Ref.
16	Adenovirus (incorporating CMV or AFP promoter)	LacZ	Hepatocellular carcinoma in woodchuck: Tumor samples Nontumor samples	—	 5–50 20–80	*20*
17	Adenovirus [incorporating the the midkine (MK) promoter]	HSV-TK, luciferase	Wilms' tumor cells (G-401) and neuroblastoma cells (SK-N-SH)	>15 <15	—	*21*
18	Adenovirus	HSV-TK, LacZ	Administered to rats glioma cells as: Infusion (5×10^9 pfu, 150 µL, 1 µL/min) Infusion (5×10^9 pfu, 50 µL) Infusion (5×10^9 pfu, 3 × 50 µL)		 40 5 25	*22*
19	Adenovirus	CD, UPRT, and CD + UPRT	Human colon cancer cells, SW 480 Human breast cancer cells, SK-BR-3 Human pancreas cancer cells, PANC-1 Human colon cancer cells, LoVo, all at MOI 20 Melanoma cancer cells, B16F0 (MOI 200)	96.2±0.8 99.0±0.4 91.7±2.5 92.3±1.9 12.6±2.5	—	*23*

33

Table 1 *(continued)*
In Vitro and In Vivo Transduction Efficiencies

No.	Delivery vector	Gene delivered	Type of cells infected	In vitro (%)	In vivo (%)	Ref.
20	Adenovirus (incorporating CMV promoter)	CD	Type of cells transduced at : MOI 10: Colo320, WiDr, HCT116, LoVo, T84 MOI 10-100: HT29, Colo620, SkCo-1CC35 (murine) MOI 100–1000: Colo205 MOI > 1000MCA26 (murine)	50[a]	—	*24*
21	Adenovirus, lentivirus, Semliki forest virus, and Sindbis virus	HSV-TK	Human prostate carcinoma lines: DU-145, LN-CaP and PC-3 transfected with: adenovirus lentivirus Semliki forest virus Sindbis virus	23–53 29–39 0.6–3.7 0.1–3.6	— —	*25*
22	Retrovirus (recombinant retroviruses bearing the ecotropic envelope or the feline endogenous virus RD114 envelope)	HSV-TK, *LacZ*	Human rabdomyosarcoma cells, TE 671, colorectal carcinoma cells SW620, CACO2, breast carcinoma MDA MD-361 and Kaposi derived sarcoma KS Y-1	33–57 (46±47)	—	*26*

Table 1 (*continued*)
In Vitro and In Vivo Transduction Efficiencies

No.	Delivery vector	Gene delivered	Type of cells infected	In vitro (%)	In vivo (%)	Ref.
23	Retrovirus (replicative defective STK vector)	HSV-TK, IL-2	Osteosarcoma cells MNNG and MLM	79–91	0.9–14.6 (average: 6.6)	27
24	Retrovirus	Carboxypeptidase A, LacZ	Murine squamous cell carcinoma, SCCVII	~50		28
			Human squamous cell carcinoma, UMSCC6	25–30		
			Human breast cancer cells, MCF-7	25–30		
25	Retrovirus	HSV-TK	Rauscher virus induced T-cell lymphoma, RAM	17–20	—	29
26	Retrovirus, plasmids + Fugene 6	EGFP, HSV-TK+EFGP and CYP 4B1 + EFGP	Rat glioma cell line 9L	59	—	30
			Human glioma cell line U87	10		
27	Plasmids + electroporation	NR (nitroreductase)	Human Burkitt lymphoma cells, Jijoye cells, and EBV-positive marmoset B cells, B95-8	2–5	—	31
28	Plasmids + electroporation	NR	Human hepatocellular carcinoma cells, HepG2	—	0.1	32
29	Plasmids + electroporation	IL-2, IL-12	Metastasising subline of melanoma, B16.F10	—	3–8	33
			Same without elecroporation		0.1	

35

Table 1 *(continued)*
In Vitro and In Vivo Transduction Efficiencies

No.	Delivery vector	Gene delivered	Type of cells infected	In vitro (%)	In vivo (%)	Ref.
30	Adeno-associated virus (AAV)	HSV-TK, *LacZ*	A293 cells Squamous cell carcinoma line from a human maxillary sinus cancer, NKO-1	~100 64	—	*34*
31	Adenovirus (transfected) macrophages)	CYP2B6, LacZ	Breast cancer cells spheroids	>80	—	—

CMV, cytomegalovirus; CYP, cytochrome P450; DEAE-dextran, diethylaminoethyl-dextran; DOTAP, 1,2-dioleoyloxy-3-(trimethyl ammonium)propane; EBV, Epstein–Barr virus; EGFP, enhanced green fluorescent protein; GM-CSF, granulocyte-macrophage colony stimulating factor; HCC, human hepatocellular carcinoma cells; HRP, horseradish peroxidase; HSV-TK, herpes simplex virus–thymidine kinase; HVJ, hemagglutinating virus of Japan; IL, interleukin; MK, midkine; MOI, multiplicity of infections; PAAD, polyamidoamine dendrimer; PEI, polyethyleneamine; PBMNC, peripheral blood mononuclear cells; SCLC, small-cell lung cancer cells; UPRT, uracil phosphoribosyltransferase.

*a*Estimated by using LacZ expressing vector.

2.1. Bacteria as Vectors

Bacterial vectors have been developed for use in gene therapy. One example, *Salmonella typhimurium*, localizes to melanoma tumors following systemic injection in mice (*see* Chapter 3). The wild-type pathogen led to death in the mice, whereas attenuated, hyperinvasive auxotropic mutants (by deletion of the *mbH* gene leading to lipid A metabolism) showed specific melanoma targeting following intravenous (iv) administration, with tumor : liver ratios in the range of 250 : 1 to 9000 : 1. When inoculated into C57BL6 mice bearing B16F10 melanomas, the tumor growth was suppressed and prolonged animal survival resulted. A *Salmonella* vector containing the thymidine kinase (TK) gene under the control of a β-lactamase secretion signal was developed and following ganciclovir (GCV) treatment showed efficacy in in vivo systems *(35,36)*

Other bacteria, such as *Clostridium acetobutylicum* and *Bifidobacterium longum* have been shown selectively to germinate and grow in hypoxic regions of tumors after iv injections. An accumulation ratio tumor : liver of greater than 10^3 was reported for *Bifidobacterium (37)*. *Bifidum* bacteria harboring marker genes were constructed and this gene delivery system was claimed to be tumor-specific and nontoxic.

The spores of the anaerobic, apathogenic bacteria *Clostridium* were shown to germinate and proliferate only in tumors. To obtain an efficient infiltration of *Clostridium* in the tumor, at least 10^7 spores had to be systemically administered. In tumors, stable concentrations of 10^9 colony-forming units/g (cfu/g) were found. In normal tissues, the concentrations ranged between 10^4 and 10^6 cfu/g and decreased with time *(38)*. *Clostridium* was genetically engineered to express tumor necrosis factor-α (TNF-α) and cytosine deaminase (CD) genes. The specificity of *Clostridia* was further improved by using a radiation-induced promoter to control the therapeutic genes *(38,39)*

2.2. Viral Vectors

This category of vectors presents a number of advantages, especially in terms of transfection efficiencies with respect to other categories (*see* **Table 1**). The main concerns are related to the hazards associated with their administration in humans. Unfortunately, gene therapy trials have shown that gene transfer remains disappointingly low, with primary tumors proving more resistant than in animal models *(40)*. Nontumor cells may also become infected during the transduction procedures. However, both conceptual and practical progress has been made recently to overcome these deficiencies.

2.2.1. CAR Independent Delivery

The lack of coxsachie and adenovirus receptors (CARs) in many primary tumor cells was identified as the main cause of their resistance to transfection with adenoviral vectors. For instance, CAR deficiency seems to be a near-universal feature of epithelial neoplasms *(40)*. To date, adenoviruses have been used widely because they can be produced in high titers, can infect many different cell types, and can produce a transient expression of the transgene (*see* Chapters 4 and 5). This led to the development of adenoviral vectors capable of "CAR-independent delivery" by retargeting to alternative receptors selectively expressed on tumor cells (*see* Chapter 4).

One strategy is based on retargeting using antiadenoviral fiber antibodies. A typical example is the development of the EpCAM-targeted adenoviral vector. EpCAM is a surface antigen that is overexpressed in the majority of adenocarcinomas compared to the normal epithelial counterparts. The vector was targeted to EpCAM through a bispecific antibody conjugate antiEpCAM/antiknob. Targeting ratios between 0.6 and 5.9 were achieved on clinical samples of gastric and esophageal cancers *(41)*. Using a similar strategy, retargeting to other cellular receptors including integrins, α-folate receptor, and epidermal growth factor receptor (EGFR) has been achieved (*see* Chapter 4). A potential disadvantage of this approach is the uncertain stability of the virus conjugates as well as the complexity of the system.

An alternative strategy uses a genetically modified targeting viral particle. Insertion of an Arg-Gly-Asp (RGD) motif into the HI loop of the adenoviral fiber knob resulted in efficient CAR-independent vectors by promoting the binding of the virus to integrins *(42)*. The resulting vector, Ad-luc-RGD, containing a recombinant fiber RGD protein and expressing luciferase revealed efficient CAR-independent infection of pancreatic carcinoma cells *(42)*.

2.2.2. Replication-Selective Viruses

A different way of enhancing gene transfer is to make use of post-transductional amplification (i.e., to employ replicating viral vectors) *(40,43,45)* (*see* Chapter 5). A variety of viruses has been employed, including adenoviruses *(46)* and herpes viruses *(45)*. An antitumor effect can be achieved directly by the conditionally replicative viruses or "oncolytic viruses." These vectors spread and proliferate within the tumor and, therefore, the transgene may also be extended both temporarilly and anatomically. Another advantage of this approach is that the replicating viruses can deliver therapeutic transgenes called "armed" replicating viruses, thus enhancing the potential for the eradication of the tumor *(43)*.

In a study using an HSV-replication competent vector containing *LacZ* as marker gene, a transfection efficiency in vivo in U87D glioma cells of 40% was demonstrated (*see* **Table 1**) as compared to 10% for the nonreplicative vector counterpart. LacZ transfection was stable for 14 d for the replicative vector, whereas it decreased sharply after 3 d for the nonreplicative vector *(15)*. Recombinant HSV replicative virus is capable of infecting many types of cell, allowing insertion of large DNA sequences or multiple genes. Antiviral drugs are capable of controlling the infection. G-207 is a second-generation conditionally replicating recombinant HSV-1 virus designed for clinical use in malignant brain tumors. The vector also had a *LacZ* inserted and harbored an intact *TK* gene. Gene therapy using this vector followed by GCV administration generated conflicting results, despite the high sensitivity of the transfected cells to the drug. GCV may induce the death of the G-207-infected cells and also generates a bystander effect (BE). Furthermore, GCV-mediated cell death may elicit a favorable immune response against tumor cells, thus enhancing the overall antitumor effect. On the other hand, the drug can inhibit G-207 replication, thus preventing the spread of the virus and its oncolytic effect. Phosphorylated GCV can produce the premature termination of the replicating DNA strands and affect both viral and genomic DNA syntheses *(45,47)*. These opposing mechanisms of action support the observation that treatment with GCV, following the administration of the replicative-competent HSV-1, does not enhance its antitumor effect in certain situations *(47)*.

Other GDEPT systems may benefit from the use of this vector. Introduction of cytochrome P450 CYP2B1 gene into the HSV-1 vector showed that cyclophosphamide (CPA) had a minimal effect on the viral infection and enhanced the antitumor effect of the virus *(43,48)*. Similar results were obtained with the HSV-1yCD (CD, cytosine deaminase) vector in conjunction with 5-fluorocytosine (5-FC) treatment, where the antitumor effect was augmented and the virus replication was unaffected *(49)*.

Replication-selective adenoviruses have also been engineered *(44)*. The most well known is ONYX-015, which has a deletion in the adenovirus E1B region enabling it to replicate preferentially in tumor cells (*see* Chapter 5). There are reports that the insertion of the TK gene in this vector (AdTK^{RC}) followed by GCV administration augmented the antitumor effect with respect to the virus alone in melanoma, cervical, and colon carcinoma xenografts *(50,51)*. However, later work could not confirm the augmentation of the effect following GCV treatment *(52–54)*. Although data suggesting that the addition of the TK gene in the replicating virus is not beneficial, the concept of "armed" replicating viruses is likely to have benefits using other GDEPT systems.

2.2.3. Promoter-Specific Expression

One way to achieve targeting specificity towards cancer cells is the use of tissue-specific promoters. This procedure is also known as tissue-targeted expression *(55,56)* (*see* Chapter 19). If a tumor cell overexpresses a particular protein because of increased specific transcriptional activity of its promoter (rather than gene duplication), and a therapeutic gene is inserted downstream of this promoter, then introduction of this DNA sequence into these tumor cells should allow specific expression of the gene. Here, normal tissue that is also transduced would express much lower levels of the gene product and express none in an ideal system. This methodology (transcriptional selectivity) does not enhance transfection efficiency, but it is able to increase the expression of a therapeutic gene in cancer cells and to prevent or minimize the expression of the same gene in normal (surrounding) cells.

A number of promoters has already been investigated with positive results: for example, α-fetoprotein (AFP) promoter to target hepatocellular carcinoma, prostate-specific antigen (PSA) to target prostate cancer, Willebrandt factor to target endothelial cells, DF3 MUC-1 promoter to target breast cancer cells, tyrosinase promoter to target melanoma cells, JC virus promoter and myelin-based promoter to target glioma cells, prs-9 promoter to target rabdomyosarcoma cells, c-erbB2 promoter to target breast, pancreatic, and non-small-cell lung cancer (NSCLC) cells, and the osteocalcin promoter to target osteosarcoma *(55)*.

Recently the midkine promoter (MK) was suggested for the treatment of pediatric tumors (Wilms tumor and neuroblastoma). MK is a newly identified heparin-binding growth factor that is transiently expressed in the early stages of retinoic acid-induced differentiation of embryonal carcinoma cells and is overexpressed in many human malignant tumors. A recombinant replication-defective adenovirus containing the TK gene under the control of the MK promoter followed by GCV administration achieved high activity in Wilms tumors (G-401) and neuroblastoma (SK-N-SH). In contrast with adenoviral vectors harboring the *TK* gene under control of the cytomegalovirus (CMV) promoter, the system did not produce any liver toxicity following GCV administration *(21)*. The promoter of the vascular endothelial growth factor (VEGF) that is activated by hypoxia was found to be useful in killing highly metastatic Lewis lung carcinoma A11 cells under hypoxic conditions. A retroviral vector was constructed harboring the HSV-TK gene under the control of the VEGF promoter *(57)*.

Several examples showed that the use of enhancers in conjunction with specific promoters in viral constructs may be beneficial. Placing a 1455-bp PSA-enhancer sequence upstream of either the PSA or the glandular kallicrein promoter (hKLK2) increased the expression of the marker gene in the PSA-positive prostate cancer cell line LNCaP by 20-fold. Tandem duplication of the PSA enhancer increased expression to 50-fold whilst retaining tissue specificity. Furthermore, expression of all enhancer constructs was increased 100-fold above basal levels when induced with dihydrotestosterone. Adenoviral vectors produced on this basis and harboring either the epidermal growth factor promoter (EGFP) or the *nitroreductase (NR)* genes were evaluated in LNCaP cells, showing selective expression in PSA-positive cells *(58)*. On a similar basis, a hypoxia-inducible enhancer (a fragment of a human VEGF containing a hypoxia-responsive element) was coupled to an AFP promoter in a retroviral vector with an *HSV-TK* gene. After transfection into hepatoma cells and following exposure to 1% O_2 and GCV, specific toxicity was reported *(59)*.

Recently, the L-plastin promoter has been proposed for use in gene therapy. It belongs to a family of genes encoding actin-binding proteins. Infection of ovarian carcinoma cells (OvCar-5 and SK-OV-3) with the recombinant replication-defective adenovirus containing the CD gene under the control of the L-plastin promoter followed by 5-FC treatment proved to be effective both in vitro and in vivo *(18)*.

The latency-associated promoter (LAP) was proposed for sustaining long-term expression in neurones. However, in vivo data indicate that although the HSV-1-LAP vector can drive the expression of the TK gene in a variety of central nervous system (CNS) neurones, there is a slow downregulation of the promoter *(60)*.

The Myc-Max-binding motif (which activates the transcription of an adjacent promoter) was proposed for the treatment of small cell lung cancer, which overexpressed *myc*-family oncogenes *(17)*. A Cre/loxP approach was also suggested in conjunction with the CD/5-FC suicide gene therapy system for the treatment in vivo of gastric carcinoma models *(61)*.

Finally, the osteocalcin promoter has been used in a conditionally replication-competent adenoviral vector. The recombinant Ad-OC-E1a vector harboring the osteocalcin promoter proved to be effective in inhibiting the growth of PSA-producing and nonproducing human prostate cancer cell lines *(62)*.

2.3. Nonviral and Viral/Nonviral Hybrid Vectors

The alternative to viral vectors are the nonviral strategies *(6,63)* (*see* Chapters 7 and 8). These include transfection procedures such as injection of naked DNA and the use of physical devices such as gene guns, jet injection, and electroporation *(64)*. However, more common systems are based on noncovalent complexes of carrier molecules and plasmid DNA. Such systems are suitable for systemic gene delivery to tumors and/or metastases. The development of such carrier molecules is difficult because a number of biological barriers must be overcome. Major advantages are linked to safety and the fact that large expression cassettes can be transferred by this procedure. Using a plasmid in conjunction with electroporation, a transfection efficiency in vivo of 3–8% was obtained as compared to 0.1% for the same plasmid without electroporation *(32,33)*. However, the approach is plagued by low transfection efficiencies, especially in vivo. Also, differences in gene expression between rodents and human have been reported.

The main categories of nonviral vectors used in gene delivery are those forming complexes with DNA. These include lipoplexes (such as cationic lipids or cytofectins) and polyplexes (such as poly-L-lysine [PLL], polyethyleneimine [PEI], peptides, dextrans, and dendrimers). For the lipoplexes, transfection efficiencies in vitro in the range 0.2–35% have been reported *(6,8,10)*.

An exciting development has been to combine the viral and nonviral strategies. One possibility is to use a viral/nonviral hybrid vector. Accordingly liposomes in conjunction with the hemagglutinating Japan virus (HVJ liposomes) were constructed. These liposomes showed low immunogenicity and good in vivo transfection ability (*see* **Table 1**). The in vivo transfection efficiency in male SCID mice bearing hepatocellular carcinoma tumors (HuH7 cells) was 19.7±6% *(7)* The same system was used to transfer the CD gene to nude mice bearing BXPC3 human pancreatic tumor xenografts. A transfection efficiency of approx 30% was measured at day 3 (using *LacZ* as marker gene), but at day 7, almost no positive β-galactosidase cells were found *(65)*. After administration of repeated doses of 5-FC and also HVJ-CD liposomes, the tumor size was reduced by 72% at day 28.

Progress in the design of anionic HVJ liposomes has been made recently. In contrast to cationic liposomes, which do not penetrate tissues because of their net positive charge and large size, the HVJ-AVE anionic liposomes can penetrate tissues and exhibit higher efficiency of transfection. Recently, HVJ-AVE anionic liposomes with the envelope that mimics the human immunodeficiency virus (HIV) have been constructed and the *LacZ* gene was transfected by intrathecal administration to the CNS in primates. Transfection efficiencies of 29–59% in neurons were reported *(11)*.

An alternative strategy uses polycations to increase the adenoviral mediated expression of the transgenic protein. Complexation of adenovirus harboring the *LacZ* gene with PEI allows the selective transfection of biliary epithelia via biliary canulation. In vivo administration of 1×10^9 pfu of adenovirus cocomplexed with PEI led to >80% infected epithelial cells, whereas adenovirus alone infected <5% *(12)*.

Finally, a variety of ligands has been examined for their liposome-targeting abilities, including folates and transferrins. Folate-containing cationic liposomes were optimized for the systemic delivery of the *p53* gene to mice carrying JSQ-3 xenografts derived from tumors of the nasal vestibule, which had failed radiation therapy. Transfection efficiencies of 40–50% were achieved after systemic administration of the vector *(5)*.

In summary, a wide range of vectors has been developed that can be used for suicide gene therapy, with a large number of optimized parameters, such as CAR retargeting, replication and promoter selectivity, and hybrid vectors. When the optimized vectors are combined with the best gene suicide therapy systems, efficacy in vivo has been demonstrated.

References

1. Glorioso, J. C., De Luca, N. A., and Fink, D. J. (1995) Development and application of of herpes simplex virus vector for gene therapy. *Annu. Rev. Microbiol.* **49**, 675–710.
2. Vile, R. G., Diaz, R. M., Miller, N., Tuszyanski, A., and Russell, S. G. (1995) Tissue specific gene expression from Mo-MLV retroviral vectors with hybrid LTRs containing the murine tyrosine enhancer/promoter. *Virology* **214**, 307–313.
3. Kremer, E. J. and Perricaudet, M. (1995) Adenovirus and AAV mediated gene transfer. *Br. Med. Bull.* **51**, 31–44.
4. Spooner, R. A., Deonarain, M. P., and Epenetos, A. A. (1995) DNA vaccination for cancer treatment. *Gene Ther.* **2**, 173–180.
5. Xu, L., Pirollo, K. F., Rait, A., Murray, A. L., and Chang E. H. (1999) Systemic p53 gene therapy in combination with radiation results in human tumor regression. *Tumor Target.* **4**, 92–104.
6. Schatzlein, A. G. (2001) Non-viral vectors in cancer gene therapy: principles and progress. *Anti-Cancer Drug Des.* **12**, 275–304.
7. Hasegawa, H., Shimada, M., Yonemitsu, Y., et al. (2001) Preclinical and therapeutic utility of HVJ liposomes as a gene transfer vector for hepatocellular carcinoma using herpes simplex virus thymidine kinase. *Cancer Gene Ther.* **8**, 252–258.
8. Bentires-Alj, M., Helin, A.-C., Lechanteur, C., et al. (2000) Cytosine deaminase suicide gene therapy for peritoneal carcinomatosis. *Cancer Gene Ther.* **7**, 20–26.
9. Greco, O., Folkes, L. K., Wardman, P., Tozer, G. M., and Dachs, G. U. (2000) Development of a novel enzyme/prodrug combination for gene therapy of cancer: horseradish peroxidase/indole-3-acetic acid. *Cancer Gene Ther.* **7**, 1414–1420.
10. Harada, Y., Iwai, M., Tanaka, S., et al. (2000) Highly efficient suicide gene expression in hepatocellular carcinoma cells by Epstein–Barr virus-based plasmid vectors combined with polyamidoamine dendrimer. *Cancer Gene Ther.* **7**, 27–36.
11. Hagihara, Y., Saitoh, Y., Kaneda, Y., Kohmura, E., and Yoshimine, T. (2000) Widespread gene transfection into the central nervous system of primates. *Gene Ther.* **7**, 759–763.
12. Mc Kay, T. R., MacVinish, L. J., Carpenter, B., et al. (2000) Selective in vivo transfection of murine biliary ephitelia using polycation-enhanced adenovirus. *Gene Ther.* **7**, 644–652.
13. Tanaka, M., Fraizer, G. C., De La Cerda, J., Cristiano, R. J., Liebert, M., and Grossman, H. B. (2001) Connexin 26 enhances the bystander effect in HSVtk/GCV gene therapy for human bladder cancer by adenovirus/PLL/DNA gene delivery. *Gene Ther.* **8**, 138–148.
14. Majumdar, A., Zolotorev, A., Samuel, S., et al. (2000) Efficacy of herpes simplex virus thymidine kinase in combination with cytokine gene therapy in an experimental metastatic breast cancer model. *Cancer Gene Ther.* **7**, 1086–1099.
15. Ichikawa, T. and Chiocca, E. A. (2001) Comparative analysis of transgene delivery and expression in tumors inoculated with a replication-conditional or defective viral vector. *Cancer Res.* **61**, 5336–5339.
16. Meck, M. E., Wierdl, M., Wagner, L. M., et al. (2001) A virus-directed enzyme prodrug therapy approach to purging neuroblastoma cells from hematopoietic cells using adenovirus encoding rabbit carboxyl esterase and CPT-11. *Cancer Res.* **61**, 5083–5089.

17. Nishino, K., Osaki, T., Kumagai T., et al. (2001) Adenovirus-mediated gene therapy specific for small cell lung cancer cells using a myc-max binding motif. *Int. J. Cancer* **91**, 851–856.

18. Peng, X.Y., Won, J.H., Rutherford, T., et al. (2001) The use of L-plastin promoter for adenoviral-mediated , tumor-specific gene-expression in ovarian and bladder cancer cell lines. *Cancer Res.* **61**, 4405–4413.

19. Watanabe, T., Shinohara, N., Sazawa, A., et al. (2001) Adenovirus-mediated gene therapy for bladder cancer in an orthotopic model using a dominant negative H-ras mutant. *Int. J. Cancer* **92**, 712–717.

20. Bilbao, R., Gerolami, R., Bralet, M.-P., et al. (2000) Transduction efficacy, antitumoral effect, and toxicity of adenovirus-mediated herpes simplex virus thymidine kinase/ganciclovir therapy of hepatocellular carcinoma: the woodchuck animal model. *Cancer Gene Ther.* **7**, 657–662.

21. Adachi, Y., Reynods, P. N., Yamamoto, M., et al. (2000) Midkine promoter-based adenoviral vector gene delivery for pediatric solid tumors. *Cancer Res.* **60**, 4305–4310.

22. Brust, D., Feden, J., Farnsworth, J., Amir, C., Broaddus, W. C., and Valerie, K. (2000) Radiosensitization of rat glioma with bromodeoxycytidine and adenovirus expressing herpes simplex virus-thymidine kinase delivered by slow, rate-controlled positive pressure infusion. *Cancer Gene Ther.* **7**, 778–788.

23. Erbs, P., Regulier, E., Kintz, J., et al. (2000) In vivo cancer gene therapy by adenovirus-mediated transfer of a bifunctional yeast cytosine deaminase/uracil phosphoribosyltransferase fusion gene. *Cancer Res.* **60**, 3813–3822.

24. Block, A., Freund, C. T. F., Chen, S.-H., et al. (2000). Gene therapy of metastatic colon carcinoma: regression of multiple hepatic metastases by adenoviral expression of bacterial cytosine deaminase. *Cancer Gene Ther.* **7**, 438–445.

25. Loimas, S., Toppinen, M.-R., Visakorpi, T., Janne, J., and Wahlfors, D. (2001) Human prostate carcinoma cells as target for herpes simplex virus thymidine kinase-mediated suicide gene therapy. *Cancer Gene Ther.* **8**, 137–144.

26. Mavria, G. and Porter, C. D. (2001) Reduced growth in response to ganciclovir treatment or subcutaneous xenografts expressing HSV-tk in the vascular compartment. *Gene Ther.* **8**, 913–920.

27. Walling, H. W., Swarthout, G. T., and Culver, K. W. (2000) Bystander-mediated regression of osteosarcoma via retroviral transfer of the herpes simplex virus thymidine kinase and human interleukin-2 genes. *Cancer Gene Ther.* **7**, 187–196.

28. Hamstra, D. A., Page, M., Maybaum, J., and Rehemtulla, A. (2000) Expression of endogenously activated secreted or cell surface carboxypeptidase A sensitizes tumor cells to methotrexate-α-peptide prodrugs. *Cancer Res.* **60**, 657–665.

29. Rivas, C., Chandler, P., Melo, J. V., Simpson, E., and Apperley, J. F. (2000) Absence of in vitro or in vivo bystander effects in a thymidine kinase-transduced murine T-lymphoma. *Cancer Gene Ther.* **7**, 954–962.

30. Steffens, S., Frank, S., Fisher, U., et al. (2000) Enhanced green fluorescent proteinfusion proteins of herpes simplex virus type 1 thymidine kinase and cytochrome P450 4B1: applications for prodrug-activating gene therapy. *Cancer Gene Ther.* **7**, 806–812.

31. Westphal, E.-M., Ge, J., Catchpole, J. R., Ford, M., and Kennedy, S. C. (2000) The nitroreductase/CB1954 combination in Eptein–Barr virus-positive B cell lines: Induction of bystander killing in vitro and in vivo. *Cancer Gene Ther.* **7**, 97–106.

32. Djeha, A. H., Hulme, A., Dexter, M. T., et al. (2000) Expression of *Escherichia coli* B nitroreductase in established human tumor xenografts in mice results in potent antitumoral and bystander effects upon systemic administration of CB1954. *Cancer Gene Ther.* **7**, 721–731.

33. Lohr, F., Lo, D. Y., Zaharoff, D. A., et al. (2001) Effective tumor therapy with plasmid cytokines combined with in vivo electroporation. *Cancer Res.* **61**, 3281–3284.

34. Kanazawa, T., Urabe, M., Mizukami, H., et al. (2001) γ-Rays enhance rAAV-mediated transgene expression and cytocidal effect of AAV-HSV-tk/ganciclovir on cancer cells. *Cancer Gene Ther.* **8**, 99–106.

35. Kirn, D. (2000) Replication-selective microbiological agents: figthing cancer with targeted germ warfare. *J. Clin. Investig.* **105**, 837–839.

36. Pawelek, J. M., Low, K. B., and Bermudes, D. (1997) Tumor-targeted Salmonella as a novel anticancer vector. *Cancer Res.* **57**, 4537–4544.

37. Yazawa, K., Fujimori, M., Amano, J., Kano, Y., and Taniguchi, S. (2000) Bifidobacterium longum as a delivery system for cancer gene therapy: selective localization and growth in hypoxic tumors. *Cancer Gene Ther.* **7**, 269–274.

38. Nuyts, S., Theys, J., Landuyt, W., Van Mellaert, L., Lambin, P., and Anne, J. (2001) Increasing specificity of anti-tumour therapy: cytotoxic proteins delivery by non-pathogenic Clostridia under regulation of radio-induced promoter. *Anticancer Res.* **21**, 857–862.

39. Nuyts, S., Van Mellaert, L., Theys, J., Landuyt, W., Lambin, P., and Anne, J. (2001) The use of radiation-induced bacterial promoters in anaerobic-conditions: a means to control gene expression in Clostridium-mediated gene therapy. *Radiat. Res.* **155**, 716–723.

40. Curiel, D. T., Gerritsen, W. R., and Krul, M. R. (2000) Progress in cancer gene therapy. *Cancer Gene Ther.* **7**, 1197–1199.

41. Heideman, D. A. H., Snijders, P. J. F., Craanen, M. W., et al. (2001) Selective gene delivery toward gastric and esophageal adenocarcinoma cells via EpCAM-targeted adenoviral vectors. *Cancer Gene Ther.* **8**, 342–351.

42. Wesseling, J. C., Bosma, P. J., Krasnykh, V., et al. (2001) Improved gene transfer efficiency to primary and established human pancreatic carcinoma target cells via epidermal growth factor receptor and integrin-targeted adenoviral vector. *Gene Ther.* **8**, 969–976.

43. Hermiston, T. (2000) Gene-delivery from replication-selective viruses: arming guided missiles in the war against cancer. *J. Clin. Investig.* **105**, 1169–1172.

44. Heise, C. and Kirn, H. D. (2000) Replication-selective adenoviruses as oncolytic agents. *J. Clin. Investig.* **105**, 847–851.

45. Martuza, R. L. (2000) Conditionally replicating herpes vector for gene therapy. *J. Clin. Investig.* **105**, 841–846.

46. Kirn, D. (2001) Clinical research results with dI 1520 (ONYX-015), a replication selective adenovirus for the treatment of cancer: what have we learned? *Gene Ther.* **8**, 89–98.

47. Todo, T., Rabkin, S. D., and Martuza, R. L. (2000) Evaluation of ganciclovir-mediated enhancement of the antitumoral effect in oncolytic, multimutated herpes simplex virus type 1 (G207) therapy of brain tumor. *Cancer Gene Ther.* **7**, 939–946.

48. Aghi, M., Chou, T. C., Suling, K., Breakefield, X. O., and Chiocca, I. A. (1999) Multimodal cancer treatment mediated by a replicating oncolytic virus that delivers the oxazaphosphorine/rat cytochrome P450 2B1 and ganciclovir/herpes simplex virus thymidine kinase gene therapies. *Cancer Res.* **59**, 3861–3865.

49. Nakamura, H., Mullen, J. T., Chanrasekhar, S., Pawlik, T. M., Yoon, S. S., and Tanabe, K. K. (2001) Multimodality therapy with a replication-conditional herpes simplex virus 1 mutant that express yeast cytosine deaminase for intratumoral conversion of 5-fluorocytosine tom 5-fluorouracil. *Cancer Res.* **61**, 5447–5452.

50. Wildner, O., Morris, J. C., Vahanian, N. N., Ford H., Jr., Ramsey, W. J., and Blaese, R. M. (1999) Adenoviral vectors capable of replication improve the efficacy of HSVtk/GCV suicide gene therapy of cancer. *Gene Ther.* **6**, 57–62.

51. Wildner, O. and Morris, J. C. (2000) The role of the E1B 55 kDa gene product in oncolytic adenoviral vectors expressing herpes simplex virus-tk: assessment of antitumor efficacy and toxicity. *Cancer Res.* **60**, 4167–4174.

52. Freytag, S. O., Rogulski, K. R., Paielli, D. L., Gilbert, J. D., and Kim, J. H. (1998) A novel three-pronged approach to kill cancer cells selectively: concomitant viral, double suicide gene, and radiotherapy. *Hum. Gene Ther.* **9**, 1323–1333.

53. Rogulski, K. R., Wing, M. S., Paielli, D. L., Gilbert, J. D., Kim J. H., and Freytag, S. O. (2000) Double suicide gene therapy augments the antitumor activity of a replication-competent lytic adenovirus through enhanced cytotoxicity and radiosensitization. *Hum. Gene Ther.* **11**, 67–76.

54. Lambright, E.S., Amin, K., Wiewrodt, R., et al. (2001) Inclusion of the herpes simplex thymidine kinase gene in a replicating adenovirus does not augment antitumor efficacy. *Gene Ther.* **8**, 946–953.

55. Dachs, G. U., Dougherty, G. J., Stratford, I. J., and Chaplin, D. J. (1997) Targeting gene therapy for cancer. *Oncol. Res.* **9**, 313–325.

56. Spear, M. A. (1998) Gene therapy of gliomas: receptors and transcriptional targeting. *Anticancer Res.* **18**, 3223–3232.

57. Koshikawa, N., Takenaga, K., Tagawa, M., and Sakiyama, S. (2000) Therapeutic efficacy of the suicide gene driven the promoter of vascular endothelial growth factor gene against hypoxic tumor cells. *Cancer Res.* **60**, 2936–2941.

58. Latham, J. P. F., Searle, P. F., Mautner, V., and James, N. D. (2000) Prostate-specific antigen promoter/enhancer driven gene therapy for prostate cancer: construction and testing of a tissue specific adenovirus vector. *Cancer Res.* **60**, 334–341.

59. Ido, A., Uto, H., Moriuchi, A., et al. (2001) Gene therapy targeting for hepatocellular carcinoma: selective and enhanced suicide gene expression regulated by a hypoxia-inducible enhancer linked to a human a-fetoprotein promoter. *Cancer Res.* **61**, 3016–3021.

60. Scarpini, C. G., May, J., Lachman, R. H., et al. (2001) Latency associated promoter transgene expression in the central nervous system after stereotaxic delivery of replication-defective HSV-1-based vectors. *Gene Ther.* **8**, 1057–1071.

61. Ueda, K., Iwahashi, M., Nakamori, M., et al. (2001) Carcinoembryonic antigen-specific suicide gene therapy of cytosine deaminase/5-fluoro-cytosine enhanced by the Cre/loxP system in the orthotopic gastric carcinoma model. *Cancer Res.* **61**, 6158–6162.

62. Matsubara, S., Wada, Y., Gardner, T. A., et al. (2001) A conditional replication-competent vector, Ad-OC-E1a, to cotarget prostate cancer and bone stroma in an experimental model of androgen-independent prostate cancer bone metastasis. *Cancer Res.* **61**, 6012–6019.

63. Miller, A.D. (1998) Cationic liposomes for gene therapy. *Angew. Chem. Int. Ed.* **37**, 1768–1785.

64. Luo, D. and Salzman, W. M. (2000) Synthetic DNA delivery systems. *Nature Biotechnol.* **18**, 33–37.

65. Kanyama, H., Tomita, N., Yamano, T., et al. (2001) Usefulness of repeated intratumoral gene transfer using hemagglutinating virus of Japan-liposome method for cytosine deaminase suicide gene therapy. *Cancer Res.* **61**, 14–18.

3

Construction of VNP20009

A Novel, Genetically Stable Antibiotic-Sensitive Strain of Tumor-Targeting Salmonella for Parenteral Administration in Humans

Kenneth Brooks Low, Martina Ittensohn, Xiang Luo, Li-Mou Zheng, Ivan King, John M. Pawelek, and David Bermudes

1. Introduction

The engineering of tumor-targeting *Salmonella* strains bearing a high degree of both attenuation and tumor inhibition is a recently developed approach to vector-based treatment of cancer *(1,2)*. Tumor-targeted *Salmonella* have many desirable features for a tumor-selective delivery vehicle:

1. **Systemic administration.** *Salmonella* can be delivered by intravenous (iv), intraperitoneal (ip), or intratumoral (it) injection. Viral vectors largely or completely lack efficacy following systemic delivery.
2. **Replication competent.** Unlike other agents such as monoclonal antibodies, *Salmonella* replicate; thus, systemic administration of a low-dose replicates to an effective dose within the target tumor.
3. **High degree of tumor specificity.** *Salmonella* accumulate to levels hundreds to thousands of times greater within the tumor as compared to normal tissues. This allows for the potential of delivering high levels of specific therapeutic agents, such as prodrug activation enzyme systems, directly to the tumor, avoiding systemic toxicity.
4. **Broad tumor specificity.** These *Salmonella* vectors target a broad range of solid tumors, including melanoma, lung, colon, breast, renal, hepatic, and prostate tumors, independent of p53 mutations.
5. **Delivery capacity.** Live *Salmonella* are metabolically active and continuously produce active proteins while infecting tumors.
6. **Posttreatment eradication.** *Salmonella* are sensitive to antibiotics, allowing cessation of treatment or posttreatment elimination.

From: *Methods in Molecular Medicine, Vol. 90, Suicide Gene Therapy: Methods and Reviews*
Edited by: C. J. Springer © Humana Press Inc., Totowa, NJ

Although the strains of *Salmonella* developed thus far have a significant ability to selectively replicate within tumors and inhibit tumor growth, they have been generated using techniques including ultraviolet (UV) and nitrosoguanidine-derived point mutations and/or have antibiotic resistance. We have now constructed a strain with tumor-targeting and tumor-inhibition properties containing deletion mutations and lacking antibiotic resistance. This strain, VNP20009, has remained stable through extensive serial passage in vitro and remains stable after introduction into and reisolation from laboratory animals. Owing to the purine auxotrophy of the strain, it is highly attenuated, and an additional attenuation is achieved by disruption in the *msbB* gene, which alters the lipid A and greatly diminishes the potential to induce tumor necrosis factor-α (TNF-α) and cause septic shock. High-dose iv administration in laboratory animals results in minimal systemic toxicity, despite long-term persistence within tissues. This strain of *Salmonella* is the first to undergo parentral administration in human clinical trials.

Studies of genetically modified *Salmonella* strains have demonstrated both safe and effective use as oral vaccines in humans *(3–14)*. Mutations in these bacterias' metabolism or virulence factors severely limit their ability to replicate and to cause disease, yet they retain the ability to reach gut lympoidal tissue and elicit a strong immune response. That property of this normally self-limited infection is achieved without attendant symptoms for which *Salmonella* is so well known. Preliminary studies in mice of *Salmonella choleraesuis* serotype Typhimurium (*Salmonella typhimurium*) strains with specific mutations had shown that highly attenuated strains could result in minimal systemic complications yet provide protective immunity. Homologous mutations in the human-specific typhoid strains have shown that the safety profile has correlated well, although the immune stimulatory effects have not always followed the same pattern as in mice.

Tumor-targeting *Salmonella* strains have been developed that are both limited in their pathogenesis and have mutant lipopolysaccharide (LPS), which staves off induction of septic shock *(2)*, and yet have high-level intratumoral replication. These proofs of principal experiments with efficacy demonstrated in tumor-bearing mice and safety shown in both mice and pigs have used strains engineered with both antibiotic-resistance makers and UV/nitrosoguanidine mutations in key attenuating genes. Further development of tumor-targeting *Salmonella*, including preclinical toxicology in non-human primates and initiation of clinical trials in humans, necessitates the development of a strain bearing properties consistent with the principles of safety developed for vaccine strains, including the lack of antibiotic-resistance markers and deletions in attenuating mutations.

We have developed a strain of *Salmonella*, VNP20009, with the properties desirable for a live Gram-negative bacterial anticancer agent with applications in humans. First, we added a previously characterized purine deletion into the hyperinvasive strain YS72, which has served as the platform strain for previous studies *(1,2)*. YS72, however, contains a UV/nitrosoguanidine-derived purine deficiency; thus, the new strain contains a purine gene deletion. We subsequently added an *msbB* deletion and removed the internal antibiotic marker. These properties of this strain are highly stable both in vitro and in vivo *(15)*.

With regard to safety, the findings have been that high-dose iv administration of attenuated *Salmonella* results in minimal systemic toxicity despite long-term persistence within tissues *(15,16)*. Cynomologous monkeys dosed with 1×10^{10} intravenously did not die from the injection, even though this species is known to succumb to natural infections of this strain of *Salmonella*. Although all comparitors, including iv injection of wild type into monkeys or humans, are not available, these numbers are quite staggering if one compares the estimated 10^6 believed to be required for oral infection in humans; infection and severe systemic effects following iv injection levels would be expected to occur at even lower doses.

2. Materials

2.1. Bacterial Strains, Growth, and Transducing Phage

The *Salmonella* strains used included ATCC14028 (wild type), YS72 [*pur⁻ xyl⁻* hyperinvasive mutant from ATCC14028 *(1)*], YS82 [LT2 *msbB1::tet recD541::Tn10dCm hsdSA29 hsdSB121 hsdL6 metA22 metE551 trpC2 ilv-452* H1-b H2-e,n,x *fla*-66 nml(–) *rpsL120 xyl-404 galE719* (2); YS8211 (*msbB1::tet* from ATCC14028 by transduction using YS82 as donor *(2)*]. Throughout the procedures, *msbB⁺* strains were grown in Luria–Bertani (LB) broth (1% Bactotryptone/0.5% Bacto-yeast extract/1% $NaCl_2$ or LB plates containing 1.5% agar at 37°C. *msbB⁻* strains were grown in modified LB (MSBB) containing 10 g tryptone, 5 g yeast extract, 2 mL of 1 *N* $CaCl_2$, and 2 mL of 1 *N* $MgSO_4$ per liter, adjusted to pH 7 using 1 *N* NaOH. For transducing *msbB1::tet*, LB lacking NaCl (LB-0) was used, with 4 mg/L tetracycline. Transductions were performed using bacteriophage P22 (mutant HT105/1 *int*-201 *(17)*. (*See* **Note 1.**)

2.2. Tumor Cells

Tumor cells from murine and human origins were used for in vitro and in vivo experiments, including murine melanoma B16F10 (Fidler, M.D. Anderson Cancer Center), human colon cancer HTB 39 and HCT 116, human hepatoma HTB 52, human renal carcinoma CRL 1611, and human breast carcinoma BT20 (all except B16F10 were obtained from the ATCC), and maintained on the specifically recommended tissue culture medium (TCM), usually with 10% fetal bovine serum (FBS; Gibco) and 5% CO_2 in humidified air at 37°C. Antibiotics such as penicillin (Sigma) (100 units/mL) and streptomycin (Sigma) (100 µg/mL) may be added to aid in maintaining bacteria-free cultures. Mammalian cells were usually detached from the culture dish using 1% EDTA or a solution of trypsin and EDTA (Sigma).

2.3. Tumor Models

Tumor cells were thoroughly washed by successive centrifugations in phosphate-buffered saline (PBS) before implantation. Tumor cells were always inoculated in the same position (e.g., subcutaneously in the left shoulder region with 5×10^5 B16F10 for syngenic mice or 2×10^7 cells [e.g., human colon carcinoma HCT 116, human breast carcinoma BT20, human renal carcinoma CRL 1611, or human hepatoma HTB 52] for human tumor xenografts in *nu/nu* mice.

3. Methods

The derivation of VNP20009 involved seven steps, beginning with the wild-type bacteria and ending with VNP20009 (*see* **Fig. 1**).

3.1. Mutagenization and Selection of a Clone In Vitro

Salmonella typhimurium strain 14028 was purchased from the American Type Culture Collection (bovine liver isolate, 1957, CDC6516-60). This strain was grown on LB agar and a single clone was picked and designated "14028 wild type" ("wild type"). In our generation of VNP20009, we began with a strain derived from the wild type, clone YS72 (*1*), derived by an in vitro* selection for hyperinvasiveness. The selection protocol for the hyperinvasive clones is fully described by Bermudes et al. (*18*).

3.2. Introduction of purI1757::Tn10 Insertion into YS72 (YS1641) and Bochner Selection to Derive Δpurl (YS1642)

1. Tn*10* Transduction of the *purI* Insertion. Using bacteriophage P22 (mutant HT105/1 *int*-201), YS72 is transduced to tetracycline resistance using strain TT11 (*purI1757*::Tn*10*; *Salmonella* Genetic Stock Center) as donor. A stock of P22 was grown on TT11 and then used to infect early log phase YS72. These bacteria were then plated to LB agar containing 10 µg/mL tetracycline (LB-tet) and incubated overnight. Antibiotic-resistant colonies were then purified by streaking them out on LB-tet and then subjected them to auxotrophy analysis using M56 plates with and without thiamine and adenine (M56: 0.037 M KH_2PO_4, 0.06 M Na_2HPO_4, 0.02% $MgSO_4 \cdot 7H_2O$, 0.2% $(NH_4)_2SO_4$, 0.001% $Ca(NO_3)_2$, 0.00005% $FeSO_4 \cdot 7H_2O$, with a carbon source [e.g., 0.1–0.3% glucose] as a sterile-filtered additive, and further supplemented with 0.16 µg/mL thiamine and 33 µg/mL adenine). Solid M56 media is made by preparing separate autoclaved 2X concentrates of the mineral salts and the agar, which are combined after sterilization. (*See* **Note 2.**)
2. Loss of the Tetracycline Marker. The resulting strain, YS1641, was subjected to a Bochner selection (*19*) to obtain a tetracycline-sensitive derivative. Bacteria were plated on agar containing 2 mg/mL fusaric acid and 25 mg/mL chlorotetracycline, and growing colonies were rechecked for tetracycline sensitivity by replica plating. This tetracycline-sensitive strain was also tested for purine auxotrophy (described in **step 1**), to ensure that the Bochner deletion did not result in restoration of purine biosynthesis, but rather was the result of the more likely event of deletion of *tet* determinant along with part of the *purI* gene. This strain (Δ*purI*⁻) was denoted YS1642.
3. Stability of Purine Auxotrophy. Strain YS1642 was further tested for reversion to purine⁺ by two methods. Method A: 100 µL of an overnight culture of YS6142 grown in LB broth (approx 2×10^9/mL) was plated to adenine-depleted media and incubated overnight. No growth was obtained on adenine minus plates. Method B: 10 mL of overnight culture (approx 2×10^{10} total) was placed in 100 mL M56 media lacking adenine and shaken for 2 d at 37°C in order to enrich for any purine⁺ revertants. One hundred microliters of this culture was then plated to M56 agar plates lacking adenine. No growth was observed; thus, this strain is shown to revert to Pur⁺ at a frequency of less than 1 in 10^{10} cells.

*In these discussions, we refer to all nonanimal experiments as in vitro, regardless of the use of live bacteria and/or mammalian cells.

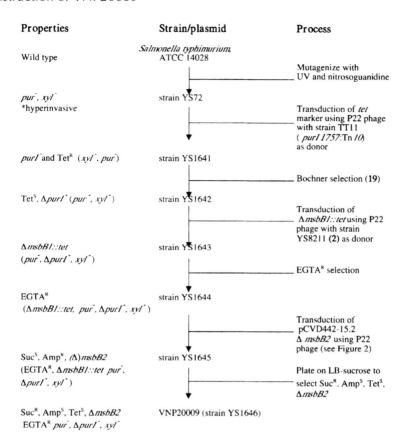

Properties	Strain/plasmid	Process

Wild type — *Salmonella typhimurium*, ATCC 14028

Mutagenize with UV and nitrosoguanidine

pur⁻, xyl⁻
*hyperinvasive — strain YS72

Transduction of *tet* marker using P22 phage with strain TT11 (*purI 1757*:Tn *10*) as donor

purI⁻ and Tet^R (*xyl⁻, pur⁻*) — strain YS1641

Bochner selection (19)

Tet^S, Δ*purI⁻* (*pur⁻, xyl⁻*) — strain YS1642

Transduction of Δ*msbB1::tet* using P22 phage with strain YS8211 (2) as donor

Δ*msbB1::tet*
(*pur⁻, ΔpurI⁻, xyl⁻*) — strain YS1643

EGTA^R selection

EGTA^R
(Δ*msbB1::tet, pur⁻, ΔpurI⁻, xyl⁻*) — strain YS1644

Transduction of pCVD442-15.2 Δ *msbB2* using P22 phage (see Figure 2)

Suc^S, Amp^R, (Δ)*msbB2*
(EGTA^R, Δ*msbB1::tet pur⁻, ΔpurI⁻, xyl⁻*) — strain YS1645

Plate on LB-sucrose to select Suc^R, Amp^S, Tet^S, Δ*msbB2*

Suc^R, Amp^S, Tet^S, Δ*msbB2*
EGTA^R *pur⁻, ΔpurI⁻, xyl⁻* — VNP20009 (strain YS1646)

*Not studied in subsequent strains

Fig. 1. Schematic depiction of the derivation of VNP20009 (i.e., strain YS1646) from wild-type *S. typhimurium* (strain ATCC 14028). *pur⁻*, auxotrophic for purines; *xyl⁻*, unable to metabolize xylose; UV, ultraviolet; *purI⁻* specifically disrupted in the purine I gene; Tet^R, resistant to tetracycline; Tet^S, sensitive to tetracycline; Δ*msbB1::tet*, a disrupted form of msbB which contains a tetracycline gene insertion; (Δ)*msbB2*, a second form of disrupted *msbB*, which does not contain an antibiotic-resistance marker; EGTA^R, resistant to ethylene glycol bis(b-aminoethyl ether)-*N,N,N′,N′*-tetraacetic acid; Suc^S, sensitive to sucrose; Suc^R, resistant to sucrose; Amp^S, sensitive to ampicillin and carbanicillin; Amp^R, resistant to ampicillin and carbanicillin.

3.3. Derivation of msbB1::tet and Transduction into YS1642 to Derive YS1643

1. Isolation of the *Salmonella msbB*. Our initial form of a disrupted *msbB* gene is described by Low et al. *(2)*. The isolation of the corresponding gene from *Salmonella* utilized low-stringency DNA/DNA hybridization of a *Salmonella* genomic DNA library carried in *Salmonella* LT2 5010. A probe for *msbB* was generated from the *Escherichia coli* plasmid pRS415-223 by digesting with *Bgl*II/*Hinc*II and isolating a 600-bp fragment that

corresponds to a portion of the coding sequence. This fragment was labeled using α^{32}P-dCTP and used to probe the *Salmonella* library at low-stringency conditions consisting of 6X sodium chloride/sodium citrate (SSC), 0.1% sodium dodecyl sulfate (SDS), 2X Denhardt's, and 0.5 % nonfat dry milk *(20)* overnight at 55°C. Strongly hybridizing colonies were purified, and plasmids were extracted and subjected to restriction digestion and *in situ* gel hybridization under the same conditions used for colony hybridization *(17)*. Further restriction digests revealed a 2-kb fragment of DNA that strongly hybridized with the probe and was sequenced at the Yale University Boyer Center using fluorescent dye termination thermal cycle sequencing.

2. Disruption of the *Salmonella msbB*. A knockout construct was generated using the cloned *Salmonella msbB* gene. The cloned gene was cut with *Sph*I and *Mlu*I, thereby removing approximately half of the *msbB* coding sequence, and the tetracycline resistance gene from pBR322 was cut with *Aat*II and *Ava*I and inserted after blunt-ending using the Klenow fragment of DNA polymerase I. The knockout disruption was accomplished by homologous recombination *(21)* where the construct was linearized and transformants of *Salmonella* YS501 selected by resistance to tetracycline and a polymerase chain reaction (PCR)-based analysis of the structure of their *msbB* gene. PCR was used with primers, which generate a fragment inclusive of the region into which the tetracycline gene was inserted, where the forward primer is 5' GTTGACTGGGAAGGTCTGGAG 3', corresponding to bases 586–606, and the reverse primer is 5' CTGACCGCGCTCTATCGCGG 3', corresponding to bases 1465–1484. Wild-type *Salmonella msbB⁺* results in an approx 900-bp product, whereas the disrupted gene with the tetracycline insert results in an approx 1850-bp product. Several clones were obtained where only the larger PCR product was produced, suggesting that the disruption in the *msbB* gene had occurred. Southern blot analysis *(20)* was used to confirm the disruption of the chromosomal copy of *Salmonella msbB* using two independently derived clones.

3. Mobilization of the *msbB* deletion into other strains. Bacteriophage P22 transduction from the *msbB⁻ recD⁻ Salmonella* strain YS82 was used to generate ensuing clones that were tested for disruption of the *msbB⁻* gene by the PCR-based diagnostic described in **step 2**. An intermediate strain was constructed (strain YS8211 in our studies) by transducing *msbB1*::*tet* using YS82 as the donor and the wild-type 14028 as recipient. Strain YS1642 was then transduced with a *msbB1*::*tet* gene via bacteriophage P22 *(17)*, using strain YS8211 (*msbB1*::*tet*) as the donor. The *tet* gene in the *msbB1*::*tet* gene confers resistance to 5 mg/L of tetracycline. The resulting strain thus obtained was YS72 *purI*(Δ) *msbB1*::*tet* (strain YS1643 in our studies). The deletion was again confirmed by PCR assay.

3.4. Selection of a Clone (YS1644) With a Defined Level of EGTA Resistance

1. Selection for EGTA resistance. Strain YS1643, like other *msbB⁻* strains *(22)*, was found to be sensitive to 10 m*M* ethylene glycol bis(β-aminoethyl ether)-*N*,*N*,*N'*,*N'*-tetraacetic acid (EGTA). In order to facilitate phage transductions and obtain better growth properties, this strain was subjected to selection for EGTA^R on 3 m*M* EGTA. One such isolate was denoted as YS1644 and was found to have enhanced growth at physiological concentrations of NaCl. The phenotype is stable as assayed by colony uniformity on EGTA-containing agar after a number of generations of growth. (*See* **Note 3**.)

3.5. Derivation and Transduction of msbB2 (Δ)bla sacB and Transduction into YS1644 to Derive YS1645

The knockout construct used to generate the chromosomally integrated *msbB2(Δ)bla sac*B was constructed using pCVD442 *(23)*.

1. The plasmid vector was cut with *Sma*I and dephorsphorylated with calf intestinal phospatase.
2. The genomic clone of *Salmonella msbB* was cut with *Mlu*I and *Sph*I, removing approximately half of the coding sequence, blunt-end polished with Klenow polymerase, and religated.
3. A correctly ligated clone was cut with *Eco*RV and an approx 1500-bp fragment isolated and ligated into the *Sma*I site of pCVD442 to give plasmid pCVD-15.2.
4. Using *E. coli* strain SM10 λpir as a mating donor, a suicide mating was performed with *Salmonella* YS82, and the new strain designated YS8226 obtained.
5. Strain YS1644 was transduced with the (Δ)*msbB2* (*bla, sacB*) chromosomal element using YS8226 as the donor. This transduction process brings in the second version of the disrupted *msbB* gene resulting in a partial diploid, as shown in **Fig. 2**. The *bla* gene is responsible for the transcription of the enzyme β-lactamase, which metabolizes ampillicin, and was used to select transductants. The *sacB* gene is responsible for the conversion of sucrose into a toxic chemical, levan, which is lethal to the host cells, and was used to select for recombinants. The presence of the *bla* and *sacB* genes allows the selection of the Amp^R Suc^S strain (denoted as strain YS1645 in our studies), which contained both the (Δ)*msbB1::tet* and (Δ)*msbB2* genes.

3.6. Selection of a Sucrose-Resistant, Ampicillin-Sensitive, Tetracycline-Sensitive Derivative of YS1645 (Strain YS1646)

1. Strain YS1645 was plated on LB sucrose to select a Suc^R Amp^S Tet^S derivative to remove the *msbB::tet* gene and restore antibiotic sensitivity (i.e., a derivative with deletion of *msbB1::tet bla sacB* (*see* **Fig. 2**) as described by Donnenberg and Kaper *(23)* except that the LB–sucrose agar plates are made without NaCl, and the plates are incubated at 30°C. (*See* **Note 4**.)
2. After the growth of colonies on these plates, they were gridded to an LB plate and replica plated to either tetracycline-, ampicillin-, or sucrose-containing plates in order to detect the presence of a clone that lacks both the antibiotic and sucrase markers. In our studies, one such derivative was denoted as strain YS1646 (VNP20009).

3.7. Tumor Targeting of VNP20009

The resulting strain (VNP20009) was assayed for its ability to target tumors and its tumor-to-normal tissue ratio. Normal tissues primarily infected by *Salmonella* include the spleen and liver. Because of the size and accessibility of the liver, we generally use this organ as an indicator of the highest-level cfu in normal tissues.

1. C57BL6 mice were implanted subcutaneously with 5×10^5 B16F10 mouse melanoma cells and staged until the appearance of palpable tumors (approx 2 wk).
2. *Salmonella* were cultured on LB agar overnight at 37°C.

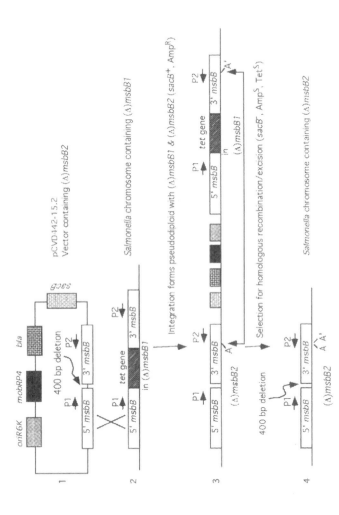

Fig. 2. Recombination processes involved in replacing the tetracycline-containing (Δ)msbB1 with the non-antibiotic-containing (Δ)msbB2. (1) pCVD442-15.2 msbB vector, which contains (Δ)msbB2, (2) homologous recombination with the (Δ)msbB1 chromosomal copy in *Salmonella* YS26, derived from YS82 (2), which contains a tetracycline-resistance determinant (*tet*) in (Δ)msbB, (3) the chromosomally integrated vector resulting in both (Δ)msbB1 and (Δ)msbB2, and (4) following sucrose-resistance selection, the genetic organization in strain VNP20009 (see process 3 for an example of possible crossover locations A and A'). *oriR6K*, the plasmid origin of replication; *mobRP4*, the mobilization element in order for this plasmid to be transferred from one strain to another; *bla*, the β-lactamase gene, which confers sensitivity to β-lactam antibiotic such as carbenicillin and ampicillin; *sacB*, the gene that confers sensitivity to sucrose. *Note:* Not drawn to scale.

54

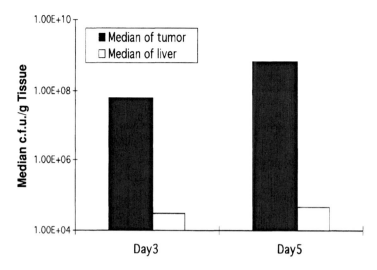

Fig. 3. Biodistribution of VNP20009 in DLD-1 human colon carcinoma xenographs in nu/nu mice. Colony forming units (cfu) were determined on d 3 and 5 in tumors and normal tissue (liver).

3. The following day they were transferred to LB broth, adjusted in concentration to optical density $OD_{600} = 0.1$ (approx 2×10^8 cfu/mL), subjected to further growth at 37°C on a rotator to $OD_{600} = 0.8$, and placed on ice.

4. Following growth, they were diluted to a concentration of 10^4 to 10^7 cfu/mL in PBS on ice, warmed to room temperature, and 0.2 mL injected intraperitoneally or intravenously into C57BL6 mice ($n = 5$-10).

5. After subsequent time periods, usually 1–7 d of infection, mice were euthanized. Tumors and livers were removed aseptically, rinsed with sterile PBS, weighed, and homogenized with LB broth at a ration of 5 : 1 (vol broth : wt tumor).

6. Serial dilutions to LB agar plates were used to determine the cfu per gram of tissue. Our results often showed tumor to liver ratios in excess of 1000 : 1 (*see* **Fig. 3**).

3.8. Tumor Inhibition by VNP20009

Experimental determination of antitumor activity follows the same general protocol for determinations of tumor-targeting described in **Subheading 3.7**. However, because of the rapid growth of many tumor models and the lack of necessity for palpable tumors at early time-points, tumors were staged earlier, usually at 5–12 d. Tumor measurements should always made by the same person in order to compensate for any individual biases and assure consistency.

1. Nude mice were implanted subcutaneously with 1×10^7 DLD1 mouse melanoma cells and staged between d 5 and d 12.

2. *Salmonella* were cultured on LB agar overnight at 37°C.

3. The following day, the bacteria were transferred to LB broth, adjusted in concentration to $OD_{600} = 0.1$ (approx 2×10^8 cfu/mL), subjected to further growth at 37°C on a rotator to $OD_{600} = 0.8$, and placed on ice.

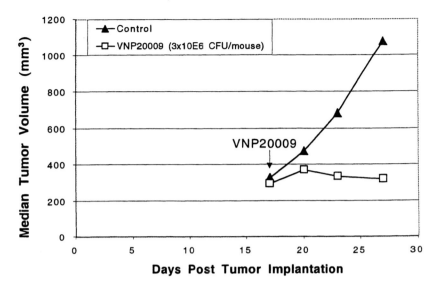

Fig. 4. Tumor inhibition of DLD-1 human colon carcinoma xenographs in nu/nu mice by VNP20009. Tumors were staged to approx 200–400 mm³, and the treatment group received 3 × 10⁶ cfu/mouse of VNP20009. Tumor volume was monitored over time.

4. Following growth, they were diluted to a concentration of 10⁴ to 10⁸ cfu/mL (usually 10⁷) in PBS on ice, warmed to room temperature, and 0.2 mL injected intraperitoneally into the nude mice (n = 5-10).

5. After the appearance of palpable tumors in any group, calipers were used to determine the volume (in mm³ = *LWH*) and the final volume adjusted by multiplying by 0.5236. Results are shown in **Fig. 4.**

3.9. Summary

VNP20009, generated as described earlier, is a highly effective tumor-targeting and tumor-inhibiting strain of *S. typhimurium. msbB⁻* strains have the advantages of lower-level stimulation of TNF-α and septic shock, which may make them particularly suited for parentral administration in humans. Vion filed an Investigational New Drug application with the Food and Drug Administration and the trial was conducted at four sites (Cleveland Clinic, Clevland, OH; National Cancer Institute, Bethesda, MD; Beth Israel-Deaconess, Boston, MA; Royal Marsden, London, UK). In earlier studies, we have used *Salmonella* as a delivery vehicle for effector genes such as the herpes simplex virus–thymidine kinase (HSV1-TK) *(18).* Future applications of VNP20009 will include the addition of effector genes, keeping in mind the requirements of stability and antibiotic sensitivity. Plasmid-based systems have now been developed that do not require antibiotic selection and are highly stable as a result of the presence of an essential gene on the plasmid *(asd)* with a corresponding deletion in the chromosome, thus requiring the presence of the plasmid for survival *(24).* Likewise, chromosomally integrated genes require no antibiotic selection and can also be highly stable. Second-generation vectors will likely take advantage of these and other gene expression systems.

4. Notes

1. Phage were grown on donor bacteria by diluting an overnight culture of the donor strain 1 : 5 in LB medium and adding P22 phage to a final concentration of 5×10^6/mL. This mixture is grown overnight with aeration and treated with a few drops of chloroform for 5 min at 37°C, and debris is removed by centrifuging for 10 min at 6000g. For transductions, this donor phage is used in a 1 : 20 phage to bacteria ratio to infect the recipient strain, which comprises a freshly growing culture at about 10^8/mL in LB broth. After a 20-min preadsorption period, dilutions are plated onto selective plates.
2. Reversion to Pur$^+$ was tested by plating 0.1 mL of an overnight culture onto minimal agar (no adenine). Whereas the leaky Pur$^-$ strains produced dozens of colonies of various sizes, the *purI*::Tn10 derivatives gave rise to no Pur$^+$ revertant colonies.
3. The EGTA resistance and its genetic stability have been described by Clairmont et al. *(15)*. The sensitivity assay is performed by incorporating EGTA into the agar plates. LB-0 media (LB lacking NaCl) as described is adjusted to neutral pH with 0.002 N (final concentration) NaOH and supplemented with either 3 or 10 mM EGTA. VNP20009 is characterized by growth on 3 mM but not on 10 mM EGTA. Genetic stability can be assayed on strains that have been serial passaged (e.g., 150 generations). Individual colonies are then patched and replica-plated and scored for the percent retaining the original phenotype.
4. With regard to transductions and subsequent sucrose resolution of partial diploids, we have sometimes found that we are unable to obtain correctly resolved clones despite repeated attempts. Resolution from independently transduced clones can sometimes overcome this problem. In addition, we have found a prescreen of partial diploid clones essential for finding those with the proper properties. The prescreen involves gridding patches of independent, partial diploids to the sucrose-containing media and growing them at 30°C. Clones with a propensity to resolve correctly have irregular "fuzzy" edges. Use of this technique allows prescreening a large number of colonies.

Acknowledgments

We wish to thank Terrence Doyle, Samuel Miller, and Keith Joiner for helpful discussions. This work was supported by Vion Pharmaceuticals.

References

1. Pawelek, J., Low, K. B., and Bermudes, D. (1997) Tumor-targeted *Salmonella* as a novel anticancer agent. *Cancer Res.* **57,** 4537–4544.
2. Low, K. B., Ittensohn, M., Le, T., et al. (1999) Lipid A mutant *Salmonella* with suppressed virulence and TNFα induction retain tumor-targeting *in vivo. Nature Biotechnol.* **17,** 37–41.
3. Angelakopoulos, H. and Hohmann, E. L. (2000) Pilot study of *phoP/phoQ*-deleted *Salmonella enterica* serovar *typhimurium* expressing *Helicobacter pylori* urease in adult volunteers. *Infect. Immun.* **68,** 2135–41.
4. Cryz, S. J. Jr, Que, J. U., Levine, M. M., Wiedermann, G., and Kollaritsch, H. (1995) Safety and immunogenicity of a live oral bivalent typhoid fever (*Salmonella typhi* Ty21a)–

cholera (*Vibrio cholerae* CVD 103-HgR) vaccine in healthy adults. *Infect. Immun.* **63**, 1336–1339.

5. Dilts, D. A., Riesenfeld-Orn, I., Fulginiti, J. P., et al. (2000) Phase I clinical trials of *aroA aroD* and *aroA aroD htrA* attenuated *S. typhi* vaccines; effect of formulation on safety and immunogenicity. *Vaccine* **18**, 1473–1484.

6. Gonzales, C., Hone, D., Noriega, F. R., et al. (1994) *Salmonella typhi* vaccine strain CVD904 expressing the circumsporozoite protein of *Plasmodium falciparum*: strain construction and safety and immunogenicity in humans. *J. Infect. Dis.* **169**, 927–931.

7. Hohmann, E. L., Oletta, C. A., and Miller, S. I. (1996) Evaluation of a *phoP/phoQ*-deleted, *aroA*-deleted live oral *Salmonella typhi* vaccine strain in human volunteers. *Vaccine* **14**, 19–24.

8. Hohmann, E. L., Oletta, C. A., Killeen, K. P., and Miller S. I. (1996) *phoP/phoQ*-deleted *Salmonella typhi* (Ty800) is a safe and immunogenic single-dose typhoid fever vaccine in volunteers. *J. Infect. Dis.* **173**, 1408–1414.

9. Kollaritsch, H., Furer, E., Herzog, C., Wiedermann, G., Que, J. U., and Cryz, S. J., Jr. (1996) Randomized, double-blind placebo-controlled trial to evaluate the safety and immunogenicity of combined *Salmonella typhi* Ty21a and *Vibrio cholerae* CVD 103-HgR live oral vaccines. *Infect. Immun.* **64**, 1454–1457.

10. Levine, M. M., Hone, D. M., Stocker, B. A. D., and Cadoz, M. (1990) New and improved vaccines against typhoid fever, in: *New Generation Vaccines*, (Woodrow, G. C. and Levine, M. M., eds.), Marcel Dekker, New York, pp. 269–287.

11. Levine, M. M., Ferreccio, C., Abrego, P., Martin, O. S., Ortiz, E., and Cryz, S. (1999) Duration of efficacy of Ty21a, attenuated *Salmonella typhi* live oral vaccine. *Vaccine* **17 (Suppl. 2)**, S22–S27.

12. Tacket, C. O., Hone, D. M., Curtiss, R., III, et al. (1992) Comparson of the safety and immunogenicity of Δ*aroC* Δ*aroD* and Δ*cya* Δ*crp Salmonella typhi* strains in adult volunteers. *Infect. Immun.* **60**, 536–541.

13. Tacket, C. O., Sztein, M. B., Losonsky, G. A., et al. (1997) Safety of live oral *Salmonella typhi* vaccine strains with deletions in *htrA* and *aroC aroD* and immune response in humans. *Infect. Immun.* **65**, 452–456.

14. Tacket, C. O., Sztein, M. B., Wasserman, S. S., et al. (2000) Phase 2 clinical trial of attenuated *Salmonella enterica* serovar *typhi* oral live vector vaccine CVD 908-htrA in U.S. volunteers. *Infect. Immun.* **68**, 1196–1201.

15. Clairmont, C., Lee, K. C., Pike, J., et al. (2000) Biodistribution and genetic stability of the novel antitumor agent VNP20009, a genetically modified strain of *Salmonella typhimurium*. *J. Infect. Dis.* **181**, 1996–2002.

16. Lee, K. C., Zheng, L.-M., Luo, X., et al. (2000) Comparative evaluation of the acute toxic effects in monkeys, pigs, and mice of a genetically engineered *Salmonella* strain (VNP20009) being developed as an antitumor agent. *Int. J. Toxicol.* **19**, 19–25.

17. Davis, R. W., Botstein, D., and Roth, J. R. (1980) *Advanced Bacterial Genetics*, Cold Spring Harbor Laboratory Press, Cold Spring Harbor, NY.

18. Bermudes, D., Low, B., and Pawelek, J. (2000) Tumor-targeted *Salmonella*: strain development and expression of the HSV TK effector gene, in: *Gene Therapy: Methods and Protocol*, (Walther, W. and Stein U. eds.), Humana, Totowa, NJ, Vol. 35, pp. 419–436.

19. Bochner, B. R., Huang, H-C., Schieven, G. L., and Ames, B. N. (1980) Positive selection for loss of tetracycline resistace. *J. Bacteriol.* **143**, 926–933.

20. Sambrook, J., Fritsch, E. F., and Maniatis, T. (1989) *Molecular Cloning: A Laboratory Manual*, 2nd ed., Cold Spring Harbor Laboratory Press, Cold Spring Harbor, NY.

21. Russell, C. B., Thaler, D. S., and Dalhlquist, F. W. (1989) Chromosomal transformation of *Escherichia coli recD-* strains with linearized plasmids. *J. Bacteriol.* **171,** 2609–2613.
22. Murray, S. R., Bermudes, D., de Felipe, K. S., and Low, K. B. (2001) Extragenic suppressors of *msbB⁻* growth defects in *Salmonella. J. Bacteriol.* **183,** 5554–5561.
23. Donnenberg, M. S. and Kaper, J. B. (1991) Construction of an *eae* deletion mutant of enteropathogenic *Escherichia coli* by using a positive-selection suicide vector. *Infect. Immun.* **59,** 4310–4317.
24. Galán, J. E., Nakayama, K., and Curtiss, R., III. (1990) Cloning and characterization of the *asd* gene of *Salmonella typhimurium*: use in stable maintenance of recombinant plasmids in *Salmonella* vaccine strains. *Gene* **94,** 29–35.

4

Nonreplicating DNA Viral Vectors for Suicide Gene Therapy

The Adenoviral Vectors

Masato Yamamoto and David T. Curiel

1. Introduction

Nonreplicative DNA viral vectors (i.e., adenovirus, herpes simplex virus, adeno-associated virus) have been widely used for suicide gene therapy against cancer because their strong and temporary expression of the transgene fit this purpose. Particularly, nonreplicating "adenoviral" vectors have been used in the largest number of clinical trials among all viral vectors. Thus, this chapter covers the adenovirus type 5-based nonreplicative vector.

Basically, the procedures to generate adenoviral vector can be categorized into two distinct methods: The first is based on the homologous recombination in mammalian cells and the second is based on the homologous recombination in *Escherichia coli*. We mainly have been using the latter system because the sequence of the adenovirus vector can be verified before generating the virus and because this procedure does not require plaque isolation.

In the case of making conventional E1/E3-deleted vectors with a transgene cassette in the E1-deleted region (*see* **Fig. 1**), we use the system reported by He et al. *(1)*. This system consists of a shuttle vector for the recombination of E1 region, pShuttle, and a adenoviral backbone plasmid, pAdEasy1. These plasmids can be purchased from Quantum Biotechnologies. As pShuttle does not have either a promoter or a polyadenylation signal for the transgene, these components should also be placed into E1-deleted region together with the transgene.

When simply aiming to achieve strong expression of the transgene, we employ the cytomegalovirus (CMV) immediate-early promoter. In this case, the direction of the expression cassette does not matter. However, in the case of promoter-based-specific

From: *Methods in Molecular Medicine, Vol. 90, Suicide Gene Therapy: Methods and Reviews*
Edited by: C. J. Springer © Humana Press Inc., Totowa, NJ

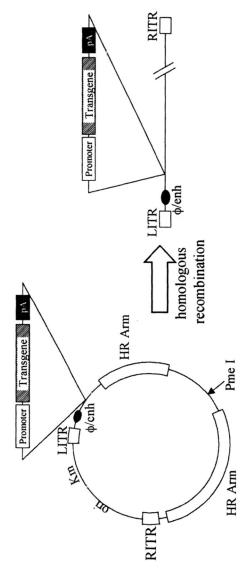

Fig. 1. Typical structure of shuttle plasmid and adenovirus vector for suicide gene therapy.

control of the expression, there is no standardized structure to give the best promoter function with respect to strength and fidelity. In our hands, the longer promoter sequences, including not only positive regulatory elements but also surrounding sequence, often give better results. We usually place the expression cassette in the "left to right" direction, but sometimes the "right to left" direction may provide better fidelity. The possible reasons for this phenomenon relate to the transcription initiation activity in the left inverted terminal-repeat (LITR) region and enhancer activity of packaging signal *(2–4)*.

In this chapter, we will cover the general protocol for adenoviral vector generation and production, basic analyses of the promoter in adenoviral construct using the luciferase expression vector, and suicide gene therapy experiments based on herpes simplex virus–thymidine kinase (HSV-TK).

2. Materials

2.1. Plasmid Construction

1. Transgene (i.e., HSV-TK, CD, luciferase).
2. Promoter (i.e., CMV promoter from pCEP4, tissue/tumor-specific promoters).
3. Polyadenylation signal (i.e., SV40 polyA from pGL3B-basic).
4. Shuttle vector (i.e., pShuttle).
5. Water bath (37°C and 50°C).
6. Spectrophotometer (for DNA quantification).
7. Agarose gel electrophoresis apparatus.
8. Gel extraction kit (Qiagen).
9. Qiagen plasmid kit (Qiagen).
10. Adenoviral backbone plasmid (pAdEasy1).
11. Electroporator.
12. SOC medium.
13. BJ5183 electro-competent cell.
14. DH5α chemical competent cell.
15. Luria–Bertani (LB)-Ampicillin (Amp) (plate and liquid).
16. LB-kanamycin (KM) (plate and liquid).
17. Glucose/Tris/EDTA solution: 50 mM glucose, 25 mM Tris-HCl, pH 8.0, 10 mM EDTA.
18. NaOH/SDS (sodium dodecyl sulfate) solution: 0.2 M NaOH, 1% SDS.
19. Potassium acetate solution: 5 M KAc, pH 4.8.
20. Restriction endonucleases for recombinant check.
21. Restriction endonuclease (*PmeI*).
22. Plate incubator and bio-shaker (30°C and 37°C, respectively).

2.2. Vector Generation

1. Restriction endonuclease (*PacI*).
2. Phenol/chloroform/isoamyl alcohol.
3. TE: 10 mM Tris-HCl, pH 8.0, 1 mM EDTA.
4. 293 Cell (ATCC).
5. Superfect (Qiagen).
6. Dulbecco's modified Eagle's medium (DMEM) (without any supplement).
7. DMEM + 5% FCS (DMEM supplemented with 5% heat-inactivated fetal calf serum and antibiotics).

8. CsCl in PBS:

   $\rho = 1.5$ Dissolve 30 g of optical grade CsCl in final 42.5 mL of phosphate-buffered saline (PBS);

   $\rho = 1.35$ Dilute 15 mL of CsCl ($\rho = 1.5$) to 21 mL with PBS;

   $\rho = 1.25$ Dilute 11 mL of CsCl ($\rho = 1.5$) to 22 mL with PBS
   (Must be sterilized by filtration).

9. Dulbecco's phosphate-buffered saline (D-PBS).
10. Glycerol (UltraPure, Gibco-BRL).
11. Dry ice.
12. Ethanol.
13. Centrifuge with swing baskets (for 50-mL and 250-mL tubes).
14. Ultracentrifuge with swing rotor (i.e., SW41Ti).
15. 5-mL Syringe.
16. Needle (23G).
17. Slide-A-Lyzer 10K (Pierce).
18. Cold room.
19. Autoclaved Eppendorf tubes.
20. −80°C Freezer.

2.3. Analyses of the Promoter Using Luciferase Expression Vector

2.3.1. In Vitro Experiment

1. Target cells.
2. Cell culture apparatus.
3. 96-Well cell culture plate.
4. Complete medium for target cells.
5. DMEM + 5% FCS.
6. Virus to be analyzed.
7. PBS.
8. Cell culture lysis buffer (CCLB, Promega).
9. Luminomater tube and compatible tube.
10. Luciferase assay system (Promega).
11. Dc protein assay (Bio-Rad).

2.3.2. In Vivo Experiment

1. Mice Xenograft model: athymic nude mice; Immunocompetent mice: C57/BL6 or Balb/c mice.
2. Anesthetics.
3. Dry ice.
4. Ethanol.
5. CCLB.
6. Luminomater tube.
7. Luciferase assay system (Promega).
8. Luminometer for 10 s.
9. Dc protein assay (Bio-Rad).

2.4. TK-GCV Experiments

2.4.1. In Vitro TK-GCV Experiments

1. Target cell lines.
2. Control cell lines.

3. Cell culture apparatus.
4. 96-Well plate.
5. DMEM + 5% FCS.
6. Complete medium.
7. Ganciclovir sodium (GCV, CYTOVENE-IV) (*see* **Note 1**).
8. PBS.
9. CellTiter 96 AQueous (Promega).
10. Plate reader with 490-nm filter.

2.4.2. In Vivo TK-GCV Experiments

1. Mice.
2. Anesthetics (ketamine [100 mg/kg wt] + xylazine [15 mg/kg wt]).
3. PBS.
4. Syringe with 23G needle (for cell inoculation).
5. Insulin syringe (281/2G, viral injection).
6. Vernier.
7. Animal operation gear.

3. Methods

3.1. Plasmid Construction

1. Subclone promoter, transgene and poly-A signal into the multicloning site of shuttle vector (i.e., pShuttle) (*see* **Fig. 1** and **Note 2**).
2. Check the construct by restriction analysis.
3. Cut 5 μg of the shuttle vector with *Pme*I (O/N).
4. Electrophorese the DNA on 1.0 % agarose gel.
5. Cut out the band and extract DNA with the gel extraction kit as described by the manufacturer (elute with H_2O).
6. Determine the DNA concentration by optical density OD_{260}.
7. Mix 500 ng of linearized shuttle vector and 100 ng of (circular) pAdEasy1.
8. Cotransform BJ5183 by electroporation (1.8 kV).
9. Add SOC medium immediately.
10. Incubate at 30°C for 30 min.
11. Plate onto LB-KM plate.
12. Incubate at 30°C (O/N or 20 h) (*see* **Note 3**).
13. Pick up small colonies and cultivate in LB-KM O/N at 30°C.
14. Mini-prep with conventional alkaline–SDS method (*see* **Note 4**).
15. Check the recombinant with restriction enzymes (usually *Bam*H1) (*see* **Note 5**).
16. Transform DH5α with correct clone's DNA.
17. Plate on LB-KM plate and incubate O/N at 30°C.
18. Pick up large colony and cultivate in LB-KM O/N at 30°C.
19. Mini-prep with conventional alkaline–SDS method and check the clone with restriction enzyme (*see* **Note 4**).
20. Inoculate the good clone onto 100 mL LB-KM and incubate O/N at 30°C.
21. Plasmid prep with plasmid kit (*see* **Note 6**).

3.2. Vector Generation

1. Cut 10 μg with *Pac*I (approx 3 h, O/N) (*see* **Note 7**).
2. Phenol/chloroform extraction, ethanol precipitation with sodium acetate, 70% ethanol rinsing and drying.

3. Dissolve in 20 μL of TE.
4. Inoculate (approx 1–2) × 10^5 per well of 293 cell on two wells of a six-well plate and incubate O/N.
5. Transfect two wells of 293 cell with linearized shuttle vector using Superfect as described by manufacturer.
6. Incubate 7–10 d until cytopathic effect (CPE) becomes apparent entirely in the wells (*see* **Note 8**).
7. Recover medium and cells into centrifuge tube, repeat freeze and thaw three times, centrifuge at 1450*g* for 10 min at 25°C and recover supernatant.
8. Infect 293 cells on a 10-cm dish with 2 mL of the lysate (*see* **Note 9**).
9. Incubate for 2 h in CO_2 incubator (rock every 15 min).
10. Add 10 mL of complete medium.
11. Incubate until getting entire CPE (approx 36–48 h).
12. Recover cells and medium.
13. Repeat **step 7**.
14. Keep half of this crude viral lysate (CLV) as seed stock.
15. Dilute the rest to 10 mL with DMEM + 5% FCS.
16. Infect 293 cells on two 15-cm dishes with 5 mL of the lysate.
17. Incubate 2 h in CO_2 incubator (rock every 15 min).
18. Add 15 mL of complete medium.
19. Incubate until getting entire CPE.
20. Recover cells and medium.
21. Repeat **step 7**.
22. Dilute CVL to 100 mL with DMEM + 5% FCS.
23. Infect 293 cells on 20 15-cm dishes with 5 mL of the lysate.
24. Incubate 2 h in CO_2 incubator (rock every 15 min).
25. Add 15 mL of complete medium.
26. Incubate until getting entire CPE.
27. Recover cells and medium into 250-mL centrifuge tube.
28. Centrifuge at 160*g*, 5 min at 4°C.
29. Remove most of the medium and resuspend the cells in 40 mL of the medium.
30. Repeat freeze and thaw three times, vortex well, centrifuge at 1450*g* for 10 min at 4°C and recover supernatant (*see* **Note 10**).
31. Put 2 mL of CsCl (ρ = 1.35) into ultracentrifuge tubes; calmly overlay with 3 mL of CsCl (ρ = 1.25) (*see* **Note 11**).
32. Carefully put 6 mL of CVL on it.
33. Adjust the height with the rest of CVL (*see* **Fig. 2**).
34. If necessary, adjust the balance with PBS.
35. Ultracentrifuge with SW41Ti rotor at 35,000 rpm, 10°C, 2 h. Brake can be used.
36. Aspirate the solution from the top to the empty capsid band (*see* **Fig. 2** and **Note 12**).
37. Recover the lower band with pipet and put it into 50-mL centrifuge tube.
38. Add CsCl (ρ = 1.35) to 23 mL and completely mix it.
39. Put it into two new ultracentrifuge tubes.
40. Ultracentrifuge with SW41Ti rotor at 35,000 rpm, 10°C, 8 h to O/N. (Do not use the brake.)
41. Recover lower band by puncture with a 23G needle (*see* **Fig. 2** and **Note 12**).
42. Dilute with equal volume of PBS+20% glycerol.
43. Put the virus into the Slide-A-Lyzer with syringe with a 23G needle.
44. Dialyze against PBS+10% glycerol (more than 200 times volume).

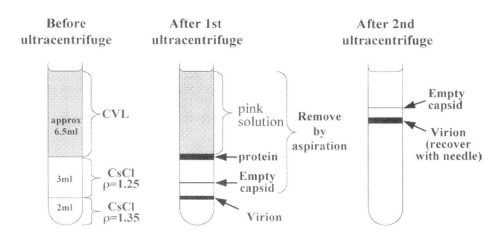

Fig. 2. Ultracentrifuge purification of adenovirus vector.

45. Change PBS+10% glycerol every 2 h, twice.
46. Recover the virus with syringe with a 23G needle.
47. Put it into autoclaved Eppendorf tube and freeze on dry ice.
48. Keep the stock at –80°C.
49. Determine the concentration (physical OD and plaque-forming unit assay) (*see* **Note 13**).

3.3. Analyses of the Promoter in Adenoviral Construct Using Luciferase Expression Vector

To analyze the function of the promoter configured in the adenoviral vector construct, we employ the luciferase gene as reporter. This method enables sensitive and wide-range detection of the transgene expression without using a radioisotope.

3.3.1. In Vitro Experiment

Ordinarily, we perform this assay at 50 multiplicity of infection (MOI) (=pfu/cell). The infectivity of the cells used for the experiments should be analyzed before studying the promoter function because the infectivity may vary in each cell.

1. Inoculate cells on 24-well plates (50,000 cells/well) (*see* **Note 14**).
2. Incubate O/N with complete medium.
3. Dilute virus to 2.5×10^7 (pfu/mL) with DMEM + 5% FCS.
4. Aspirate medium and add 100 μL of viral solution.
5. Incubate for 1 h (rock every 15 min).
6. Aspirate viral solution and add 1 mL of complete medium.
7. Incubate for 48 h.
8. Aspirate medium.
9. Carefully wash the cells with 500 μL of PBS.
10. Add 100 μL of 1× cell culture lysis buffer (CCLB, Promega).
11. Incubate 10 min at room temperature.
12. Scrape off the cells with proximal end of the 200-μL pipet tip.

13. Recover the lysate into an Eppendorf tube.
14. Vortex for 10 s.
15. Spin at 12,000 rpm for 30 s.
16. Recover supernatant into new tube.
17. Place 1 µL of lysate into the luminomater tube (*see* **Note 15**).
18. Add 20 µL of luciferase substrate (luciferase assay system, Promega) (*see* **Note 15**).
19. Measure the luminometer for 1 s (*see* **Note 15**).
20. Measure protein concentration of each sample with Dc protein assay (Bio-Rad).
21. Calculate relative light units (RLU)/mg protein.

3.3.2. In Vivo Analysis (see **Note 16**)

1. Inject 10^9 pfu of the virus into the xenograft or intravenously (*see* **Note 17**).
2. Maintain the mice for 48 h.
3. Sacrifice the mice and harvest the tumors or organs to be analyzed.
4. Freeze the organs on dry ice.
5. Grind the organ sample with mortar and pestle prechilled by dry ice–ethanol (*see* **Notes 18** and **19**).
6. Put the ground organ into the eppendorf tube (approx 500 µL).
7. Add approx 2 volumes of CCLB into the tube.
8. Vortex for 20 s.
9. Repeat freeze and thaw three times.
10. Vortex for 20 s.
11. Centrifuge at 14,000 rpm for 2 min in a microcentifuge.
12. Transfer the supernatant into a new tube and centrifuge at 14,000 rpm for 2 min.
13. Recover the supernatant.
14. Take 10 µL of lysate into the luminomater tube (*see* **Note 15**).
15. Add 200 µL of luciferase substrate (luciferase assay system, Promega) (*see* **Note 15**).
16. Measure with luminometer for 10 s (*see* **Note 15**).
17. Measure protein concentration of each sample with Dc protein assay (Bio-Rad).
18. Calculate RLU/mg protein.

3.4. Suicide Gene Therapy Experiments

3.4.1. In Vitro TK-GCV Experiments

We verify the function of the HSV-TK expressing vectors with cell lines. One point to be mentioned is that the sensitivity of the each cell against activated GCV varies. Therefore, positive and negative control vectors always must be tested in parallel with the vectors under evaluation.

1. Plate target cells onto 96-Well tissue culture plate at a density of 3000 per well.
2. Cultivate with complete medium O/N.
3. Aspirate medium.
4. Add the HSV-tk expression vectors and control vectors diluted with 50 µL of DMEM + 5% FCS.
5. Incubate for 2 h in the incubator.
6. Aspirate the virus solution.
7. Add 100 µL of complete medium containing GCV.
8. Incubate for 3–5 d.
9. Prepare standards (0, 1000, 3000, 10,000 per well) of each cell (*see* **Note 20**).
10. Analyze viable cell number with Cell Titer Kit as described by the manufacturer.

11. Convert the optical density to the number of cells.

3.4.2. In Vivo TK-GCV Experiments

Here, we describe the experiments with subcutaneous xenografts, which are most frequently used model for the therapeutic experiments. However, the model system varies with the target diseases (i.e., lung, liver, and peritoneal metastasis) (*see* **Note 21**).

1. Inoculate target cell on the frank of the nude mice (approx 10^6 cells per injection).
2. Wait until tumors develop to 6–8 mm in diameter.
3. [d 0] Inject virus into the tumor (10^9 pfu in 100 μL PBS).
4. [d 1] Start measuring the tumors.
5. [d 1–14] Administer GCV 50 mg/kg wt, intraperitoneally, twice a day.
6. [d 28] Sacrifice mice and analyze all tumor samples.

4. Notes

1. We use CYTOVENE-IV dissolved with sterile PBS.
2. Ordinarily, we place promoter, transgene, and poly-A signal in the left-to-right direction. As described in **Subheading 1.** some promoters show higher fidelity in the opposite direction. Also, some sequences in the transgene have been reported to affect promoter function *(5)*. Therefore, the design of the vector sometimes requires try and error.
3. As we are expecting clones that underwent homologous recombination in this step, smaller colonies represent such recombinants. Because the growth of those colonies is very slow, it sometimes requires 20 h before colonies become ready to be picked up.
4. As the plasmids in these clones are more than 30 kb, a spin column system may not perform well. Therefore, we are using the conventional alkaline–SDS method for this step.
5. Here, we have to check that we have the correct expression cassette in recombinants. In the case of using the pShuttle system, BamHI is convenient for this purpose. However, the enzyme may vary depending on the system. For this step, the shuttle vector used for recombination should be cut in parallel. This greatly helps the evaluation of the results.
6. This step can be performed with any plasmid purification procedure. In our hand, the EndoFree Plasmid Purification Kit (Qiagen) works best in the meaning of labor and number of generated plaques.
7. As we transfect two wells of 293 cells with 2 μg per well of *Pac*I-treated plasmid, we start from 10 μg of the plasmid, expecting the loss by phenol extraction and ethanol precipitation.
8. If the colonies appear after 14 d, they might be undesired recombinants (possibly replication competent adenovirus [RCA]).
9. Keep the rest of CVL as "seed stock" of the virus.
10. This solution is expected to be turbid and pink.
11. The overlay of the gradient must be done quietly.
12. After the first ultracentrifuge, the layers from the top to the empty capsid band are removed by aspiration. Then, the band with virion is recovered with a pipet. After the second ultracentrifuge, the band with virion is recovered with syringe and needle by puncturing the tube.
13. Physical titer by OD: 2× lysis solution: 880 μL dialysis buffer, 100 μL 10% SDS, 20 μL 100 m*M* EDTA.

    a. Add 50 μL 2× lysis solution onto 50 μL virus. (Use dialysis buffer instead of virus to make a blank tube.)
    b. Vortex, 30 s.
    c. Incubate 10 min at 56°C.

    d. Spin, 14,000 rpm with microcentrifuge.

    e. Measure the OD^{260} nm (1 OD_{250} = dilution factor 2×10^{12} virus particles/mL = 2×10^{12} virus particles/mL).

14. We always analyze positive and negative control cells in parallel with the cell lines assessed.
15. The condition of luciferase assay may vary with the cells, vectors, assay system, or luminometer. A most important point is to avoid the overscale of the RLU. This returns an unexpectable RLU number.
16. All of the procedure must conform to the institutional animal experiment guidelines, especially in the context of humane care.
17. We inject 100 µL of the virus solution diluted with PBS. We use an insulin syringe with 281/2G for intravenous or intratumoral injection because of its minimal dead volume.
18. Contamination of the ethanol into the sample may influence lusiferase assays severely.
19. Because the luciferase activity in the samples varies at most four orders of magnitude, the contamination between samples largely affect the result.
20. As the efficiency of MTS conversion varies in each cell, the OD should be converted into cell number with standard curve of the identical cell.
21. In mouse intraperitoneal administration, the range of the GCV dose on literature is 30-100 mg/kg wt, once or twice a day. All of the painful procedures must be performed under proper anesthesia.

Acknowledgments

This work was supported by grants from the National Cancer Institute (R01 CA74242, R01 CA86881, R01 CA83821), NIDDK(ROI DK 63615), US Department of Defense (DAMD 17-03-1-0104), and the Lustgarten Foundation. We thank Ramon Alemany, Cristina Balague, Kaori Suzuki, and Julia Davytova for assistance.

References

1. He, T. C., Zhou, S., da Costa, L. T., et al. (1998) A simplified system for generating recombinant adenoviruses. *Proc. Natl. Acad. Sci. USA* **95,** 2509–2514.
2. Hearing, P. and Shenk, T. (1986) The adenovirus type 5 E1A enhancer contains two functionally distinct domains: one is specific for E1A and the other modulates all early units in cis. *Cell* **45,** 229–236.
3. Steinwaerder, D. S. and Lieber, A. (2000) Insulation from viral transcriptional regulatory elements improves inducible transgene expression from adenovirus vectors in vitro and in vivo. *Gene Ther.* **7,** 556–567.
4. Hitt, M. M., Addison, C. L., and Graham, F. L. (1997) Human adenovirus vectors for gene transfer into mammalian cells. *Adv. Pharmacol.* **40,** 137–206.
5. Kurachi, S., Deyashiki, Y., Takeshita, J., et al. (1999) Genetic mechanisms of age regulation of human blood coagulation factor IX. *Science* **285,** 739–743.

5

Replication-Selective Oncolytic Adenoviruses

Gunnel Halldén, Stephen H. Thorne, Jingping Yang, and David H. Kirn

1. Introduction

Replication-selective oncolytic viruses are being developed as novel, targeted anti-cancer agents (virotherapy) *(1,2)*. Viruses have evolved to infect cells, replicate, induce cell death, release viral particles, and, finally, to spread in human tissues. Replication in tumor tissue leads to amplification of the input dose at the tumor site, whereas a lack of replication in normal tissues can result in efficient clearance and reduced toxicity. Revolutionary advances in molecular biology and genetics have led to a fundamental understanding of both the replication and pathogenicity of viruses and carcinogenesis. These advances have allowed novel agents to be engineered to enhance their safety and/or their antitumoral potency *(2,3)*. One approach to engineering adenovirus selectivity has been to complement loss-of-function mutations in cancers with loss-of-function mutations within the adenovirus genome. Many of the same critical regulatory proteins that are inactivated by viral gene products during adenovirus replication are also inactivated during carcinogenesis *(4–7)*. Because of this convergence, the deletion of viral genes that inactivate these cellular regulatory proteins can be complemented by genetic inactivation of these proteins within cancer cells *(8,9)*. This concept was proven by the E1B55kD deletion in the *dl*1520 mutant virus (Onyx-015), which is selective for cells lacking functional p53 *(8)* enabling viral replication in the majority of human cancers. Clinical trials with *dl*1520 ultimately proved the selectivity and relative safety of this approach (i.e., **refs. *10–12***). However, more efficacious adenoviruses are needed.

This chapter will review key methods and protocols for the testing and evaluation of replication-selective oncolytic adenoviruses in vitro and in vivo. We include protocols for (1) interactions with cytotoxic chemotherapy drugs in vitro, (2) imaging in live animals, and (3) a phase I/II clinical trial. Construction of viral mutants and basic

From: *Methods in Molecular Medicine, Vol. 90, Suicide Gene Therapy: Methods and Reviews*
Edited by: C. J. Springer © Humana Press Inc., Totowa, NJ

protocols in virology have previously been extensively covered and will only be referred to in this chapter (for detailed protocols, *see* **ref. 13**).

1.1. Interaction Studies in Cells in Culture: Viral Mutants in Combination With Cytotoxic Chemotherapy Drugs

Cancer therapy such as surgery, radiation, and chemotherapy are often only effective in early-stage disease, whereas metastatic cancers are rarely eliminated by single-agent therapy. Hence, low efficacy was documented with *dl*1520 as a single-agent therapy in phase I and I/II trials. However, a favorable and potentially synergistic interaction with chemotherapy was discovered in some tumor types *(11)*. Cell-culture-based models have been developed for the evaluation of viral mutants and drug interactions in vitro *(14,15)*. Conditions for supra-additive (synergistic) and subadditive (antagonistic) effects on cell death can thus be evaluated in cancer cell lines in culture prior to preclinical testing. These models can be used to evaluate if the combination with cytotoxic chemotherapy drugs could result in enhanced effects on cell death and if these interactions were dependent on the order of addition of each therapy. We performed a series of sequencing studies in both human and murine cancer cell lines testing adenoviral mutants in combination with cytotoxic drugs used in the clinic.

The methods in this chapter outline cell culture conditions for two human cell lines, LNCaP and H460, preparation of wild-type adenovirus type 5 (Ad5) and cytotoxic drugs (paclitaxel and cisplatin), the cell proliferation/killing assay (MTS assay), and analysis of virus and drug interactions by construction of isobolograms. For in-depth analysis of synergy vs antagonism, and construction and statistical significance of isobole graphs, we refer the reader to the literature *(16–18)*.

1.2. Comparing the In Vivo Distribution Patterns of Adenoviral Strains by Noninvasive Bioluminescent Imaging

In recent years, a large volume of work has focused on the problems of retargeting adenoviral strains to specific tissue types and on producing tissue-specific expression of genes from adenoviral cassettes for use in cancer gene therapy. Although much can be learned from in vitro and cell culture assays, accurate analyses of alterations in biodistribution or gene expression patterns require the use of living animals. Traditionally, this is assessed by the ex vivo examination of postmortem or biopsy samples. However, the assay of many different tissue types is time-consuming and any temporal information requires a different set of animals for each time-point. This not only requires a large number of animals, but any time-course information from individual animals is lost. Noninvasive imaging methods, such as magnetic resonance imaging (MRI) or positron-emission tomography (PET), have therefore emerged as powerful alternative tools for these studies. However, many biological processes cannot be externally monitored by these methods, as key molecules are not distinguishable, even in the presence of contrast dyes or radioactive tracers. However, the observation that biological sources of light can be detected from within a living mammal *(19)* has allowed charge-coupled device (CCD) cameras and bioluminescent reporters to be used together as an alternative means to noninvasively image whole animals *(20)*. This relatively simple and very sensitive method has increasingly been used to follow the biodistribution of viruses and bacteria within a host organism *(21–23)*. The methods involved and equipment required for the rapid screening of different adenoviral constructs by bioluminescent imaging will be covered in this chapter.

1.3. Clinical Trials: Intraarterial and Intravenous Delivery of VTP-1 Adenovirus E1A Mutant in Patients With Metastatic Colorectal Carcinoma

Definitive data are now available from numerous phase I and II clinical trials with *dl*1520, a well-characterized and well-quantitated virus *(10–12,24)*. In summary, *dl*1520 was well tolerated at the highest practical doses that could be administered (2 $\times$ 10^{12} to 2 $\times$ 10^{13} particles) by intratumoral, intraperitoneal, intraarterial, and intravenous routes. No clinically significant toxicity in the liver or other organs was notable. Flulike symptoms were the most common toxicities and were increased in patients receiving intravascular treatment. In addition to toxicity and efficacy data, it was critical to obtain biological data on viral replication, antiviral immune responses, and their relationship to antitumoral efficacy in the earliest phases of clinical research.

In this section, we will review a clinical trial protocol for a phase I/II dose escalation study in patients with inoperable 5-fluorouracil (5-FU)-resistant colorectal carcinoma liver metastasis for evaluation of a second-generation E1-region-deleted adenoviral mutant (VTP-1) *(9)*. The protocol is designed for delivery of virus either by hepatic arterial (HAI) or intravenous (iv) infusion.

2. Materials

2.1. Virus and Cytotoxic Drug Interactions in Culture

1. Dulbecco's modified Eagle's Medium (DMEM) (Invitrogen, CA, USA).
2. Fetal calf serum (FCS) (Invitrogen).
3. Sterile flat-bottom 96-well culture plates.
4. H460 cells, non-small-cell lung carcinoma cell line (ATCC, VA, USA).
5. LNCaP cells, prostate epithelial carcinoma cell line (ATCC).
6. Paclitaxel (Taxol) (Calbiochem, CA, USA).
7. Cis-platinum (Cisplatin) (Sigma-Aldrich, UK).
8. Adenovirus type 5 wild type (Ad5) and mutants.
9. Dimethyl sulfoxide (DMSO).
10. MTS assay kit, CellTiter 96 Aqueous, One Solution Cell Proliferation Assay (Promega, WI, USA).
11. Enzyme-linked immunosorbent assay (ELISA) Microplate reader equipped with a 490-nm filter.
12. Software for analysis of dose–response curves such as Prism and Excel.

2.2. Bioluminescent Imaging In Vivo

1. Plate-reading luminometer.
2. Sterile, white 96-well tissue culture plates.
3. Luciferase assay system (Promega, Madison, WI).
4. IVIS Imaging System with Living Image software (Xenogen Corp., Alameda, CA).
5. D-Luciferin or coelenterazine.
6. 70% Ethyl or methyl alcohol.
7. Cell culture lysis reagent (Promega, Madison, WI).
8. Colorimetric protein assay (Bio-Rad, Hercules, CA).

3. Methods

3.1. Interaction Studies With Paclitaxel and Cisplatin

3.1.1. Cell Culture

The LNCaP and H460 cells were grown in DMEM supplemented with 10% FCS at 37°C and kept in an atmosphere of 5% CO_2. First, cell seeding density in 96-well plates was determined so that cells were subconfluent at the end of the study, 6 d later. Early passage cells were seeded at 5×10^3 to 4×10^4 cells/well and assayed every day for 6 d by the MTS cell proliferation reagent (see below). A cell density of 1×10^4 cells/well resulted in exponential growth over time, up to 5–6 d in culture for most cell lines, including LNCaP and H460 cells (see **Note 1**).

3.1.2. Preparation of Ad5, Paclitaxel, and Cisplatin

A wide concentration range of each agent was tested to generate dose–response curves for determination of dose killing 50% of cells (EC_{50} values) including nine test concentrations each of virus and cytotoxic drugs. The concentrations were selected so that the two to three highest concentrations resulted in 100% cell killing and the two to three lowest concentrations had no effect on cell death. A reproducible and sensitive dose response was obtained with virus or drugs for 5–6 d at the following concentration ranges: for Ad5 wild-type virus 1×10^{-6} to 1×10^5 particles/cell (ppc), for paclitaxel 3×10^{-8} to 3×10^4 nM, and for cisplatin 8×10^{-7} to 2×10^2 µM. Stock solutions of the cytotoxic drugs were made and stored at –20°C; paclitaxel in methanol at 6.0 mM, and cisplatin in DMSO at 10 mM. All subsequent dilutions (5- to 10-fold) were in the incubation media; DMEM was supplemented with 2% FCS (see **Note 2**). Virus was stored at –80°C and was prepared by previously established methods (*13,25*). Viral particle concentration and plaque-forming units (pfu) were determined according to standard procedures (*13,26*).

Four different mixture ratios were included in each experiment, keeping the ratios of Ad5/drug constant for all cell lines and studies so that complete dose–response curves could be generated for each test ratio. The ratios were as follow: 3, 33, 333, and 3333 for Ad5/paclitaxel and 50, 250, 1250, and 6250 for Ad5/cisplatin.

3.1.3. Cell Killing Assay

Each experiment was carried out using 96-well plates, one plate for a complete dose–response curve including virus, one cytotoxic drug, and four mixture ratios of the combination treatment. The plates were set up in triplicate and each study repeated three times. Live cells were quantitated as an indirect measure of cell death with the tetrazolium compound reagent MTS [Owen's reagent; 3-(4,5-dimethylthiazol-2-yl)-5-(3-carboxymethoxyphenyl)-2-(4-sulfophenyl)-2*H*-tetrazolium] and an electron-coupling reagent PMS (phenazine methosulfate) supplied as a one-component solution. The MTS tetrazolium compound is converted to a soluble formazan product in aqueous solution by mitochondrial dehydrogenase enzymes found in metabolically active cells. The amount of formazan product can be quantitated after 30 min by absorbance at 490 nm and is directly proportional to the number of living cells in the well. The product is stable for up to 4 h, with an increase in absorbance over time enabling multiple readings of the same plate. Two sets of conditions were tested and evaluated for each virus and drug combination. In one study, cells were preincubated with drug before virus was added, and in the second study, cells were infected with virus prior to the addition of drug. These sequencing studies were to establish if supra-additive effects on cell death could be achieved by a specific sequence of administration. In most cases, either virus or drug was added 1 d after cell seeding, and after an additional day in culture, drug or virus was added for the remaining incubation time. It is important to consider the stability of each drug in culture when designing a new study. For example, paclitaxel is hydrolyzed within 3–4 d in aqueous solution, whereas cisplatin is relatively stable in the culture media. Therefore, the experimental design was different for the two drugs. For paclitaxel, the above protocol was followed, and both virus and paclitaxel were present throughout the remaining incubation period. However, for cisplatin, the cells were incubated with drug for 4 h while the virus was present throughout the experiment. All studies were terminated 7 d after cell seeding.

3.1.4. Sequencing Studies

Day 0: Plate cells at 1×10^4 cells/well in 96-well plates in 100 µL DMEM supplemented with 10% FCS.

Day 1: Remove media and replace with 80 µL incubation media (DMEM supplemented with 2% FCS). Make up dilutions of virus and drugs at 10 times the final concentration in incubation media (*see* **Subheading 3.1.2.**). Add 10 µL of the agent to be tested first, either virus or drug, to the respective wells.

On each plate, set up three wells as control (untreated cells + media) and three wells as blank (media only). Each experiment is performed in triplicate plates.

Day 2: Make up fresh dilutions of virus and drugs (*see* **Subheading 3.1.2.**). Add 10 µL of either drug or virus to the respective wells. For example, wells containing paclitaxel will receive 10 µL of the respective virus dilutions. Add media to wells receiving one agent only or neither virus nor drug, so that the final volume in each well is 100 µL. Incubate at 37°C and monitor plates daily.

Days 6–7: Thaw an aliquot of the MTS reagent and add 20 µL to each well to terminate the study. Incubate for 0.5–1.0 h at 37°C and measure absorbance at 490 nm. If absorbance values are low (less than 1.0 optical density [OD] units), incubate for another 0.5–1.0 h) and repeat the measurement (*see* **Note 3**). The incubation and measurement can be repeated up to 4 h after addition of reagent. Process data as described in **Subheading 3.1.5.**

3.1.5. Determination of EC$_{50}$ Values and Analysis of Additive, Supra-Additive, and Subadditive Interactions

The 490-nm absorbance data are a direct measure of live cells in each well and the proportion of cell death (expressed as percent of total cells) can be calculated using the following conversion:

$$\text{Live cell } (z) = \frac{y - \text{bl}}{c - \text{bl}}$$
$$\% \text{ Dead cells } (w) = (1 - z) \times 100$$

where y is the measurement in the test well, bl is the average of the media blank, and c is the average of control untreated cells. The average blank absorbance values from each plate (media only) is subtracted from every well and cells without treatments (control), averaged, and used as the 100% live cell reference (no cell death). Each value from treated wells can be compared to the control, averaged from the three plates, and percent dead cells calculated for each well. Data are analyzed (i.e., Prism software) and dose–response curves constructed to calculate the dose killing 50% of cells (EC_{50} values) for each condition, including virus and cytotoxic drugs alone and for each test ratio. Effects on cell death are presented both as a function of viral dose (see **Fig. 1A**) and of drug concentration (see **Fig. 1B**). To evaluate whether interactions did occur, isobole graphs can then be generated by connecting the two points for virus and drug alone, (vEC50, 0) and (0, dEC50), and by plotting the individual EC_{50} values for each condition in the same diagram (see **Fig. 2**). The combination index (CI) is used to estimate additive, supra-additive, and subadditive interactions:

$$CI = \frac{vcEC_{50}}{vEC_{50}} + \frac{dcEC_{50}}{dEC_{50}}$$

where vEC_{50} is the EC_{50} of Ad5 alone, dEC_{50} is the EC_{50} of drug alone, $vcEC_{50}$ is the EC_{50} of Ad5 at the respective combination ratio, and $dcEC_{50}$ is the EC_{50} of the drug at the respective combination ratio.

If CI >1, there is a subadditive effect; if CI <1, there is a supra-additive effect; and if CI = 1, there is no interaction (additive effect). Examples of supra-additive effects are demonstrated in **Fig. 2**, where each mixture ratio of Ad5 and cisplatin resulted in CI values <1 (data below the line of additivity).

3.2. In Vivo Viral Distribution Patterns

3.2.1. Luciferase-Expressing Adenovirus

Although methods for adenoviral construction will not be discussed in detail, the following methods describe some considerations for such constructs and their initial in vitro testing, followed by the design and application of small mammal experiments, analysis of results, and ex vivo verification (see **Note 4**).

3.2.2. Considerations for Viral Constructs

The luminescent imaging of bacterial pathogenesis in living animals normally utilizes bacteria-carrying plasmids, which encode both the luciferase enzyme and the enzymes required for the construction of its substrate, such as with the lux operon of Xenorhabdus luminescens (27). However, the limited cloning capacity of adenovirus allows only the luciferase gene itself to be inserted. Its substrate must then be administered to the host animal prior to imaging. Therefore, some thought must be given to the choice of luciferase enzyme. Firefly luciferase enzyme has been most commonly used, as its substrate (D-luciferin) is known to rapidly and evenly distribute throughout the host animal following intraperitoneal administration. Recently, however, the Renilla luciferase enzyme/protein system has also been shown to function well within mammalian hosts (28). This also has the advantage that it uses a different substrate (coelentarazine) to the Firefly system, making it possible to use two luminescent reporter genes in one host system. This opens up the possibility of studying the effects of coinfection by two micro-organisms at once or the examination of colocalization of

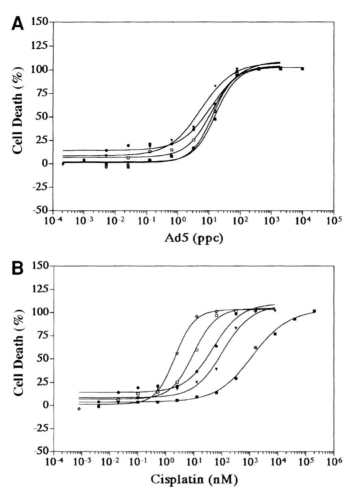

Fig. 1. Dose–response curves for LNCaP cells treated with Ad5 and cisplatin alone and at four different ratios: (**A**) as a function of viral particles/cell (ppc) and (**B**) as a function of cisplatin concentration (n*M*). Ad5 or cisplatin alone (■) and each Ad5/cisplatin mixture ratio 1–4, respectively (▼ ratio 1=50, ● ratio 2=50, □ ratio 3=1250, ◇ ratio 4=6250).

virus to specifically transfected tumor cells. It is also possible that could be used to simultaneously examine viral location as well as tissue-specific gene expression from a virally encoded promoter.

Another consideration during the design of the viral construct is the choice of the promoter. Studies looking at changes in adenoviral distribution will require a strong, constitutive promoter such as the cytomegalovirus (CMV) promoter, whereas the examination of patterns of tissue-specific gene expression are likely to incorporate specialized promoters (*see* **Note 4**). It is recommended that nonreplicating vectors are

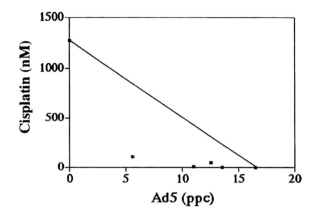

Fig. 2. Isobologram of Ad5 in combination with cisplatin, showing EC_{50} values for the four different combination ratios and for drug and virus alone shown in **Fig. 1**. The four data points under the line of additivity illustrate supra-additive interactions.

used during retargeting experiments or when looking at tissue-specific gene expression, as this will produce a more sustained and quantitative level of luciferase expression. However, replicating virus would be incorporated when comparing the kinetics of infection and clearance of different oncolytic adenoviral strains. Alternatively, the tumor cell lines themselves may be transfected with a luciferase-expressing vector in order to then examine the location and level of tumor burden *(29)*.

3.2.3. In Vitro Testing of Viral Constructs

It is first necessary to establish the level and limits of the bioluminescence produced from any viral constructs, as this technique is most powerful when directly comparing different strains. This may be done in HEK 293 cells or in a specific cell line to be studied.

1. Split cells into a tissue culture flask and leave overnight at 37°C, 5% CO_2, so that cells reach 60–80% confluence the next day; this ensures all cells will be in the same growth log phase.
2. Seed wells of a sterile, white 96-well plate at 1×10^4 cells/well in 2% FCS and incubate for a further 24 h (this may need to be varied for different cell lines in order to achieve the desired 80–90% confluence).
3. Infect wells with 10-fold serial dilutions of virus ranging from 100,000 to 0.000001 viral particles/cell (ppc) and leave for a further 17 h, include uninfected control wells.
4. Lyse cells and assay for luciferase expression (i.e., Luciferase Assay System; Promega); a plate-reading luminometer is recommended, but a cuvette-reading system can be used. A linear increase of relative light units (RLUs) with increasing ppc should be seen, up to a maximum value. If the maximum value is three or more orders of magnitude greater than the cell-only control, then efficient luciferase expression has been achieved. In addition, 50% of maximum bioluminescence produced at approx 10–100 ppc indicates efficient levels of infection (*see* **Fig. 3**).

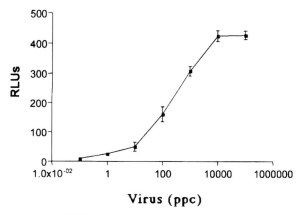

Virus (ppc)

Fig. 3. Graph showing the RLUs produced 17 h postinfection of 1×10^4 HEK 293 cells with different particles/cell (ppc) of a nonreplicating Ad5, expressing Firefly luciferase under the control of a CMV promoter. RLUs were assayed by the Luciferase Assay System, according to the manufacturer's instructions. Uninfected control cells produced 0.006 RLUs.

3.2.4. Small Mammal Studies

Several factors need to be considered when designing animal protocols and an initial small-scale study is recommended. The choice of animal subject is limited by the imaging chamber, which will only hold small rodents. Mice are preferred, as levels of light emission are dependent on tissue depth (with detection up to 1–3 cm) and a total of five mice can be imaged at any one time. If a tumor model system is being incorporated, the tumor should be located as close to the surface of the animal as possible, ideally subcutaneous or intraperitoneal.

The viral dose needs to be ascertained through pilot experiments and the route of delivery and imaging time-points will depend on what is to be examined (*see* **Notes 4–6**).

3.2.5. Imaging

1. Prepare substrate. When using D-luciferin, a fresh stock of 15 mg/mL should be made in phosphate-buffered saline (PBS) and filter-sterilized through a 0.2-μm filter. If *Renilla* luciferase enzyme is being used, coelenterazine should be made to 2 mg/mL in methanol. Also, prepare the imaging area, initialize the camera and adjust the field of view, and clean the imaging chamber with 70% ethyl alcohol.
2. Inject D-luciferin substrate at 150 mg/kg body weight or coelenterazine at 3.5 mg/kg body weight. This should be done intraperitoneally 3–5 min prior to imaging. Try to keep the start time constant between animals. It is important to perform a kinetic study to determine the optimum time of luminescence in vivo for different animal models. Firefly luciferase can be expected to be active for approx 45 min postsubstrate administration, whereas *Renilla* luciferase is active for the much shorter period of 10 min and so should be applied postanaesthetic.
3. Apply anaesthetic to the animals. Isofluorane is highly recommended, as it is nonmetabolized and the animals can be kept anesthetized for longer periods; also, the short recovery times allow for more frequent imaging. Repeated anesthesia has no discernable effect on tumor progression or viral pathogenesis.

4. Once animals have achieved a stable and safe level of anesthesia, they can be carefully placed in the imaging chamber and arranged in position for imaging. Again, observe the mice for 30–60 s to ensure that they are safely anesthetized before closing the chamber door and commencing imaging.
5. It is recommended that an initial image of 60 s exposure time and a bin level of 8 be taken. If a saturated image is produced, the exposure time can be reduced to as low as 5 s. Alternatively, a weak image may need an exposure time as long as 5 min (*see* Notes 7 and 8 for improving imaging). As a two-dimensional picture is produced, collecting several images from different angles will help ascertain the exact source of the luminescence (*see* **Fig. 4**).
6. Once satisfactory images have been produced, animals should be placed in a recovery chamber at 37°C and observed until self-righting ability has been restored.

3.2.6. Analysis of Results

The Living Image software provides a variety of options for data analysis. For example, the scale can be adjusted to clearly highlight areas of luminescence. The minimum cutoff value can be increased to remove background or decreased to pick up areas of weak bioluminescence and the maximum value altered to highlight the differences in the strength of luminescence. However, it is useful to use the same scale when comparing different groups or time-points. Regions of interest (ROIs) can also be highlighted and the luminescence produced from within these regions quantified. These can then be averaged for all of the animals within a single image and comparisons made between different groups and timepoints.

3.2.7. Ex Vivo Verification of Results

It is important to justify the accuracy of the results with some ex vivo assay. If possible, the experiment should be completed before all luminescence is lost. Animals can then be sacrificed immediately after the final image, and selected organs or tissues removed and flash frozen in liquid nitrogen for future analysis. Alternatively an extra group may be needed for sacrifice during the course of the experiment.

1. Frozen tissues can then either be ground under liquid nitrogen and suspended in a small volume (1 mL) of cell culture lysis reagent (Promega) or thawed and homogenized on ice in 0.5 mL of lysis reagent for at least 5 min before a further 0.5 mL is added.
2. Suspensions are then freeze–thawed three times in $N_2(l)/37°C$ cycles.
3. Centrifuge suspensions (3 min, 10,000g, 4°C) to remove cellular matter.
4. Remove two 100-µL aliquots from each sample; one is then used to calculate the protein content by Bradford assay (Bio-Rad, Hercules, CA) (*30*) and the other used to assay RLUs produced with the Luciferase Assay System (*see* **Subheading 3.2.3.**). The relative proportion of light emitted between different tissues and groups should mirror the relative levels of bioluminescence seen in the final image. This can then be used to justify imaging comparisons between different groups and time-points (*see* **Table 1**).

Fig. 4. Images of BALB/c mice following injection with 1×10^{10} particles of the adenovirus described and used in Fig. 3. Injection was initially via the tail vein with mice imaged 24 h later, (**A**) from the side or (**B**) from above (10 s exposure; bin 2). Strongest bioluminescence is seen emanating from the liver, this was later verified ex vivo (*see* **Table 1**). This was repeated for an intraperitoneal injection, with images taken 3 d postinjection, again from (**C**, p.82) the side or (**D**) above (30 s exposure; bin 8). This time the spleen appears to be the major target organ and, again, this is verified ex vivo in **Table 1**.

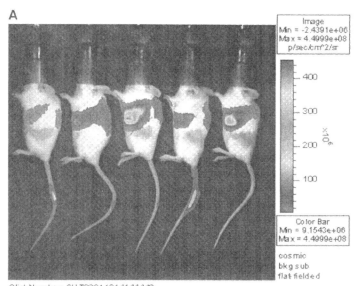

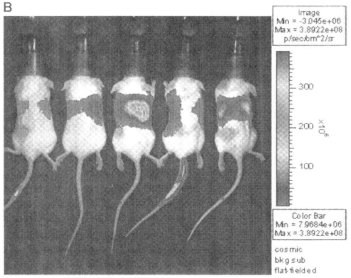

Fig. 4 *(continued on next page)*

C

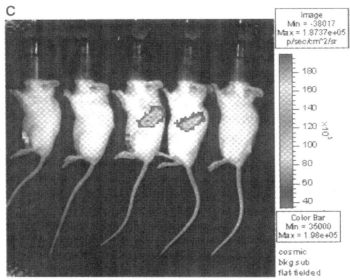

ClickNumber: SH T20011214154435
Acq Date: Fri, Dec 14, 2001
Acq Time: 15:44:47, 30 sec.
Bin: 8, FOV: 20, f# 1
Camera: IVIS 34 IC RF, SI 620 SITE

D

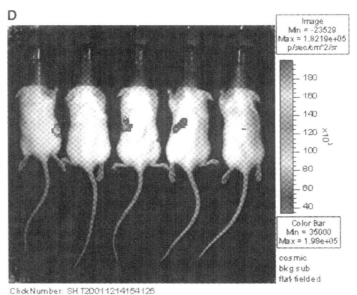

ClickNumber: SH T20011214154125
Acq Date: Fri, Dec 14, 2001
Acq Time: 15:41:38, 30 sec.
Bin: 8, FOV: 20, f# 1
Camera: IVIS 34 IC RF, SI 620 SITE

Fig. 4 *(continued from page 81)*

Table 1
Relative Luminescence from Ex Vivo Tissue Samples

	Bioluminescence (RLUs/μg protein)	
Organ	Tail vein injection	Intraperitoneal injection
Liver	301.2	12.5
Spleen	7.2	78.5
Lungs	3.5	1.7

Note: Relative levels of luminescence produced from ex vivo tissue samples (tissue removed 7 d postinjection, from the animals shown in **Fig. 4**). Protein was first extracted from the tissue and quantitated by Bradford assay, and the luminescence measured with the Luciferase Assay System. All values are the average of five samples.

3.3. Clinical Trial Protocol: Phase I/II Dose Escalation Study in Patients With Liver Metastasis

3.3.1 Study Rationale

Colorectal carcinoma liver metastases are an excellent target for adenoviral therapies. Progression in the liver is a major clinical problem, with almost all of the patients dying from colon cancer having developed liver metastasis at some point. Once the metastatic tumor deposit(s) in a patient are deemed surgically unresectable, the standard chemotherapy regimen (5-FU/leucovorin and irinotecan) results in minimal impact on survival duration. Less than 5% will live more than 2 yr. Novel therapies that can reduce the intrahepatic tumor load are needed.

Adenovirus has a natural tropism for the liver and local–regional control should benefit patients without significant extrahepatic metastases. Previous trials have shown that colorectal cancers can be readily infected following intravascular delivery and that this mode of delivery was safe and feasible for attenuated viruses *(12)*. Intravenous infusion is the preferred mode of administration because it is minimally invasive and inexpensive and the potential for systemic tumor control is maximized. However, intravenous delivery is highly inefficient, the likelihood of antibody neutralization is high, and it is possible that virus delivery to tumors is not sufficient to result in efficacy. Therefore, targeted hepatic arterial perfusion needs to be evaluated as well. This method should markedly improve delivery while decreasing contact time with neutralizing antibodies, although this mode of delivery can be expensive and requires an invasive procedure. It is essential to identify the pros and cons of each mode of administration as early as possible in the clinical research and development process (*see* **Note 9**).

3.3.2. Primary Study Objectives

To determine the following:

1. The safety/toxicity profile and maximum tolerated dose (MTD)/maximum feasible dose (MFD) by hepatic arterial (HAI) or intravenous (iv) infusion (*see* **Note 10**).

2. The level and duration of viral replication and shedding into the bloodstream following HAI or iv infusion.
3. The cytokine and antibody-mediated immune response following HAI or iv infusion (cycle 1 vs 3; *see* **Table 2**).

3.3.3. Secondary Study Objectives

To determine the following:

1. The antitumoral efficacy in patients with 5-FU-refractory tumors.
2. The pharmacokinetics of virus following HAI or iv infusion.

3.3.4. Study Population: Inclusion Criteria

Patients must meet all of the following criteria (*see* **Note 9**):

1. Histological or cytological confirmation of metastatic colorectal carcinoma.
2. Intrahepatic metastasis not resectable for potential cure.
3. Age $\geq$ 18 yr.
4. Tumor resistance to 5-FU and/or 5-FU and irinotecan defined as progressive disease within $\leq$ 6 mo after 5-FU-based chemotherapy.
5. Expected survival of at least 3 mo.
6. Measurable tumor by radiographic scanning.
7. Women of childbearing potential and nonvasectomized men must agree to use a double barrier of contraception method during the treatment period.
8. Karnovsky performance status scale (KPS) $\geq$ 70.
9. Patients' laboratory results must lie within the following parameters; granulocyte count $\geq$ 1000/mm^3, platelets $\geq$ 100,000/mm^3, serum creatinine $\leq$ 2 mg/dL, bilirubin $\leq$ 2 mg/dL, alanine aminotransferase (ALT), aspartate aminotransferase (AST), and alkaline phosphatase $\leq$ 3 times the upper limit of normal, albumin $\geq$ 3 g/dL, prothrombin time (PT) and activated partial thromboplastin time (APTT) $\leq$ 1.5 times the upper limit of normal.

3.3.5. Study Population: Exclusion Criteria

The presence of any of the following excludes a patient from entering the study: >50% replacement of the liver by cancer, severe comorbid disease that makes completion of study treatment and follow-up unlikely, esophageal variceal bleeding within 8 wk of the screening visit, an ongoing active infection or a documented history of human immunodeficiency virus (HIV) infection; concomitant hematological malignancy; treatment with any investigational agent, radiotherapy, chemotherapy, or surgery within 4 wk prior to the screening visit; antiviral therapy within 4 wk prior to the screening visit; pregnant or lactating females; inability or unwillingness to give informed consent.

3.3.6. Assignment to Treatment Arm and Dose Cohort

1. Patients without a hepatic arterial (HA) catheter *in situ* will be assigned to treatment arm A and will receive iv VTP-1; patients with a HA catheter *in situ* will be assigned to treatment arm B and will receive HAI VTP-1.
2. Each eligible patient will be enrolled into one of four dose cohorts (during phase I dose escalation) or the MTD/MFD (during phase II) on one arm (either A or B).

Table 2
Activity Schedule for VTP-1 Clinical Trial

Study day	B	1	2	3	4	5	8	10	12	15[a]
						Cycle day				
Consent form signed	X									
VTP-1 injection		X								
Inpatient		X	X							
Outpatient				X	X	X	X	X	X	X
Medical history	X	X[b]					X	X		
Physical exam[c]	X	X[b,d]	X							X
Tumor biopsy	X					X				
Blood draw for										
Routine labs[e]	X	X[b]	X	X	X		(X)[f]			X
CD3, CD4, CD8	X							X		
QPCR for virus	X	X[g]		X	X	X	X	X	X	X
Plaque assay for virus	(X)			(X)		(X)	(X)			
Cytokines by ELISA	X	X[g]		X	X	X	X	X	X	X
Urine specimen										
Routine urinalysis	X									
Urine or serum pregnancy test	X									
QPCR for virus	(X)			X		X	X	X	X	X
Imaging studies[h]										
CT or US (other)	X									X
Chest radiograph	X			X		X	X	X	X	X
Functional imaging						(X)				

B, baseline prior to treatment.

[a]Blood draws/tests, physical exams, medical history/adverse effects reporting for d 15 of the previous cycle may serve as d 1 pretreatment data for the subsequent cycle (if <7 d apart).

[b]Obtained prior to treatment.

[c]Including vital signs, Karnofsky Performance Status (KPS) and weight.

[d]Vital signs to be obtained posttreatment as follows (minimum): every 15 min × 4; then hourly × 4; if not significant (>15%) change from baseline (for blood pressure [BP], respiratory rate [RR], heart rate [HR]), then monitor per hospital ward routine—if significant change has occurred continue to check at least every hour until significant change has resolved.

[e]Complete blood count (CBC) with differential, platelets; prothrombin time (PT)/partial thromboplastin time (PTT), international normalization ratio (INR); electrolytes, blood urea nitrogen (BUN), C-reactive protein; liver function tests (including aspartate aminotransferase (AST), alanine aminotransferase (ALT), γ-glutamyl transpeptidase (CGT), total and direct bilirubin, lactic dehydrogenase (LDH) and carcino-embryonic antigen (CEA).

[f](X) indicates optional.

[g]Obtained prior to (baseline) and following treatment on d 1 at these times: 5 min, 10 min, 30 min, 60 min, 90 min, 120 min, 180 min, 360 min, 12 h, 24 h.

[h]CT, computed tomography scan; US, ultrasound.

3.3.7. Phase I Dose-Escalation Scheme

1. VTP-1 (range: 10^{11} to 3×10^{12} viral particles) will be administered by a single iv injection (arm A) or a single hepatic arterial infusion (arm B) on the first day of each cycle. Intravenous injections and hepatic arterial infusions of VTP-1 must be administered by a physician or a registered nurse trained in the administration of this treatment. Patients will be treated and initially followed as inpatients.

2. Each patient will initially receive up to three cycles of single agent viral treatment given at 2-weekly intervals followed by a computerized tomography (CT) scan 2 wk after cycle 3 (i.e., wk 6; *see* **Table 2**).

3. If this scan demonstrates a complete or partial response (CR or PR) or stable disease (SD), the viral cycles and radiographic evaluation will be repeated.

4. Patients will receive repeat treatment at the same dose if they have no dose-limiting toxicity (DLT) with cycle 1 (*see* **Note 10**). Patients experiencing a DLT will be eligible for repeat treatment at the previous (lower) dose level. If a DLT occurs in cohort 1, it will be determine what dose (if any) would be administered during subsequent treatments.

Phase I Dose Escalation:

Cohort 1:	1×10^{11} particles
Cohort 2:	3×10^{11} particles
Cohort 3:	1×10^{12} particles (MFD for phase II)
Cohort 4:	3×10^{12} particles

5. Viral doses will be escalated independently between patients on arm A and arm B. During the phase I portion on each treatment arm, the dose will be escalated from 10^{11} to 10^{12} particles in half-log increments (four levels) with one patient per dose level unless a $\geq$ grade 2 toxicity is observed. When this has been recorded, three to six patients will be entered per dose cohort.
6. Each patient will be enrolled sequentially into treatment cohorts with at least a 2-wk interval between each cohort to allow an adequate assessment of toxicity. Dose escalation will be based on the toxicity seen with the first cycle of therapy.
7. If DLT is observed in a cohort, up to six patients will be enrolled at that dose level. Patients will be enrolled until a second DLT occurs (which defines the toxic dose) or until six patients are enrolled at that dose level; at least a 1-wk interval between treatment of each of these patients will be required. If a second DLT is not experienced in that cohort, dose escalation will continue.
8. The MTD or MFD (if an MTD is not reached) will be used for each treatment arm during the phase II trial segment to further evaluate safety and efficacy.

3.3.8. Phase II

Phase I data will be reviewed prior to initiation of the phase II trial segment. If appropriate based on safety and biological end-point data, the phase II segment of the trial will commence. The MTD or MFD (if an MTD is not reached) will be used for each treatment arm during the phase II trial segment to further evaluate safety and efficacy. The MFD for phase II is 10^{12} particles. This dose resulted in tumor infection and antitumoral efficacy in previous trials with a similar adenovirus.

During this phase, 14 patients will be treated on each arm initially. If an objective response is demonstrated on either arm, enrollment may continue up to a total of 25 patients on that arm. If either (1) no objective tumor responses are seen in the first 14 patients treated or (2) intolerable toxicity is encountered at any time, the enrollment on that arm will be halted.

3.3.9. Trial Assessment (see **Table 2**)

1. Evaluation of safety and toxicity, and MTD (or MFD) and DLT. Refer to guidelines such as the National Cancer Institute Canada Common Toxicity Criteria (NCI–CTC) for definitions (*see* **Note 10**).
2. Radiographic scanning to assess tumor size either by computed tomography (CT) or ultrasound scanning (US), but the method must be consistent throughout the trial for each individual patient.

3. Viral replication and shedding into the bloodstream and/or urine can be assessed by quantitative polymerase chain reaction (Q-PCR). The detection limit is approx 10^4 genomes/mL. In order to determine whether these genomes are infectious, the concentration of plaque-forming units (pfu) should also be determined using a limiting dilution assay ($TCID_{50}$). Plasma and urine to be collected posttreatment as described in **Table 2**.

4. To demonstrate the tissue site(s) of replication, core biopsies can be obtained (if deemed safe and feasible) under radiographic guidance of one to two liver metastases, normal liver (optional), and extrahepatic metastatic disease sites (optional) during cycle 1. The biopsies may be analyzed for evidence of viral replication, cellular infiltration, and apoptosis by histology.

5. Immune response assessment: Acute inflammatory cytokines can be measured in serum (i.e., interferons [IFs], tumor necrosis factors [TNFs], and interleukins [ILs]) by ELISA or Q-PCR.

6. Neutralizing antibody titer for test virus can be determined by plaque assays performed in the presence of serially diluted patient serum.

7. Pharmacokinetics: Blood samples collected at different time-points after viral infusion (i.e., 5 min to 24 h) for determination of viral replication and clearance over time by Q-PCR.

4. Notes

1. For the interaction studies, the incubation time with virus and drugs might have to be varied dependent on the growth characteristics of each cell line. Also, cell lines extremely sensitive to viral mutants might only be kept in culture for 3–4 d postinfection.

2. All dilutions should be made fresh just prior to use. We found that potency of both virus and cytotoxic drugs decreased when stored at dilute concentrations in culture media. Paclitaxel stock solution in methanol is only stable for 1 mo when stored at $-20°C$.

3. Fetal calf serum from some sources can interfere with the MTS proliferation assay resulting in very high absorbance values for media alone. This problem can be solved by replacing the incubation media with serum-free DMEM prior to the addition of the MTS reagent. Ideally, the blank value should give a reading of 0.2 OD units and untreated control cells between 1.0 and 2.0 OD units to enable the generation of a sensitive dose–response curve with test samples spread between the blank and control. The MTS proliferation reagent is light sensitive and should be stored in smaller aliquots to be thawed only once. Store at $-20°C$.

4. Luciferase expression from a CMV promoter will produce good imaging at an adenoviral dose as low as 10^8 particles/mouse. Transfected tumor cells have previously been shown to be detectable from only a few hundred cells injected subcutaneously (approx 1 mm deep) *(29)*. However, this is also dependent on the type of bioluminescent reporter, the surrounding physiology of the animal and the depth of the luminescence.

5. Any route of delivery that achieves infection is feasible, although it should be remembered that some peripheral expression is usually seen at the site of injection. This may affect the results, especially if organ-specific injection is used. Also, intraperitoneal injection is likely to produce some general infection in the intraperitoneal cavity, which could then mask tissue-specific expression elsewhere.

6. It will require at least 3 h for adenovirally encoded luciferase to be expressed postinjection, and we have found that even a nonreplicating virus can still be clearly detected 7 d postinjection.

7. Although weak images can be improved by increasing the exposure time (up to a maximum of 5 min), this also increases the background noise. In order to keep background to

a minimum, the imaging area should be thoroughly cleaned before each use (feces, urine, food and bedding have all been shown to act as sources of luminescence). The mice themselves may also be cleaned prior to imaging. In addition, when black mice are used, their fur has been shown to scatter photons; thus, images may be improved if the fur is first removed by shaving or with a depilatory.

8. If the source of luminescence is too strong, regions of the image may become saturated, thus preventing quantification. This may be solved by simply reducing the exposure time of the image (down to a minimum of 5 s). However, if saturation is still found, then it may be necessary to also reduce the bin value (down to 4 or 2). Finally, if one area of particularly strong luminescence is masking the surrounding regions, it may be possible to shield this part of the animal (i.e., with black cloth or paper).

9. A number of ethical, legal, and regulatory considerations have to be addressed prior to initiation of a clinical trial. It is the responsibility of the investigator that the study be conducted in accordance with the Declaration of Helsinki and in compliance with all applicable laws and regulations of the locale and country where the study is conducted. For example, protocols have to be approved by the Gene Therapy Advisory Committee (UK), the Recombinant DNA Advisory Committee (USA), the Medicines Control Agency (UK), the Food and Drug Administration (USA), and other local authorities such as institutional review boards and ethics committees.

10. The MTD is defined as the dose immediately below the dose at which two patients experience a DLT after their first treatment. DLT is defined as any one of the following: grade 4 toxicity of any duration attributed to treatment or grade 3 toxicity lasting ≥ 5 d attributed to treatment (excluding flulike symptoms for adenovirus). For toxicity definition, see NCI–CTC. The MFD is based on manufacturing yields, usually 10^{12} to 10^{13} for adenovirus.

Acknowledgments

The following individuals have been instrumental in making this chapter possible: Nick Lemoine, Lynda Hawkins, Patricia Ryan, Yaohe Wang, Arthi Anand, Jianghui Meng, Tom Wickham, Darlene Jenkins, Harpreet Wasan, Nagy Habib, and Charles Coombes.

References

1. Kirn, D., Martuza, R. L. and Zwiebel, J. (2001) Replication-selective virotherapy for cancer: biological principles, risk management and future directions. *Nature Med.* **7(7),** 781–787.
2. Hawkins, L. K., Lemoine, N. R., and Kirn, D. (2002) Oncolytic biotherapy: a novel therapeutic platform. *Lancet Oncol.* **3,** 17–26.
3. Heise, C. and Kirn, D. (2000) Replication-selective adenoviruses as oncolytic agents. *J. Clin. Investig.* **105,** 847–851.
4. Barker, D. D. and Berk, A. J. (1987) Adenovirus proteins from both E1B reading frames are required for transformation of rodent cells by viral infection and DNA transfection. *Virology* **156,** 107–121.
5. Nielsch, U., Fognani, C., and Babiss, L. E. (1991) Adenovirus E1A–p105(Rb) protein interactions play a direct role in the initiation but not the maintenance of the rodent cell transformed phenotype. *Oncogene* **6(6),** 1031–1036.
6. Sherr, C. J. (1996) Cancer cell cycles. *Science* **274,** 1672–1677.
7. Olson, D. C. and Levine, A. J. (1994) The properties of p53 proteins selected for the loss of suppression of transformation. *Cell Growth Differ.* **5(1),** 61–71.

8. Bischoff, J. R., Kirn, D. H., Williams, A., et al. (1996) An adenovirus mutant that replicates selectively in p53-deficient human tumor cells. *Science* **274**, 373–376.
9. Heise, C., Hermiston, T., Johnson, L., et al. (2000) An adenovirus E1A mutant that demonstrates potent and selective anti-tumoral efficacy. *Nature Med.* **6(10)**, 1134–1139.
10. Nemunaitis, J., Ganly, I., Khuri, F., et al. (2000) Selective replication and oncolysis in p53 mutant tumors with ONYX-015, an E1B-55kD gene-deleted adenovirus, in patients with advanced head and neck cancer: as phase II trial. *Cancer Res.* **60**, 6359–6366.
11. Khuri, F. R., Nemunaitis, J., Ganly, I., et al. (2000) A controlled trial of intratumoral ONYX-015, a selectively-replicating adenovirus, in combination with cisplatin and 5-fluorouracil in patients with recurrent head and neck cancer. *Nature Med.* **6**, 879–885.
12. Reid T., Galanis E., Abbruzzese J., et al. (2001) Intra-arterial administration of a replication-selective adenovirus (dl1520) in patients with colorectal carcinoma metastatic to the liver: a phase I trial. *Gene Ther.* **8(21)**, 1618–1626.
13. Wold, W .S. (ed.) (1999) *Adenovirus Methods and Protocols.* Humana, Totowa, NJ.
14. Yu, D. C., Chen, Y., Dilley, J., et al. (2001) Antitumor synergy of CV787, a prostate cancer-specific adenovirus, and paclitaxel and docetaxel. *Cancer Res.* **61**, 517–525.
15. Nielsen, L. L., Gurnani, M., Shi, B., et al. (2000) Derivation and initial characterization of a mouse mammary tumor cell line carrying the polyomavirus middle T antigen: utility in the development of novel cancer therapeutics. *Cancer Res.* **60**, 7066–7074.
16. Steel, G. G. and Peckham, M. J. (1979) Exploitable mechanisms in combined radiotherapy–chemotherapy: the concept of additivity. *Int. J. Radiat. Oncol. Biol. Phys.* **5**, 85–91.
17. Aoe, K., Kiura, K., Ueoka, H., et al. (1999) Effect of docetaxel with cisplatin or vinorelbine on lung cancer cell lines. *Anticancer Res.* **19**, 291–300.
18. Osaki, S., Nakanishi, Y., Takayama, K., et al. (2000) Alteration of drug chemosensitivity caused by the adenovirus-mediated transfer of the wild-type p53 gene in human lung cancer cells. *Cancer Gene Ther.* **7(2)**, 300–307.
19. Contag, C. H., Contag, P. R., Mullins, J. I., Spilman, S. D., Stevenson, D. K., and Benaron, D. A. (1995) Photonic detection of bacterial pathogens in living hosts. *Mol. Microbiol.* **18**, 593–603.
20. Contag, P. R., Olomu, I. N., Stevenson, D. K., and Contag, C. H. (1998) Bioluminescent indicators in living animals. *Nature Med.* **4**, 245–247.
21. Francis, K.P., Joh, D., Bellinger-Kawahara, C., Hawkinson, M. J., Purchio, T. F., and Contag, P. H. (2000) Monitoring bioluminescent *Staphylococcus aureus* infections in living mice using a novel *luxABCDE* construct. *Infect. Immun.* **68**, 3594–3600.
22. Francis, K. P., Yu, J. Bellinger-Kawahara, C., et al. (2001) Visualizing pnuemococcal infections in the lungs of live mice using *Streptococcus pneumoniae* transformed with a novel Gram-positive lux transposon. *Infect. Immun.* **69**, 3350–3358.
23. Burns, S. M., Joh, D. Francis, K. P., et al. (2001) Revealing the spatiotemporal patterns of bacterial infectious diseases using bioluminescent pathogens and whole body imaging. *Contrib. Microbiol.* **9**, 71–88.
24. Kirn, D. (2001) Oncolytic virotherapy for cancer with the adenovirus dl1520 (Onyx 015): results of phase I and II trials. *Expert Opin. Biol. Ther.* **1(3)**, 525–538.
25. Green, M. and Wold, W. S. (1979) Human adenoviruses: growth, purification, and transfection assay. *Meth. Enzymol.* **58**, 425–435.
26. Tollefson, A. E., Scaria, A., Hermiston, T. W., Ryerse, J. S., Wold, L. J., and Wold, W. S. (1996) The adenovirus death protein (E3-11.6K) is required at very late stages of infection for efficient cell lysis and release of adenovirus from infected cells. *J. Virol.* **70(4)**, 2296–2306.

27. Frackman, S. Anhalt, M., and Nealson, K. H. (1990) Cloning, organization, and expression of the bioluminescence genes of *Xenorhabdus luminescens. J. Bacteriol.* **172,** 5767–5773.
28. Bhaumik, S. and Gambhir, S.S. (2002) Optical imaging of *Renilla* luciferase reporter gene expression in living mice. *Proc. Natl. Acad. Sci. USA* **99,** 377–382.
29. Sweeney, T. J. Mailander, V. Tucker, A. A. et al. (1999) Visualizing the kinetics of tumor-cell clearance in living animals. *Proc. Natl. Acad. Sci. USA* **96,** 12,044–12,049.
30. Bradford, M. M. (1976) A rapid and sensitive method for the quantitation of microgram quantities of protein utilizing the principle of protein-dye binding. *Anal. Biochem.* **72,** 248–254.

6

Retroviral Vectors for Suicide Gene Therapy

Colin Porter

1. Introduction

A recombinant retroviral vector is one of many available options for effecting gene transfer. To date, this type of vector has been most widely used and is involved in more than a third of current gene therapy trials, many of which are for delivery of suicide genes in the context of cancer treatment *(1)*. Many issues that may impinge upon the choice of vector are specific to individual applications. However, in general, retroviral vectors may be chosen for reasons of their relatively high efficiency of gene delivery, the stable integration of the transgene delivered, and their immunological "silence." A distinction exists between vectors based on murine leukemia virus (MLV) and those derived from lentiviruses, such as human immunodeficiency virus (HIV). MLV vector gene delivery is restricted to proliferating target cells *(2)*, resulting from a requirement for breakdown of the nuclear membrane, whereas HIV vectors can additionally infect nondividing cells. Lentiviral vectors are in their relative infancy and will not be considered further in this chapter. Depending on the proposed application, it will be necessary to consider whether this proliferation requirement for MLV vectors is advantageous or not. Efficacy shown by several of the suicide enzyme/prodrug systems, such as HSV thymidine kinase (HSV-TK) and gancyclovir, is similarly dependent on cell proliferation.

1.1. Vector Design

Once the decision to use retroviral vectors has been taken, the first critical step is vector design. The scientific literature contains a bewildering array of different retroviral vector designs, reflecting different system requirements. Key issues to consider include the desirability of a drug-selectable marker gene, whether expression of more than one gene is required and the necessity for tissue-dependent, cell-type-dependent, or condition-dependent transcriptional control. The simplest system for experimental manipulation is to use a vector expressing a single transgene under the control of a consitutively active promoter alongside a selectable marker. At the other

From: *Methods in Molecular Medicine, Vol. 90, Suicide Gene Therapy: Methods and Reviews*
Edited by: C. J. Springer © Humana Press Inc., Totowa, NJ

extreme would be a vector lacking a means of selection and with a requirement for transcriptional specificity for the transgene: the experimental methods employed to generate such a vector are more involved. For each of these options, there is still a variety of design alternatives *(3)*.

The simpler strategies are usually more likely to succeed. Vectors possessing multiple transcription units are less likely to generate high titers and are more prone to instability. One identified issue is the potential for promoter interference *(4)*. This could be particularly problematic in the case where selective pressure for strong expression of a selectable marker downregulates expression of the gene of interest. Strategies dependent on transcriptional control are therefore more likely to succeed in the absence of a closely linked strong transcriptional unit for selection. However, vector design is highly empirical and it is not always possible to generalize such findings.

1.2. Vector Packaging System

A second important step is the choice between stable vs transient virus production. The vector is constructed as a plasmid and transfected into a packaging cell equipped to provide the viral gene products necessary for viral assembly, vector packaging, and infectivity (products of the viral *gag*, *pol*, and *env* genes) *(3)*. Stable transfection enables a one-off generation of a producer cell clone that can be thoroughly characterized with regard to titer of virus production and suitability for clinical application if this is desired, but it has the disadvantage that selection and screening to identify a good producer clone is time-consuming. Alternatively, some or all of the packaging functions may be provided by transient cotransfection with the vector. This process is much more rapid but needs to be repeated whenever virus is required and, therefore, requires repeated quality control. Further deciding factors would be whether the protocol requires the delivery of cell-free virus or of the virus producer cells themselves, and the scale of virus production required.

Additional choices at the level of the packaging system include the species origin of the cells to be used and the viral tropism that is required. The most widely used transient systems are based on the human embryonic kidney 293 cell line because of its high efficiency of transfection. Stable packaging cells have traditionally been developed from murine 3T3 fibroblasts. However, viruses produced from such cells are unstable in human serum, in contrast to those generated from the more recently developed human packaging cell lines *(5)*. There are several MLV tropisms available as a result of the choice of the envelope protein expressed in the packaging cells. The ecotropic (E) envelope enables infection of murine but not human cells, whereas the amphotropic (A) envelope allows infection of both. That from gibbon ape leukemia virus (GALV) or an endogenous feline virus (RD114) give entry to human but not murine cells. A further dualtropic envelope (10A1) can use receptors for either A or GALV. For intended human application, most vectors to date have used the A envelope, although there is evidence that GALV or RD114 may be superior for hematopoietic cell targets *(6)*. A further pantropic option is to pseudotype the vector with the nonretroviral coat protein from vesicular stomatitis virus (VSV-G), although this is restricted to the use of transient packaging because of its toxicity toward expressing cells *(7)*.

Stable packaging cells express each of the *gag*, *pol*, and *env* genes. Some do so from a single transfected unit, whereas others have split the *gag/pol*, and *env* functions on separate plasmids *(8)*, thus providing greater protection from the possibility of recombination between the packaging and vector constructs to generate an unwanted replication-competent (helper) retrovirus.

1.3. Characterization of Vector Performance

For stable packaging cells, a large number of individual clones following transfection of the vector will need to be screened in order to identify one of sufficiently high titer of virus production. Once a recombinant retroviral vector producer system has been established, the next step is to determine the vector titer and to confirm integrity of the delivered construct. Other quality controls may be performed, such as an assay to confirm absence of helper virus. Finally, the function of the transgene following delivery to relevant target cells can be ascertained.

Titer can readily be determined for vectors possessing selectable markers following infection of target cells. There may also be functional means appropriate for some vectors (e.g., those leading to cell surface protein expression). A definitive determination that does not rely on either and is therefore essential for vectors that do not express a selectable marker is to quantitate proviral DNA content by Southern blot analysis. This also allows verification of the integrity of the provirus. If necessary, titer can be improved by vector concentration.

1.4. Vector Application

How the vector is applied will depend on the experimental system or intended therapeutic approach and the nature of the target cells. For example, a gene therapy approach aimed at purging bone marrow might be performed ex vivo by simply exposing the cells to virus. Alternatively, the intention might be to deliver virus to tumors by direct injection. Other applications might call for the use of stable producer cells in vivo.

2. Materials

1. Retroviral plasmid appropriate to vector design. Vectors based on LNCX, the Babe series of plasmids or MFG (*see* **Fig. 1A**) have been widely used and are available within the academic community. Additionally, Clontech markets a useful series of vectors. This includes LXSN and the LRCX series for dual expression of insert (X) and one of several selectable markers (R, N=Neo^R) under the control of the long terminal repeat (LTR) (L), the cytomegalovirus (CMV) immediate early promoter (C), or the SV40 promoter (S). Also available is SIR, for disabling the long terminal repeats (LTR) activity by enhancer deletion to permit insertion of the target gene plus promoter of choice, and LXIN, in which the LTR controls expression of both insert and Neo^R by virtue of an internal ribosome entry site.
2. Molecular-biology reagents and enzymes for vector construction by manipulation of retroviral plasmid and preparation of DNA for transfection, agarose gel electrophoresis, and so forth.
3. Retroviral packaging cell system for stable or transient vector production. Some of the more widely used packaging cells are listed in **Table 1**. Many of these are available from the American and European cell line repositories or directly from the laboratories where they were constructed. Additionally, Clontech markets the dualtropic packaging line, as well as 293-cell-based transient ecotropic, amphotropic, and pantropic systems.

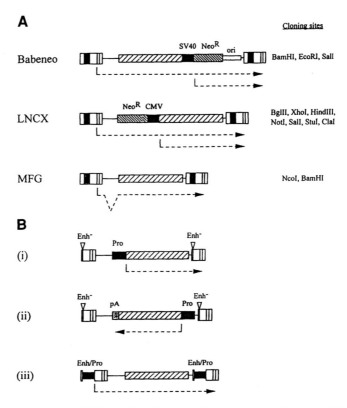

Fig. 1. Retroviral vectors. (**A**) Examples of commonly used vectors. Babeneo *(9)* and LNCX *(10)* confer Neo^R controlled by the SV40 enhancer/promoter or LTR, respectively. The therapeutic gene is driven by the LTR or CMV enhancer/promoter. MFG *(11)* simply expresses the therapeutic gene from the LTR. The tripartite LTR structure is indicated, with the viral enhancer within U3 highlighted. The expected transcripts (dashed lines) are indicated below, spliced in the case of MFG. Also given are the restriction sites suitable for gene insertion. (**B**) Three strategies for achieving tissue-specific expression using inserted promoters and/or enhancers (solid box) and deletion of the viral enhancer. The structure of the provirus in the infected cell is shown, as are the expected transcripts.

4. Cell culture reagents, including Dulbecco's modified Eagles' medium (DMEM), fetal calf serum (FCS), trypsin (0.05% in 0.02% EDTA), phosphate-buffered saline (PBS), OptiMEM (Life Technologies, product code 31985-047).

5. Disposable plastics for cell culture, including 10-cm plates, 24-well multidish plates, triple-layer T175 flasks (Nunc, cat. no. 132867), cryotubes, 15-mL and 50-mL polypropylene centrifuge tubes.

6. General chemicals: methanol, ethanol, sodium dodecyl sulfate (SDS), EDTA, sodium acetate, sodium azide.

7. Ca$_3$(PO$_4$)$_2$ transfection reagents: 2X HBS (274 mM NaCl, 42 mM HEPES, 1.5 mM Na$_2$HPO$_4$, 10 mM KCl, 13 mM D-glucose, pH 7.05) and 2 M CaCl$_2$.

Table 1
Packaging Cell Systems

Packaging cell line	Parental cell line[a]	Nature of constructs[b]	Drug selection[c]	Tropism/envelope	Availability[d]	Ref.
A. Packaging cell lines for stable virus production						
PA317	3T3	Single	HSV-TK	Amphotropic	ATCC, ECACC	*12*
GP + E-86	3T3	Split	gpt	Ecotropic	ATCC	*8*
GP + envAm12	3T3	Split	gpt, hygro	Amphotropic	ATCC	*13*
PG13	3T3	Split	HSV-TK, dhfr	GALV	ATCC, ECACC	*14*
FLY-A13	HT1080[e]	Split	bsr, phleo	Amphotropic	ECACC	*15*
-RD18				RD114		
PT67	3T3	Split	HSV-TK, dhfr	10A1 (Dualtropic)	ATCC, Clontech	*16*
B. Packaging cell lines for transient virus production						
Phoenix-Eco -Ampho	293	Split	hygro	Ecotropic Amphotropic	ATCC[f]	*17*
EcoPack™	293	Split	neo, hygro bleo, puro	Ecotropic Amphotropic	Clontech	
AmphoPack™						

Note: The table lists some of the more widely used and/or readily available packaging cell systems. For a more exhaustive listing of published systems and details of the packaging constructs used, see **ref. 3**.

[a]The choice of murine (3T3) or human (HT1080, TE671, 293) parental cell has implications for virus sensitivity or resistance, respectively, in the presence of human serum.

[b]*gag–pol* and *env* functions are either contained on a single plasmid or split between two.

[c]gpt, HSV-TK, hygro, dhfr, bsr, bleo/phleo, puro: drug-resistance marker genes xanthine–guanine phosphoribosyltransferase, herpes simplex virus–thymidine kinase, hygromycin B phosphotransferase, dihydrofolate reductase, blasticidin S deaminase, bleomycin (phleomycin)-binding protein, puromycin N-acetyltransferase, respectively.

[d]ATCC, ECACC: American Type Culture Collection (see www.atcc.org), European Collection of Cell Cultures (see www.ecac.org), respectively.

[e]Equivalent packaging cells based on the parental human rhabdomyosarcoma TE671 cell line have also been developed for ecotropic, amphotropic, and RD114-enveloped viruses: TE FLY-MO, A, RD.

[f]Requires prior agreement with originator (see www.stanford.edu/group/nolan).

8. G418 (Geneticin, Life Technologies, product code 11811-031), 100 mg/mL stock in PBS.
9. 3MM filter paper (Whatman).
10. Disposable syringes and sterile 0.45-μm filter units.
11. Polybrene, 8 mg/mL stock in PBS.
12. Giemsa stain: 5% Giemsa, 50% methanol.
13. Yeast tRNA, 10 mg/mL stock in diethylpyrocarbonate (DEPC)-treated water.
14. Proteinase K, 10 mg/mL stock (in DEPC-treated water for vector RNA preparation).
15. Phenol : chloroform : isoamyl alcohol (25 : 24 : 1, v/v), Tris-equilibrated.
16. Chloroform : isoamyl alcohol (24 : 1 v/v).
17. Slot-blotting apparatus.
18. Blotting membrane (e.g., Hybond-N [Amersham International]).
19. 20X SSPE: 3.6 M NaCl, 0.2 M sodium phosphate, 0.02 M EDTA, pH 7.7.
20. Formamide, deionized.
21. 50X Denhardt's solution: 1% bovine serum albumin (BSA), 1% Ficoll, 1% polyvinyl pyrollidone.
22. Salmon-sperm DNA, sonicated and denatured.
23. Random-primed radiolabeling kit and [α^{32}P]dCTP.
24. 20X SSC: 3 M NaCl, 0.3 M sodium citrate, pH 7.0.
25. X-ray film, cassette, and intensifying screens.
26. DNA lysis buffer: 10 mM Tris-HCl, pH 8.0, 10 mM EDTA, 10 mM NaCl, 2% SDS.
27. RNAseA, 10 mg/mL stock.
28. TE: 10 mM Tris-HCl, 1 mM EDTA, pH 8.0.
29. Denaturation solution (1.5 M NaCl, 0.5 M NaOH) and neutralization solution (1.5 M NaCl, 1 M Tris-HCl, pH 7.4) for Southern blotting.
30. Hybridization buffer (Sigma, product code H-7033) for (pre)hybridization of Southern blots.
31. Lipofectamine transfection reagent (Life Technologies, product code 18324).
32. Tangential flow ultrafiltration apparatus (Minitan-S, Millipore) and filtration membranes (300-kDa cutoff; Millipore, product code PLMK OMS10).
33. Ultrafree-15 centrifugal filter units (100-kDa cutoff; Millipore, product code UFV2 BHK).

3. Methods

3.1. Design and Construction of Recombinant Retroviral Vector Plasmid

The first step in construction is obtaining a suitable backbone vector for molecular cloning. These are plasmids containing proviruses from which nonessential sequences have been removed. At each end is a LTR, the tripartite U3-R-U5 structure of which reflects the presence of sequences repeated at (R) and unique to (U) the ends of the RNA vector genome. Between the LTRs are a sequence essential for RNA packaging and one or more cloning sites suitable for insertion, and there may also be various combinations of selectable marker and internal promoter.

The choice of vector will dictate to a large extent the means of insertion of the coding sequence for the gene to be delivered. The majority of vectors possess a suitable unique *Bam*HI (or compatible *Bgl*II) restriction site; thus, it is often convenient to prepare the insert with flanking *Bam*HI sites. Vectors such as BabeNeo, LNCX, or MFG are common examples for relatively uncomplicated strategies (*see* **Fig. 1A**). The first two are designed to express the transgene from the constitutively active LTR or internal CMV enhancer/promoter in concert with a Neo^R selectable marker under the control of internal SV40 enhancer/promoter or LTR, respectively. MFG is designed for optimal expression from the LTR and does not possess a selectable marker.

If the required vector properties include expression from a tissue-specific promoter (e.g., that for a tumor-specific marker or responsive to a particular condition, such as hypoxia), then such sequences will also need to be cloned into the vector. Specific expression can be achieved either by inclusion of an internal promoter adjacent to the transgene or by modification of the LTR transcriptional specificity (*see* **Fig. 1B**). When placed internally, this may be in the same sense as retroviral transcription or in the reverse orientation, in which case the inserted cassette should include a polyadenylation site for efficient transcription termination. Such strategies will likely necessitate deletion of the wild-type LTR activity, often achieved by deletion or replacement between the ligation-compatible *Nhe*I and *Xba*I restriction sites flanking the retroviral enhancer. The modifications are made in the 3' LTR such that they are duplicated to the 5' LTR upon vector integration in the target cell, where they become effective (*see* **Note 1**).

Clearly, it is impossible to generalize with regard to cloning strategy because there are so many design variables. However, the end point of this process should be the generation of a plasmid containing a provirus structure for transfection into the packaging cells. Transcription will produce a polyadenylated mRNA beginning with the R and U5 regions of the 5' LTR and adjacent packaging sequence, and ending with the U3 (which may be modified, as discussed earlier) and R regions of the 3' LTR. These encompass the essential cis-acting sequences necessary for packaging, reverse transcription, and provirus integration.

3.2. Generation of Vector Producer Cells

As with vector design, the eventual application will determine the choice of stable vs transient virus production, the chosen tropism, and the use of murine or human cells. Some of the most commonly used packaging systems are listed in **Table 1**.

3.2.1. Establishing a High-Titer Stable Producer Cell Clone
3.2.1.1. TRANSFECTION AND SELECTION

This section describes transfection of adherent packaging cells with vector plasmid DNA using the $CaPO_4$ coprecipitation technique. Other variations or techniques of comparable efficiency, such as lipofection, would be equally valid.

1. From a confluent 10-cm plate of packaging cells, set up a 1 : 10 passage (approx 5×10^5 cells) in a fresh 10-cm plate, using 10 mL growth medium (DMEM/FCS). Incubate at 37°C under 5% CO_2 overnight.
2. Replace the medium with 10 mL fresh medium about 4 h prior to the addition of DNA.
3. Prepare transfection mix, as follows. Combine 10 µg plasmid DNA (*see* **Note 2**) and 50 µL of 2 *M* $CaCl_2$ with water to a total 400 µL. Add this dropwise and with continual mixing to an equal volume of 2X HBS. Using a pipet, bubble several volumes of air through the mixture to mix thoroughly and encourage formation of a fine precipitate. Allow this to stand for 30 min at room temperature, by which time a slight opacity should be apparent.

4. Add the transfection mix dropwise and evenly to the cells without disturbance of the medium and return the cells to the incubator overnight.
5. Gently remove the medium (*see* **Note 3**), replace with 10 mL fresh growth medium, and incubate overnight.
6. Trypsinize the cells and replate at 1 : 5, 1 : 10, and 1 : 20 passages in growth medium containing the appropriate drug to select for transfected cells (*see* **Note 4**). For plasmids encoding Neo^R, this is 1 mg/mL G418.
7. Continue to incubate the cells in the presence of the drug for 2 wk, replacing medium at intervals. Gross cell loss but the survival of proliferating colonies of cells should become apparent. Macroscopically visible colonies should be readily seen, each one being a transfected cell clone.
8. Remove medium, wash the cells with PBS, and drain the plate. Working quickly, place on each colony a small (e.g., 2 mm × 2 mm) square of Whatman 3MM filter paper soaked in trypsin solution used for passaging cells. One to two minutes later, remove the filter paper with attached cells (apply slight pressure in the process) and place it into 1 mL DMEM/FCS in a well of a 24-well plate. Repeat this process for at least 50 clones per vector construct (*see* **Note 5**).
9. When individual clones reach confluence (how long this takes can vary widely), trypsinize the cells, and expand to continue culture in 10-cm plates.
10. Once the cells are approaching confluence, replace the medium with 5 mL fresh DMEM/ FCS and incubate overnight. Remove the virus-containing supernatant and filter through a 0.45-μm filter unit. This can be used fresh or stored at –80°C prior to use. Trypsinize and cryopreserve the cells.

3.2.1.2. Titer Determination Using a Selectable Marker

Of the clones established, many will produce a virus of low or intermediate titer, and relatively few will be of significant titer. For vectors encoding a selectable marker, these can readily be screened by titration, infection, and selection of target cells. Those encoding histochemically identifiable gene products (such as β-galactosidase) or cell surface antigens *(18)* can also be screened in this way. In the case of vectors encoding suicide genes, it is possible to use a similar approach, judging the best clones to be those that lead to the greatest losses of viability upon treatment of infected cells with the prodrug.

1. From a confluent 10-cm plate of target cells (e.g., NIH3T3 fibroblasts), set up a 1 : 10 passage (approx 5 × 10^5 cells) in fresh 10-cm plates, using 10 mL growth medium (DMEM/FCS). Incubate at 37°C under 5% CO_2 overnight.
2. Replace the medium with 2 mL fresh medium and add 2.5 μL of 8 mg/mL polybrene.
3. Add 0.5 mL virus-containing supernatant or serial 10-fold dilutions in medium; mix and return the cells to the incubator for 4 h.
4. Add 7.5 mL fresh medium and incubate for a further 48 h (*see* **Note 6**).
5. Trypsinize the infected cells (and uninfected control cells) and replate at 1 : 10 into medium containing the appropriate drug (e.g., 1 mg/mL G418 in the case of vectors carrying the Neo^R gene).
6. Continue to incubate the cells in the presence of the drug for 2 wk, replacing medium at intervals. Macroscopically visible colonies should be readily seen.
7. Count the colonies of resistant cells. This can be aided by draining the medium and staining the cells for 30 min with 2.5 mL Giemsa stain.

8. The titer (infectious units/mL) can be determined from the product of the number of colonies and the virus dilution used, multiplied by 20 (because of the use of 0.5 mL virus and the 1 : 10 cell split), and divided by 4 (approximating the cell number expansion subsequent to infection and prior to splitting into selection) (*see* **Note 7**).

3.2.1.3. PRELIMINARY SCREENING OF VIRUS PRODUCER CLONES

This and the next protocol provide a general means of identifying and quantitating vector titer without dependence on the nature of the genes encoded. The following is a preliminary screen based on levels of vector RNA packaged into virus particles.

1. Combine 1 mL of 10% SDS, 0.4 mL of 0.25 *M* EDTA, and 0.2 mL of 10 mg/mL yeast tRNA (a carrier for precipitation of the viral RNA) in DEPC-treated water and 1 mL of 10 mg/mL proteinase K in DEPC-treated water. This provides enough lysis mix for 40 samples.
2. Add 65 μL lysis mix to 435 μL virus-containing producer clone supernatant in a microcentrifuge tube and incubate for 45 min at 37°C.
3. Extract using an equal volume of phenol : chloroform and centrifuge to separate the phases.
4. Remove the upper phase to a fresh tube and extract with chloroform.
5. Remove 0.4 mL from the upper phase and add 40 μL of 3 *M* sodium acetate, pH 5.2, and 1 mL ethanol. Store at –20°C overnight to precipitate the RNA.
6. Pellet the RNA using a refrigerated microcentrifuge at 13,000g for 20 min. The pellet should be easily visible.
7. Pour off the supernatant, dry the pellet under vacuum, and dissolve the RNA in 50 μL DEPC-treated water.
8. Assemble a slot-blot apparatus with a piece of nylon membrane (e.g., Hybond-N) prewetted in water. Flush the wells with water and draw through under vacuum.
9. Pipet each 50-μL sample (or dilution) to a slot of the manifold and leave 30 min before applying the vacuum.
10. Remove and air-dry the membrane. Fix the RNA by ultraviolet (UV) illumination or baking for 2 h at 80°C.
11. Prehybridize the membrane in 5X SSPE, 50% formamide, 5X Denhardt's solution, 0.5% SDS for 1–2 h at 42°C. Add denatured salmon-sperm DNA to 20 μg/mL and a ^{32}P-radio-labeled random-primed probe specific for the DNA inserted into the vector. Hybridize overnight at 42°C.
12. Rinse the membrane twice in 2X SSC, 0.1% SDS and wash sequentially at 42°C in 2X SSC, 0.1% SDS, and 1X SSC, 0.1% SDS for two times 15 min at each stringency.
13. Remove the membrane, sandwich between sheets of 3MM filter paper to remove surface liquid, and wrap in cling film.
14. Expose the membrane to X-ray film in a cassette fitted with intensifying screens, overnight at –80°C. The clones providing the highest viral titres can readily be identified as those giving the strongest hybridizing signals.

3.2.1.4. DETERMINATION OF VIRUS TITER FROM PROVIRUS COPY NUMBER

Southern blot analysis of DNA prepared from cells infected with varying amounts of virus is a general means to measure the efficiency of delivery of the transgene. The technique is quantitative but labor intensive. Although it can be used as the sole screen, in practice a preliminary screen (*see* **Subheading 3.2.1.3.**) is usually performed and this method is used to choose between relatively few preselected clones. Because the technique can provide an analysis of the integrity of the provirus, it is also a useful experiment to perform for clones selected by functional means (*see* **Subheading 3.2.1.2.**).

3.2.1.4.1. INFECTION OF TARGET CELLS

1. From a confluent 10-cm plate of target cells (e.g., NIH3T3 fibroblasts), set up a 1 : 10 passage (approx 5×10^5 cells) in fresh 10-cm plates, using 10 mL growth medium (DMEM/FCS). Incubate at 37°C under 5% CO_2 overnight.
2. Replace the medium with 2 mL fresh medium and add 2.5 µL of 8 mg/mL polybrene.
3. Add 0.5 mL virus-containing supernatant or dilution in medium; mix and return the cells to the incubator for 4 h.
4. Add 7.5 mL fresh medium and incubate for a further 2–3 d, until confluent (*see* **Note 6**).
5. From a parallel plate, trypsinize and count the cells to determine the number present at the point of infection.
6. When confluent, trypsinize the infected cells (and uninfected control cells), remove into medium, and pellet, using polypropylene tubes. Wash the cell pellet with PBS (*see* **Note 8**).

3.2.1.4.2. PREPARATION OF GENOMIC DNA

1. Resuspend the cell pellet and add 2 mL DNA lysis buffer. Add proteinase K to 100 µg/mL and incubate at 55°C for 3 h.
2. Extract using an equal volume of phenol : chloroform. Mix gently, by inversion, for 5 min and centrifuge for 10 min to separate the phases.
3. Using a wide-bore pipet (or cut-off pipet tip), gently remove the upper phase to a fresh tube and extract again.
4. Remove the upper phase as before and add 10 µL of 10 mg/mL RNAse A. Incubate for 30 min at 37°C.
5. Extract, as in **step 2**, with phenol : chloroform.
6. Remove the upper phase and add 0.1 volume of 3 *M* sodium acetate, pH 5.2, and 2.5 volumes of ethanol. Gently mix by inversion. The precipitating high-molecular-weight genomic DNA should be apparent, slowly condensing to a cotton-wool appearance.
7. With a pipet tip, fish out the condensed precipitate and place into 0.5 mL of 70% ethanol in a microcentrifuge tube.
8. Briefly spin in a microcentrifuge and pour off the supernatant. Allow the pellet to air-dry at room temperature.
9. Add 100 µL TE, pH 8.0, and allow the DNA to dissolve overnight at 4°C.
10. Using a cut-off pipet tip, gently resuspend the dissolved DNA and remove a 5-µL aliquot. Dilute this into 0.5 mL TE and measure the optical density at 260 and 280 nm, using a quartz cuvet. From the optical density OD_{260}, determine the concentration of DNA (an absorbance of 1.0 for a 10-mm path length corresponds to 50 µg/mL).

3.2.1.4.3. SOUTHERN BLOT ANALYSIS

1. Digest 10 µg each DNA overnight in a total volume of 60 µL, using 40 units of an appropriate restriction enzyme (*see* **Note 9**). Include DNA prepared from control (uninfected) cells. Also include quantitation standards, consisting of such control DNA plus plasmid DNA representing, for example, 0.1–1 gene copy number equivalents per diploid genome. The amount (in µg) for single-copy equivalence is calculated by dividing the size of the plasmid in basepairs by the genome size (6×10^9 basepairs) and multiplying by 10.
2. Separate the digested DNA overnight by agarose gel electrophoresis, using, for example, 0.7% agarose. Stain and photograph the gel, using a ruler to record the positions of the size markers.

3. Denature and neutralize the gel (1 h each step) prior to overnight capillary transfer to a nylon membrane (e.g., Hybond-N), using 20X SSC.
4. Wash the membrane briefly in 2X SSC, air-dry, and fix the DNA by UV illumination or baking for 2 h at 80°C.
5. Prehybridize the membrane for 1 h at 65°C. Add a ^{32}P-radiolabeled random-primed probe specific for the DNA inserted into the vector and hybridize the membrane overnight at 65°C.
6. Rinse the membrane twice in 2X SSC, 0.1% SDS and wash sequentially at 65°C in 2X SSC, 0.1% SDS, and 0.2X SSC, 0.1% SDS for two times 15 min at each stringency.
7. Remove the membrane and sandwich between sheets of 3MM filter paper to remove surface liquid and wrap in cling film.
8. Expose the membrane to X-ray film in a cassette fitted with intensifying screens, overnight at at –80°C. Repeat for shorter/longer exposures, as required.
9. Estimate provirus copy number by comparison of signal intensity with the standards. The titer (infectious units/mL) can be determined from the product of the number of cells at the time of infection and the copy number equivalence (giving the number of infection events) multiplied by 2 (because of the use of 0.5 mL virus) and the virus dilution used (*see* **Note 7**).

3.2.2. Transient Virus Production

The following protocol describes the use of 293-based transient packaging cells, including the Phoenix and Clontech systems. Ecotropic and amphotropic versions of these cells are available. The viral genes are stably integrated so that provision of the vector DNA is all that is necessary to generate the virus. Other systems require that the *env* or both the *env* and the *gag–pol* packaging constructs are simultaneously transfected.

1. Seed 293-based packaging cells at 5×10^5 cells per 10-cm plate in 10 mL growth medium (DMEM/FCS) and incubate at 37°C under 5% CO_2 until 70–80% confluent.
2. Dilute 20 µg plasmid DNA in 0.8 mL OptiMEM and combine with 80 µg Lipofectamine transfection reagent also diluted in 0.8 mL OptiMEM. Incubate at room temperature for 15 min.
3. Add a further 6.4 mL OptiMEM and use to replace the medium on a plate of cells to be transfected. Incubate for 5 h at 37°C and replace supernatant with 10 mL growth medium.
4. Replace the medium toward the end of the second day for overnight harvest of virus-containing supernatant 48 h after the addition of DNA. Filter the supernatant through a 0.45-µm filter unit.
5. Determine the virus titer as described earlier (*see* **Subheadings 3.2.1.2.** and **3.2.1.4.**).

3.3. Preparation and Characterization of Retroviral Vectors

3.3.1. Vector Preparation

1. If using a stable producer cell system, thaw the cell stock corresponding to the clone identified as having the highest titer. The cells should be expanded and several further early-passage frozen stocks generated. In practice, this can be combined with medium-scale preparation of the vector.
2. Grow the producer cells until approaching confluence and change the medium for the smallest volume that is adequate, typically 5 mL when using 10-cm plates. Growth medium (DMEM/FCS) or serum-free medium (OptiMEM) may be used and give equivalent titers.

3. Incubate overnight at 37°C and then remove the virus-containing supernatant. Trypsinize and cryopreserve the cells.
4. Filter through a 0.45-μm filter unit and freeze the vector preparation in aliquots at –80°C.
5. For subsequent vector preparations from stable producer cell clones, it is advisable not to use cells that are late passage, because high titer is not always sustained and extended culture also favors the appearance of helper virus.

3.3.2. Vector Characterization

The titer of each vector preparation should be determined using the protocols described in **Subheadings 3.2.1.2.** and **3.2.1.4.** Even if not required for titration, it is advisable to use the Southern blot protocol for the initial vector preparation to verify that delivery and provirus integration occur without unexpected deletions or rearrangements. It is also advisable to test the virus-containing supernatant to confirm the absence of replication-competent (helper) retrovirus, although this is unlikely to occur when using packaging cells with split *gag/pol* and *env* functions.

3.3.2.1. SCREENING FOR HELPER VIRUS

This method relies on the use of a cell line with an integrated provirus that can be mobilized in the presence of *gag/pol* and *env* gene products provided by a helper virus (*see* **Note 10**). Both the indicator and assay cells should be appropriate for the vector tropism employed.

1. Infect a suitable indicator cell line with the vector preparation, as described in **Subheading 3.2.1.4.1., steps 1–4**.
2. When confluent, harvest the supernatant and filter using a 0.45-μm filter unit. The supernatant will contain mobilized indicator virus if the original vector preparation contains helper virus. For increased sensitivity, the infected indicator cells can be passaged and grown longer before assaying the medium, in order to allow propagation of any helper virus.
3. Infect a suitable target cell line with the supernatant, as **step 1**, and assay for the indicator gene (e.g., histochemical stain for β-galactosidase, or split into G418-containing medium for Neo^R).

3.3.3. Concentration of Retroviral Vectors

For some applications, it may be beneficial to concentrate vector preparations. An important consideration when concentrating retroviruses is that the envelope proteins are easily shed, with resultant reduced infectivity. Alternative protocols are provided, each of which is preferable to concentration by ultracentrifugation, for which recovery is not quantitative. It is also worth bearing in mind that although the concentration will increase titer as determined by limiting dilution, there are examples of coconcentrating inhibitory material that, at least in vitro, negate this enhancement when using the concentrate *(19)*. This effect, when present, is probably dependent on both the producer cell type and the nature of the target cell. Aliquots preconcentration and postconcentration should be titered to determine the efficiency of recovery.

3.3.3.1. CONCENTRATION USING LOW-SPEED CENTRIFUGATION

1. Centrifuge 10–15 mL vector preparation at 2500*g* for 12–14 h at 4°C.
2. Gently discard the supernatant and add 0.5 mL OptiMEM.
3. Incubate at 4°C for 30–60 min and gently resuspend prior to use.

3.3.3.2. CONCENTRATION BY TANGENTIAL-FLOW ULTRAFILTRATION

This method works by concentrating material unable to pass under pressure through a membrane of 300 kDa molecular-weight size limit. Continuous flow of the medium containing the virus tangential to the membrane prevents the accumulation of such material at the membrane surface, which would otherwise prevent further concentration.

1. Prepare approx 500 mL virus in OptiMEM and filter (0.45 μm) as usual (*see* **Note 11**).
2. Assemble Millipore Minitan-S ultrafiltration apparatus, flush the system with water at pump speed setting 8 with an inlet pressure gauge reading of 5 psi and perform the integrity test. Flush the system by circulating PBS for several minutes. The rate of filtrate accumulation should be 40–50 mL/min.
3. Recirculate the virus preparation, adjusting the outlet clamp to maintain the inlet pressure. The filtration rate will be lower than for PBS and will drop as concentration proceeds. Continue until about 30 mL remains (after approx 1 h).
4. Reduce speed to setting 3, adjust pressure, and continue until about 20 mL remains (*see* **Note 12**).
5. Recirculate for 2 min with no back-pressure, then remove inlet tube from liquid and allow concentrated virus to exit the system.
6. Measure final volume and filter (0.45 μm) to ensure sterility.
7. Flush the system with 0.1 *M* NaOH, then switch off the pump and leave in place for 15 min to clean the membrane, before flushing with water. For immediate reuse, the system should be re-equilibrated with PBS as in **step 2**. Alternatively, disassemble and store the membrane at 4°C in 0.1% sodium azide.

3.3.3.3. SMALL-SCALE CONCENTRATION BY CENTRIFUGAL ULTRAFILTRATION

This is effectively a small-scale version of the previous protocol, with the membrane orientated vertically to maximize the filtration area. The largest molecular-weight size limit available is 100 kDa.

1. Insert Millipore Ultrafree-15 centrifugal filtration unit into 50-mL centrifuge tube.
2. Prepare filter unit by rinsing with 70% ethanol, followed by PBS, and then washing through with 10 mL PBS by centrifugation at 2000*g* for 10 min.
3. Add 15 mL virus preparation and centrifuge at 2000*g* until the desired final volume (e.g., 0.5–1 mL) is reached (approx 8 min).

3.4. Application of Retroviral Vectors for Cancer Gene Therapy

The use of retroviral vectors for gene delivery to cell lines in vitro has been discussed in **Subheadings 3.2.1.2.** and **3.2.1.4.1.** Populations or clones of cells containing the provirus can be enriched by drug selection (e.g., G418 for Neo[R]-containing vectors), fluoresence-activated cell sorting, or limiting dilution and functional assay, as appropriate for the vector in use. Similar approaches can be used for ex vivo transduction of cells that can readily be removed from the body, such as hematopoietic cells. Function in terms of reduced cell viability or clonogenic potential can be assessed following prodrug exposure, as detailed elsewhere in this volume.

For in vivo delivery to tumors, the virus can be administered by direct intratumoral injection. Some experimental protocols call for the delivery of virus producer cells to allow for a period of virus production in vivo. This might involve coinjection of irradiated producer cells and tumor cells *(20)*. More relevant to cancer treatment is delivery after tumor establishment, such as via the hepatic portal vein in order to seed producer cells into the liver for the treatment of colorectal metastases *(21)* or by stereotactic intratumoral injection into the brain for malignant glioma *(22)*. The latter is currently undergoing phase III clinical trial. Prodrug is administered after a delay of several days to allow time for transduction and expression. Systemic delivery awaits the development of efficient means of achieving specificity by manipulation of virus targeting *(23)*. Because of the wide variety of potential uses, it is not possible to give generalized application protocols in this chapter.

4. Notes

1. Long-terminal-repeat modification is complicated by the duplication of restriction sites at each end of the vector, necessitating recovery of partially digested DNA fragments for molecular cloning. Suitable restriction sites within the U3 region (which contains the viral enhancer and promoter) of the MLV LTR include *Nhe*I, *Xba*I, and *Sac*I.
2. If the plasmid DNA does not itself encode a selectable marker, within or without the retroviral vector sequences, then a selectable plasmid should be included at 10-fold lower molarity to enable cotransfection. This might commonly be 0.5 μg pSV2neo.
3. After overnight incubation with the transfection mix, a fine precipitate should be visible under the microscope, overlying the adherent cells.
4. This is variable, depending on the experimental requirements. In practice, it is usual to passage to different degrees to account for potential variation in the tranfection efficiency. If the intention is to isolate individual clones, it is advisable to use a harder split and make several replicates. In contrast, if a bulk transfected population is required, then a lower split and few replicates are likely to be adequate. Bulk populations can be useful for comparing different vector constructs and are relatively easy to prepare, but yield lower titers of virus than those attainable using selected clones.
5. There are various alternative means of isolating individual clones, such as the use of cloning rings. With practice, the method described can be performed quickly with little opportunity for cross-contamination.
6. Alternatively, remove the medium and replace with 10 mL fresh medium. This may be necessary for target cells that do not tolerate extended contact with polybrene.
7. In fact, this calculation underestimates titer by a factor of 2 because the provirus integrates into only one of the postmitotic daughter cell nuclei resulting from an infected cell.
8. If required, the cell pellet can be frozen at this point for later preparation upon thawing.
9. Restriction enzymes that cut once within each LTR and not elsewhere provide the most information regarding provirus integrity. *Nhe*I, *Sac*I, and *Kpn*I are often suitable.
10. A cell clone harboring provirus with wild-type LTRs and expressing β-galactosidase or Neo^R is suitable. A more stringent variation of the helper assay is to test for *gag/pol* or

env helper functions independently. This requires an indicator cell containing provirus and *env* or *gag/pol* sequences, respectively.

11. The required incubator space can be minimized by using six triple-layer 175-cm² flasks with 25 mL OptiMEM per level, giving 450 mL final harvest.
12. It is important to avoid the introduction of air and consequent frothing, which results in the loss of titer. Twenty milliliters is the minimum final retentate volume because of the internal system capacity.

References

1. www.wiley.co.uk/genetherapy/clinical.
2. Miller, D. G., Adam, M. A., and Miller, A. D. (1990) Gene transfer by retrovirus vectors occurs only in cells that are actively replicating at the time of infection. *Mol. Cell Biol.* **10,** 4239–4242.
3. Collins, M. K. L. and Porter, C. D. (1999) Retroviral vectors, in *Blood Cell Biochemistry Volume 8: Hematopoiesis and Gene Therapy* (Fairbairn, L. J. and Testa, N. G., eds.), Kluwer Academic/Plenum, New York, pp. 57–88.
4. Emerman, M. and Temin, H. (1984) Genes with promoters in retrovirus vectors can be independently suppressed by an epigenetic mechanism. *Cell* **39,** 459–467.
5. Takeuchi, Y., Cosset, F.-L., Lachmann, P. J., Okada, H., Weiss, R. A., and Collins, M. K. L. (1994) Type C retrovirus inactivation by human complement is determined by both the viral genome and producer cell. *J. Virol.* **68,** 8001–8007.
6. Porter, C. D., Collins, M. K. L., Tailor, C. S., et al. (1996) Comparison of efficiency of infection of human gene therapy target cells via four different retroviral receptors. *Hum. Gene Ther.* **7,** 913–919.
7. Emi, N., Friedmann, T., and Yee, J. K. (1991) Pseudotype formation of murine leukaemia virus with the G protein of vesicular stomatitis virus. *J. Virol.* **65,** 1202–1207.
8. Markowitz, D., Goff, S., and Bank, A. (1988) A safe packaging line for gene transfer: separating viral genes on two different plasmids. *J. Virol.* **82,** 1120–1124.
9. Morgenstern, J. P. and Land, H. (1990) Advanced mammalian gene transfer: high titre retroviral vectors with multiple drug selection markers and a complementary helper-free packaging cell line. *Nucleic Acids Res.* **18,** 3587–3596.
10. Miller, A. D. and Rosman, G. J. (1989) Improved retroviral vectors for gene transfer and expression. *BioTechniques* **7,** 980–990.
11. Ohashi, T., Boggs, S., Robbins, P., et al. (1992) Efficient transfer and sustained high expression of the human glucocerebrosidase gene in mice and their functional macrophages following transplantation of bone marrow transduced by a retroviral vector. *Proc. Natl. Acad. Sci. USA* **89,** 11,332–11,336.
12. Miller, A. D. and Buttimore, C. (1986) Redesign of retrovirus packaging cell lines to avoid recombination leading to helper virus production. *Mol. Cell. Biol.* **6,** 2895–2902.
13. Markowitz, D., Goff, S., and Bank, A. (1988) Construction and use of a safe and efficient amphotropic packaging cell line. *Virology* **167,** 400–406.
14. Miller, A. D., Garcia, J. V., Suhr, N. V., Lynch, C. M., Wilson, C., and Eiden, M. V. (1991) Construction and properties of retrovirus packaging cells based on gibbon ape leukemia virus. *J. Virol.* **65,** 2220–2224.
15. Cosset, F.-L., Takeuchi, Y., Battini, J. L., Weiss, R. A., and Collins, M. K. L. (1995) High titre packaging cells producing recombinant retroviruses resistant to human serum. *J. Virol.* **69,** 7430–7436.
16. Miller, A. and Chen, F. (1996) Retrovirus packaging cells based on 10A1 murine leukemia virus for production of vectors that use multiple receptors for cell entry. *J. Virol.* **70,** 5564–5571.

17. www.stanford.edu/group/nolan.

18. Strair, R. K., Towle, M. J., and Smith, B. R. (1988) Recombinant retroviruses encoding cell surface antigens as selectable markers. *J. Virol.* **62,** 4756–4759.

19. Slingsby, J. H., Baban, D., Sutton, J., et al. (2000) Analysis of 4070A envelope levels in retroviral preparations and effect on target cell transduction efficiency. *Hum. Gene Ther.* **11,** 1439–1451.

20. Mavria, G. and Porter, C. D. (2001) Reduced growth in response to ganciclovir treatment of subcutaneous xenografts expressing HSV-tk in the vascular compartment. *Gene Ther.* **8,** 913–920.

21. Hurford, R. K., Dranoff, G., Mulligan, R. C., and Tepper, R. I. (1995) Gene therapy of metastatic cancer by in vivo gene targeting. *Nature Genet.* **10,** 430–435.

22. Ram, Z., Culver, K. W., Walbridge, S., Blaese, R. M., and Oldfield, E. H. (1993) In situ retroviral-mediated gene transfer for the treatment of brain tumours in rats. *Cancer Res.* **53,** 83–88.

23. Russell, S. J., and Cosset, F.-L. (1999) Modifying the host range properties of retroviral vectors. *J. Gene Med.* **1,** 300–311.

7

Nonviral Liposomes

Andrew D. Miller

1. Introduction

Cationic liposome/micelle-based systems have come closer to providing clinically effective gene delivery than any other chemical nonviral delivery systems to date. These systems are formed from either a single synthetic cationic amphiphile (known as a cytofectin; *cyto* for cell and *fectin* for transfection [i.e., gene delivery and expression]) or, more commonly, from the combination of a cytofectin and a neutral lipid such as dioleoyl L-α-phosphatidylethanolamine (DOPE) or cholesterol (Chol) (*see* **Fig. 1**). There are at least 40 cationic liposome/micelle systems that have been reported to mediate nucleic acid delivery to cells, of which a number have been commercialized (*see* **Table 1**) *(1–25)*. More are being reported all the time, but in each case, the key ingredient is the cytofectin used. The structures of a number of representative diverse cytofectins are shown (*see* **Fig. 1**). Although hydrophobic regions are reasonably similar, polar linkers and cationic head groups vary quite substantially. Typically, cytofectin and neutral lipid components are mixed together in an appropriate mole ratio and then induced or formulated into unilammellar vesicles by any one of a number of methods, including reverse-phase evaporation (REV) and dehydration–rehydration (DRV) *(1,2)* (*see* **Table 1**). Alternatively, cytofectins may be assembled into micellar structures after being dispersed in water or aqueous organic solvents *(1,2)* (*see* **Table 1**). Unilammellar vesicles or micelles may then be combined with nucleic acids to form cationic liposome/micelle–nucleic acid complex (lipoplex; LD) mixtures consisting of nanometric complex structures that are able to deliver nucleic acids into cells (*see* **Fig. 2** on p. 108–111). Once formed, these nanometric complexes are competent to enter cells, usually by endocytosis triggered by nonspecific interactions between complexes and the cell surface proteoglycans of adherent cells (*see* **Fig. 2**). Once inside, a proportion of the bound nucleic acids escapes from early endosomes into the cytoplasm, performing a therapeutic function there as in the case of mRNA (path B; **Fig. 2**), or trafficks to the nucleus to perform a therapeutic function there, as in the case of DNA (path C; **Fig. 2**).

From: *Methods in Molecular Medicine, Vol. 90, Suicide Gene Therapy: Methods and Reviews*
Edited by: C. J. Springer © Humana Press Inc., Totowa, NJ

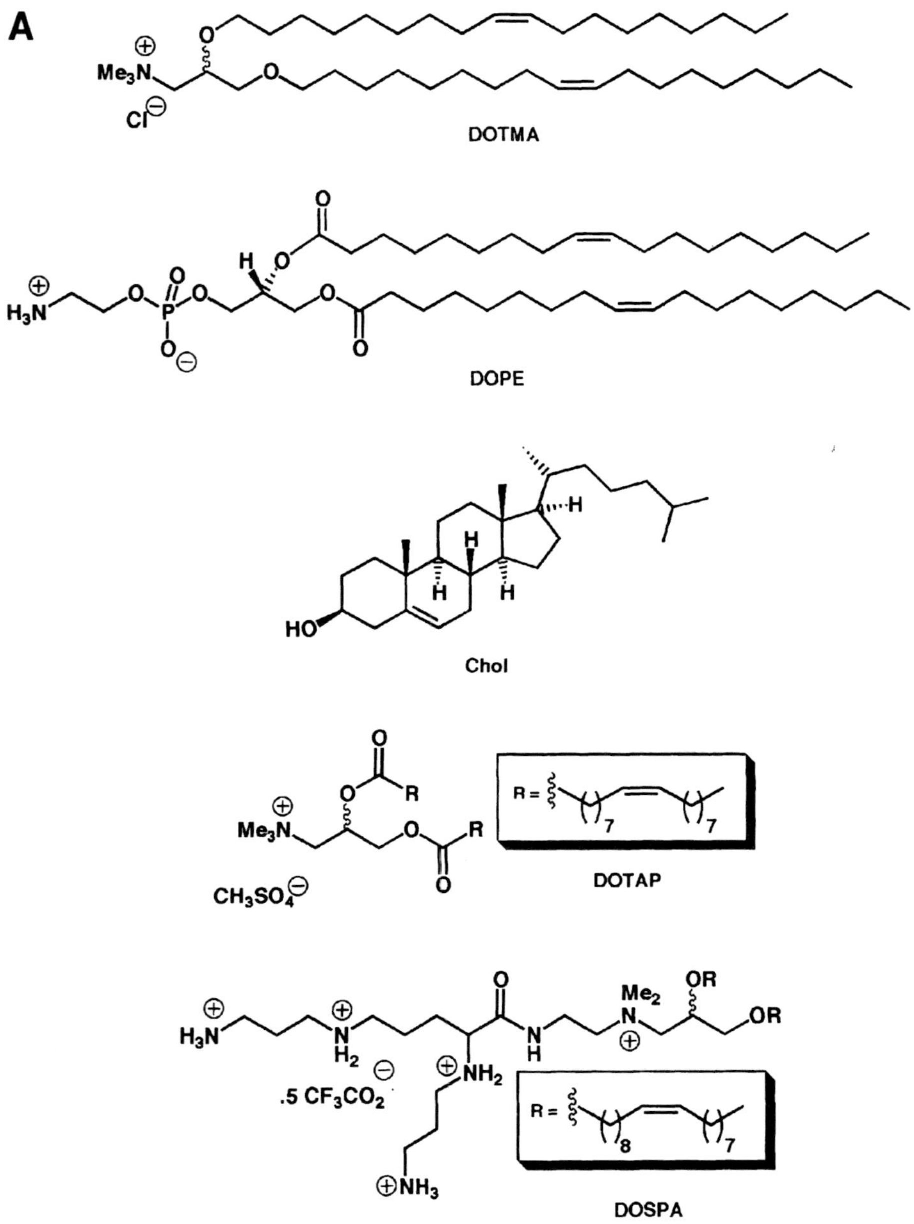

A

DOTMA

DOPE

Chol

DOTAP

DOSPA

Fig. 1(A)

Fig. 1. (**A–D**) Summary of structures of the main cytofectins and neutral lipids as described in the text and in **Table 1**, p.112.

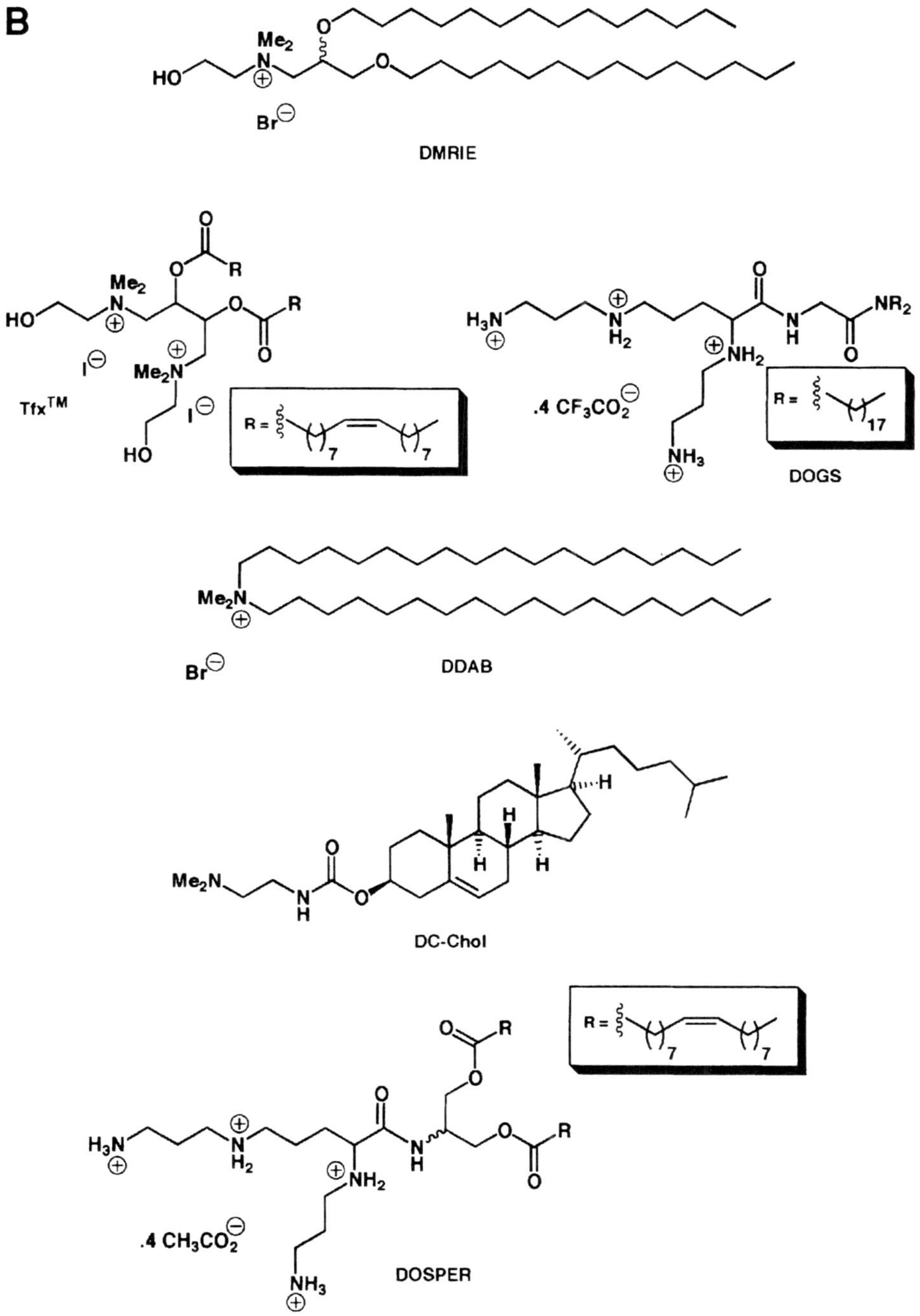

B

DMRIE

Tfx™

DOGS

DDAB

DC-Chol

DOSPER

Fig. 1(B)

Fig. 1(C)

Fig. 1(D)

Table 1
Selection of Significant Cationic Liposome/Micelle Systems

Cytofectin	Formulation	Trade name/manufacturer	Ref.
Commercialized			
DOTMA	DOTMA/DOPE 1 : 1 (w/w)	Lipofectin™/Gibco-BRL	*3*
DOTAP	DOTAP	DOTAP/Roche Molecular	*4*
DOSPA	DOSPA/DOPE 3 : 1 (w/w)	LipofectAMINE™/Gibco-BRL	*5*
DMRIE	DMRIE/Chol 1 : 1 (m/m)	DMRIE-C/Gibco-BRL	*6*
Tfx	Tfx/DOPE (Tfx-10, -20, -50)	Tfx™/Promega	*7*
DOGS	Micelle	Transfectam®/Promega	*8*
DDAB	DDAB/DOPE 1 : 2.5 (w/w)	LipofectACE™/Gibco-BRL	*10*
DC-Chol	DC-Chol/DOPE 6 : 4 (m/m)	DC-Chol/Sigma	*11*
DOSPER	DOSPER	DOSPER/Roche Molecular	*12*
Not commercialized			
RPR 120535	Micelle		*14*
Cholic acid hexamine	Cholic acid hexamine/DOPE 1 : 1 (w/w)		*15*
GL-67	GL-67/DOPE 1 : 2 (m/m)		*16*
CTAP	CTAP/DOPE 1 : 2 (m/m), 6:4 (m/m)		*17*
BGTC	BGTC/DOPE 3 : 2 (m/m)		*19*
DOTIM	DOTIM/Chol 1 : 1 (m/m) or DOTIM/DOPE 1:1 (m/m)		*20*
SAINT	SAINT/DOPE 1 : 1 (w/w)		*21*
DODAC	DODAC/DOPE 1 : 1 (m/m)		*22*
Lipid-glycoside	Lipid-glycoside		*23*
DC-6-14	DC-6-14/DOPE/Chol 4 : 3 : 3 (m/m/m)		*24*
EG316	EG316/Chol 1 : 1 (w/w)		*25*

Abbreviations:

w/w: weight ratio; m/m: mol ratio; DOPE, dioleoyl-L-α-phosphatidylethanolamine; DOTMA, *N*-[1-(2,3-dioleyloxy)propyl]-*N*,*N*,*N*-trimethyl ammonium chloride; DOTAP, 1,2-dioleyloxy-3-(trimethylammonio)propane; DOSPA, 2,3-dioleyloxy-*N*-[2-(sperminecarboxamido)ethyl]-*N*,*N*-dimethyl-1-propanaminium trifluoroacetate; DMRIE, 1,2-dimyristyloxypropyl-3-dimethylhydroxyethylammonium bromide; DOGS, dioctadecylamidoglycylspermine; DDAB, dimethyldioctadecylammonium bromide;DC-Chol,3β-[*N*-(*N'N'*-dimethylaminoethane)carbamoyl]cholesterol; DOSPER, 1,3-dioleoyloxy-2-(6-carboxyspermyl)propylamide; CTAP, ¹⁵-cholesteryloxycarbonyl-3,7,12-triazapentadecane-1,15-diamine; BGTC, bis-guanidinium-tren-cholesterol; DOTIM, 1-[2-(oleoyloxy)ethyl]-2-oleyl-3-(2-hydroxyethyl)imidazolinium chloride; SAINT, synthetic amphiphiles interdisciplinary; DODAC, dioleyldimethylammonium chloride; DC-6-14, *O*,*O'*-ditetradecanoyl-*N*-(α-trimethylammonioacetyl)diethanolamine chloride; EG316, diolyl 2-(trimethylphosphonio)ethylphosphonate iodide.

This process is seductively simple but is, in reality, deeply inefficient. The problems of cationic liposome-mediated gene delivery are legion *(1,2,26)*. LD complexes formed from cationic liposomes and nucleic acids are difficult to formulate reproducibly. They are susceptible to aggregation, unstable in biological fluids (e.g., high salt and serum), difficult to store long term, and do not mediate reproducible transfections in vivo, ex vivo, and even in vitro. Moreover, LD complexes are not cell-type-specific; they slow to enter cells (hours), prone to endosome entrapment, and are only weak facilitors of DNA entry into the cell nucleus. In spite of these problems, some cationic liposome systems have found favor in clinical trials, not the least for topical lung delivery in cystic fibrosis clinical trials *(27,28)*. Furthermore, there has been a steady stream of recent reports concerning the application of simple LD systems to deliver genes in vivo—for instance to brain, tumors, fetuses, nasal passages, inflamed joints, and skin *(29–42)*. However, in general there has been a growing realization that current simple LD systems are unlikely to be of routine clinical use without further adaptation. Consequently, there has been a substantive effort made over the last few years to characterize the main barriers to efficient transfection in vitro and in vivo, as well as an effort to determine the most appropriate LD physical parameters for optimal transfection. In doing this, there has been an implicit hope that ways could be found to adapt LD systems, thereby ensuring suitability for clinical use.

2. Barriers to Efficient Transfection

There have been an impressive number of studies in the last few years aimed at understanding the barriers to efficient LD transfection in vitro and in vivo. Many of these barriers are fearsome. Studies clearly show that topical lung delivery is beset by problems from mucus *(43)*, intravenous (iv) and intraarterial (ia) delivery by serum components such as acidic serum albumin proteins, low-density lipoprotein (LDL), macroglobulins, and other low-molecular-weight components *(44–49)*. In short, mucus consists of mucins, amphiphilic lipoproteins that readily disrupt the structural integrity of LD complexes, thereby preventing LD transfection. In serum, transfection efficiency is impaired by hydrophobic, negatively charged proteins such as serum albumin that associate with LD complexes, thereby inhibiting direct cellular uptake, as well as opsonize complexes for reticulo-endothelial system (RES) scavenging *(49)*. Alternatively, low-molecular-weight lipids like oleic acid (OA) and large glycosides like heparin readily disrupt the structural integrity of LD complexes by displacing nucleic acids and lipid components, thereby directly impairing transfection efficiency *(49)*. If this were not enough, cationic systems are known to activate complement *(50)*, and bacterially derived plasmid DNA, most usually used to prepare LD complexes, now appears to be immunogenic eliciting immune responses from so-called unmethylated CpG islets whether delivered by the topical lung route or intravenously *(51–54)*. These myriad problems ensure that LD complexes especially delivered intravenously have short circulation times (less than minutes) in biological fluids and generally poor in vivo transfection efficiencies. A direct consequence of short circulation times is the classic first-pass effect. After iv injection of LD complexes, gene expression in the lung is typically 100-fold greater than in other organs such as the liver or

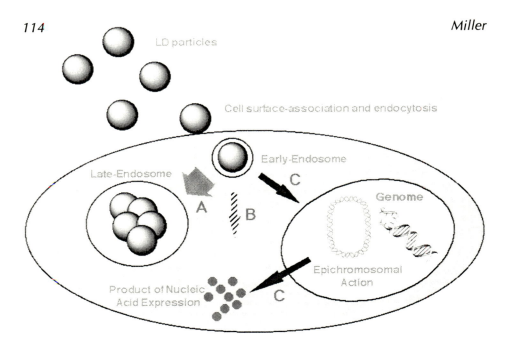

Fig. 2

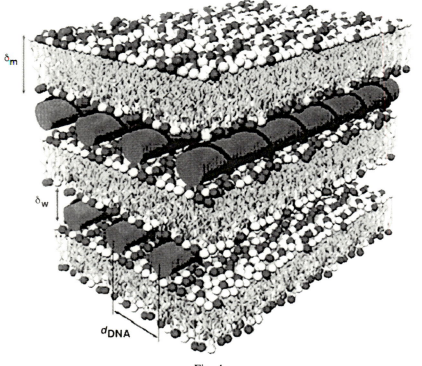

Fig. 4

spleen *(55)*. This is mainly because the pulmonary circulation is the first capillary bed that LD complexes will encounter postinjection, and enlarged serum-disrupted LD complexes will readily deposit in this lung microvasculature *(55–57)*, possibly anchored by association with heparin proteoglycans on the pulmonary endothelial surface *(58)*.

However, even assuming that in vivo stability problems can be resolved, recent in vitro transfection studies have revealed other highly significant barriers to efficient transfection once the plasma membrane of cells has been accessed. In addition to the well-known problems of slow endocytosis and late endosome entrapment (*see* preceding), there has been some impressive evidence to show the vulnerability of exogeneous DNA to cytosolic nucleases following DNA escape from early endosome compartments *(59)*. Furthermore, studies involving fluorescence correlation spectroscopy have also revealed plasmid DNA to bind extensively to immobile cellular obstacles (cytoskeleton) in the cytosol, thereby severely impeding intracellular migration of DNA toward the nucleus *(60)*. Even at the nuclear envelope, significant barriers are found. Tseng et al. *(61)* have provided convincing evidence that LD complexes are unable to promote DNA entry within the nuclear envelope without the intervention of the M-phase in the cell cycle when the nuclear membrane is partially dismantled to allow mitosis and cell division to take place. Otherwise, the nuclear pore complexes appear unable to support facile entry of large plasmid DNA into the nucleus. The complexity of these pore complexes is only now being appreciated, and accessing the nuclear volume via these pore complexes should be regarded as one of the most severe barriers to somatic cell LD transfection *(62–66)*.

◄ Fig. 2. Diagram showing process of LD complex cell entry. LD particles that have not succumbed to aggregation and/or serum inactivation associate with the cell surface and enter usually by endocytosis. The majority in early endosomes become trapped in late endosomes (path A) and the nucleic acids fail to reach the cytosol. A minority are able to release their bound nucleic acids into the cytosol. Path B is followed by RNA that acts directly in the cytosol. Path C is followed by DNA that enters the nucleus in order to act. The diagram is drawn making the assumption that plasmid DNA has been delivered, which is expressed in an epichromosomal manner. Reproduced from **ref. 26** with the permission of BIOS Scientific Publishers Ltd.

◄ Fig. 4. Schematic diagram of the proposed local arrangement of LD complexes. The DNA molecules are represented as rods (blue). The head groups of anionic/zwitterionic lipids are shown as white spheres, those of cytofectins are shown as red spheres. Cytofectins are more concentrated near the DNA. The notation δ_m refers to bilayer thickness, δ_w to interbilayer separation, and d_{DNA} to DNA interaxial spacing. The magnitude of d_{DNA} was observed to increase from approx 25 to 60 Å as the cationic liposome/DNA (positive/negative charge) ratio increased from less than to more than 1. Reprinted with permission from **ref. 74**. Copyright 1997 American Association for the Advancement of Science.

3. Transfection Structure–Activity Studies

Biophysical structure–activity studies designed to understand the structures of LD complexes and their relationships to LD transfection efficiency have been numerous. Unfortunately, the diversity of cytofectin structures, LD systems, and biological targets has resulted in considerable inconsistency in the results reported by the research groups concerned. For instance, LD transfection in vivo is quite often reported to be optimal when the positive/negative charge ratio of the LD mixture is greater than 1 *(34,45,47)*. For LD transfection in vitro, the optimal positive/negative charge ratio may be much higher than 1 *(8,67)*, but, more frequently, the optimal ratio is reported to be closer to 1 *(6,68–70)*. However, recently described transfection studies clearly show that optimal in vitro LD transfection of COS-7 cells and in vivo LD transfection of Balb/c mice lungs requires LD mixtures with an overall positive/negative charge ratio of <1 *(18)*. This observation has been supported by the results of others *(71)*.

Similarly diverse views exist concerning the structures of LD complexes optimal for transfection. In some circumstances, LD mixtures optimal for in vitro transfection appear to be heterogeneous and polydisperse, consisting of a variety of structures all in dynamic equilibrium *(72,73)*. These structures have been variously identified and described by a number of researchers and they include multilammellar lipid/nucleic acid clusters (>100 nm in diameter) *(74–78)*, perhaps with some surface-associated nucleic acids *(79)*, thinly lipid-coated DNA nucleic acid strands *(80)*, and free nucleic acids *(76)*. These structural observations have led to a substantive debate concerning the relative importance of each of these structural entities for efficient in vitro transfection. However, LD mixtures optimal for in vitro transfection do not necessarily have to be so heterogeneous and polydisperse. Recent studies using sophisticated cryo-electron microscopy have clearly demonstrated that LD mixtures optimal for in vitro and in vivo transfection may actually consist of discrete LD particles (60–250 nm in diameter) exhibiting bilammellar perimeters and striations with a periodicity of 4.2±2 nm (*see* **Fig. 3**) *(18)*. Small-angle X-ray scattering (SAXS) and other cryo-electron microscopy studies of LD mixtures have revealed similar periodicities of approx 6.5 and 3.5 nm that have been shown to result from the encapsulation of DNA molecules in regular periodic arrays within a multilammellar LD assembly *(74,75,81–83)* (*see* **Fig. 4** on p. 114). Therefore, the observed LD particles are most likely composed in a similar way. Hence, in this case at least, optimal LD transfection in vitro and in vivo must be mediated primarily by these discrete, multilammellar LD particles *(18)*. The significance of discrete LD particles for optimal transfection has been supported by the results of at least one other published study comparing LD structure with in vivo transfection efficacy *(84)*. Evidence then suggests that the regular multilamellar bilayer structure ($L\alpha_I$) of LD particles should undergo a phase change in the endosome-forming inverted hexagonal-phase structures (H_{II}) that may disrupt endosome membranes and faciliate nucleic acid escape into the cytosol *(85)*. Lipids like DOPE are well known to prefer H_{II} phases under physiological conditions of temperature and pH, and the $L\alpha_I{\rightarrow}H_{II}$ phase transition has been widely implicated as a key facilitator of membrane-fusion and membrane-disruption events.

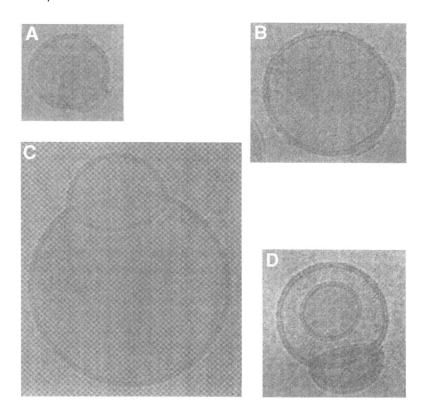

Fig. 3. Cryo-electron microscopy images of LD particles. These LD particles were formed after the combination of N^1-cholesteryloxycarbonyl-3,7-diazanonane-1,9-diamine CDAN/ DOPE cationic liposomes and plasmid DNA in the [cytofectin]/[nucleotide] ([cyt]/[nt]) mole ratio of 0.6, optimal for in vitro and in vivo lung transfection. Final lipid concentration was 0.17 mM. Original magnification is 200,000× (1 cm = 50 nm). Reproduced from **ref. *18*** by permission of the Royal Society of Chemistry.

General biophysical structure–activity studies have generated a number of possible correlations among LD structure, physical attributes, and transfection efficiency. For instance, Akao et al. *(86)* have suggested that successful gene delivery will occur when the phase-transition temperature, T_c, of the cationic liposome formulation is less than 37°C. However, this has not been supported by more recent studies *(87)*, although lower phase-transition temperatures appear to be helpful in some cases *(88)*. Other authors have suggested a proportional relationship between the zeta potential of cholesterol-based cationic liposomes and their gene delivery efficiency *(89)*. Once again, such a suggestion has not been supported by more recent studies *(18)*. Still others have systematically cataloged the deleterious effects of electron-withdrawing groups in cytofectin head groups on transfection efficiency *(90)*. However, the inescapable conclusion is that most biophysical structure–activity studies are of only limited value providing few conclusions of general utility that have been confirmed by independent studies involving a variety of different LD systems. Moreover, there have been few attempts to derive unifying biophysical parameters able to account for differences in LD transfection efficiency in vitro and in vivo.

One exception may be found in the work of Stewart et al. *(18)*, who studied the physical properties of a systematic series of cationic liposomes and their corresponding LD mixtures. Liposomes were formulated from DOPE and cholesterol-based polyamine cytofectins such as N^{15}-cholesteryloxycarbonyl-3,7,12-triazapentadecane-1,15-diamine (CTAP) and N^1-cholesteryloxycarbonyl-3,7-diazanonane-1, 9-diamine (CDAN) *(see* **Fig. 1)**. Successful in vivo transfection was linked to the ability of cationic liposome systems to (1) efficiently neutralize, condense, and encapsulate nucleic acids into LD particles and (2) present unprotonated amine functional groups (pK_a <8) at neutral pH with the capacity for endosome buffering, thereby facilitating nucleic acid escape from endosome compartments into the cytosol after cell entry. By contrast, successful in vitro transfection was linked to inefficient neutralization, condensation, and encapsulation of nucleic acids and the presence of unprotonated amine functional groups. Critically, both main factors were observed to be under the control of the cytofectin polyamine head-group structure. The inclusion of "natural" propylene and butylene spacings between the amine functional groups of head groups appeared to promote efficient neutralization, condensation, and encapsulation of nucleic acid. The inclusion of "unnatural" ethylene spacings appeared to promote the reverse effect but was simultaneously a successful means of lowering amine pK_a values from 9–10 to below 8. Assuming that inefficient neutralization, condensation, and encapsulation of nucleic acids is also indicative of unstable LD complexes, Turek et al. *(91)* appear to have corroborated these findings in part by showing unstable LD complexes to be optimal for in vitro transfection. Similarly, Zuidam and Barenholz *(92)* have also reported LD transfection in vitro to be most efficient with unstable LD complexes.

4. Ternary Transfection Systems

Unfortunately, there has been a marked inability to capitalize on the wealth of biophysical data and an increasingly sophisticated understanding of the LD transfection process (as described earlier) to derive clinically useful binary LD systems. Accordingly, there have been a number of recent trends moving away from traditional binary toward ternary LD systems. A number of ternary systems have been described over the past few years in which the cationic character of the cationic liposome/micelle is supplemented by an additional cationic entity designed to assist nucleic acid condensation and encapsulation as well as to enhance transfection. Cationic entities that have been used include protamine *(46,93–101)*, poly-L-lysine *(102,103)*, spermidine *(104)*, lipopolylysine *(105)*, histone proteins *(106)*, chromatin proteins *(107)*, human histone-derived peptides *(108)*, L-lysine-containing synthetic peptides *(109)*, not to mention a histidine/lysine (H-K) copolymer *(110)*. However, with the arguable exception of protamine-based ternary LD systems, few of the other reported systems have been shown to make much impression on the problems of LD transfection and the barriers to efficient transfection described earlier. Liposome : polycation : DNA or, more specifically, lipid : protamine : DNA (LPD) systems have been largely formulated using 3β-[N-(N',N'-dimethylaminoethane)carbamoyl]cholesterol (DC-Chol)/DOPE or 1,2-dioleoyloxy-3-(trimethylammonio)propane (DOTAP)/Chol cationic liposomes, or DOTAP micelles (see **Fig. 1**). DOTAP-based LPD systems were found to give much more efficient and much less variable transfection in vivo than was observed with DOTAP-mediated transfection *(94)*. DOTAP/Chol-based LPD systems were even more effective and were found to formulate into discrete particles (approx 135±42 nm) *(95)*. However, such particles were readily modified by serum, causing gradual vector disintegration, release of DNA, and probable RES scavenging *(46,95)*. Released DNA was also noted to be susceptible to extracellular nuclease digestion. Of additional concern, LPD was found to promote a systemic, Th1-like innate immune response in mice, much more appropriate for a DNA vaccine than for gene therapy *(97)*. However, the general impression given is that LPD systems could have a role to play clinically for the passive delivery of genes to lung endothelial cells but are not appropriate for targeted gene delivery to other tissues *(46)*.

Other ternary LD systems have tried to introduce alternative approaches and/or functionality in order to try and find more credible solutions. For instance, there have been attempts to combine binary LD systems with microspheres *(111,112)*, replication-deficient adenovirus *(113)*, and fusogenic peptides like GALA or HA2 intended to promote disruption of early endosome membranes and enhance DNA release into the cytosol *(114–116)*. Intriguingly, whereas fusogenic peptides do appear to enhance in vitro LD transfection, this enhancement becomes rather modest when an excess of cationic liposome/micelle is used to prepare LD complexes, suggesting that cytofectins themselves may have fusogenic behavior with respect to endosome membranes *(117,118)*. Perhaps for this reason, Budker et al. *(119)* were motivated to develop a simple fusogenic cationic liposome system formulated from cytofectins with imidazole and 4-aminopyridyl head groups that are only partially protonated at neutral pH and fully protonated under mildly acidic pH conditions (pH 5–6), giving acceptable in vitro transfection efficiencies.

Alternatively, peptides consisting of an oligo-L-lysine moiety linked to a moiety specific for cell surface integrin proteins have been combined with LD systems *(120–122)*. In the latter case, credible enhancements of at least an order of magnitude in in vitro transfection have been observed over and above the results of binary LD transfection owing to the involvement of integrin-mediated cell uptake *(121,122)*. Furthermore, enhancements to in vivo transfection have been reported as well, but the mechanism of enhancement does not appear to be integrin-receptor dependent in this case *(120)*. There has been some apparent success in using neoglycolipids as targeting agents inserted into LD complexes. For instance, Behr and coworkers reported in vitro galactose-receptor-mediated uptake into hepatoma cells of LD complexes formulated with a triantennary galactolipid *(67)*. More recently, Kawakami et al. have suggested liver targeting in vivo using LD complexes formulated with a mannosyl neoglycolipid as targeting agent, although mannosyl-induced LD stabilization leading to longer circulation times could well be sufficient explanation to account for these results too *(123,124)*.

Transferrin has become a very popular agent for combining with binary LD systems on the basis that transferrin-receptor-mediated uptake may enhance transfection owing to the fact that receptors are found routinely at the surface of vascular endothelial cells associated with tumors or the blood–brain barrier and are rapidly internalized upon binding transferrin *(115,125–127)*. However, although in vitro and ex vivo transfection is enhanced relative to binary LD transfection, the mechanism is quite clearly transferrin-receptor independent, the protein instead acting primarily to promote endosome disruption and subsequent escape of complexed DNA into the cytosol *(115,125)*. In addition, transferrin is an acidic protein, negatively charged at neutral pH. Accordingly, the association of transferrin with binary LD systems seems to reduce the overall positive charge and simultaneously provides a combined steric and electronic barrier to biological fluid components, allowing in vitro transfection to take place, even in 60% serum. In the latter context, human serum albumin (HSA) has been deliberately combined with binary LD systems in order to create negatively charged, sterically protected complexes appropriate for in vitro transfection in the presence of up to 30% serum and even for lung or spleen transfection in vivo *(128)*. Even lectin proteins have been used to promote in vitro transfection *(129)*. Whether or not any of the ternary LD complexes described in this section have any meaningful clinical use remains unproven given the very limited nature of the in vivo transfection data so far presented in these cases.

5. Platform Technologies

Given the difficulties faced in making meaningful progress in bringing LD systems to clinical readiness in gene therapy, the only solution must be to set up properly defined, stable systems that can be easily upgraded in very clearly defined ways—in other words, nonviral vector platform technologies. Currently, there are regrettably few systems that could be described as nonviral vector platform technologies developed around cationic liposome/micelle systems. The above-described LPD systems could fit into this category provided that further developments continue to be made and innovations introduced. In addition, there are two other systems of potential interest, namely the new liposome : mu : DNA (LMD) system and the more established stabilized plasmid–lipid particles (SPLP) systems.

The LMD system is a ternary LD system built around the mu (μ) peptide associated with the condensed core complex of the adenovirus. Mature adenovirus consists of an icosahedral, nonenveloped capsid particle (approx 90 nm) enclosing a core complex that consists of a linear dsDNA viral genome (approx 36 kbp) noncovalently associated with two cationic proteins (proteins V [pV] and VII [pVII]) and a 19-residue cationic peptide known as μ *(130,131)*. There is as yet no clear picture concerning the core structure, and little understanding of the relative contributions of pV, pVII, and μ peptide to the process by which viral DNA is delivered into the host cell nucleus. However, evidence begins to suggest that pVII and μ peptide are most tightly associated with viral DNA, whereas pV may play a role in assisting the delivery of the adenovirus core complex into the host cell nucleus *(132,133)*. The μ peptide results from the cleavage of a 79-residue precursor protein by adenovirus-encoded proteinase and contains no known nuclear localization signal but has powerful DNA condensing properties *(130)*, sufficient for the peptide to enhance routine cationic liposome-mediated transfection in vitro *(134)*.

In comparison with LD systems, homogeneous LMD particles (120±30 nm) can be formulated reproducibly that are amenable to long-term storage at −80°C and stable up to a plasmid DNA concentration of 5 mg/mL (nucleotide concentration 15 mM), a concentration appropriate for facile use in vivo *(135)*. Using LD systems, nucleotide concentrations >4 mM are difficult to achieve owing to ready LD particle aggregation above this concentration threshold *(16–18)*. Moreover, LMD transfections appear to be significantly more time and dose efficient in vitro than LD transfections. LMD transfection times as short as 10 min and DNA doses as low as 0.001 μg/well result in significant gene expression, whereas LD transfections typically require transfection times of several hours (up to 24 h) and plasmid DNA doses of approx 1 μg/well. Most importantly, LMD transfections will also take place in the presence of biological fluids (e.g., up to 100% serum), conditions typically intractable to LD transfections, suggesting that the LMD formulation exhibits an additional element of stability. Preliminary studies carried out by confocal microscopy on dividing tracheal cells suggest that endocytosis is not a significant barrier to LMD transfection in comparison to LD transfection. There is every possibility that both cytofectin and even the μ peptide are exercising considerable fusogenic behavior with respect to early endosome membranes *(116–118)*. However, plasmid DNA does not appear to enter the nucleus of growth-arrested cells, suggesting that the nuclear pore complex remains a significant barrier to LMD transfection. In vivo, LMD transfection of lung was up to sixfold more dose efficient than transfection with GL-67 : DOPE : DMPE-PEG$_{5000}$ (1 : 2 : 0.05 m/ m/m) (one of the best nonviral vector systems reported to date for lung transfection; DMPE = dimyristoylphosphatidylethanolamine). LMD has been called an artificial viruslike nanoparticle (VNP) on the basis that cryo-electron microscopy shows LMD particles to consist of a mu : DNA (MD) particle encapsulated within a cationic bilammellar liposome (*see* **Fig. 5**). Because these particles are self-assembled with ease from simple peptide, cationic liposome and plasmid DNA components, they should be upgraded in a modular fashion with relative ease for future specific applications of interest. For instance, there should be little difficulty in introducing appropriate cell targeting and stabilizing functionality into the lamellar outer coat. Similarly, additional functionality should be added to the MD core with ease so as to promote more efficient intracellular trafficking of plasmid DNA, in particular to try to facilitate plasmid DNA entry into the nucleus *(135)*.

A common feature of neutral and anionic liposomes used for drug delivery is often the inclusion of polyethylene glycol (PEG) lipids in liposomal bilayers that simultaneously provide a steric barrier to interaction with biological fluid components and prevent uptake of liposomal vesicles by cells of the RES *(1,136)*. Hong et al. reported one of the first attempts to use PEG lipids to stabilize LD complexes *(104)*. In this instance, dimethyldioctadecylammoniumbromide (DDAB)/Chol cationic liposome-based LD particles were stabilized for storage by inclusion of N-[ω-methoxypoly(oxyethylene)-α-oxycarbonyl]-DSPE (PEG-PE; DSPE = distearoylphosphatidylethanolamine) and

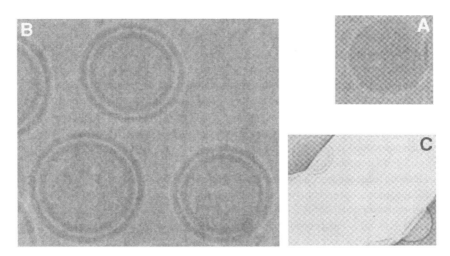

Fig. 5. Cryo-electron microscopy images of LMD particles. **(A)** mu : DNA (MD) particle (1 cm = 48 nm); **(B)** liposome : mu : DNA (LMD) particles prepared with DC-Chol/DOPE cationic liposomes and plasmid DNA particle (1 cm = 48 nm); **(C)** an LMD particle fractured between the inner and outer leaflets of the first of the two bilayers that surround the higher density MD core particle (1 cm = 114 nm). (Reproduced from **ref. 135** with permission from Nature Publishing Group.)

partially stabilized in the circulation in vivo. However, >1 mol% of PEG-PE proved sufficient to reduce lung in vivo transfection efficacy to a fraction of the transfection level mediated by DDAB/Chol cationic liposomes alone, indicative of a necessary compromise between a requirement to include PEG-PE for stabilization purposes countered by a requirement to keep levels modest in order to avoid steric blocking of LD transfection. SPLP systems represent a considerable technical advance over the stabilized LD system reported by Hong et al. and have the virtue of being well defined and characterized systems like LMD. Whereas LMD shows impressive transfection efficiency, SPLP systems are less efficacious but do show impressive stability in vivo. Plasmid DNA has been shown to be trapped within very well-defined SPLP particles stabilized by PEG moieties attached to the particles by a ceramide anchor.

The first-generation SPLP system contained DOPE (84 mol%), low levels (6 mol%) of cationic lipid dioleyldimethylammonium chloride (DODAC), and quite high levels of PEG-ceramide with an arachidoyl acyl group (PEG-CerC$_{20}$) (10 mol%) *(137)*. The surface tenacity of PEG-CerC$_{20}$ ($t_{1/2}$ >13 d) proved such an intractable steric barrier to transfection that PEG-CerC$_{20}$ was replaced by PEG-CerC$_8$ ($t_{1/2}$ <1.2 min) with an octanoyl acyl group. Plasmid DNA entrapment was then accomplished by a detergent dialysis procedure employing octylglucoside (OGP) and a dialysis medium dosed with citrate (100 mM) and NaCl (120–140 mM), providing ionic strength sufficient to enhance cationic lipid incorporation into SPLP particles during the entrapment process (55–70% efficient). Free plasmid DNA was removed by passage over a DEAE ion-exchange column and empty vesicles by sucrose-density gradient centrifugation, giving second-generation DOPE : DODAC : PEG-CerC$_8$ SPLP particles containing DODAC (24–30 mol%) and PEG-CerC$_8$ (15 mol%) (diameter approx 100±40 nm) *(138)*. In vitro and in vivo SPLP transfection was found to be comparable or moderately better than DODAC/DOPE-mediated transfection. These levels are still low and much progress needs to be made, but the most important aspect is the very structural integrity of the SPLP particles (no changes in size or DNA encapsulation at 4°C for 5 mo) and the real practical and handling advantages of such a controlled system with regard to scale-up, manufacturing, and storage in common with LMD. Very recently, Shi and Pardridge reported a variation of SPLP in the form of an immuno-cationic liposome system based around very low-ratio cationic liposomes doped with PEG-PE variants—one for stabilization and one for the covalent attachment of an antibody specific for the blood–brain barrier (BBB) transferrin receptor *(139)*. Good circulation times were reported and some encapsulated plasmid DNA did appear to be delivered successfully across the BBB, resulting in transgene expression in neurological tissue. However, lung, spleen, and liver all showed significant transgene expression as well.

6. Alternative Lipid-Based Transfection Systems

In recent times, frustration with cationic liposome/micelle-based systems has precipitated a revival of interest in neutral or anionic-lipid-based transfection systems. Nucleic acid delivery systems mostly likely will be effective in vivo if they can be made "triggerable" (i.e., stable and nonreactive in extracellular fluids but unstable once recognized and internalized by target cells in the target organ of choice). With the exception of SPLP systems, cationic liposome/micelle-based transfection systems err on the side of instability in the presence of extracellular fluids, as described earlier. In contrast, liposome systems composed of neutral or anionic lipids have much longer circulation times and very different clearance profiles compared to systems composed with cytofectins. Neutral liposomes have been successfully applied as carriers for anticancer drugs and antibiotics to achieve lower toxicities, altered distributions, and higher drug efficacies than unencapsulated drugs *(140)*. In addition, neutral or anionic liposomes passively accumulate in tumors and sites of inflammation where vasculature is malformed or permeabilized, and retargeting strategies have been applied with some success, in comparison with cationic systems *(140)*.

Simple neutral liposome-based transfection systems have two clear disadvantages compared with cytofectin-based systems: little capacity to achieve any appreciable level of transfection and highly inefficient encapsulation or entrapment of negatively charged nucleic acids in particles small enough for administration in vivo. Solutions to both problems have been actively sought over the past few years. For instance, efficient methods have been developed for the encapsulation of oligodeoxynucleotides (ODNs) into small (100–200 nm) neutral liposomes *(141–143)*, and even an efficient means of plasmid DNA encapsulation into small neutral liposomes has been described *(140)*. The problem of transfection using such neutral liposome-encapsulated nucleic acids still needs to be properly addressed, but incorporation of the ever-growing available range of endosmolytic peptides such as GALA and pH-sensitive, membrane-lytic polymers may provide part of the solution to this problem *(116,144)*, alongside the use of ligands such as transferrin, mentioned earlier.

At around the time of inception of cationic liposome-mediated nucleic acid delivery, pH-sensitive immunoliposomes were being evaluated for gene delivery in vivo *(145)*. The term "pH-sensitive" liposome can be interpreted very broadly *(144)*, but the majority of reported systems are comprised of DOPE and titratable anionic acidic lipids such as cholesteryl hemisuccinate (CHEMS), OA, or diacylsuccinylglycerol (*see* **Fig. 6**), lipids that are all negatively charged at neutral pH. These acidic lipids are thought to stabilize the normal lamellar bilayer structure ($L\alpha_I$) of liposomes by harnessing forces of electrostatic repulsion to prevent DOPE molecules from associating to form inverted hexagonal-phase structures (H_{II}). However, if these liposomes become internalized into cells by endocytosis, protonation of the anionic acidic lipids is thought to remove the constraint of electrostatic repulsion and vesicles become destabilized as DOPE molecules revert to H_{II} structures, promoting membrane fusion/disruption and thereby allowing endosome escape of any liposome-associated molecules such as nucleic acids. Simple pH-sensitive liposome systems without antibodies or other such functionalities mediate transfection quite weakly compared with simple cationic liposome systems *(146)*, underlining the necessity of combining pH-sensitive liposome systems with ligands for targeting/cell uptake enhancement if measurable transfection is to be obtained. In spite of early promise *(145,147–149)*, the primary limitation of pH-sensitive liposome systems (viz. highly inefficient encapsulation or entrapment of negatively charge plasmid DNA) has proved a difficult limitation to overcome. Shorter ODNs appear to encapsulate into pH-sensitive liposomes more readily perhaps than plasmid DNA *(150)*, but on the whole, passive encapsulation of DNA into anionic liposomes usually requires the use of a high concentration of lipids to increase the "entrapped volume" leading to the generation of excessive levels of empty liposomes (entrapment efficiency <20%). Common approaches to improving encapsulation, including freeze–thaw, polycarbonate membrane extrusion, and/or sonication, can damage DNA severely too *(151)*.

Accordingly, Lee and Huang *(151)* attempted to circumvent this problem while attempting to benefit from the use of pH-sensitive liposomes, by designing a novel folate-targeted liposome-entrapped polycation-condensed DNA system known as LPDII. In this, DNA was first complexed to poly-L-lysine in the ratio 1 : 0.75 (w/w) and then entrapped into folate-targeted pH-sensitive anionic liposomes composed of DOPE/CHEMS/folate-PEG-DOPE 6 : 4 : 0.01 (m/m/m) via charge interaction, giving small particles (74±14 nm). Folate, like transferrin described earlier, has proved a durable ligand for transfection studies owing to the prevalence of folate receptors in tumors and frequent demonstrations of folate-mediated macromolecule delivery to tumor cells in vitro and to xenograft tumor cells in vivo *(152)*. At low lipid-to-DNA ratios, positively charged LPDII particles behaved as cationic LD complexes exhibiting folate-independent in vitro transfection. At high ratios, folate-dependent in vitro transfection was clearly observed *(151)*. A number of variations of LPDII have since been reported. These include replacing CHEMS with *N*-citraconyl-DOPE (C-DOPE) (*see* **Fig. 6**) *(153)* or OA *(154)*, replacing poly-L-lysine with polyethylenimine (PEI) *(154)* or protamine sulfate *(155)*, using transferrin in place of folate *(156)*, or even replacing the pH-sensitive liposome coat with an anionic artificial viral envelope

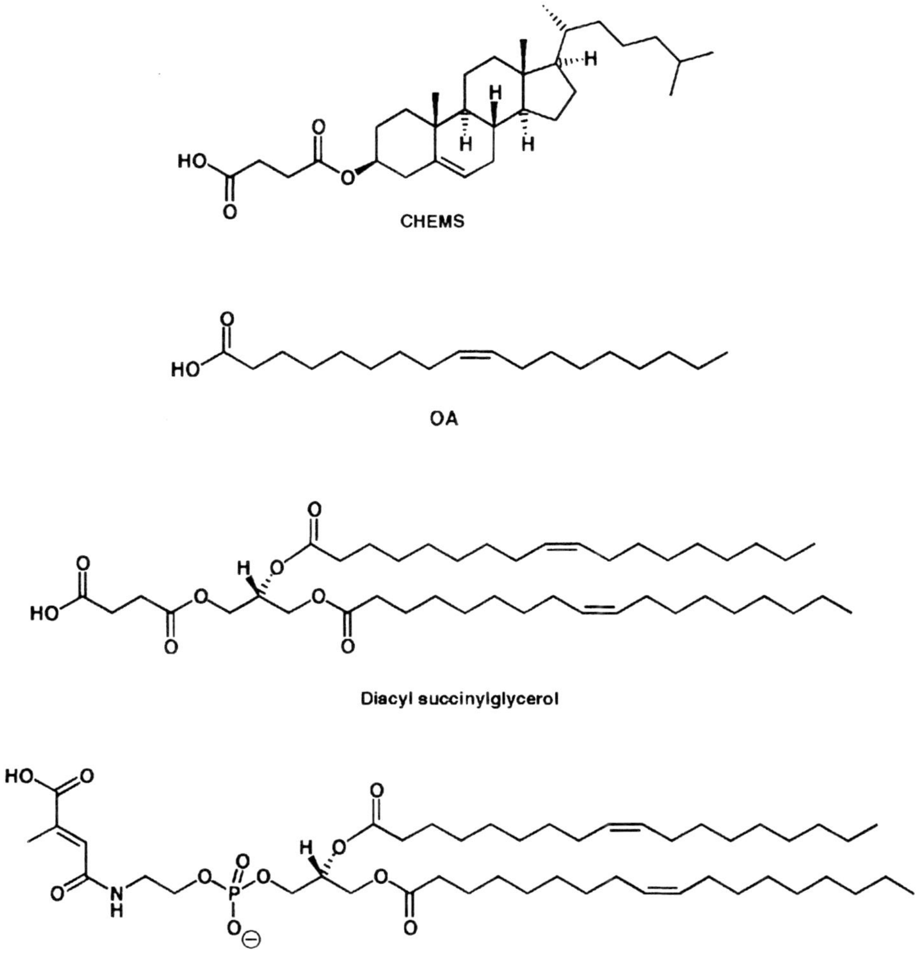

Fig. 6. Summary of structures of the main lipids for pH-sensitive liposome systems.

(AVE) formulation *(155)* (see below). In all cases, there remain to be convincing demonstrations that LPDII-like systems will transfect in vivo. The principle of precondensing nucleic acids with a cationic agent followed by encapsulation by a negatively charged liposome system has also been developed by other research groups. For instance, histones H2A or H1 *(157,158)*, spermidine *(159)*, or spermine *(160)* have all been reported to be effective precondensing agents prior to encapsulation by anionic liposome systems. Once again, little in vivo transfection data appear to have been provided for these systems. An interesting new variation on this principle has been to prepare LD complexes and coat them with sufficient anionic succinylated poly(glycidol) to produce particles with a net negative charge able to transfect cells in vitro with the assistance of transferrin, even in the presence of serum *(161)*.

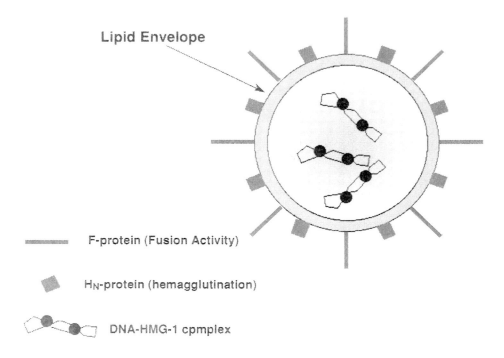

Fig. 7. Diagram showing structure of HVJ-liposome system. Reproduced from **ref. 26** with the permission of BIOS Scientific Publishers Ltd.

If in vivo data are largely absent from a discussion about LPDII and LPDII-like transfection systems, the same cannot be said to be true of the hemagglutinating virus of Japan (HVJ)-liposome system. This system may be described as a virosome, a term originally coined in reference to combinations of liposomes and various virus glyco-proteins but now more generally used to refer to various types of viral/nonviral hybrid vector system. The HVJ-liposome system is prepared from a combination of ultravio-let (UV)-irradiated virions of the HVJ (Sendai virus) and liposomes in which are en-capsulated nucleic acids complexed with the high mobility group 1 (HMG-1) protein *(162,163)*. The HMG-1 protein is there to assist nuclear access and localization of delivered nucleic acids as well as promoting gene stabilization within the nuclear envelope *(162,164)*. Although negatively charged and approx 350–500 nm in size, HVJ liposomes themselves have been used in an impressive range of local systemic and anticancer applications in vivo involving both ODN and plasmid DNA delivery *(162,163,165,166)*. One major reason for the success of HVJ liposomes is the pres-ence of the hemagglutinin-neuraminidase (H_N) and fusion (F) glycoproteins in the liposome bilayer (*see* **Fig. 7**). These are fusogenic proteins that allow HVJ liposomes to interact with cell surface sialic residues, fuse with the cell membrane, and then release encapsulated nucleic acids directly into the cytoplasm, bypassing endocytosis altogether *(163)*. For this reason, HVJ liposomes have also been called fusogenic liposomes *(167)*. An HVJ cationic liposome system based on the cytofectin DC-Chol has been reported able to transfect various mammalian cell types in vitro 100- to 800-fold more effectively than conventional HVJ liposomes *(168)*. In addition, HVJ cationic liposomes prepared with the cytofectin N-(α-trimethylammonioacetyl)-didodecyl-D-glutamate chloride (TMAG) (*see* **Fig. 1**) have proved able to mediate delivery of nucleic acids to tracheal and bronchiolar epithelial cells in vivo with reasonable efficiency *(169)*. Further in vivo applications of HVJ cationic liposomes have also been described *(162,170)*. Finally, there have been some interesting reports concerning in vivo gene delivery by HVJ-AVE liposomes *(171,172)* assembled from anionic AVE liposomes with a lipid composition similar to that of HIV retroviral envelopes *(173,174)*. These appear to be modestly more efficacious than conventional HVJ liposomes.

The clear success of HVJ liposomes has resulted in a number of interesting developments associated with the fusogenic proteins F and H_N. For instance, F virosomes have been described consisting of reconstituted HVJ viral envelopes containing only the F protein that were able to mediate efficient gene delivery to liver cells in vitro and in vivo *(175,176)*. Alternatively, a system has been described involving the combination of neutral liposomes and poly-L-lysine-condensed DNA with samples of F and H_N proteins extracted from purified HVJ *(177)*; this is somewhat LPDII-like in character. Kondoh et al. *(178)* have outlined something similar for ODN delivery. Neither of these two systems has been evaluated in vivo. Of additional interest are a number of recently reported cationic virosome systems. These include DODAC-containing virosomes prepared with the influenza membrane fusion protein hemagglutinin *(179)* and used to deliver genes to cells in vitro, cationic lipid-reconstituted influenza-virus envelopes used to deliver ODNs to cells in vitro *(180)*, and LD complexes prepared from N-[1-(2,3-dioleyloxy)propyl]-N,N,N-triethyl ammonium chloride (DOTMA)/DOPE cationic liposomes and plasmid DNA doped with the partially purified G glycoprotein of the vesicular stomatitis virus envelope (VsV-G) *(181)*.

7. Future Prospects

Platform technologies like LMD and SPLP systems are the only meaningful way forward for cationic liposome/micelle-based systems. These systems provide a firm foundation in terms of reproducible formulation, long-term storage, and transfection outcomes, a foundation that allows for careful and scrupulous development toward clinical applications. They represent well-characterized, well-understood transfection vehicles constructed from a primary toolkit of well-defined chemical entities. Given this foundation, future development may then be performed in a sequential and logical fashion, making modular adaptations to the primary vehicle with new toolkits of novel chemical entities designed to engage a chosen clinical application. Each new toolkit will need to be derived from a thorough understanding and analysis of the barriers to efficient transfection. Given the arrival of proper platform technologies, cationic liposome/micelle-based systems should now stand a realistic chance of becoming sound vector technologies for clinical gene therapy in the future. Of the other nonviral liposome systems, HVJ liposomes and related systems appear to be powerful local gene delivery agents. However, whether these may become adapted for distal delivery remains to be seen. Moreover, these virosome systems are not well characterized and may well be difficult to prepare in bulk, obviating their potential use as platform gene therapy technologies.

References

1. Miller, A. D. (1998) Cationic liposomes for gene therapy. *Angew. Chem. Int. Ed.* **37,** 1768–1785.
2. Miller, A. D. (1998) Cationic liposome systems in gene therapy. *Curr. Res. Mol. Ther.* **1,** 494–503.
3. Felgner, P. L., Gadek, T. R., Holm, M., et al. (1987) Lipofection: a highly efficient, lipid-mediated DNA-transfection procedure. *Proc. Natl. Acad. Sci. USA* **84,** 7413–7417.
4. Leventis, R. and Silvius, J. R. (1990) Interactions of mammalian cells with lipid dispersions containing novel metabolizable cationic amphiphiles. *Biochim. Biophys. Acta* **1023,** 124–132.
5. Gebeyehu, G., Jessee, J. A., Valentina, C., and Hawley-Nelson, P. (1993) Cationic lipids. In US-05334761, GIBCO/BRL.
6. Felgner, J. H., Kumar, R., Sridhar, C. N., et al. (1994) Enhanced gene delivery and mechanism studies with a novel series of cationic lipid formulations. *J. Biol. Chem.* **269,** 2550–2561.
7. Nantz, M. H., Bennett, M. J., and Malone, R. W. (1996) Cationic transport reagents. In US-05527928, Promega.
8. Behr, J. P., Demeneix, B., Loeffler, J. P., and Perez-Mutul, J. (1989) Efficient gene transfer into mammalian primary endocrine cells with lipopolyamine-coated DNA. *Proc. Natl. Acad. Sci. USA* **86,** 6982–6986.
9. Kunitake, T., Okahata, Y., Tamaki, K., Kumamaru, F., and Takayanagi, M. (1977) Formation of the bilayer membrane from a series of quaternary ammonium salts. *Chem. Lett.* 387–390.
10. Kunitake, T., Nakashima, N., Shimomura, M., et al. (1980) Unique properties of chromophore-containing bilayer aggregates: enhanced chirality and photo-chemically induced morphological change. *J. Am. Chem. Soc.* **102,** 6642–6644.
11. Gao, X. and Huang, L. (1991) A novel cationic liposome reagent for efficient transfection of mammalian cells. *Biochem. Biophys. Res. Commun.* **179,** 280–285.
12. Dodds, E., Dunckley, M. G., Naujoks, K., Michaelis, U., and Dickson, G. (1998) Lipofection of cultured mouse muscle cells: a direct comparison of Lipofectamine and DOSPER. *Gene Ther.* **5,** 542–551.
13. Pitard, B., Aguerre, O., Airiau, M., et al. (1997) Virus-sized self-assembling lamellar complexes between plasmid DNA and cationic micelles promote gene transfer. *Proc. Natl. Acad. Sci. USA* **94,** 14,412–14,417.
14. Byk, G., Dubertret, C., Escriou, V., et al. (1998) Synthesis, activity, and structure–activity relationship studies of novel cationic lipids for DNA transfer. *J. Med. Chem.* **41,** 224–235.
15. Walker, S., Sofia, M. J., Kakarla, R., et al. (1996) Cationic facial amphiphiles: a promising class of transfection agents. *Proc. Natl. Acad. Sci. USA* **93,** 1585–1590.
16. Lee, E. R., Marshall, J., Siegel, C. S., et al. (1996) Detailed analysis of structures and formulations of cationic lipids for efficient gene transfer to the lung. *Hum. Gene Ther.* **7,** 1701–1717.
17. Cooper, R. G., Etheridge, C. J., Stewart, L., et al. (1998) Polyamine analogues of 3β-[N-(N',N'-dimethylamino-ethane)carbamoyl]cholesterol (DC-Chol) as agents for gene delivery. *Chem. Eur. J.* **4,** 137–152.

18. Stewart, L., Manvell, M., Hillery, E., et al. (2001) Physico-chemical analysis of cationic liposome–DNA complexes (lipoplexes) with respect to in vitro and in vivo gene delivery efficiency. *J. Chem. Soc., Perkin Trans.* 2, 624–632.
19. Vigneron, J. P., Oudrhiri, N., Fauquet, M., et al. (1996) Guanidinium–cholesterol cationic lipids: efficient vectors for the transfection of eukaryotic cells. *Proc. Natl. Acad. Sci. USA* **93**, 9682–9686.
20. Solodin, I., Brown, C. S., Bruno, M. S., et al. (1995) A novel series of amphiphilic imidazolinium compounds for in vitro and in vivo gene delivery. *Biochemistry* **34**, 13537–13544.
21. van der Woude, I., Wagenaar, A., Meekel, A. A., et al. (1997) Novel pyridinium surfactants for efficient, nontoxic in vitro gene delivery. *Proc. Natl. Acad. Sci. USA* **94**, 1160–1165.
22. Vitiello, L., Bockhold, K., Joshi, P. B., and Worton, R. G. (1998) Transfection of cultured myoblasts in high serum concentration with DODAC : DOPE liposomes. *Gene Ther.* **5**, 1306–1313.
23. Bessodes, M., Dubertret, C., Jaslin, G., and Scherman, D. (2000) Synthesis and biological properties of new glycosidic cationic lipids for DNA delivery. *Bioorg. Med. Chem. Lett.* **10**, 1393–1395.
24. Ishiwata, H., Suzuki, N., Ando, S., Kikuchi, H., and Kitagawa, T. (2000) Characteristics and biodistribution of cationic liposomes and their DNA complexes. *J. Controlled Rel.* **69**, 139–148.
25. Floch, V., Loisel, S., Guenin, E., et al. (2000) Cation substitution in cationic phosphonolipids: a new concept to improve transfection activity and decrease cellular toxicity. *J. Med. Chem.* **43**, 4617–4628.
26. Miller, A. D. (1999) Nonviral delivery systems for gene therapy, in *Understanding Gene Therapy* (Lemoine, N. R., ed.), Bios Scientific, Oxford, pp. 42–69.
27. Caplen, N. J., Alton, E. W., Middleton, P. G., et al. (1995) Liposome-mediated CFTR gene transfer to the nasal epithelium of patients with cystic fibrosis. *Nature Med.* **1**, 39–46.
28. Alton, E. W. F. W., Stern, M., Farley, R., et al. (1999) Cationic lipid-mediated CFTR gene transfer to the lungs and nose of patients with cystic fibrosis: a double-blind placebo-controlled trial. *Lancet* **353**, 947–954.
29. Birchall, J. C., Marichal, C., Campbell, L., Alwan, A., Hadgraft, J., and Gumbleton, M. (2000) Gene expression in an intact ex-vivo skin tissue model following percutaneous delivery of cationic liposome-plasmid DNA complexes. *Int. J. Pharm.* **197**, 233–238.
30. Anwer, K., Meaney, C., Kao, G., et al. (2000) Cationic lipid-based delivery system for systemic cancer gene therapy. *Cancer Gene Ther.* **7**, 1156–1164.
31. Gaensler, K. M. L., Tu, G. H., Bruch, S., et al. (1999) Fetal gene transfer by transuterine injection of cationic liposome–DNA complexes. *Nature Biotechnol.* **17**, 1188–1192.
32. Hyde, S. C., Southern, K. W., Gileadi, U., et al. (2000) Repeat administration of DNA/liposomes to the nasal epithelium of patients with cystic fibrosis. *Gene Ther.* **7**, 1156–1165.
33. Mohr, L., Yoon, S. K., Eastman, S. J., et al. (2001) Cationic liposome-mediated gene delivery to the liver and to hepatocellular carcinomas in mice. *Hum. Gene Ther.* **12**, 799–809.
34. Schwartz, B., Benoist, C., Abdallah, B., et al. (1995) Lipospermine-based gene transfer into the newborn mouse brain is optimized by a low lipospermine/DNA charge ratio. *Hum. Gene Ther.* **6**, 1515–1524.
35. Zhu, N., Liggitt, D., Liu, Y., and Debs, R. (1993) Systemic gene expression after intravenous DNA delivery into adult mice. *Science* **261**, 209–211.
36. Rogy, M. A., Auffenberg, T., Espat, N. J., et al. (1995) Human tumor necrosis factor receptor (p55) and interleukin 10 gene transfer in the mouse reduces mortality to lethal endotoxemia and also attenuates local inflammatory responses. *J. Exp. Med.* **181**, 2289–2293.

37. Liu, Y., Liggitt, D., Zhong, W., Tu, G., Gaensler, K., and Debs, R. (1995) Cationic liposome-mediated intravenous gene delivery. *J. Biol. Chem.* **270**, 24,864–24,870.
38. Thierry, A. R., Lunardi-Iskandar, Y., Bryant, J. L., Rabinovich, P., Gallo, R. C., and Mahan, L. C. (1995) Systemic gene therapy: biodistribution and long-term expression of a transgene in mice. *Proc. Natl. Acad. Sci. USA* **92**, 9742–9746.
39. Stephan, D. J., Yang, Z. Y., San, H., et al. (1996) A new cationic liposome DNA complex enhances the efficiency of arterial gene transfer in vivo. *Hum. Gene Ther.* **7**, 1803–1812.
40. Zhu, J., Zhang, L., Hanisch, U. K., Felgner, P. L., and Reszka, R. (1996) A continuous intracerebral gene delivery system for in vivo liposome-mediated gene therapy. *Gene Ther.* **3**, 472–476.
41. Wright, M. J., Rosenthal, E., Stewart, L., et al. (1998) β-Galactosidase staining following intracoronary infusion of cationic liposomes in the in vivo rabbit heart is produced by microinfarction rather than effective gene transfer: a cautionary tale. *Gene Ther.* **5**, 301–308.
42. Fellowes, R., Etheridge, C. J., Coade, S., et al. (2000) Amelioration of established collagen induced arthritis by systemic IL-10 gene delivery. *Gene Ther.* **7**, 967–977.
43. Kitson, C., Angel, B., Judd, D., et al. (1999) The extra- and intracellular barriers to lipid and adenovirus-mediated pulmonary gene transfer in native sheep airway epithelium. *Gene Ther.* **6**, 534–546.
44. Litzinger, D. C., Brown, J. M., Wala, I., et al. (1996) Fate of cationic liposomes and their complex with oligonucleotide in vivo. *Biochim. Biophys. Acta* **1281**, 139–149.
45. Liu, F., Qi, H., Huang, L., and Liu, D. (1997) Factors controlling the efficiency of cationic lipid-mediated transfection in vivo via intravenous administration. *Gene Ther.* **4**, 517–523.
46. Li, S., Tseng, W. C., Stolz, D. B., Wu, S. P., Watkins, S. C., and Huang, L. (1999) Dynamic changes in the characteristics of cationic lipidic vectors after exposure to mouse serum: implications for intravenous lipofection. *Gene Ther.* **6**, 585–594.
47. Yang, J. P. and Huang, L. (1997) Overcoming the inhibitory effect of serum on lipofection by increasing the charge ratio of cationic liposome to DNA. *Gene Ther.* **4**, 950–960.
48. Yang, J. P. and Huang, L. (1998) Time-dependent maturation of cationic liposome-DNA complex for serum resistance. *Gene Ther.* **5**, 380–387.
49. Zelphati, O., Uyechi, L. S., Barron, L. G., and Szoka, F. C., Jr. (1998) Effect of serum components on the physico-chemical properties of cationic lipid/oligonucleotide complexes and on their interactions with cells. *Biochim. Biophys. Acta* **1390**, 119–133.
50. Plank, C., Mechtler, K., Szoka, F. C., Jr., Wagner, E. (1996) Activation of the complement system by synthetic DNA complexes: a potential barrier for intravenous gene delivery. *Hum. Gene Ther.* **7**, 1437–1446.
51. Dow, S. W., Fradkin, L. G., Liggitt, D. H., Willson, A. P., Heath, T. D., and Potter, T. A. (1999) Lipid–DNA complexes induce potent activation of innate immune responses and antitumor activity when administered intravenously. *J. Immunol.* **163**, 1552–1561.
52. Li, S., Wu, S. P., Whitmore, M., Loeffert, E. J., et al. (1999) Effect of immune response on gene transfer to the lung via systemic administration of cationic lipidic vectors. *Am. J. Physiol.* **276**, L796–L804.
53. McLachlan, G., Stevenson, B. J., Davidson, D. J., and Porteous, D. J. (2000) Bacterial DNA is implicated in the inflammatory response to delivery of DNA/DOTAP to mouse lungs. *Gene Ther.* **7**, 384–392.
54. Pasquini, S., Deng, H., Reddy, S. T., Giles-Davis, W., and Ertl, H. C. (1999) The effect of CpG sequences on the B cell response to a viral glycoprotein encoded by a plasmid vector. *Gene Ther.* **6**, 1448–1455.

55. Osaka, G., Carey, K., Cuthbertson, A., et al. (1996) Pharmacokinetics, tissue distribution, and expression efficiency of plasmid [^{33}P]DNA following intravenous administration of DNA/cationic lipid complexes in mice: use of a novel radionuclide approach. *J. Pharm. Sci.* **85,** 612–618.

56. Song, Y. K., Liu, F., Chu, S., and Liu, D. (1997) Characterization of cationic liposome-mediated gene transfer in vivo by intravenous administration. *Hum. Gene Ther.* **8,** 1585–1594.

57. Hofland, H. E., Nagy, D., Liu, J. J., Spratt, K., Lee, Y. L., Danos, O., and Sullivan, S. M. (1997) In vivo gene transfer by intravenous administration of stable cationic lipid/DNA complex. *Pharm. Res.* **14,** 742–749.

58. Mounkes, L. C., Zhong, W., Cipres-Palacin, G., Heath, T. D., and Debs, R. J. (1998) Proteoglycans mediate cationic liposome–DNA complex-based gene delivery in vitro and in vivo. *J. Biol. Chem.* **273,** 26,164–26,170.

59. Lechardeur, D., Sohn, K. J., Haardt, M., et al. (1999) Metabolic instability of plasmid DNA in the cytosol: a potential barrier to gene transfer. *Gene Ther.* **6,** 482–497.

60. Lukacs, G. L., Haggie, P., Seksek, O., Lechardeur, D., Freedman, N., and Verkman, A. S. (2000) Size-dependent DNA mobility in cytoplasm and nucleus. *J. Biol. Chem.* **275,** 1625–1629.

61. Tseng, W. C., Haselton, F. R., and Giorgio, T. D. (1999) Mitosis enhances transgene expression of plasmid delivered by cationic liposomes. *Biochim. Biophys. Acta* **1445,** 53–64.

62. Wente, S. R. (2000) Gatekeepers of the nucleus. *Science* **288,** 1374–1377.

63. Aronsohn, A. I. and Hughes, J. A. (1998) Nuclear localization signal peptides enhance cationic liposome-mediated gene therapy. *J. Drug Target.* **5,** 163–169.

64. Neves, C., Escriou, V., Byk, G., Scherman, D., and Wils, P. (1999) Intracellular fate and nuclear targeting of plasmid DNA. *Cell. Biol. Toxicol.* **15,** 193–202.

65. Subramanian, A., Ranganathan, P., and Diamond, S. L. (1999) Nuclear targeting peptide scaffolds for lipofection of nondividing mammalian cells. *Nature Biotechnol.* **17,** 873–877.

66. Zanta, M. A., Belguise-Valladier, P., and Behr, J. P. (1999) Gene delivery: a single nuclear localization signal peptide is sufficient to carry DNA to the cell nucleus. *Proc. Natl. Acad. Sci. USA* **96,** 91–96.

67. Remy, J. S., Kichler, A., Mordvinov, V., Schuber, F., and Behr, J. P. (1995) Targeted gene transfer into hepatoma cells with lipopolyamine-condensed DNA particles presenting galactose ligands: a stage toward artificial viruses. *Proc. Natl. Acad. Sci. USA* **92,** 1744–1748.

68. Alton, E. W. F. W., Middleton, P. G., Caplen, N. J., et al. (1993) Non-invasive liposome-mediated gene delivery can correct the ion transport defect in cystic fibrosis mutant mice. *Nature Genet.* **5,** 135–142.

69. McQuillin, A., Murray, K. D., Etheridge, C. J., et al. (1997) Optimization of liposome mediated transfection of a neuronal cell line. *Neuroreport* **8,** 1481–1484.

70. Fife, K., Bower, M., Cooper, R. G., et al. (1998) Endothelial cell transfection with cationic liposomes and herpes simplex-thymidine kinase mediated killing. *Gene Ther.* **5,** 614–620.

71. Son, K. K., Patel, D. H., Tkach, D., and Park, A. (2000) Cationic liposome and plasmid DNA complexes formed in serum-free medium under optimum transfection condition are negatively charged. *Biochim. Biophys. Acta* **1466,** 11–15.

72. Labat-Moleur, F., Steffan, A. M., Brisson, C., et al. (1996) An electron microscopy study into the mechanism of gene transfer with lipopolyamines. *Gene Ther.* **3,** 1010–1017.

73. Zabner, J., Fasbender, A. J., Moninger, T., Poellinger, K. A., and Welsh, M. J. (1995) Cellular and molecular barriers to gene transfer by a cationic lipid. *J. Biol. Chem.* **270,** 18,997–19,007.

74. Radler, J. O., Koltover, I., Salditt, T., and Safinya, C. R. (1997) Structure of DNA-cationic liposome complexes: DNA intercalation in multilamellar membranes in distinct interhelical packing regimes. *Science* **275**, 810–814.

75. Lasic, D. D., Strey, H., Stuart, M. C. A., Podgornik, R., and Frederik, P. M. (1997) The structure of DNA–liposome complexes. *J. Am. Chem. Soc.* **119**, 832–833.

76. Gustafsson, J., Arvidson, G., Karlsson, G., and Almgren, M. (1995) Complexes between cationic liposomes and DNA visualized by cryo-TEM. *Biochim. Biophys. Acta* **1235**, 305–312.

77. Gershon, H., Ghirlando, R., Guttman, S. B., and Minsky, A. (1993) Mode of formation and structural features of DNA-cationic liposome complexes used for transfection. *Biochemistry* **32**, 7143–7151.

78. Hui, S. W., Langner, M., Zhao, Y. L., Ross, P., Hurley, E., and Chan, K. (1996) The role of helper lipids in cationic liposome-mediated gene transfer. *Biophys. J.* **71**, 590–599.

79. Eastman, S. J., Siegel, C., Tousignant, J., Smith, A. E., Cheng, S. H., and Scheule, R. K. (1997) Biophysical characterization of cationic lipid: DNA complexes. *Biochim. Biophys. Acta* **1325**, 41–62.

80. Sternberg, B., Sorgi, F. L., and Huang, L. (1994) New structures in complex formation between DNA and cationic liposomes visualized by freeze-fracture electron microscopy. *FEBS Lett.* **356**, 361–366.

81. Schmutz, M., Durand, D., Debin, A., Palvadeau, Y., Etienne, A., and Thierry, A. R. (1999) DNA packing in stable lipid complexes designed for gene transfer imitates DNA compaction in bacteriophage. *Proc. Natl. Acad. Sci. USA* **96**, 12,293–12,298.

82. Xu, Y., Hui, S. W., Frederik, P., and Szoka, F. C., Jr. (1999) Physicochemical characterization and purification of cationic lipoplexes. *Biophys. J.* **77**, 341–353.

83. Pitard, B., Oudrhiri, N., Vigneron, J. P., et al. (1999) Structural characteristics of supramolecular assemblies formed by guanidinium-cholesterol reagents for gene transfection. *Proc. Natl. Acad. Sci. USA* **96**, 2621–2626.

84. Densmore, C. L., Giddings, T. H., Waldrep, J. C., Kinsey, B. M., and Knight, V. (1999) Gene transfer by guanidinium–cholesterol: dioleoylphosphatidyl-ethanolamine liposome–DNA complexes in aerosol. *J. Gene Med.* **1**, 251–264.

85. Koltover, I., Salditt, T., Radler, J. O., and Safinya, C. R. (1998) An inverted hexagonal phase of cationic liposome-DNA complexes related to DNA release and delivery. *Science* **281**, 78–81.

86. Akao, T., Nakayama, T., Takeshia, K., and Ito, A. (1994) Design of a new cationic amphiphile with efficient DNA-transfection ability. *Biochem. Mol. Biol. Int.* **34**, 915–920.

87. Balasubramaniam, R. P., Bennett, M. J., Aberle, A. M., Malone, J. G., Nantz, M. H., and Malone, R. W. (1996) Structural and functional analysis of cationic transfection lipids: the hydrophobic domain. *Gene Ther.* **3**, 163–172.

88. Bennett, C. F., Mirejovsky, D., Crooke, R. M., et al. (1998) Structural requirements for cationic lipid mediated phosphorothioate oligonucleotides delivery to cells in culture. *J. Drug Target.* **5**, 149–162.

89. Takeuchi, K., Ishihara, M., Kawaura, C., Noji, M., Furuno, T., and Nakanishi, M. (1996) Effect of zeta potential of cationic liposomes containing cationic cholesterol derivatives on gene transfection. *FEBS Lett.* **397**, 207–209.

90. Nantz, M. H., Li, L., Zhu, J., Aho-Sharon, K. L., Lim, D., and Erickson, K. L. (1998) Inductive electron-withdrawal from ammonium ion headgroups of cationic lipids and the influence on DNA transfection. *Biochim. Biophys. Acta* **1394**, 219–223.

91. Turek, J., Dubertret, C., Jaslin, G., Antonakis, K., Scherman, D., and Pitard, B. (2000) Formulations which increase the size of lipoplexes prevent serum-associated inhibition of transfection. *J. Gene Med.* **2,** 32–40.
92. Zuidam, N. J. and Barenholz, Y. (1999) Characterization of DNA–lipid complexes commonly used for gene delivery. *Int. J. Pharm.* **183,** 43–46.
93. Sorgi, F. L., Bhattacharya, S., and Huang, L. (1997) Protamine sulfate enhances lipid-mediated gene transfer. *Gene Ther.* **4,** 961–968.
94. Li, S. and Huang, L. (1997) In vivo gene transfer via intravenous administration of cationic lipid–protamine–DNA (LPD) complexes. *Gene Ther.* **4,** 891–900.
95. Li, S., Rizzo, M. A., Bhattacharya, S., and Huang, L. (1998) Characterization of cationic lipid–protamine–DNA (LPD) complexes for intravenous gene delivery. *Gene Ther.* **5,** 930–937.
96. Li, B., Li, S., Tan, Y., et al. (2000) Lyophilization of cationic lipid–protamine-DNA (LPD) complexes. *J. Pharm. Sci.* **89,** 355–364.
97. Whitmore, M., Li, S., and Huang, L. (1999) LPD lipopolyplex initiates a potent cytokine response and inhibits tumor growth. *Gene Ther.* **6,** 1867–1875.
98. Chesnoy, S. and Huang, L. (2000) Structure and function of lipid–DNA complexes for gene delivery. *Annu. Rev. Biophys. Biomol. Struct.* **29,** 27–47.
99. Dokka, S., Toledo, D., Shi, X., Ye, J., and Rojanasakul, Y. (2000) High-efficiency gene transfection of macrophages by lipoplexes. *Int. J. Pharm.* **206,** 97–104.
100. Birchall, J. C., Kellaway, I. W., and Gumbleton, M. (2000) Physical stability and in-vitro gene expression efficiency of nebulised lipid–peptide–DNA complexes. *Int. J. Pharm.* **197,** 221–231.
101. Mizuarai, S., Ono, K., You, J., Kamihira, M., and Iijima, S. (2001) Protamine-modified DDAB lipid vesicles promote gene transfer in the presence of serum. *J. Biochem.* **129,** 125–132.
102. Gao, X. and Huang, L. (1996) Potentiation of cationic liposome-mediated gene delivery by polycations. *Biochemistry* **35,** 1027–1036.
103. Vitiello, L., Chonn, A., Wasserman, J. D., Duff, C., and Worton, R. G. (1996) Condensation of plasmid DNA with polylysine improves liposome-mediated gene transfer into established and primary muscle cells. *Gene Ther.* **3,** 396–404.
104. Hong, K., Zheng, W., Baker, A., and Papahadjopoulos, D. (1997) Stabilization of cationic liposome–plasmid DNA complexes by polyamines and poly(ethylene glycol)–phospholipid conjugates for efficient in vivo gene delivery. *FEBS Lett.* **400,** 233–237.
105. Zhou, X. and Huang, L. (1994) DNA transfection mediated by cationic liposomes containing lipopolylysine: characterization and mechanism of action. *Biochim. Biophys. Acta* **1189,** 195–203.
106. Fritz, J. D., Herweijer, H., Zhang, G., and Wolff, J. A. (1996) Gene transfer into mammalian cells using histone-condensed plasmid DNA. *Hum. Gene Ther.* **7,** 1395–1404.
107. Namiki, Y., Takahashi, T., and Ohno, T. (1998) Gene transduction for disseminated intraperitoneal tumor using cationic liposomes containing non-histone chromatin proteins: cationic liposomal gene therapy of carcinomatosa. *Gene Ther.* **5,** 240–246.
108. Schwartz, B., Ivanov, M. A., Pitard, B., et al. (1999) Synthetic DNA-compacting peptides derived from human sequence enhance cationic lipid-mediated gene transfer in vitro and in vivo. *Gene Ther.* **6,** 282–292.
109. Vaysse, L. and Arveiler, B. (2000) Transfection using synthetic peptides: comparison of three DNA-compacting peptides and effect of centrifugation. *Biochim. Biophys. Acta* **1474,** 244–250.

110. Chen, Q. R., Zhang, L., Stass, S. A., and Mixson, A. J. (2000) Co-polymer of histidine and lysine markedly enhances transfection efficiency of liposomes. *Gene Ther.* **7,** 1698–1705.
111. Dass, C. R., Walker, T. L., Kalle, W. H. J., and Burton, M. A. (2000) A microsphere–liposome (microplex) vector for targeted gene therapy of cancer. II. In vivo biodistribution study in a solid tumor model. *Drug Deliv.* **7,** 15–19.
112. Dass, C. R., Walker, T. L., Kalle, W. H. J., and Burton, M. A. (1999) A microsphere-lipoplex (microplex) vector for targeted gene therapy of cancer. I. Construction and in vitro evaluation. *Drug Deliv.* **6,** 259–269.
113. Stecenko, A., King, G., Torii, K., et al. (2000) Enhancement of liposome-mediated gene transfer to human airway epithelial cells by replication-deficient adenovirus. *Exp. Lung Res.* **26,** 179–201.
114. Simoes, S., Slepushkin, V., Gaspar, R., de Lima, M. C., and Duzgunes, N. (1998) Gene delivery by negatively charged ternary complexes of DNA, cationic liposomes and transferrin or fusigenic peptides. *Gene Ther.* **5,** 955–964.
115. Simoes, S., Slepushkin, V., Pires, P., Gaspar, R., de Lima, M. P., and Duzgunes, N. (1999) Mechanisms of gene transfer mediated by lipoplexes associated with targeting ligands or pH-sensitive peptides. *Gene Ther.* **6,** 1798–1807.
116. Drummond, D. C., Zignani, M., and Leroux, J. (2000) Current status of pH-sensitive liposomes in drug delivery. *Prog. Lipid Res.* **39,** 409–460.
117. Kamata, H., Yagisawa, H., Takahashi, S., and Hirata, H. (1994) Amphiphilic peptides enhance the efficiency of liposome-mediated DNA transfection. *Nucleic Acids Res.* **22,** 536–537.
118. Kichler, A., Mechtler, K., Behr, J. P., and Wagner, E. (1997) Influence of membrane-active peptides on lipospermine/DNA complex mediated gene transfer. *Bioconjug. Chem.* **8,** 213–221.
119. Budker, V., Gurevich, V., Hagstrom, J. E., Bortzov, F., and Wolff, J. A. (1996) pH-sensitive, cationic liposomes: a new synthetic virus-like vector. *Nature Biotechnol.* **14,** 760–764.
120. Jenkins, R. G., Herrick, S. E., Meng, Q. H., et al. (2000) An integrin-targeted non-viral vector for pulmonary gene therapy. *Gene Ther.* **7,** 393–400.
121. Cooper, R. G., Harbottle, R. P., Schneider, H., Coutelle, C., and Miller, A. D. (1999) Peptide mini-vectors for gene delivery. *Angew. Chem. Int. Ed.* **38,** 1949–1952.
122. Colin, M., Maurice, M., Trugnan, G., et al. (2000) Cell delivery, intracellular trafficking and expression of an integrin-mediated gene transfer vector in tracheal epithelial cells. *Gene Ther.* **7,** 139–152.
123. Kawakami, S., Sato, A., Nishikawa, M., Yamashita, F., and Hashida, M. (2000) Mannose receptor-mediated gene transfer into macrophages using novel mannosylated cationic liposomes. *Gene Ther.* **7,** 292–299.
124. Kawakami, S., Sato, A., Yamada, M., Yamashita, F., and Hashida, M. (2001) The effect of lipid composition on receptor-mediated in vivo gene transfection using mannosylated cationic liposomes in mice. *Stp Pharm. Sci.* **11,** 117–120.
125. da Cruz, M. T. G., Simoes, S., Pires, P. P. C., Nir, S., and de Lima, M. C. P. (2001) Kinetic analysis of the initial steps involved in lipoplex–cell interactions: effect of various factors that influence transfection activity. *Biochim. Biophys. Acta* **1510,** 136–151.
126. de Ilarduya, C. T., and Duzgunes, N. (2000) Efficient gene transfer by transferrin lipoplexes in the presence of serum. *Biochim. Biophys. Acta* **1463,** 333–342.
127. Tan, P. H., King, W. J., Chen, D., et al. (2001) Transferrin receptor-mediated gene transfer to the corneal endothelium. *Transplantation* **71,** 552–560.

128. Simoes, S., Slepushkin, V., Pires, P., Gaspar, R., de Lima, M. C. P., and Duzgunes, N. (2000) Human serum albumin enhances DNA transfection by lipoplexes and confers resistance to inhibition by serum. *Biochim. Biophys. Acta* **1463**, 459–469.

129. Yanagihara, K. and Cheng, P. W. (1999) Lectin enhancement of the lipofection efficiency in human lung carcinoma cells. *Biochim. Biophys. Acta* **1472**, 25–33.

130. Anderson, C. W., Young, M. E., and Flint, S. J. (1989) Characterization of the adenovirus 2 virion protein, mu. *Virology* **172**, 506–512.

131. Hosokawa, K. and Sung, M. T. (1976) Isolation and characterization of an extremely basic protein from adenovirus type 5. *J. Virol.* **17**, 924–934.

132. Chatterjee, P. K., Vayda, M. E., and Flint, S. J. (1985) Interactions among the three adenovirus core proteins. *J. Virol.* **55**, 379–386.

133. Matthews, D. A. and Russell, W. C. (1998) Adenovirus core protein V interacts with p32— a protein which is associated with both the mitochondria and the nucleus. *J. Gen. Virol.* **79**, 1677–1685.

134. Murray, K. D., Etheridge, C. J., Shah, S. I., et al. (2001) Enhanced cationic liposome-mediated transfection using the DNA-binding peptide μ (mu) from the adenovirus core. *Gene Ther.* **8**, 453–460.

135. Tagawa, T., Manvell, M., Brown, N., et al. (2002) Characterisation of LMD virus-like nanoparticles self-assembled from cationic liposomes, adenovirus core peptide μ (mu) and plasmid DNA. *Gene Ther.* **9**, 564–576.

136. Lasic, D. D. and Papahadjopoulos, D. (1995) Liposomes revisited. *Science* **267**, 1275–1276.

137. Wheeler, J. J., Palmer, L., Ossanlou, M., et al. (1999) Stabilized plasmid-lipid particles: construction and characterization. *Gene Ther.* **6**, 271–281.

138. Zhang, Y. P., Sekirov, L., Saravolac, E. G., et al. (1999) Stabilized plasmid-lipid particles for regional gene therapy: formulation and transfection properties. *Gene Ther.* **6**, 1438–1447.

139. Shi, N. Y. and Pardridge, W. M. (2000) Noninvasive gene targeting to the brain. *Proc. Natl. Acad. Sci. USA* **97**, 7567–7572.

140. Bailey, A. L. and Sullivan, S. M. (2000) Efficient encapsulation of DNA plasmids in small neutral liposomes induced by ethanol and calcium. *Biochim. Biophys. Acta* **1468**, 239–252.

141. Thierry, A. R., Rahman, A., and Dritschilo, A. (1993) Overcoming multidrug resistance in human tumor cells using free and liposomally encapsulated antisense oligodeoxynucleotides. *Biochem. Biophys. Res. Commun.* **190**, 952–960.

142. Stuart, D. D., Kao, G. Y., and Allen, T. M. (2000) A novel, long-circulating, and functional liposomal formulation of antisense oligodeoxynucleotides targeted against MDR1. *Cancer Gene Ther.* **7**, 466–475.

143. Stuart, D. D. and Allen, T. M. (2000) A new liposomal formulation for antisense oligodeoxynucleotides with small size, high incorporation efficiency and good stability. *Biochim. Biophys. Acta* **1463**, 219–229.

144. Gerasimov, O. V., Boomer, J. A., Qualls, M. M., and Thompson, D. H. (1999) Cytosolic drug delivery using pH- and light-sensitive liposomes. *Adv. Drug. Deliv. Rev.* **38**, 317–338.

145. Wang, C. Y. and Huang, L. (1987) pH-sensitive immunoliposomes mediate target-cell-specific delivery and controlled expression of a foreign gene in mouse. *Proc. Natl. Acad. Sci. USA* **84**, 7851–7855.

146. Legendre, J. Y. and Szoka, F. C., Jr. (1992) Delivery of plasmid DNA into mammalian cell lines using pH-sensitive liposomes: comparison with cationic liposomes. *Pharm. Res.* **9**, 1235–1242.

147. Wang, C. Y. and Huang, L. (1989) Highly efficient DNA delivery mediated by pH-sensitive immunoliposomes. *Biochemistry* **28**, 9508–9514.

148. Holmberg, E. G., Reuer, Q. R., Geisert, E. E., and Owens, J. L. (1994) Delivery of plasmid DNA to glial cells using pH-sensitive immunoliposomes. *Biochem. Biophys. Res. Commun.* **201**, 888–893.

149. Geisert, E. E., Jr., Del Mar, N. A., Owens, J. L., and Holmberg, E. G. (1995) Transfecting neurons and glia in the rat using pH-sensitive immunoliposomes. *Neurosci. Lett.* **184**, 40–43.

150. Ropert, C., Lavignon, M., Dubernet, C., Couvreur, P., and Malvy, C. (1992) Oligonucleotides encapsulated in pH sensitive liposomes are efficient toward Friend retrovirus. *Biochem. Biophys. Res. Commun.* **183**, 879–885.

151. Lee, R. J. and Huang, L. (1996) Folate-targeted, anionic liposome-entrapped polylysine-condensed DNA for tumor cell-specific gene transfer. *J. Biol. Chem.* **271**, 8481–8487.

152. Wang, S. and Low, P. S. (1998) Folate-mediated targeting of antineoplastic drugs, imaging agents, and nucleic acids to cancer cells. *J. Control. Release* **53**, 39–48.

153. Reddy, J. A. and Low, P. S. (2000) Enhanced folate receptor mediated gene therapy using a novel pH-sensitive lipid formulation. *J. Control. Release* **64**, 27–37.

154. Guo, W. J. and Lee, R. J. (2000) Efficient gene delivery using anionic liposome-complexed polyplexes (LPDII). *Biosci. Rep.* **20**, 419–432.

155. Welz, C., Neuhuber, W., Schreier, H., Repp, R., Rascher, W., and Fahr, A. (2000) Nuclear gene targeting using negatively charged liposomes. *Int. J. Pharm.* **196**, 251–252.

156. Feero, W. G., Li, S., Rosenblatt, J. D., et al. (1997) Selection and use of ligands for receptor-mediated gene delivery to myogenic cells. *Gene Ther.* **4**, 664–674.

157. Balicki, D. and Beutler, E. (1997) Histone H2A significantly enhances in vitro DNA transfection. *Mol. Med.* **3**, 78–787.

158. Hagstrom, J. E., Sebestyen, M. G., Budker, V., Ludtke, J. J., Fritz, J. D., and Wolff, J. A. (1996) Complexes of non-cationic liposomes and histone H1 mediate efficient transfection of DNA without encapsulation. *Biochim. Biophys. Acta* **1284**, 47–55.

159. Ibanez, M., Gariglio, P., Chavez, P., Santiago, R., Wong, C., and Baeza, I. (1996) Spermidine-condensed DNA and cone-shaped lipids improve delivery and expression of exogenous DNA transfer by liposomes. *Biochem. Cell. Biol.* **74**, 633–643.

160. Shangguan, T., Cabral-Lilly, D., Purandare, U., et al. (2000) A novel *N*-acyl phosphatidylethanolamine-containing delivery vehicle for spermine-condensed plasmid DNA. *Gene Ther.* **7**, 769–783.

161. Kono, K., Torikoshi, Y., Mitsutomi, M., et al. (2001) Novel gene delivery systems: complexes of fusigenic polymer-modified liposomes and lipoplexes. *Gene Ther.* **8**, 5–12.

162. Kaneda, Y. (1999) Development of a novel fusogenic viral liposome system (HVJ-liposomes) and its applications to the treatment of acquired diseases. *Mol. Membr. Biol.* **16**, 119–122.

163. Yonemitsu, Y., Alton, E. W., Komori, K., Yoshizumi, T., Sugimachi, K., and Kaneda, Y. (1998) HVJ (Sendai virus) liposome-mediated gene transfer: current status and future perspectives (review). *Int. J. Oncol.* **12**, 1277–1285.

164. Kaneda, Y., Iwai, K., and Uchida, T. (1989) Increased expression of DNA cointroduced with nuclear protein in adult rat liver. *Science* **243**, 375–378.

165. Morishita, R., Gibbons, G. H., Kaneda, Y., Ogihara, T., and Dzau, V. J. (1994) Pharmacokinetics of antisense oligodeoxyribonucleotides (cyclin B1 and CDC 2 kinase) in the vessel wall in vivo: enhanced therapeutic utility for restenosis by HVJ-liposome delivery. *Gene* **149**, 13–19.

166. Aoki, M., Morishita, R., Higaki, J., et al. (1997) In vivo transfer efficiency of antisense oligonucleotides into the myocardium using HVJ-liposome method. *Biochem. Biophys. Res. Commun.* **231**, 540–545.

167. Nakanishi, M., Mizuguchi, H., Ashihara, K., et al. (1999) Gene delivery systems using the Sendai virus. *Mol. Membr. Biol.* **16**, 123–127.

168. Saeki, Y., Matsumoto, N., Nakano, Y., Mori, M., Awai, K., and Kaneda, Y. (1997) Development and characterization of cationic liposomes conjugated with HVJ (Sendai virus): reciprocal effect of cationic lipid for in vitro and in vivo gene transfer. *Hum. Gene Ther.* **8**, 2133–2141.

169. Yonemitsu, Y., Kaneda, Y., Muraishi, A., Yoshizumi, T., Sugimachi, K., and Sueishi, K. (1997) HVJ (Sendai virus)-cationic liposomes: a novel and potentially effective liposome-mediated technique for gene transfer to the airway epithelium. *Gene Ther.* **4**, 631–638.

170. Uehara, T., Honda, K., Hatano, E., et al. (1999) Gene transfer to the rat biliary tract with the HVJ-cationic liposome method. *J. Hepatol.* **30**, 836–842.

171. Hagihara, Y., Saitoh, Y., Kaneda, Y., Kohmura, E., and Yoshimine, T. (2000) Widespread gene transfection into the central nervous system of primates. *Gene Ther.* **7**, 759–763.

172. Tsujie, M., Isaka, Y., Nakamura, H., Kaneda, Y., Imai, E., and Hori, M. (2001) Prolonged transgene expression in glomeruli using an EBV replicon vector system combined with HVJ liposomes. *Kidney Int.* **59**, 1390–1396.

173. Chander, R. and Schreier, H. (1992) Artificial viral envelopes containing recombinant human immunodeficiency virus (HIV) gp160. *Life Sci.* **50**, 481–489.

174. Schreier, H., Ausborn, M., Gunther, S., Weissig, V., and Chander, R. (1995) (Patho)physiologic pathways to drug targeting: artificial viral envelopes. *J. Mol. Recogn.* **8**, 59–62.

175. Ramani, K., Bora, R. S., Kumar, M., Tyagi, S. K., and Sarkar, D. P. (1997) Novel gene delivery to liver cells using engineered virosomes. *FEBS Lett.* **404**, 164–168.

176. Ramani, K., Hassan, Q., Venkaiah, B., Hasnain, S. E., and Sarkar, D. P. (1998) Site-specific gene delivery in vivo through engineered Sendai viral envelopes. *Proc. Natl. Acad. Sci. USA* **95**, 11,886–11,890.

177. Ponimaskin, E., Bareesel, K. K. H., Markgraf, K., et al. (2000) Sendai virosomes revisited: reconstitution with exogenous lipids leads to potent vehicles for gene transfer. *Virology* **269**, 391–403.

178. Kondoh, M., Matsuyama, T., Suzuki, R., et al. (2000) Growth inhibition of human leukemia HL-60 cells by an antisense phosphodiester oligonucleotide encapsulated into fusogenic liposomes. *Biol. Pharm. Bull.* **23**, 1011–1013.

179. Schoen, P., Chonn, A., Cullis, P. R., Wilschut, J., and Scherrer, P. (1999) Gene transfer mediated by fusion protein hemagglutinin reconstituted in cationic lipid vesicles. *Gene Ther.* **6**, 823–832.

180. Waelti, E. R. and Gluck, R. (1998) Delivery to cancer cells of antisense L-myc oligonucleotides incorporated in fusogenic, cationic-lipid-reconstituted influenza-virus envelopes (cationic virosomes). *Int. J. Cancer* **77**, 728–733.

181. Abe, A., Miyanohara, A., and Friedmann, T. (1998) Enhanced gene transfer with fusogenic liposomes containing vesicular stomatitis virus G glycoprotein. *J. Virol.* **72**, 6159–6163.

8

Peptide- and Polymer-Based Gene Delivery Vehicles

Richard Brokx and Jean Gariépy

1. Introduction

The goal of suicide gene therapy is the specific expression of a toxic gene in cancer cells. In order to achieve this objective, vehicles and transfection strategies must be designed to specifically deliver suicide genes to the desired cells. Up to now, the use of bacteria and other micro-organisms, viruses, and nonviral liposomes as well as the transfection of naked DNA have all been explored as methods of introducing foreign DNA into cells. This chapter describes the use of peptides, proteins, and polymers in the formulation of nonviral transfection agents. A number of recent reviews have outlined the advantages and disadvantages of nonviral systems to deliver therapeutic agents *(1–3)* and genes *(4–9)*. One advantage of these vectors over viral systems is the diversity of agents that can be used. Unlike viruses, which often lack cell specificity, the potential exists to tailor the delivery of peptide- or polymer-based vectors to target cells of interest. On the other hand, viruses are advantageous in that they have evolved to use natural mechanisms to enter cells and their DNA is packaged to induce the expression of foreign genes. The efficient delivery and expression of novel genes can also be achieved with nonviral systems. Many of the agents discussed in this chapter, however, remain under development and are not commercially available. Nonetheless, there exists a great potential for the use of peptide- and polymer-based delivery agents in clinical applications.

Ideally, nonviral transfection agents should mimic viruses in terms of four properties *(9)*: the compaction of DNA, the recognition of such complexes by cells (i.e., binding to cell surface receptors), their internalization into intracellular vesicles and their subsequent release from these vesicles into the cytosol, and, finally, their localization into the nucleus of cells. Peptide- and polymer-based vehicles can, to some extent, act as virus mimics. The simplest are commercially available cationic polymers *(10)*, which function to compact DNA and give it a positive charge, allowing entry into cells. As such, they are nonspecific in the cells they target, but are often

From: *Methods in Molecular Medicine, Vol. 90, Suicide Gene Therapy: Methods and Reviews*
Edited by: C. J. Springer © Humana Press Inc., Totowa, NJ

used in conjunction with other targeting molecules to increase their transfection efficiency. Other targeting molecules that are used include short peptide sequences, which are internalized by cells. Peptides are advantageous in that they can be assembled readily by solid-phase peptide synthesis. However, peptide synthesis on a large scale, such as in pharmaceutical applications, is expensive. Moreover, current synthetic methodologies typically limit the length of synthetic peptides to less than 80–100 amino acids, so the targeting sequences that can be chosen must be relatively short. One consequence of this limitation is that peptide sequences coding for cell targeting or subcellular localization must be kept to a minimum. The efficiency of transfection may be increased by exploiting the concept of multivalency, as exemplified in the design of "loligomers" *(2,11–13)*. Alternatively, bacterially expressed chimeric proteins have been developed as cell-targeting nonviral transfection systems. These constructs are generally "mix-and-match" designs. The importance of simple polycations as DNA delivery agents will first be discussed.

2. Polycations

The stability and size of DNA molecules represent two important challenges in transfecting cells with naked DNA. Plasmids are stable at 4°C or below 0°C, but naked DNA is susceptible to cleavage at room temperature because of the labile nature of the phosphodiester backbone. Moreover, naked DNA is particularly susceptible to nucleases in the context of in vivo experiments. The half-life of DNA plasmids in blood plasma or the cytosol of cells is typically of the order of hours *(9)*. In addition, DNA forms highly extended, hydrated structures because of the high negative charge of the phosphodiester backbone (even supercoiled DNA structures are quite "relaxed" in relation to proteins) that are unable to effectively cross cell membranes. In the cell, however, the extended structure and instability of DNA is controlled by the efficient condensation of DNA into nucleosomal complexes. Polycationic proteins such as histones as well as other nucleosomal proteins have, in fact, been found to compact DNA in vitro and can serve as transfection agents *(14–16)*. Simpler, synthetic polycations can substitute for nucleosomal proteins in enabling DNA entry into cells. The efficacy of polycations in facilitating gene transfer has been discussed in a number of recent reviews *(17–19)*. Polycations that have been used in the literature include poly-L-lysine and other poly-amino acids, polyethyleneimine, cationic dendrimers, and other molecules. The most widely used polycation in transfection experiments today is poly-L-lysine.

2.1. Poly-L-lysine

Poly-L-lysine (PLL) was originally employed as a drug delivery vehicle *(20)*. It was later used as a carrier for oligonucleotides (**ref.** *21* and references therein). Synthetic oligonucleotides have been chemically conjugated to PLL with a mean molecular weight (MW) of 14 kDa. In order to achieve the desired biological effect, the covalently attached DNA had to be released from the PLL carrier, which purportedly occurred through the action of hydrolases in the nucleus *(21)*. Chemical linkages between plasmids and PLL are not generally needed, as these two molecular entities are essentially polymers of opposite charges and can readily form noncovalently associated complexes at physiological pH. The ratio of DNA to PLL is important and is usually expressed in terms of a "charge ratio" of lysine to nucleotide. For DNA, each nucleotide carries a charge of −1 at physiological pH because of its phosphate group, whereas every ε-amino group of PLL represents a +1 charge. Optimal charge ratios for transfection vary among reports, but they usually favor a net cationic charge ratio (i.e., more lysine amino groups than phosphates) in order for DNA to be completely compacted and the DNA : polycation conjugate to be attracted to negative groups on the surface of cells *(22)*. A charge ratio of 1.5 (lysine : nucleotide) has been suggested to be the most efficient at DNA transfection *(23)*. It was also found that transfection with PLL is dependent on cell surface proteoglycans *(23)*. This is not surprising because the positively charged PLL : DNA complexes would be attracted to the negatively charged sulfate groups of the proteoglycans. It could also explain why transfection with PLL varies among different cell types, because different cells present different subsets of surface proteoglycans.

Internalization of PLL : DNA complexes by cells is thought to occur by absorptive endocytosis, a general phenomenon by which cationic molecules are imported into cells (*see* **Fig. 1**). The complexes are internalized in vesicles often referred to as endosomes. For gene expression to occur, DNA has to be released from such endosomal compartments and ultimately reach the nucleus. Achieving effective levels of transfection may thus require the use of endosomolytic agents, such as chloroquine *(10)*. The intracellular trafficking of PLL and its complexes with drugs or DNA remain a significant challenge to solve before PLL can be used in gene therapy.

2.2. Polyethyleneimine

Polyethyleneimine (PEI) *(18,24)* and related structures are synthetic polymers with a much higher charge density than polyamino acids like PLL. PEI can be synthesized as either linear or branched polymers (*see* **Fig. 2**). Most transfection studies report the use of a branched form of PEI *(18)*. A transfection agent termed ExGen™500, based on a linear form of PEI, has also been reported to be effective and is available commercially *(24,24)*. Like PLL, PEI enables DNA entry into cells at slightly cationic charge ratios of about 1.5 *(26)*. Because of the high density of amino groups in PEI, however, only about every sixth group is protonated and, thus, a ratio of about nine nitrogens per phosphate (N : P) is needed to achieve a charge ratio of 1.5. [A convenient conversion figure for these calculations is that a 10 : 1 N : P ratio is equal to a PEI : DNA weight ratio of 1.29 : 1 *(27)*]. This high number of unprotonated amino groups enables the highly charged PEI to possess buffering capacity even at acidic pHs. PEI can thus act to neutralize the acidic environment present in endosomal or lysosomal vesicles (pH of 4.5–5). This property, often referred to as a "proton sponge" effect, protects DNA from digestion by nucleases, which are generally most active at low pH. This "proton sponge" effect also results in the influx of water and chloride counterions into endosomes in order to maintain osmotic and charge balances, causing the rupture of endosome/lysosome vesicles and releasing DNA into the cytoplasm. As a consequence, lysosomolytic agents such as chloroquine are not needed for transfection with PEI.

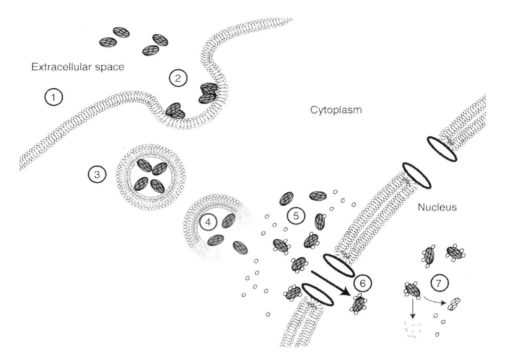

Fig. 1. Absorptive endocytosis of condensed DNA by eukaryotic cells. The positively charged polycation : DNA complexes are attracted to the negatively charged cell membrane (step 1). This triggers invagination of the cell membrane (step 2) and the eventual internalization of coated vesicles (step 3). A fraction of the vesicles burst (step 4), releasing their contents into the cytoplasm. The complexed DNA then enters the nucleus, either by passive diffusion or, as depicted, by recognition of the complex by nuclear transport proteins, shown as small open ovals (step 5), then active transport into the nucleus through nuclear pores (step 6). Once inside the nucleus, the DNA : polycation complex is degraded and the DNA is released (step 7).

2.3. Polyamidoamine Dendrimers

Another class of polycationic molecules that has been used as transfection agents is the cationic dendrimer *(28)*, highly branched synthetic macromolecules. The synthesis of these molecules starts with a "core" amine molecule, such as ammonia, onto which monomer building blocks are then added to create branches with new amino groups. These arms then serve as seed locations for the addition of more building blocks in the next round (or "generation") of synthesis. Each successive generation doubles the number of branches and thus the number of amino groups. The number of generations can be carefully controlled, resulting in macromolecules of a defined size (*see* **Fig. 2**). Their shape is spherical, with a high concentration of positive charges on the surface. For example, a generation-8 polyamidoamine (PAMAM) dendrimer from an ammonia core has a molecular weight of 17.5 kDa, 768 positive charges, and a diameter of 92 Å *(29)*. The dimensions of such dendrimers are similar to those of proteins.

Polyamidoamine dendrimers can efficiently aid the transport of DNA into cells with results that compare favorably to liposomal transfection reagents *(28,30,31)*. The structures of DNA : dendrimer complexes have not been investigated, nor have PAMAM dendrimers been compared directly to PLL or PEI in transfection experiments. The spherical shape of these dendrimers, with charges being presented only on their surface, would suggest that they may not be as effective at packing DNA than cationic polymers. Indeed, an enhancement in transfection efficiency was observed for dendrimers after they had been partially degraded by heat treatment *(32)*. This phenomenon may be the result of the increased flexibility of the degraded dendrimers and enhanced ability to compact DNA.

2.4. Other Polycations

In addition to PLL, PEI, and dendrimers, other polycations and cationic polypeptides have been used to transfect eukaryotic cells. Other polyamino acids have been used in transfections *(10)* but none have become as popular as PLL. There are also versions of polycations that have been modified to reduce their toxicity. Grafted polymers of neutral hydrophilic compounds have been useful in decreasing the toxicity of PLL *(33)* and PEI *(34)* while maintaining their efficiency in transfection. For example, a crosslinked PEI–polyalcohol hydrogel product called NanoGel is available commercially from Supratek Inc. (Laval, Quebec, Canada) *(35)*, although it is still under development as a general transfection reagent. Nevertheless, such polymers represent a second generation of drug and DNA delivery vehicles that are starting to address and incorporate desirable features lacking in PLL and PEI.

There are also several peptide sequences that can induce intracellular transport *(36)* and thus can play the role of polycations. Popular examples include peptides based on the homeodomain of the *Drosophila* transcription factor Antennapedia *(37–39)* and the arginine-rich HIV-1 Tat domain *(40,41)*. HIV-Tat-like "peptoid" polymers *(42)* have also been reported containing building blocks that are not susceptible to the action of peptide hydrolases. It has been suggested that arginine-rich peptides may not enter cells by absorptive endocytosis but rather by fusing with cell membranes *(37–39)*, which means that the issue of endosomal retention (*see* **Subheading 4.**) may be avoided. This mechanism remains to be proven and the level of DNA transfection achieved with arginine-rich peptides suggests results similar to that reported for PLL. Surprisingly, a direct comparison of arginine-rich peptides to PLL and PEI in terms of transfection vehicles has not yet been reported and is somewhat needed to assess their distinguishing features.

2.5. Polycations: Practical Considerations

Apart from the important charge ratio of DNA to polycations, there are important variables to consider when designing protocols in polycation-mediated gene delivery. One variable is the molecular-weight range of the polycation preparation selected. The heterogeneity in each preparation (i.e., the range of molecular weights within a particular preparation) is also an issue. PLL is available from different suppliers in differing molecular weights. For example, Sigma (St. Louis, MO, USA) supplies PLL

A

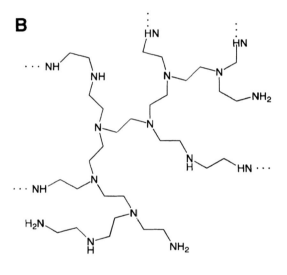

B

C

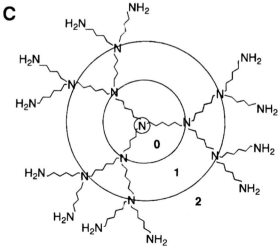

Fig. 2

at molecular weights ranging from approx 1 kDa to > 300 kDa. It must be remembered that PLL is often used as a reagent to promote adhesion of cells and tissues to solid substrates. This additional role for PLL represents an issue because molecular weights of PLL above 10 kDa have proven useful both as a synthetic substrate for attaching cells to plates as well as for DNA transfection.

In the case of PEI, there are three suppliers that are most commonly cited in the literature *(18)*: Sigma sells a product with a reported average (weight average) molecular weight of 750 kDa, whereas Polysciences (Warrington, PA, USA), and Fluka (Milwaukee, WI, USA) sell preparations with molecular weights of up to 1 million Daltons. The PEI polymers with larger weights (> 100 kDa) represent the preferred ones for transfection. PEI with molecular weights below 10 kDa are ineffective as transfection agents *(18,43)*.

Transfection efficiency with PEI can also vary with the supplier of the product, with polydispersity (i.e., heterogeneity in size) and the degree of branching posing the greatest problems. Most reports suggest the use of more highly branched PEI preparations as being effective in transfections. Interestingly, a linear PEI preparation is also sold specifically for transfections and in vivo DNA delivery (ExGen™500; Fermentas) *(24)*. Most PEI products, if not explicitly labeled as linear, are branched, and their structures should be confirmed with the supplier. With the polydispersity issue, one study *(44)* reported that more polydisperse (Polysciences; MW 70 kDa, as opposed to Fluka, MW 600 kDa–1000 kDa) preparations are more efficient in transfecting DNA into a human endothelial cell line in serum-containing medium. This result could be linked to the ability of smaller PEI molecules to "plug holes" in larger PEI : DNA complexes. This feature may be further exploited by intentionally adding small "plug" PEI molecules (Polysciences, MW 10 kDa) after the initial formation of complexes between DNA and higher-molecular-weight PEI polymers *(44)*.

The method by which polycation : DNA complexes are prepared represents an additional issue. Two important factors to be considered are the ability of polycations

---

◄   Fig. 2. Structure of polycations used for DNA delivery to mammalian cells. (**A**) Poly-L-lysine (PLL), a linear polyamino acid. The primary amino groups of PLL are typically fully charged at pH 7.0. (**B**) Polyethyleneimine (PEI). PEI can be produced either in a linear form or with varying degrees of branching. A highly branched form is shown. PEI has a high density of amino groups (every third atom in the polymer chain is a nitrogen atom) and, moreover, branched PEI has primary, secondary, and tertiary amino groups; as a consequence of these two factors, not all amino groups in PEI are protonated at physiological pH. Thus, PEI is effective as a "proton sponge," buffering the low pH of endosomes, leading to osmotic swelling and eventual rupture of endosomal vesicles. (**C**) Polyamidoamine (PAMAM) dendrimer. Dendrimers are constructed by successive additions of starting materials in "generations," making progressively larger molecules. Shown is a generation 2-(G2) PAMAM dendrimer; the successive generations are numbered in the figure. Typical PAMAM dendrimers used in transfections are G8. Only the terminal amino groups in PAMAM dendrimers are charged; these molecules assume a spherical shape, with all of the charged amino groups on the surface.

and DNA to form insoluble aggregates and the toxicity of uncomplexed polycations. Polylysine : DNA complexes tend to aggregate when polycations and DNA are mixed together, yielding cloudy solutions or white precipitates. These aggregates will be retained by 0.2- or 0.45-μm filters generally used to sterilize samples. Two major methods have been suggested to avoid aggregation. The first is to use physiological salt concentrations (i.e., 150 mM NaCl) but limit solutions to less than 20 μg/mL DNA; the second is to prepare complexes in a high-salt solution (up to 2 M NaCl) and then slowly dialyze the sample to a lower salt concentration *(19)*. The first method is much simpler because it avoids dialysis steps, but the low DNA concentrations used mean that larger volumes are needed for transfection. Moreover, even at 150 mM NaCl, the large size of the DNA : PLL complexes limits their penetration into tissues and uptake by cells. PEI : DNA complexes have also been prepared by mixing solutions at 20 μg/ mL DNA and 150 mM NaCl *(26)*. PEI : DNA complexes prepared by this method are apparently smaller, mostly below 50 nm in diameter *(45)*, which may be another reason for the higher efficiency of PEI over PLL in gene transfer. Another problem with polycation-mediated gene transfer is the toxicity of the polycation : DNA preparations. PEI : DNA complexes are thought to be more toxic than PLL : DNA complexes, but this is still under debate. One approach to reducing the toxicity of these complexes is to remove any free PEI by centrifuging the preparations (e.g., at 10,000g for 30 min) and then resuspending the complexes in PEI-free medium *(44)*. The toxicity of PEI represents a major hurdle to its use in gene therapy. The development of DNA-carrier polymers that have less toxic side effects than PEI and other polycations currently available remains the subject of much ongoing research.

3. Cell Targeting and Introduction of Cell Specificity

Polycations such as PLL and PEI function well to protect DNA from nucleases and allow efficient entry of DNA into cells. However, these complexes are not specific for the types of cell they transfect and, thus, it is not possible to specifically target cells using these methodologies. Targeted gene delivery is a major objective of gene therapy *(8)*, and the creation of a "magic bullet" to effectively and specifically kill cancer cells is the primary goal of suicide gene cancer therapy. One relatively simple method of targeting gene expression to one area in an organism is to include tissue- or organ-specific promoters or transcription elements in the DNA vector *(46)*. This approach has been explored by several groups with different DNA elements. This avenue of research will not be discussed in this chapter. One important parameter affecting the outcome of this strategy is that all tissues in the body be transfected prior to the tissue-specific expression of a suicide gene. Potentially, large amounts of the transfection agent may thus have to be administered to achieve the desired effect. This limitation has important negative implications for gene therapy if the transfection agent happens to be toxic and/or expensive.

Another method of targeting cells is to directly administer the DNA : vector complex to the affected area. For example, there has been some success with administering PEI : DNA aerosols to the lung *(27)*. Local delivery via intratumoral injection is also possible. However, the success of this approach lies in addressing the issue of poor penetration of large polycation : DNA complexes into solid tumors. This problem arises because of the high interstitial pressure frequently observed in poorly vascularized tumor masses. Ex vivo gene therapy may represent an option in cases where cancer patients are aggressively treated with high-dose chemotherapy, necessitating stem cell transplants. In this context, graft cells recovered from the patient could be transfected with a toxic gene and then replaced into the patient to selectively kill cancer cells *(17)*. In terms of purging methods, less laborious negative selection methods are available as well as positive selection approaches based on the preferential expansion and recovery of stem cells.

None of the above delivery strategies systemically target DNA complexes to specific cell or tissue types. A promising approach for achieving a more targeted delivery is to attach receptor-specific ligands to PEI, PLL, or other polycations *(5,19,47,48)*. The mechanism of internalization of the DNA : vector conjugate is also altered from absorptive endocytosis to receptor-mediated endocytosis. The overexpression of specific cell surface receptors such as the epidermal growth factor (EGF) receptor *(49)*, the transferrin receptor *(50)*, and the folate-binding receptor *(51,52)* has been observed on cancer cells, suggesting that their natural ligands can be used for receptor-mediated transfection. Alternatively, galactose has served as a targeting ligand for asialoglycoprotein receptors on hepatocytes *(53–56)*. Cell surface proteins have also been targeted with antibodies conjugated to polycations such as PLL *(19)*. Although specific ligands have been shown to specifically target cell types in in vitro studies, their use in designing effective gene therapy reagents faces several hurdles in terms of crossreactivity and homogeneity of preparation. Synthesis and characterization conditions leading to the production of stable, homogeneous ligand–polycation copolymer preparations need to be established if such bioconjugates are to be used in clinical applications. Additionally and more importantly, what needs to be addressed in the design of these conjugates is a strategy that would allow DNA : polymer complexes to escape from endosomes and be transported to the nucleus.

4. Endosomal Escape

In order to express a suicide gene in a target cell, it is first necessary to direct the localization of a DNA plasmid to the nucleus. Two separate intracellular events must occur to ensure the routing of DNA to this cellular compartment. The first event is the escape of DNA : vehicle complexes from endosomes into the cytoplasm, and the second step is nuclear import. The release of DNA complexes from vesicular compartments such as endosomes remains a major hurdle in designing DNA delivery vehicles *(57,58)*. The efficiency of endosomal escape by currently used nonviral polycation : DNA complexes is low, with most of the imported plasmid conjugates never reaching the cytoplasm, let alone the nucleus. The complexes are eventually broken down in endosomes and other vesicles, with DNA being degraded by endosomal nucleases *(9)*. Two strategies have been exploited to allow the release of DNA : vehicle complexes from vesicular compartments. The first approach is based on the concept of osmolytic rupture, where the nature of the polycation used may allow it to be further protonated in endosomes. This mechanism would operate when the pH in the vesicular compartment is lowered, such as in the case of endosomes. More precisely, pH levels can range from about 6.5 in early endosomes to pH 5 or lower in late endosomes/lysosomes. The increased protonation state of particular polycations under this acidic pH range would result in the influx of ions into the endosomal compartment to counterbalance the buffering capacity of the polycation itself. The influx, which includes counterions such as chloride ions to maintain charge balance and water molecules to maintain osmotic balance inside these vesicles, is expected to result in the rupture and release of endosomal contents into the cytoplasm. Polycations can be selected on the basis of their relative protonation states at neutral and low pH. For example, polyethylenenimines have an impressive potential to be protonated within the lower pH ranges found in endosomes, making them very effective "proton sponges" in inducing osmolytic rupture *(26)*. In contrast, PLL has a poor "proton sponge" potential, and, therefore, in PLL-mediated transfections, the polyplexes are often coadministered with weak bases such as chloroquine *(19)*, an agent able to produce a similar effect. Unfortunately, the toxicity of chloroquine precludes its use in in vivo applications. Imidazole derivatives also display ionizable groups that can produce a "proton sponge" effect at endosomal pH levels. Histidine, one of the building blocks of peptides and proteins, represents the only amino acid harboring an imidazole side chain. It has been reported that various copolymers of histidine and lysine, as well as synthetic imidazole-containing polymers, have the ability to not only compact DNA but also to transfect cells more efficiently than PLL alone *(59–62)*. Moreover, they are less toxic to cells than PEI.

The second mechanism by which endosomes and lysosomes can be ruptured is through membrane disruption *(57,63)*. Endosomolytic peptide sequences are found in bacterial toxins and viral proteins. These peptides tend to be hydrophobic in character and their sequences also contain a number of acidic residues, as opposed to the basic groups found in polycations, which are protonated as the pH is lowered in the endosome. This event results in the peptide sequence becoming less ionic and more hydrophobic as a function of acidic pH, enabling it to fuse with and disrupt the membrane of the endosome, releasing its contents into the cytoplasm. These endosomolytic or fusogenic peptides include sequences derived from influenza virus hemagglutinin HA-2 *(63,64)* and their variants *(65,66)*, and larger translocation domains from *Pseudomonas* exotoxin A *(67,68)* and diptheria toxin *(69,70)* (Table 1). Such sequences could potentially be inserted into protein-based gene carrier systems for use in vivo.

The two discussed processes for endosomal escape may occur simultaneously to some degree in most cases. PLL and PEI do have some limited hydrophobic character and, in addition, will interact through their charged groups with the negatively charged lipids of biological membranes. Fusogenic peptides, in addition to fusing to membranes, also bind protons, which results in osmotic swelling that aids in promoting endosomal lysis. An example of a peptide where both events probably occur to a significant degree is a histidine-containing variant of HA-2 *(65)*. The histidine residues act as a "proton sponge," whereas the underlying sequence fuses with the endosomal membrane.

Table 1
Some Fusogenic Peptide Sequences Used Successfully for Gene Delivery
in the Literature

Name	Sequence	Ref.
HA-2$_{1-20}$	GLFEAIAGFIENGWEFMIDG	*64*
	(residues 1–20 of hemagglutinin A)	
JTS-1	GLFEALLELLESLWELLLEA	*66*
H5WYG	GLFHAIAHFIHGGWHGLIHGWYG	*65*
ETA$_{252-366}$	Residues 252–366 of *Pseudomonas*	*67,68*
	exotoxin A	
DT$_{195-383}$	Residues 195–383 of diptheria toxin	*69,70*

Note: The first three (all derived from the N-terminal fusogenic sequence of hemagglutinin A) were made synthetically, whereas the other two were used in the context of larger modular proteins.

The present generation of endosomolytic compounds, whether they are a "proton sponge" or are fusogenic in nature, also have undesirable properties as potential DNA carriers. For instance, the toxicity to chloroquine and PEI toward eukaryotic cells has resulted in the need to develop less toxic variants of these compounds, whereas the immunogenicity of fusogenic peptides, given that they are derived from bacterial and viral proteins, remain to be addressed more completely if these vehicles are to be used commercially. In addition, fusogenic peptides may be toxic to a broad range of eukaryotic cells as a result of their action on plasma membranes prior to their import into endosomes. The large size of many fusogenic sequences also makes them poor candidates for peptide synthesis. Finally, their hydrophobic character often results in poorly soluble peptides, making them difficult to handle in practical applications. Some of these problems can be avoided by including the fusogenic sequences in larger chimeric proteins, thereby protecting them from aggregation, and by coadministering these constructs with polycations. At present, however, most of the studies in gene therapy do not employ fusogenic peptides but rather rely on the intrinsic low levels of endosomal lysis by polycations. In summary, a major limiting factor in the efficiency of most nonviral vectors is the release of plasmid DNA from endosomal compartments.

5. Nuclear Targeting

The import and retention of the DNA vector within the nucleus of a cell represents another important routing event to encode in a delivery vehicle. This compartmentalization event can be achieved if the DNA complexes can efficiently traverse the nuclear envelope. Passive diffusion of molecules into the nucleus through nuclear pores can occur—the pores are 9 nm in diameter, allowing macromolecules less than about 50 kDa in size to enter freely *(71)*. This size limit is much lower than the expected mass of most polycation : DNA complexes. However, particles up to 25 nm in diameter can be actively transported into the nucleus *(71)*, and polycation : DNA complexes can enter the nucleus by this route. In addition, DNA : carrier complexes could also possibly enter the nucleus as the nuclear envelope breaks down during cell division. This could be an important route of entry for cancer cells (*see* final paragraph, this subheading). Proteins that normally reside in the nucleus of cells tend to contain one or more nuclear localization signals (NLSs) *(2,72)* or are associated with proteins routed to the nucleus. Nuclear import of proteins that contain NLSs takes place through recognition of the NLS by cytosolic proteins called importins, which deliver the protein to the nuclear pore complex *(72)*, where the proteins then enter the nucleus. One common characteristic of most NLSs is the presence of several cationic residues within their sequence, suggesting that polycation : DNA complexes, having the general characteristics of NLSs, may be recognized by importins and actively transported to the nucleus. However, this structural analogy may not be valid because noncationic residues have also been shown to be important for the activity of nuclear localization signals *(73)*.

When designing a specific DNA transport vector, it is thus desirable to take advantage of naturally occurring NLSs to direct DNA to the nucleus, rather than simply relying on the general properties of polycations like PLL and PEI. A popular NLS sequence encompasses residues 124–135 (Thr-Pro-Pro-Lys-Lys-Lys-Arg-Lys-Val-Glu-Asp-Pro) of the SV40 large T-antigen *(13,74)*. It possesses several cationic residues and represents a relatively short sequence, two desirable features when making synthetic conjugates. This NLS sequence alone is sufficient to direct molecules, including DNA conjugates, to the nucleus of cells *(74,76)*. Another interesting putative NLS is a 30-amino-acid peptide derived from a lupus-related monoclonal anti-DNA antibody, which is internalized and accumulates in the nuclei of 3T3 and CCL39 cells *(77)*.

The inclusion of nuclear localization sequences is an important improvement to a DNA carrier vehicle. However, the presence of an efficient NLS may not be necessary to target DNA to the nucleus of cancer cells. In proliferating cells such as cancer cells, it is possible for large molecules, such as plasmid DNA and DNA complexes, to reach the nucleus as the nuclear membrane disassembles during cell division. If the cytoplasmic half-life of the DNA complexes exceeds the time-scale of cell division, DNA complexes could potentially be entrapped in the nuclei of both daughter cells following the reassembly of the nuclear envelope. Thus, in suicide gene cancer therapy, it might be desirable in some instances to actually decrease the efficiency of nuclear localization of the carrier vehicle. This strategy would partly limit the expression of the suicide gene to proliferating cells, making it more specific for cancer cells. It remains to be seen if a suicide gene carrier can actually be attenuated in this way to reduce side effects while maintaining its efficacy.

6. Constructing a Nonviral DNA Carrier

Several features required of a DNA carrier to effectively transfect cells have been discussed and there is now a need to integrate these parameters into practical assemblies. These features include DNA protection and condensation, targeting of the construct to specific cells, internalization of the construct, release from the endosome, and transport of the DNA to the nucleus. Because many of these functions can be addressed using peptide sequences, one design approach would be to assemble them either into synthetic scaffolds *(2,78)* or recombinant modular proteins *(70)*, where each domain inserted into these peptide-based templates would perform a different task needed of a DNA carrier vehicle. The architecture of naturally occurring bacterial toxins such as *Pseudomonas* exotoxin A (ETA) *(67,68)* and diptheria toxin (DT) *(70)* represent vivid examples of this modular single-chain assembly concept. ETA and DT are multitasking protein assemblies with clearly defined functional domains. They have the ability to specifically bind to receptors on mammalian cells. Following their internalization and sequestration into endosomes, they are able to escape this vesicular compartment to reach the cytosol through the action of their endosomolytic domain (also referred to as a translocation domain). Finally, both toxins possess an ADP-mono-ribosyltransferase enzymatic activity acting on a cytosolic substrate. The enzyme transfers ADP-ribose from NAD to elongation factor 2, inactivating the factor and thus inhibiting protein synthesis. By replacing the natural cellular recognition domains with an antibody domain that binds a receptor overexpressed in cancer cells, the targeting function of the toxin can be changed such that it attacks cancer cells. Additionally, the catalytic domain of the toxin could be replaced with a DNA-binding sequence such as the DNA-binding domain from the yeast transcription factor GAL4. This domain binds a specific DNA sequence with high affinity. This sequence could be inserted on the desired piece of target DNA, enabling the new modular protein to carry DNA into cancer cells. However, this detoxified protein toxin would still not effectively condense DNA. One solution to this problem would be to preform the complex between the modular protein and plasmid and then to mix the protein : DNA complex with PLL or PEI. The cationic polymer would condense the DNA efficiently while preserving the specific cell-binding feature of the DNA carrier protein *(67,68,70)*. The retained translocation domain of the toxin would enable the complex to escape from the endosome. The efficiency of routing to the nucleus could also be improved by including a nuclear localization signal into the protein scaffold.

The multivalent display of functional domains and their effective presentation on a scaffold represent two important parameters that can enhance properties of DNA transfection vehicles such as their receptor-binding avidity and cell-routing functions. For instance, the GAL4 DNA-binding domain associates with its DNA element as a dimer. With a tandem repeat of the GAL4 DNA target sequence per plasmid, each DNA molecule can associate with two dimers (four monomers in total) of the GAL4 DNA-binding domain, and thus there are four cell surface receptor-binding motifs bound by each DNA molecule. This multivalent arrangement would result in higher binding avidity for the plasmid DNA vehicle to its target cells. A number of bacterial toxins such as Shiga toxin, cholera toxin, and the *Escherichia coli* heat-labile enterotoxin *(79,80)* already display pentamers of cell-targeting motifs. Their general AB_5 subunit organization includes a catalytically active A chain that is noncovalently associated to a pentamer of identical B-subunits that presents multiple receptor-binding sites. Other routing features such as endosomal lysis and nuclear targeting can also be enhanced by presenting multiple copies of such signals on the delivery vehicle. One simple method of increasing the valency of interaction of the modular proteins with plasmid

DNA would be to introduce more GAL4 DNA-binding domains into the plasmid. This strategy would place constraints on the types of sequences that can be introduced into the plasmid. In the case of PLL conjugates incorporating galactose and transferrin, the level of multivalency can be partly controlled by conjugating several targeting molecules to each PLL molecule. The final ratio of components integrated in these conjugates will depend on the concentration of each element present in the reaction vessel and the coupling conditions (19,56). Unfortunately, protein conjugation reactions are often difficult to control in solution, resulting in heterogeneous populations of PLL constructs. This issue must be addressed if PLL conjugates are to be used in future therapeutic applications.

One unique approach to designing multivalent DNA targeting molecules is the concept of loligomers (2,11), which are branched, synthetic peptides containing identical, multifunctional arms. The synthesis of loligomers is based on the strategy of assembling multiple antigenic peptides (MAPs) on a branched lysine scaffold (81–83). Briefly, loligomers are constructed by solid-phase synthesis, where arms are created by the successive additions of identically protected lysine residues. In solid-phase peptide synthesis, linear peptides are assembled by protecting the side-chain ε-amino groups of lysine residues with a different protecting group than its backbone α-amino group, ensuring that successive additions of amino acids are made only in a linear fashion along the backbone. In contrast, the simultaneous deprotection of the two amino groups of lysine would result in the subsequent addition of the following amino acid at both positions and the creation of two branches on the peptide. A molecule with eight arms is produced after three successive branching steps with lysine residues. The branches are then extended using conventional solid-phase peptide synthesis, with each branch incorporating the same signals. The structure of a typical loligomer molecule is shown in **Fig. 3**. It has eight identical branches, each containing a pentalysine cellular import signal (referred to as a cytoplasmic translocation signal [CTS]) and a NLS derived from the SV40 T-antigen (74). This loligomer is able to effectively transfer DNA to the nucleus of cultured mammalian cells (12,13), with a much greater efficiency than linear peptides harboring the same routing sequences. As illustrated in **Fig. 3**, nucleus-directing loligomers have a high amount of positively charged residues, owing to both their CTS and NLS sequences. The high content of lysine and arginine residues in their sequence gives them properties similar to cationic homopolymers such as PLL and PEI. The simple mixing of a loligomer with DNA results in the condensation of the DNA and charge neutralization. However, a loligomer : DNA charge ratio greater than 1 is needed for optimal transfection (discussed later in this paragraph). Entry of DNA : loligomer complexes is proposed to occur through absorptive endocytosis (see **Fig. 1**) (12), in a similar fashion to PLL. Branched peptide vehicles harboring other import signals, such as polyarginine tails, were comparable to polylysine sequences at promoting the internalization of DNA (Kawamura and Gariépy, unpublished results); the arginine-rich HIV Tat translocation domain (40), however, was found to be not as efficient. A similar comparison of the effectiveness of lysines and arginines was also found in a peptide system with two branches (84). A loligomer : DNA weight ratio of 0.5 is sufficient to complex plasmid DNA and retard

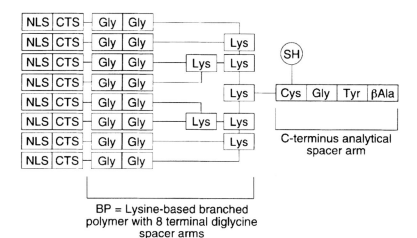

BP = Lysine-based branched
polymer with 8 terminal diglycine
spacer arms

Fig. 3. Structure of "loligomer 4," a loligomer used in DNA delivery to cultured mammalian cells. Loligomer 4 has eight identical arms as a result of branching brought on by the successive additions of bifunctional lysine residues. The analytical core includes a tyrosine residue for quantitation purposes and a cysteine residue to be used potentially for coupling chemical groups via its unique thiol. The eight identical arms consist of a NLS derived from residues 124–135 of the simian virus (SV40) T-antigen (sequence APPKKKRKVEDP in one-letter code) and a cytoplasmic translocation signal (CTS; sequence KKKKK). Loligomer 4 has a molecular weight of 17.5 kDa and a charge of +72.

its mobility in agarose gels *(13)*. The conversion factor for the loligomer : DNA weight ratio to a loligomer : DNA charge ratio is 1.5. Thus, at a weight ratio of 0.5, the net charge of the complexes is still actually slightly negative, but not enough to allow the DNA to proceed through an agarose gel. It must be remembered that the DNA intercalating ethidium dye used to visualize the band also carries a positive charge. In contrast to the electrophoresis experiments, a loligomer : DNA weight ratio of 3 : 1 is most optimal for transfection *(12,13)*, which corresponds to a charge ratio of 4.5, significantly higher than the optimal charge ratios for PLL- or PEI-mediated transfection. A possible reason for this difference might be that the first charge equivalents of the loligomer neutralize and compact the DNA, but the addition of more loligomers ensures the presentation of exposed import and NLS sequences, which induce internalization and target the complex to the nucleus of cells.

As with PLL : DNA and PEI : DNA complexes, the escape of loligomer : DNA complexes from endosomes is inefficient. However, the presence of a true NLS on each branch of the loligomer molecule ensures that each complex that escapes the endosome is targeted to the nucleus. Thus, loligomers represent an overall increase in efficiency. Also, because loligomers are synthetic, it may be possible to introduce a small fusogenic sequence into the loligomers to induce endosomal lysis. All known fusogenic sequences are both long and hydrophobic, features that are not attractive in terms of their inclusion into loligomers. A simpler approach to increase the efficiency of escape of loligomers from the endosome is to coadminister loligomers with endosomolytic agents, such as PEI or chloroquine. PEI would also bind to DNA, thereby reducing the amount of loligomers needed to neutralize DNA. Thus, presumably less loligomer would be needed to transfect cells. The co-usage of a specific DNA transport protein and PLL to transfect cells has already been discussed. Loligomers have not yet been used as in vivo gene delivery agents. A protocol is presented next for the preparation of loligomer : DNA complexes that could potentially be used in gene therapy.

7. Protocol for Gene Delivery With Loligomers
7.1. Loligomer Preparation

At the moment, nucleus-directed loligomers *(13)* are not commercially available as a transfection reagent. Loligomers can be prepared by conventional solid-phase peptide synthesis. The complete procedure for synthesis is not presented here, but the production of branched peptides has been discussed in more detail in the literature *(11,81–83)*. An important practical consideration is that in order to avoid overcrowding as a consequence of branching, loligomers must be synthesized on a resin with a low level of loading, typically around 0.1 mmol/g. As already mentioned, branches are produced by the placement of lysine residues with identical protecting groups. Apart from that, the procedures that are used are identical to those used for synthesis of linear peptides. Currently, we use a protocol based on 9-fluorenylmethyloxycarbonyl (Fmoc)-protected amino acids and di-Fmoc($N\alpha$, $N\varepsilon$)-L-lysine to create the branches. Loligomers have been synthesized on an Applied Biosystems 431A peptide synthesizer using a manufacturer's protocol with double coupling steps to ensure complete coupling of each residue. Deprotection of side chains was carried out after cleavage of the loligomer from the resin. The preparation is then analyzed by reverse-phase high-performance liquid chromatography (RP-HPLC). The high positive charge and the branched nature of loligomers make them difficult to analyze by mass spectrometry. Quantitative amino acid analysis is the method of choice to determine the composition of these peptides. A β-alanine residue is included in the C-terminal core of the loligomer to provide a convenient internal standard to enable quantitation of the number of branches per loligomer molecule. They can be stored as lyophilized powders at –20°C or lower for long periods.

7.2. Increasing the Versatility of the Loligomer Platform Design for In Vivo Use

Branched peptides will need to be homogeneous and pure for in vivo uses. These criteria will be difficult to meet for loligomers in light of inherent synthesis inefficiencies associated with the assembly of branched peptides by solid-phase methods. Specifically, each branching step during loligomer synthesis effectively doubles the level of substitution on the support and subsequently results in chain crowding and reduced coupling efficiency in later steps during synthesis. The compounding of inefficient coupling steps results in sequence heterogeneity (as amino acid deletions) affecting each arm. These synthesis problems are difficult to characterize by mass spectrometry or amino acid analyses. Branched peptides are also difficult to purify by standard chromatographic methods. A sequential synthesis approach can be used to alleviate these problems *(85–87)*. More precisely, a short, branched peptide scaffold (BrCH$_2$CO-Glu)$_4$K$_2$KGßA as well as individual linear peptides representing arms would all be constructed by solid-phase synthesis, thus simplifying the subsequent purification and characterization steps. Each arm would be prepared with a C-terminal lysine residue modified with an ε-*N-S*-acetylmercaptoacetyl (SAMA) group. In a second step performed in solution, arms would then be attached to the small, branched scaffold via Lys-*Nε-S* CH$_2$CO-Glu linkages to complete the synthesis. This approach suggests that long arms (>50 residues) could be prepared and purified prior to their assembly on the peptide scaffold.

7.3. Preparation of Loligomer: DNA Complexes

A protocol for using nucleus-directed loligomers has been described in **ref. *13***. Briefly, a solution of loligomer (approx 1 mg/mL) is first prepared in phosphate-buffered saline (PBS). The concentration of loligomer in this solution is determined either by ulraviolet (UV) absorbance spectroscopy or using a protein assay kit (Bio-Rad). Plasmids are dissolved in water and their concentration in solution determined by UV absorbance (a 50-µg/mL solution of double-stranded DNA has an absorbance of 1.0 at 260 nm). A minimal weight ratio of loligomer to plasmid for transfection studies can be initially determined from gel shift experiments. This minimal ratio would correspond to the amount of loligomer needed to fully complex and retard the electrophoretic migration of plasmid DNA into an agarose gel. A good starting condition would be to dispense 10 µg each of loligomer and DNA into a microcentrifuge tube, mix, and adjust the final volume of the mixture to 50 µL with PBS. When mixing the loligomer and DNA, it is important to calculate and dispense the amount of PBS needed into the tube first. Plasmid DNA is then added, followed by the loligomer solution, and the tube is then mixed immediately. These steps will ensure that DNA and the loligomer do not form insoluble precipitates. Following the mixing step, tubes are left to stand at room temperature for 10 min. Loligomer : DNA complexes prepared by this method can then be used for DNA delivery by resuspending cells in media and simply exposing them to these peptide–DNA complexes for 4 h or longer. The presence or absence of fetal calf serum in the medium does not affect the level of cellular import.

8. Conclusions

Peptide-based polymers and polycations represent simpler, costeffective, and potentially less immunogenic classes of gene delivery agents than viruses. Additionally, such nonviral systems have fewer limitations on the length of DNA that can be introduced into cells than viral packaging. Currently, the two major challenges of these nonviral gene delivery systems are their lack of specificity with regard to gene delivery to cell and tissue types and their inefficient escape from endosomes. Significant advances are currently being made to provide solutions to both of these parameters. With these questions answered, polycations, proteins, and peptide-based polymers can challenge viruses as the most favored transfection agents.

References

1. Frankel, A. E., Kreitman, R. J., and Sausville, E. A. (2000) Targeted toxins. *Clin. Cancer Res.* **6,** 326–334.
2. Gariepy, J. and Kawamura, K. (2001) Vectorial delivery of macromolecules into cells using peptide-based vehicles. *Trends Biotechnol.* **19,** 21–28.
3. Moghimi, S. M. and Rajabi-Siahboomi, A. R. (2000) Recent advances in cellular, sub-cellular and molecular targeting. *Adv. Drug Deliv. Rev.* **41,** 129–133.
4. Kabanov, A. (1999) Taking polycation gene delivery systems from in vitro to in vivo. *Pharm. Sci. Technol. Today* **2,** 365–372.
5. Anwer, K., Bailey, A., and Sullivan, S.M. (2000) Targeted gene delivery: a two-pronged approach. *Crit. Rev. Ther. Drug Carrier Syst.* **17,** 377–424.
6. Cristiano, R. J. (1998) Targeted, non-viral gene delivery for cancer gene therapy. *Front. Biosci.* **3,** D1161–D1170.
7. Kouraklis, G. (1999) Progress in cancer gene therapy. *Acta Oncol.* **38,** 675–683.
8. Peng, K. W. (1999) Strategies for targeting therapeutic gene delivery. *Mol. Med. Today* **5,** 448–453.
9. Mahato, R. I. (1999) Non-viral peptide-based approaches to gene delivery. *J. Drug Target.* **7,** 249–268.
10. Pouton, C. W., Lucas, P., Thomas, B. J., Uduehi, A. N., Milroy, D. A., and Moss, S. H. (1998) Polycation–DNA complexes for gene delivery: a comparison of the biopharmaceutical properties of cationic polypeptides and cationic lipids. *J Control. Release* **53,** 289–299.
11. Sheldon, K., Liu, D., Ferguson, J., and Gariepy, J. (1995) Loligomers: design of de novo peptide-based intracellular vehicles. *Proc. Natl. Acad. Sci. USA* **92,** 2056–2060.
12. Singh, D., Kiarash, R., Kawamura, K., LaCasse, E. C., and Gariepy, J. (1998) Penetration and intracellular routing of nucleus-directed peptide-based shuttles (loligomers) in eukaryotic cells. *Biochemistry* **37,** 5798–5809.
13. Singh, D., Bisland, S.K., Kawamura, K., and Gariepy, J. (1999) Peptide-based intracellular shuttle able to facilitate gene transfer in mammalian cells. *Bioconjug. Chem.* **10,** 745–754.
14. Bottger, M., Vogel, F., Platzer, M., Kiessling, U., Grade, K., and Strauss, M. (1988) Condensation of vector DNA by the chromosomal protein HMG1 results in efficient transfection. *Biochim. Biophys. Acta* **950,** 221–228.
15. Demirhan, I., Hasselmayer, O., Chandra, A., Ehemann, M., and Chandra, P. (1998) Histone-mediated transfer and expression of the HIV-1 tat gene in Jurkat cells. *J. Hum. Virol.* **1,** 430–440.
16. Zaitsev, S. V., Haberland, A., Otto, A., Vorob'ev, V. I., Haller, H., and Bottger, M. (1997) H1 and HMG17 extracted from calf thymus nuclei are efficient DNA carriers in gene transfer. *Gene Ther.* **4,** 586–592.
17. Garnett, M. C. (1999) Gene-delivery systems using cationic polymers. *Crit. Rev. Ther. Drug Carrier Syst.* **16,** 147–207.
18. Godbey, W. T., Wu, K. K., and Mikos, A. G. (1999) Poly(ethylenimine) and its role in gene delivery. *J Control. Release* **60,** 149–160.
19. Wagner, E., Ogris, M., and Zauner, W. (1998) Polylysine-based transfection systems utilizing receptor-mediated delivery. *Adv. Drug Deliv. Rev.* **30,** 97–113.
20. Ryser, H. J. and Shen, W. C. (1978) Conjugation of methotrexate to poly(L-lysine) increases drug transport and overcomes drug resistance in cultured cells. *Proc. Natl. Acad. Sci. USA* **75,** 3867–3870.

21. Leonetti, J. P., Degols, G., and Lebleu, B. (1990) Biological activity of oligonucleotide-poly(L-lysine) conjugates: mechanism of cell uptake. *Bioconjug. Chem.* **1,** 149–153.
22. Singh, A. K., Kasinath, B. S., and Lewis, E. J. (1992) Interaction of polycations with cell-surface negative charges of epithelial cells. *Biochim Biophys Acta* **1120,** 337–342.
23. Mislick, K. A. and Baldeschwieler, J. D. (1996) Evidence for the role of proteoglycans in cation-mediated gene transfer. *Proc. Natl. Acad. Sci. USA* **93,** 12,349–12,354.
24. Horbinski, C., Stachowiak, M. K., Higgins, D., and Finnegan, S. G. (2001) Polyethyleneimine-mediated transfection of cultured postmitotic neurons from rat sympathetic ganglia and adult human retina. *BMC Neurosci.* **2,** 2.
25. Lemkine, G. F. and Demeneix, B. A. (2001) Polyethylenimines for in vivo gene delivery. *Curr. Opin. Mol. Ther.* **3,** 178–182.
26. Boussif, O., Lezoualc'h, F., Zanta, M. A., et al. (1995) A versatile vector for gene and oligonucleotide transfer into cells in culture and in vivo: polyethylenimine. *Proc. Natl. Acad. Sci. USA* **92,** 7297–7301.
27. Gautam, A., Densmore, C. L., Xu, B., and Waldrep, J. C. (2000) Enhanced gene expression in mouse lung after PEI-DNA aerosol delivery. *Mol. Ther.* **2,** 63–70.
28. Kukowska-Latallo, J. F., Bielinska, A. U., Johnson, J., Spindler, R., Tomalia, D. A., and Baker, J. R., Jr. (1996) Efficient transfer of genetic material into mammalian cells using Starburst polyamidoamine dendrimers. *Proc. Natl. Acad. Sci. USA* **93,** 4897–4902.
29. Tomalia, D.A., Baker, H., DeWald, J., et al. (1985) A new class of polymers: Starburst dendritic molecules. *Polym. J.* **17,** 117–132.
30. Harada, Y., Iwai, M., Tanaka, S., et al. (2000) Highly efficient suicide gene expression in hepatocellular carcinoma cells by epstein-barr virus-based plasmid vectors combined with polyamidoamine dendrimer. *Cancer Gene Ther.* **7,** 27–36.
31. Maruyama-Tabata, H., Harada, Y., Matsumura, T., et al. (2000) Effective suicide gene therapy in vivo by EBV-based plasmid vector coupled with polyamidoamine dendrimer. *Gene Ther.* **7,** 53–60.
32. Tang, M. X., Redemann, C. T., and Szoka, F. C., Jr. (1996) In vitro gene delivery by degraded polyamidoamine dendrimers. *Bioconjug. Chem.* **7,** 703–714.
33. Toncheva, V., Wolfert, M. A., Dash, P. R., et al. (1998) Novel vectors for gene delivery formed by self-assembly of DNA with poly(L-lysine) grafted with hydrophilic polymers. *Biochim. Biophys. Acta* **1380,** 354–368.
34. Nguyen, H. K., Lemieux, P., Vinogradov, S. V., et al. (2000) Evaluation of polyether-polyethyleneimine graft copolymers as gene transfer agents. *Gene Ther.* **7,** 126–138.
35. Shin, Y., Chang, J. H., Liu, J., Williford, R., and Exarhos, G. J. (2001) Hybrid nanogels for sustainable positive thermosensitive drug release. *J. Control. Release* **73,** 1–6.
36. Schwartz, J. J. and Zhang, S. (2000) Peptide-mediated cellular delivery. *Curr. Opin. Mol. Ther.* **2,** 162–167.
37. Derossi, D., Joliot, A. H., Chassaing, G., and Prochiantz, A. (1994) The third helix of the Antennapedia homeodomain translocates through biological membranes. *J. Biol. Chem.* **269,** 10,444–10,450.
38. Derossi, D., Calvet, S., Trembleau, A., Brunissen, A., Chassaing, G., and Prochiantz, A. (1996) Cell internalization of the third helix of the Antennapedia homeodomain is receptor-independent. *J. Biol. Chem.* **271,** 18,188–18,193.
39. Derossi, D., Chassaing, G., and Prochiantz, A. (1998) Trojan peptides: the penetratin system for intracellular delivery. *Trends Cell. Biol.* **8,** 84–87.
40. Vives, E., Brodin, P., and Lebleu, B. (1997) A truncated HIV-1 Tat protein basic domain rapidly translocates through the plasma membrane and accumulates in the cell nucleus. *J Biol Chem* **272,** 16,010–16,017.

41. Eguchi, A., Akuta, T., Okuyama, H., et al. (2001) Protein transduction domain of HIV-1 Tat protein promotes efficient delivery of DNA into mammalian cells. *J. Biol. Chem.* **276,** 26,204–26,210.

42. Wender, P. A., Mitchell, D. J., Pattabiraman, K., Pelkey, E. T., Steinman, L., and Rothbard, J. B. (2000) The design, synthesis, and evaluation of molecules that enable or enhance cellular uptake: peptoid molecular transporters. *Proc. Natl. Acad. Sci. USA* **97,** 13,003–13,008.

43. Godbey, W. T., Wu, K. K., and Mikos, A. G. (1999) Size matters: molecular weight affects the efficiency of poly(ethylenimine) as a gene delivery vehicle. *J. Biomed. Mater. Res.* **45,** 268–275.

44. Godbey, W. T., Wu, K. K., Hirasaki, G. J., and Mikos, A. G. (1999) Improved packing of poly(ethylenimine)/DNA complexes increases transfection efficiency. *Gene Ther.* **6,** 1380–1388.

45. Dunlap, D. D., Maggi, A., Soria, M. R., and Monaco, L. (1997) Nanoscopic structure of DNA condensed for gene delivery. *Nucleic Acids Res.* **25,** 3095–3101.

46. Nettelbeck, D. M., Jerome, V., and Muller, R. (2000) Gene therapy: designer promoters for tumour targeting. *Trends Genet.* **16,** 174–181.

47. Kircheis, R., Kichler, A., Wallner, G., et al. (1997) Coupling of cell-binding ligands to polyethylenimine for targeted gene delivery. *Gene Ther.* **4,** 409–418.

48. Kircheis, R., Schuller, S., Brunner, S., et al. (1999) Polycation-based DNA complexes for tumor-targeted gene delivery in vivo. *J. Gene Med.* **1,** 111–120.

49. Cohen, B. D., Siegall, C. B., Bacus, S., et al. (1998) Role of epidermal growth factor receptor family members in growth and differentiation of breast carcinoma. *Biochem. Soc. Symp.* **63,** 199–210.

50. Trowbridge, I. S. and Shackelford, D. A. (1986) Structure and function of transferrin receptors and their relationship to cell growth. *Biochem. Soc. Symp.* **51,** 117–129.

51. Sudimack, J. and Lee, R. J. (2000) Targeted drug delivery via the folate receptor. *Adv. Drug Deliv. Rev.* **41,** 147–162.

52. Wang, S. and Low, P. S. (1998) Folate-mediated targeting of antineoplastic drugs, imaging agents, and nucleic acids to cancer cells. *J. Control. Release* **53,** 39–48.

53. Erbacher, P., Roche, A. C., Monsigny, M., and Midoux, P. (1995) Glycosylated polylysine/DNA complexes: gene transfer efficiency in relation with the size and the sugar substitution level of glycosylated polylysines and with the plasmid size. *Bioconjug. Chem.* **6,** 401–410.

54. Hashida, M., Takemura, S., Nishikawa, M., and Takakura, Y. (1998) Targeted delivery of plasmid DNA complexed with galactosylated poly(L-lysine). *J Control. Release* **53,** 301–310.

55. Kawakami, S., Yamashita, F., Nishikawa, M., Takakura, Y., and Hashida, M. (1998) Asialoglycoprotein receptor-mediated gene transfer using novel galactosylated cationic liposomes. *Biochem. Biophys. Res. Commun.* **252,** 78–83.

56. Nishikawa, M., Takemura, S., Takakura, Y., and Hashida, M. (1998) Targeted delivery of plasmid DNA to hepatocytes in vivo: optimization of the pharmacokinetics of plasmid DNA/galactosylated poly(L-lysine) complexes by controlling their physicochemical properties. *J. Pharmacol. Exp. Ther* **287,** 408–415.

57. Wagner, E. (1999) Application of membrane-active peptides for nonviral gene delivery. *Adv Drug Deliv Rev* **38,** 279–289.

58. Plank, C., Zauner, W., and Wagner, E. (1998) Application of membrane-active peptides for drug and gene delivery across cellular membranes. *Adv. Drug Deliv. Rev.* **34**, 21–35.

59. Benns, J. M., Choi, J. S., Mahato, R. I., Park, J. S., and Kim, S. W. (2000) pH-sensitive cationic polymer gene delivery vehicle: *N*-Ac-poly(L-histidine)-graft-poly(L-lysine) comb shaped polymer. *Bioconjug. Chem.* **11**, 637–645.

60. Midoux, P. and Monsigny, M. (1999) Efficient gene transfer by histidylated polylysine/pDNA complexes. *Bioconjug. Chem.* **10**, 406–411.

61. Pack, D.W., Putnam, D., and Langer, R. (2000) Design of imidazole-containing endosomolytic biopolymers for gene delivery. *Biotechnol. Bioeng.* **67**, 217–223.

62. Putnam, D., Gentry, C.A., Pack, D.W., and Langer, R. (2001) Polymer-based gene delivery with low cytotoxicity by a unique balance of side-chain termini. *Proc. Natl. Acad. Sci. USA* **98**, 1200–1205.

63. Plank, C., Oberhauser, B., Mechtler, K., Koch, C., and Wagner, E. (1994) The influence of endosome-disruptive peptides on gene transfer using synthetic virus-like gene transfer systems. *J. Biol. Chem.* **269**, 12,918–12,924.

64. Wagner, E., Plank, C., Zatloukal, K., Cotten, M., and Birnstiel, M. L. (1992) Influenza virus hemagglutinin HA-2 N-terminal fusogenic peptides augment gene transfer by transferrin–polylysine–DNA complexes: toward a synthetic virus-like gene-transfer vehicle. *Proc. Natl. Acad. Sci. USA* **89**, 7934–7938.

65. Midoux, P., Kichler, A., Boutin, V., Maurizot, J. C., and Monsigny, M. (1998) Membrane permeabilization and efficient gene transfer by a peptide containing several histidines. *Bioconjug. Chem.* **9**, 260–267.

66. Gottschalk, S., Sparrow, J. T., Hauer, J., et al. (1996) A novel DNA–peptide complex for efficient gene transfer and expression in mammalian cells. *Gene Ther.* **3**, 48–57.

67. Fominaya, J. and Wels, W. (1996) Target cell-specific DNA transfer mediated by a chimeric multidomain protein. Novel non-viral gene delivery system. *J. Biol. Chem.* **271**, 10,560–10,568.

68. Fominaya, J., Uherek, C., and Wels, W. (1998) A chimeric fusion protein containing transforming growth factor-alpha mediates gene transfer via binding to the EGF receptor. *Gene Ther.* **5**, 521–530.

69. Fisher, K. J. and Wilson, J. M. (1997) The transmembrane domain of diphtheria toxin improves molecular conjugate gene transfer. *Biochem. J.* **321(Pt. 1)**, 49–58.

70. Uherek, C., Fominaya, J., and Wels, W. (1998) A modular DNA carrier protein based on the structure of diphtheria toxin mediates target cell-specific gene delivery. *J. Biol. Chem.* **273**, 8835–8841.

71. Gorlich, D. and Mattaj, I. W. (1996) Nucleocytoplasmic transport. *Science* **271**, 1513–1518.

72. Jans, D. A., Xiao, C. Y., and Lam, M. H. (2000) Nuclear targeting signal recognition: a key control point in nuclear transport? *Bioessays* **22**, 532–544.

73 Makkerh, J. P., Dingwall, C., and Laskey, R. A. (1996) Comparative mutagenesis of nuclear localization signals reveals the importance of neutral and acidic amino acids. *Curr. Biol.* **6**, 1025–1027.

74. Kalderon, D., Roberts, B. L., Richardson, W. D., and Smith, A. E. (1984) A short amino acid sequence able to specify nuclear location. *Cell* **39(3 Pt. 2)**, 499–509.

75. Chan, C. K. and Jans, D. A. (1999) Enhancement of polylysine-mediated transferrinfection by nuclear localization sequences: polylysine does not function as a nuclear localization sequence. *Hum. Gene Ther.* **10**, 1695–1702.

76. Chaloin, L., Vidal, P., Lory, P., et al. (1998) Design of carrier peptide-oligonucleotide conjugates with rapid membrane translocation and nuclear localization properties. *Biochem. Biophys. Res. Commun.* **243**, 601–608.
77. Avrameas, A., Ternynck, T., Gasmi, L., and Buttin, G. (1999) Efficient gene delivery by a peptide derived from a monoclonal anti-DNA antibody. *Bioconjug. Chem.* **10**, 87–93.
78. Tuchscherer, G., Grell, D., Mathieu, M., and Mutter, M. (1999) Extending the concept of template-assembled synthetic proteins. *J. Pept. Res.* **54**, 185–194.
79. Merritt, E. A. and Hol, W. G. (1995) AB5 toxins. *Curr. Opin. Struct. Biol.* **5**, 165–171.
80. Sandvig, K. and van Deurs, B. (2000) Entry of ricin and Shiga toxin into cells: molecular mechanisms and medical perspectives. *EMBO J* **19**, 5943–5950.
81. Tam, J. P. (1988) Synthetic peptide vaccine design: synthesis and properties of a high-density multiple antigenic peptide system. *Proc. Natl. Acad. Sci. USA* **85**, 5409–5413.
82. Tam, J. P. (1996) Recent advances in multiple antigen peptides. *J Immunol. Meth.* **196**, 17–32.
83. Tam, J. P. and Spetzler, J. C. (1997) Multiple antigen peptide system. *Methods Enzymol.* **289**, 612–637.
84. Plank, C., Tang, M. X., Wolfe, A. R., and Szoka, F. C., Jr. (1999) Branched cationic peptides for gene delivery: role of type and number of cationic residues in formation and in vitro activity of DNA polyplexes [published erratum appears in Hum Gene Ther **10**, 2272 (1999)]. *Hum. Gene Ther.* **10**, 319–332.
85. Brugghe, H. F., Timmermans, H. A., Van Unen, L. M., et al. (1994) Simultaneous multiple synthesis and selective conjugation of cyclized peptides derived from a surface loop of a meningococcal class 1 outer membrane protein. *Int. J. Pept. Protein Res.* **43**, 166–172.
86. Drijfhout, J. W., Bloemhoff, W., Poolman, J. T., and Hoogerhout, P. (1990) Solid-phase synthesis and applications of N-(S-acetylmercaptoacetyl) peptides. *Anal. Biochem.* **187**, 349–354.
87. Drijfhout, J. W. and Bloemhoff, W. (1991) A new synthetic functionalized antigen carrier. *Int. J. Pept. Protein Res.* **37**, 27–32.

9

Design of Prodrugs for Suicide Gene Therapy

Dan Niculescu-Duvaz, Ion Niculescu-Duvaz, and Caroline J. Springer

1. Introduction

A major problem for cancer treatment is the presence of toxic side effects associated with chemotherapeutic agents that limit their efficacy. Alternatively, this can be regarded as the limitation of the dose of drug available to a patient before major general toxicity occurs, with consequent decrease in tumor cell killing and reduced chances of cure. A novel approach designed to circumvent this problem and increase the local concentration of cytotoxic drug at the tumor site with fewer and less drastic systemic side effects is gene-directed enzyme prodrug therapy (GDEPT).

This chapter addresses the design and selection of prodrugs for GDEPT. Several enzyme/prodrug systems have been described and are in different stages of development, from in vitro preclinical studies *(1)* to phase III clinical trials *(2)*. Different enzymes from various sources have been used in conjunction with prodrugs having different mechanisms of activation and action. Despite much chemical diversity, there are a number of common requirements for prodrugs in GDEPT that have been reviewed previously *(3–10)*.

A prodrug designed for a GDEPT system should be a good substrate for the activating enzyme. Favorable characteristics of prodrugs for GDEPT include efficient prodrug activation even at low concentration of prodrug (low K_M) and rapid conversion of the prodrug to the active drug (high k_{cat}) *(3,10)*. The prodrug should not be a substrate for any endogenous enzyme, in order to avoid cytotoxic activation outside the tumor in normal tissues *(5,10)*. Good physiological stability of prodrug is required to prevent premature release of cytotoxic drug or deactivation of the prodrug before it reaches the expressed enzyme. A suitable pharmacokinetic profile in terms of bioavailability, biodistribution, area under the curve (AUC), and half-life in plasma is necessary. The cytotoxicity differential between prodrug and drug should be as high as possible to allow a comfortable therapeutic window. A minimum of 100-fold differential is considered by some authors *(3,10)* to be necessary for significant therapeu-

From: *Methods in Molecular Medicine, Vol. 90, Suicide Gene Therapy: Methods and Reviews*
Edited by: C. J. Springer © Humana Press Inc., Totowa, NJ

tic gains, although lower values have been reported to produce good biological effects *(11–13)*. With the emergence of replicatively competent viral vectors, bacterial vectors, and engineered macrophages, the interaction between prodrug and vector is also a consideration. The prodrug should not release a drug that kills the vector prematurely. On the other hand, prodrugs can be used to control the spread and adverse responses resulting from these new vectors *(14,15)*.

The released drug should also fulfill a number of criteria. Ideally, it should be active against both dividing and quiescent cells *(3,5,16)*. Examples of drugs fulfilling this requirement are: alkylating agents, 6-methylpurine and 2-fluoroadenine *(17,18)*. Its cytotoxicity should be as high as possible in order to overcome potential limitations in prodrug penetration of tumors and in the capacity of the activation mechanism *(19)*. A bystander effect (BE) is compulsory for the drug, as only a percentage of tumor cells will be transfected or transduced and will therefore express the activating enzyme. Following activation of prodrug, the drug has to effect the killing of both the enzyme-expressing and the neighboring non-enzyme-expressing tumor cells. This BE is based on the diffusion or transport of the drug from the formation site to the neighbor cells. A highly diffusible drug is likely to mount a stronger BE. In order to both diffuse freely in the interstitial space and to cross the cells' membranes, the drug should ideally be a neutral, uncharged compound. This last requirement does not apply if a different mechanism of BE or active transport of drug is involved. However, if a drug is too diffusible and stable, leakage into the general circulation will occur, with corresponding systemic toxicity. For this reason, the half-life of the drug should be optimized, in order to achieve the right compromise between tumor diffusion and prevention of systemic escape *(3,10,20)*. A suggested range of suitable half-life is from many seconds to several minutes *(16,21)*. Drugs that are acting directly without the requirement for extra endogenous enzymatic activation steps have an advantage in circumventing potential resistance because of low expression of endogenous enzyme, discussed previously.

The requirements for prodrugs and drugs discussed previously are general and valid also for other targeted enzyme–prodrug therapies [tumor-activated prodrugs *(9)*, bioreductive prodrugs *(19,21–24)* (*see* Chapter 2), antibody-directed enzyme prodrug therapy (ADEPT) *(25,26)* (*see* Chapter 26), and polymer-directed enzyme prodrug therapy (PDEPT) *(27)*].

Some aspects of prodrug design are specific, dependent on the location of the expressed enzyme. For most GDEPT systems reported to date, the enzyme is expressed intracellularly. Consequently, the prodrugs should be able to cross the cell membrane, either by passive diffusion or by active transport. Therefore, the drug generated needs to cross two membranes in order to produce a BE. This could be a drawback, especially for active drugs like ganciclovir triphosphate, which can only be transported between cells by gap junctions. If the expressed enzyme is tethered on the outer membrane of the cells *(12,28,29)* (*see* Chapter 14) or secreted *(28,30)* (*see* Chapter 15), this requirement is waived. The prodrugs should then be hydrophilic or charged, unlike those for internally expressed enzymes. Prodrugs can be used that are deactivated based on cellular exclusion. They are likely to achieve a more substantial BE, but the possibility of drug leakage into the general circulation is higher *(7)*. Even for internally expressed enzymes, the subcellular localization has an influence on the BE, kinetics, and efficiency of cell killing *(31)* and is a factor to be borne in mind in choosing or designing prodrugs.

2. Sources of Prodrugs for GDEPT: Selection and Design

Two ways of developing prodrugs for GDEPT have been investigated so far. The first is based on known prodrugs with various spectra of activity: antiviral [ganciclovir (GCV) *(32)*, acyclovir (ACV) *(33)*, (*E*)-5-(2-bromovinyl)-2'deoxyuridine (BVDU) *(34)*, 6-methoxypurine arabinoside (ara-M) *(35)*], antibacterial [6-methylpurine-2'-deoxyribonucleoside (6-MePdR) *(36)*, 6-thioxanthine (6-TX) *(37)*], antiparasitic [allopurinol *(38)*], antifungal [5-fluorocytosine (5-FC) *(39)*], and antitumoral [5'-deoxy-5-fluorouridine (5'-DFUR) *(40)*, arabinosylcytosine (ara-C) *(41)*, cyclophosphamide and ifosfamide (CP and IF) *(42)*, mitomycin C (MMC) *(43)*, irinotecan (CPT11) *(44)*, edatrexate *(45)*, tirapazamine *(46)*], or compounds that are known to produce toxic metabolites but are poorly—or not—activated in tumors [selenomethionine (SeMet) *(47)*, 4-ipomeanol (4-IP) *(48)*, 2-aminoanthracene (2-AA) *(49)*, 2,4-dinitro-5-aziridinyl-benzamide (CB1954) *(50)*, indole-3-acetic acid (IAA) *(51)*, acetaminophen *(52)*]. Transfection of the tumor with the corresponding activating enzyme achieves the tumor-selective cytotoxic effect.

The first generation of enzyme/prodrug systems used well-known anticancer prodrugs in clinical use. The advantage was that their behavior, kinetics, and pharmacokinetics were already known and some of them are approved as drugs by the regulatory authorities. This was useful for establishing the proof of principle that GDEPT systems were working. Once the proof of principle for the initial enzyme/prodrug pair has been established, this "lead" prodrug can be used as such for preclinical/clinical studies or further development of the prodrug (similar to lead optimization) can be carried out. Two main routes of prodrug optimization have been explored:

- Screening other similar drugs/compounds as potential substrates for the activating enzyme and for improved prodrug profile [e.g., new nucleotides for herpes simplex virus-thymidine kinase (HSV-TK) *(53)* or purine nucleotide phosphorylase (PNP) *(18)*]
- Developing chemistry around the lead prodrug to generate tailored prodrugs with better efficacy in GDEPT [e.g., mustard nitroreductase (NR) prodrugs based on the CB1954 structure *(54)*]

The second route for the generation and development of enzyme/prodrug systems starts from enzymes with no prior prodrug substrate known. However, the specificity for the natural substrates and the structural requirements is well researched. The enzyme should catalyze a reaction with distinct substrate specificity, but should allow modifications in certain parts of the substrate without large alteration of the activation kinetics. This site of accepted variability is exploited either to attach a known drug to the enzyme specifier or to modify the substrate in a convenient way such that it will generate a cytotoxic drug following enzymatic activation. The generation of the initial lead prodrug, as well as further development for optimization, requires *de novo* chemical synthesis. Examples of enzymes for which prodrugs have been designed and synthesized for GDEPT include nitroreductase *(54)*, carboxypeptidase G2 (CPG2) *(55,56)*, β-glucuronidase (β-gluc) *(29)*, β-galactosidase (β-Gal) *(57)*, carboxypeptidase A (CPA) *(28)*, phosphatase *(58)*, and tyrosinase *(59)*. The generated drugs are nitrogen mustards *(54,55,60,61)*, anthracyclines *(29,56,57)*, etoposide *(58)*, methotrexate *(28,62)*, enediyenes *(63)*, amino-*seco*-CBI-TMI *(64)*, and pyrrolobenzodiazepines *(65)*.

The border between these two approaches is not always well defined. For example, the main prodrug used for NR, CB1954, was first discovered and used as an alkylating agent. Its propensity as an NR substrate was discovered later *(66)*, and further design and syntheses of prodrugs for GDEPT, some with very different structures from the lead compound, were carried out *(54,63)*. The prodrugs targeted to tyrosinase, now proposed as a GDEPT system, were first developed as compounds for the treatment of melanoma *(67–71)*.

Prodrug development has also been carried out for therapies that are alternative enzyme-directed prodrug therapies to GDEPT. Examples are CPG2, CPA, NR, β-Gal, β-gluc, and phosphatase, all of which were previously employed for antibody-directed enzyme prodrug therapy (ADEPT) *(26)* (*see* Chapter 26), tyrosinase for melanoma-directed enzyme prodrug therapy (MDEPT) *(70,71)*, and DT-diaphorase, P450 reductase and NR for bioreductive prodrugs *(23,24,72)* (*see* Chapter 27). Some of these prodrugs have already been used in GDEPT and the potential application of the others has been suggested. With the advent of the secreted and surface-tethered enzymes, the prodrugs developed for ADEPT become suitable for GDEPT. Therefore, although not reviewed in depth, some of this prodrug development work will be mentioned to illustrate common aspects of prodrug design. In order to optimize the profile and expand the range of prodrugs for a GDEPT system, either screening of known compounds/drugs or tailoring the prodrug to overcome potential shortcomings (low differential, insufficient cytotoxicity of the released drug, poor kinetics of activation, pharmacological profile, etc.) can be carried out.

3. Current Enzyme/Prodrug System for GDEPT

Recently, a table containing the main 20 GDEPT systems was published *(73)* (*see also* Chapter 1). A few further systems are alkaline phosphatase/etoposide phosphate, releasing etoposide *(58)*, horseradish peroxidase/indole-3-acetic acid *(1)*, tyrosinase/hydroxyphenylpropanol and *N*-acetyl-4-*S*-cysteaminylphenol *(59)*, linamarase/linamarin, releasing hydrogen cyanide *(74)*, and folylpolyglutamyl synthetase/edatrexate, producing edatrexate polyglutamate *(75,76)*.

4. Tailored Prodrugs for GDEPT

There are several advantages in designing specific prodrugs for a GDEPT system over using known drugs:

- There is potentially a much larger range of drugs that can be released from prodrugs, with different mechanisms of action suitable for a particular cancer type.
- The parameters required for an efficient GDEPT prodrug can be optimized by systematic chemical derivatization, crystallographic studies, and quantitative structure-activity relationships (QSAR); such parameters are: cytotoxicity differential, stability, kinetics of activation, lipophilicity/transport inside the cells, the bystander effect, and pharmacological profile.

Many tailored prodrugs for GDEPT try to take advantage of both types of approach. The prodrug is derived from a known antitumor drug, modified to become deactivated and a substrate for the foreign enzyme. Examples are anthracyclines, 5-fluorouracil, methotrexate, and etoposide prodrugs. Other prodrugs have a more radical design: both the prodrug and the released drug are new entities with respect to clinical use. This category takes advantage of cytotoxic moieties that cannot be used as systemic drugs because of undesired side effects, but that become relatively nontoxic following suitable derivatization to prodrug. Activation of these prodrugs by the expressed enzyme releases the cytotoxic moiety locally, at the tumor site, minimizing side effects. Examples of this class are alkylating agents, pyrrolobenzodiazepines, enedyines, and amino-*seco*-cyclopropylindoles.

5. Classification of Prodrugs According to the Enzymatic Reaction of Activation

Prodrugs can be activated by several types of enzymatic reaction.

5.1. Reactions Catalyzed by Hydrolases

5.1.1. Hydrolytic Scission

Several GDEPT systems rely on the hydrolysis of an amide, carbamate, urea, glycosidic ether, or phosphoric ester bond in the prodrug to generate a toxic drug (*see* **Figs. 1–4**). The popularity of this reaction for GDEPT is due to the ease of drug deactivation by acylation, alkylation, or phosphorylation. A requirement is the presence of a "handle" functional group that allows the attachment of the enzyme specifier. The most common "handles" for functional groups are: amino, hydroxy (alcohol or phenol), and carboxy. Concomitant with the attachment role, the functional group conjugation should deactivate the drug.

Deactivation by conversion of a carboxyl group to an amide was used to generate prodrugs for CPG2 and CPA (*see* **Fig. 1**). Following activation by CPG2, the electron-withdrawing amide (Hammett constant, $\sigma_p=0.38$) of the benzoic acid mustard prodrug N-{4-[(2-chloroethyl)(2-mesyloxyethyl)amino]benzoyl}-L-glutamic acid (CMDA) was converted to the electron donating negatively charged carboxylate ($\sigma_p=-0.20$), increasing the electron density at the *para* nitrogen and consequently activating the nitrogen mustard *(77)*. For CPA, the cleavage of the dipeptide bond in MTX-α-Phe prodrug releases methotrexate (MTX), which inhibits dihydrofolate reductase *(78)*.

It was found that a urea or a carbamate linkage between glutamic acid and an aromatic nucleus could also be cleaved by CPG2 *(79)*. This property has been used to generate prodrugs from the more potent 4-amino and 4-hydroxy nitrogen mustards (*see* **Fig. 2**) *(20)*. Another example of carbamate cleavage to generate a toxic phenol drug is the activation of irinotecan to the toxic metabolite SN38 by rabbit carboxylesterase (*see* **Fig. 2**) *(80)*.

The conversion of phenols and alcohols to phosphate esters is one of the most commonly used methods to increase the solubility of drugs. Cleavage by various phosphatases regenerates the active drugs. This strategy was used in one of the first examples of ADEPT *(81)*, and etoposide phosphate was also proposed for GDEPT *(58)* (*see* **Fig. 3**).

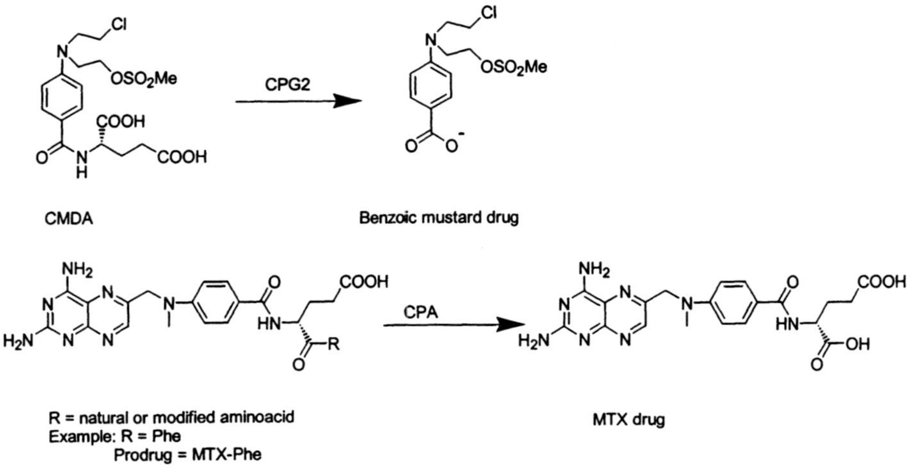

CMDA   Benzoic mustard drug

R = natural or modified aminoacid   MTX drug
Example: R = Phe
         Prodrug = MTX-Phe

Fig. 1. Prodrugs activated by hydrolysis of an amide bond.

Prodrugs for glycosidases such as β-glucuronidase, α-galactosidase, and linamarase have been synthesized for ADEPT and GDEPT. The specifying carbohydrate is linked directly or via a linker to the hydroxy or amino group of the drug. The hydroxy group can be aliphatic (82), aromatic [from a phenol nitrogen mustard (83)] (see Fig. 4), or hemiacetal (as in the cyanhydrine functionality of the linamarase prodrug) (74). The amino group is connected as a carbamate directly or via a self-immolative linker (84).

5.1.2. Hydrolytic Functional Group Transformation

The hydrolysis of the amino group of 5-fluorocytosine (5-FC) to a hydroxy group by cytosine deaminase converts the nontoxic 5-FC prodrug to the anticancer drug 5-fluorouracil (5-FU) (see Fig. 5) (85).

5.2. Activation by Nucleoside Phosphorylation

Modified nucleoside prodrugs are converted by the expressed enzyme to nucleoside monophosphate (NMP) and then by endogenous enzymes to nucleoside triphosphate (NTP), generally the ultimate active drugs (see Fig. 6). NTPs are used as substrates for polymerases, being inserted in DNA/RNA where they act as terminators for chain elongation. Other mechanisms of action have also been suggested—for example, involvement of mitogen-activated protein (MAP) kinase (86), Fas/FasL-mediated apoptosis (87), and thymidine synthase (TS) inhibition. Potential onset of resistance as a result of the low activity of endogenous kinases can be circumvented by coexpressing further enzymes in the NMP to NTP pathway (e.g., guanylate cyclase) (88).

Example of nucleoside prodrugs activated by phosphorylation are presented in **Fig. 6**.

5.3. Activation by Reductases

The main three chemical classes activated by reduction are nitroaromatics, quinones, and N-oxides. Reduction of an aromatic nitro group to hydroxylamino is per-

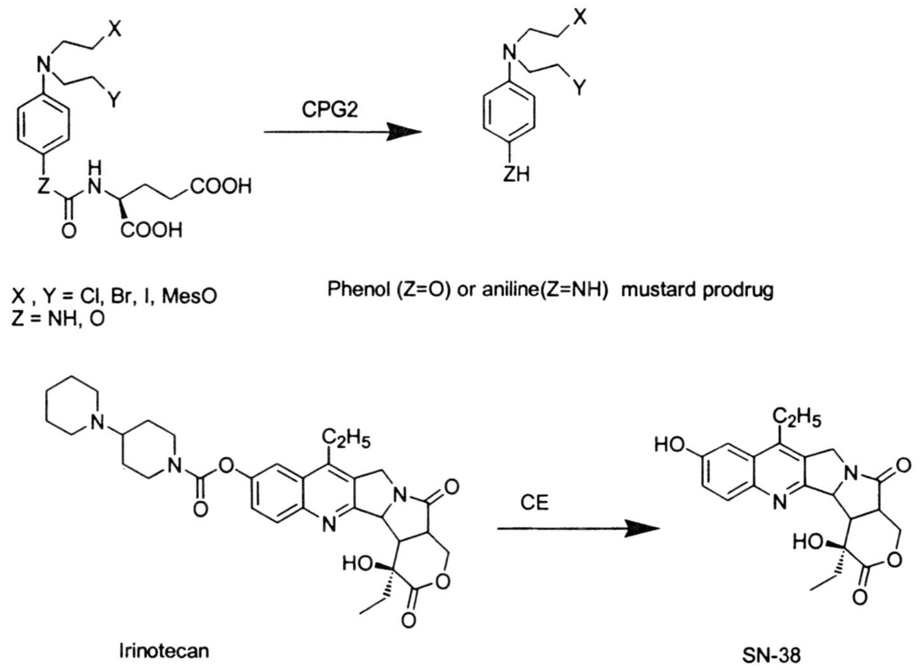

X , Y = Cl, Br, I, MesO   Phenol (Z=O) or aniline(Z=NH) mustard prodrug
Z = NH, O

Irinotecan   SN-38

Fig. 2. Prodrugs activated by hydrolysis of a carbamate or urea bond.

formed efficiently by *E. coli* NR, much faster than the human DT-diaphorase *(66)*. The formation of –NHOH acts as an electronic switch from the electron-withdrawing nitro to the electron-donating –NHOH, activating effectors such as nitrogen mustards *(54)* or triggering fragmentation of self-immolative prodrugs with the generation of active drug. Another role of the –NHOH group formed is to generate the second alkylating moiety, converting a weakly monoalkylating prodrug CB1954 to a potent difunctional metabolite (*see* **Fig. 7**).

Reduction of quinones by DT-diaphorase can be a one-electron or two-electron process. Mitomycin C (MMC) activated by DT-diaphorase has been proposed for GDEPT. Upon reduction of MMC by either mechanism, DNA damage and alkylation occurs (*see* **Fig. 8**) *(72)*.

N-oxides can also be reduced to reactive intermediates or active drugs. A one-electron reduction of tirapazamine by DT-diaphorase or P450 reductase generates a TPZ radical, which abstracts a hydrogen from DNA, inducing single- and double-strand breaks (*see* **Fig. 9**) *(72)*.

Another N-oxide prodrug, AQ4N, has a different mechanism of activation. The N-oxide in AQ4N serves both to mask the basicity of the two tertiary amino groups, potential sites of interaction with DNA, and to ensure exclusion of prodrug from cells. Following four-electrons reduction, the drug AQ4 is a potent topoisomerase II inhibitor (*see* **Fig. 9**) *(9)*.

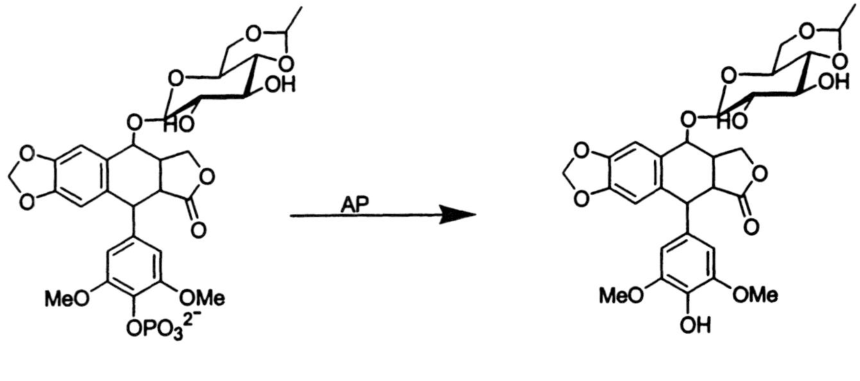

Etoposide phosphate   Etoposide

Fig. 3. Prodrugs activated by hydrolysis of a phosphate ester bond.

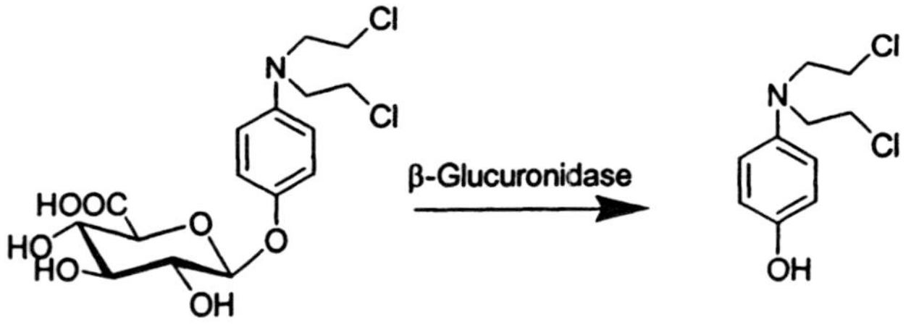

Cleavage of glycosyl phenol prodrug   Phenol nitrogen mustard

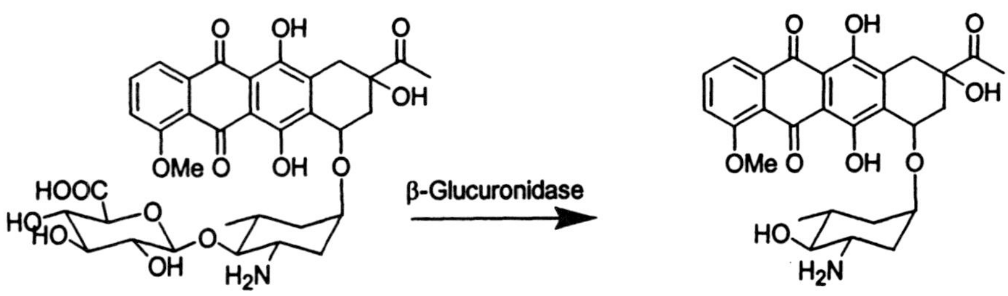

Cleavage of glycosyl alcohol prodrug   Epirubicin

Fig. 4. Prodrugs activated by hydrolysis of an aromatic or aliphatic glycosyl bond.

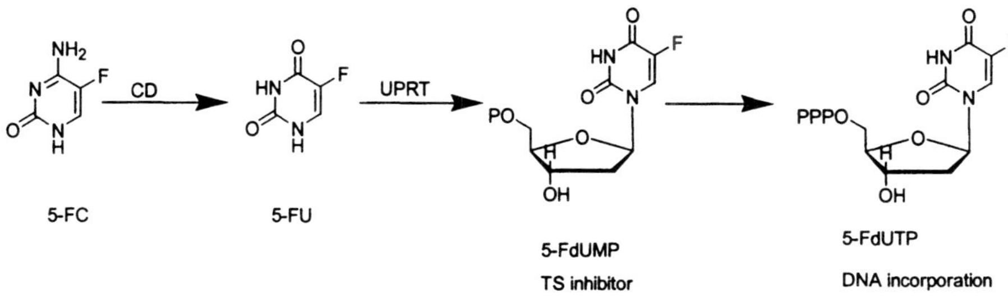

Fig. 5. Activation of 5-FU by hydrolytic group conversion.

Both, tirapazamine (TPZ) *(89)* and AQ4N *(23)* have been proposed as prodrugs for the cytochrome P450/P450 reductase GDEPT system in combination with cyclophosphamide.

5.4. Activation by Oxidases

A heterogenous range of substrates has been proposed as prodrugs activated by oxidation. The main oxidative enzymes used in GDEPT are cytochrome P450, horseradish peroxidase, and D-amino acids oxidase.

Cyclophosphamide (CP) and ifosfamde (IF) are activated by C-hydroxylation. The 4-hydroxy-CP or -IF are unstable and fragment with the formation of acrolein and phosphoramide mustard, a DNA alkylating agent *(17)*. Ipomeanol is activated by formation of an epoxide and subsequent DNA alkylation *(90)*. 2-Aminoanthracene and *p*-acetaminophen *(52)* are activated by formation of reactive quinones (*see* **Fig. 10**).

A plant hormone, 2-indoleacetic acid, was found to generate toxic species when activated by horseradish peroxidase (radicals under anoxic conditions, α,β-unsaturated Michael acceptors in oxic conditions). The system is currently being investigated for GDEPT (*see* **Fig. 11**) *(1)*.

Oxidation of D-amino acids (e.g., D-alanine) by D-amino acids oxidase produce H_2O_2. In the presence of traces of metal ions present in the cells, H_2O_2 forms highly cytotoxic hydroxyl radicals that are reactive with DNA, lipids, and proteins *(91)*.

5.5. Ribosyl Transfer

This reversible reaction has been employed in GDEPT in two ways. Transfer of ribosyl to 6-thioguanine has been achieved by xanthine-guanine phosphoribosyltransferase (XGPRT) to generate a toxic nucleotide (*see* **Fig. 12**) *(92)*. Removal of ribosyl from relatively nontoxic nucleosides by purine nucleotide phosphorylases generates a toxic purine (6-Me-purine, 2-F-adenine) (*see* **Fig. 12**) *(18)*.

5.6. Prodrugs Activated by α,β-Elimination

This reaction is catalyzed by lyases. In GDEPT, methioninase have been used to generate the toxic methylselenol from selenomethionine (*see* **Fig. 13**) *(93)*.

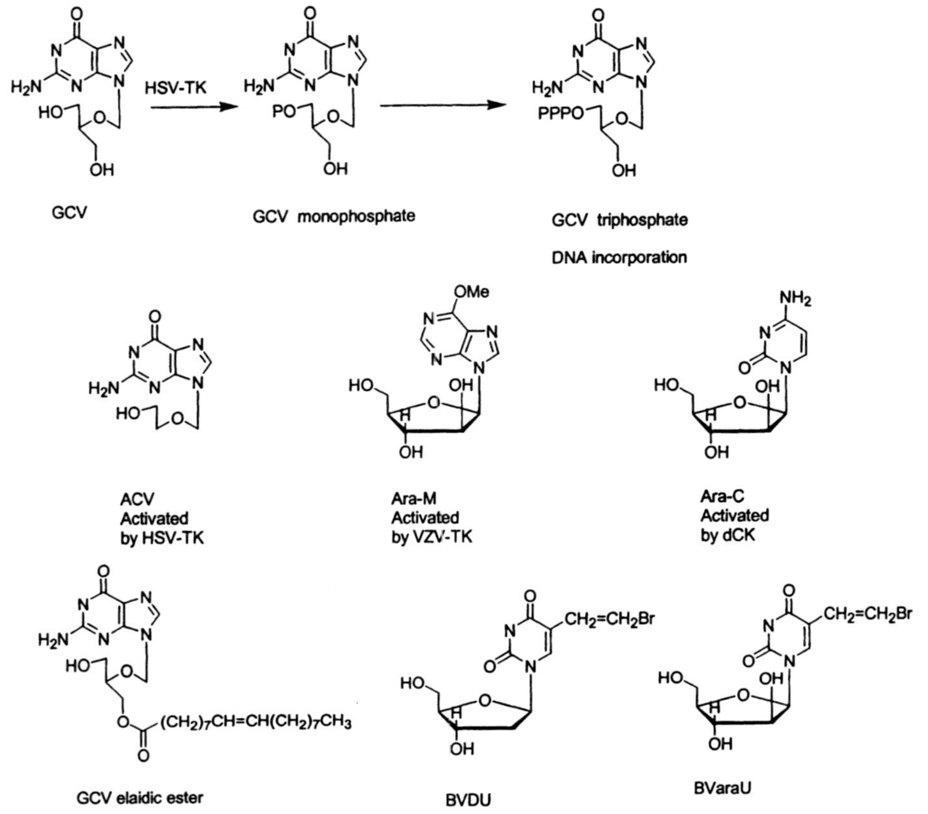

GCV   GCV monophosphate

GCV triphosphate

DNA incorporation

ACV
Activated
by HSV-TK

Ara-M
Activated
by VZV-TK

Ara-C
Activated
by dCK

GCV elaidic ester

BVDU

BVaraU

Fig. 6. Prodrugs activated by phosphorylation.

6. Direct Prodrugs and Self-Immolative Prodrugs

The general structure of a prodrug has been described using a modular model. The prodrugs are formed from a trigger, a linker, and an effector. The trigger provides specificity and is metabolized by the expressed enzyme. The linker deactivates the effector until the trigger is metabolized and transmits the effect of activation from trigger to effector. The effector is the active drug *(19)*.

According to the mechanism of drug release, the prodrugs can be classified into two classes:

- Direct prodrugs
- Self-immolative prodrugs or pro-prodrugs

A similar classification has been proposed by Carl et al. *(94)* in bipartate and tripartate prodrugs.

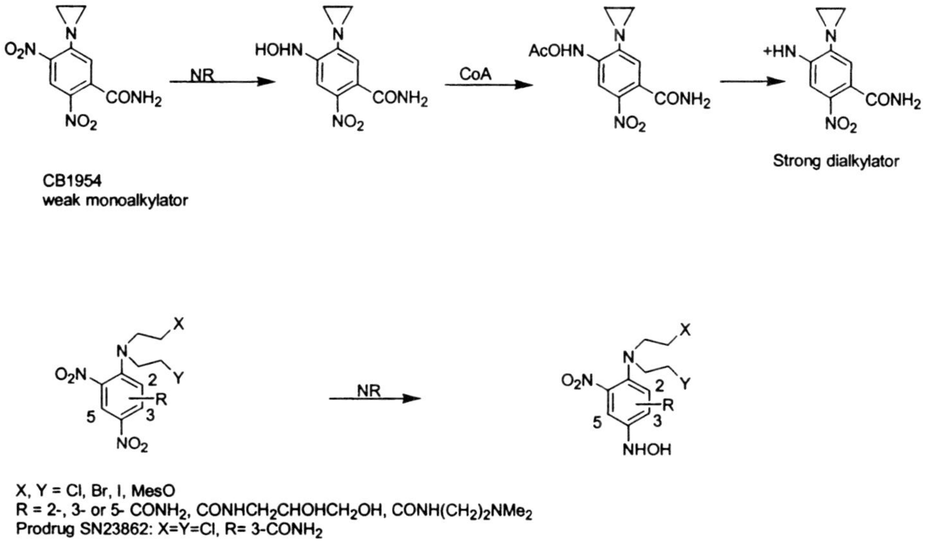
NR
CoA
CB1954
weak monoalkylator
Strong dialkylator
NR
X, Y = Cl, Br, I, MesO
R = 2-, 3- or 5- CONH2, CONHCH2CHOHCH2OH, CONH(CH2)2NMe2
Prodrug SN23862: X=Y=Cl, R= 3-CONH2

Fig. 7. Prodrugs activated by reduction of a nitro group by nitroreductase.

6.1. Direct Prodrugs

The direct prodrugs are prodrugs for which the enzymatic activation and the formation of active drug coincide. The activation of the prodrug is a one-step mechanism. For these prodrugs, the linker is missing (e.g., ganciclovir) or is part of the effector (e.g., CB1954). Most of the prodrugs described so far in this chapter are direct prodrugs.

The activation of direct prodrugs can occur in two ways:

1. Functional group modification, where the trigger/specifier moiety is converted by the enzyme but remains attached forming part of the active drug. The reduction of the 4-nitro group in prodrug SN23862 (*see* **Fig. 7**) generates the more cytotoxic 4-amino or 4-hydroxylamino mustard. Following activation, the deactivating group that was formerly the nitro remains part of the drug as the activating amino or hydroxylamino moiety. Phosphorylation of a hydroxy group in a series of nucleoside-like prodrugs generates monophosphate substrates for endogenous kinases. Hydrolytic deamination of 5-fluorocytosine generates the drug 5-fluorouracil, differing from 5-FC by the 4-hydroxy group instead of 4-amino. Oxidation of ipomeanol by CYP450 produces a reactive epoxide on the furan ring, responsible for alkylation of cellular nucleophiles.
2. Cleavage of the specifier with release of drug. For direct prodrugs, the specifier also has the role of deactivating the drug until cleavage. This method has been used to convert known drugs to prodrugs by attaching the drugs to an enzyme specifier. Examples of such specifiers are β-glucuronyl for β-glucuronidase, β-galactosyl for β-galactosidase, glutamate for CPG2, phosphate for phosphatases, and various amino acids for CPA.

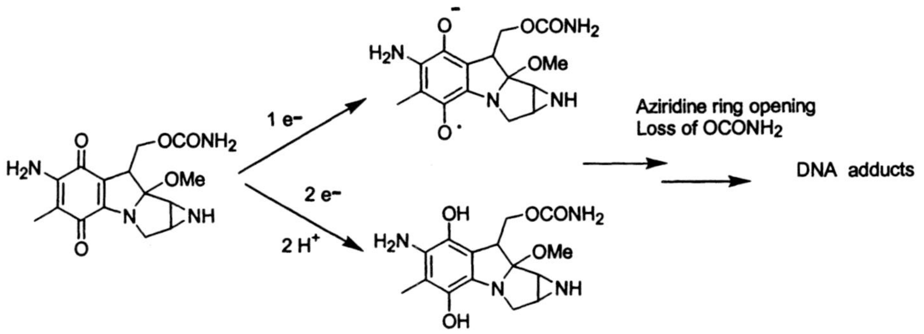

Fig. 8. Mitomycin C activated by reduction of a quinone by DT-diaphorase.

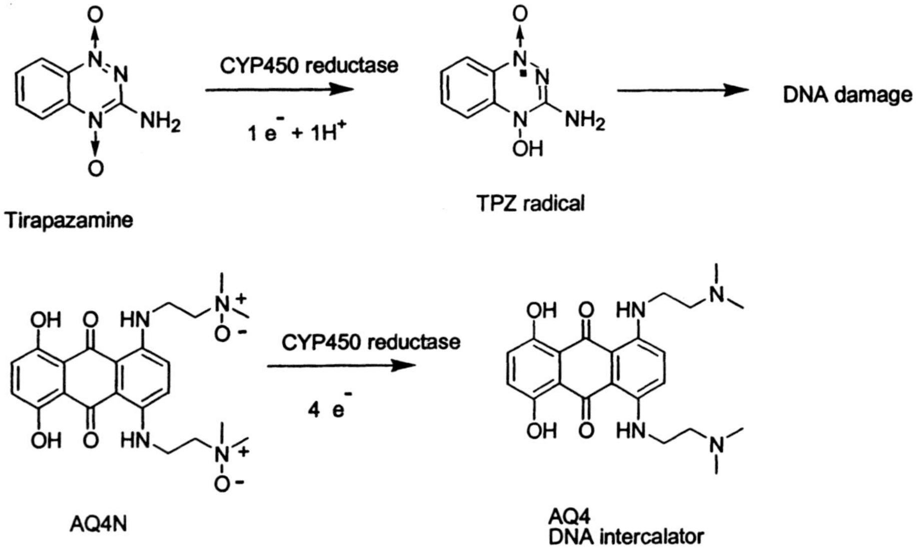

Fig. 9. Prodrugs activated by reduction of N-oxides by CYP450 reductase.

A potential problem with direct prodrugs is the rather strict substrate structural requirements for some of the activating enzymes. For CPG2, the glutamic acid must be connected to an aromatic ring, via an amide, urea, or carbamate linkage. The substitution allowed on the aromatic ring without drastic decrease in kinetics of activation is quite limited. This narrows the range of suitable drugs that fulfill the structural requirements of CPG2 that can be made into substrates for the enzyme. Aromatic nitrogen mustards are an example of drugs that can be converted to prodrugs for CPG2.

Even for enzymes with a broader acceptance of substrates, another potential problem is the slow kinetics of activation because of the proximity of the bulky drug to the

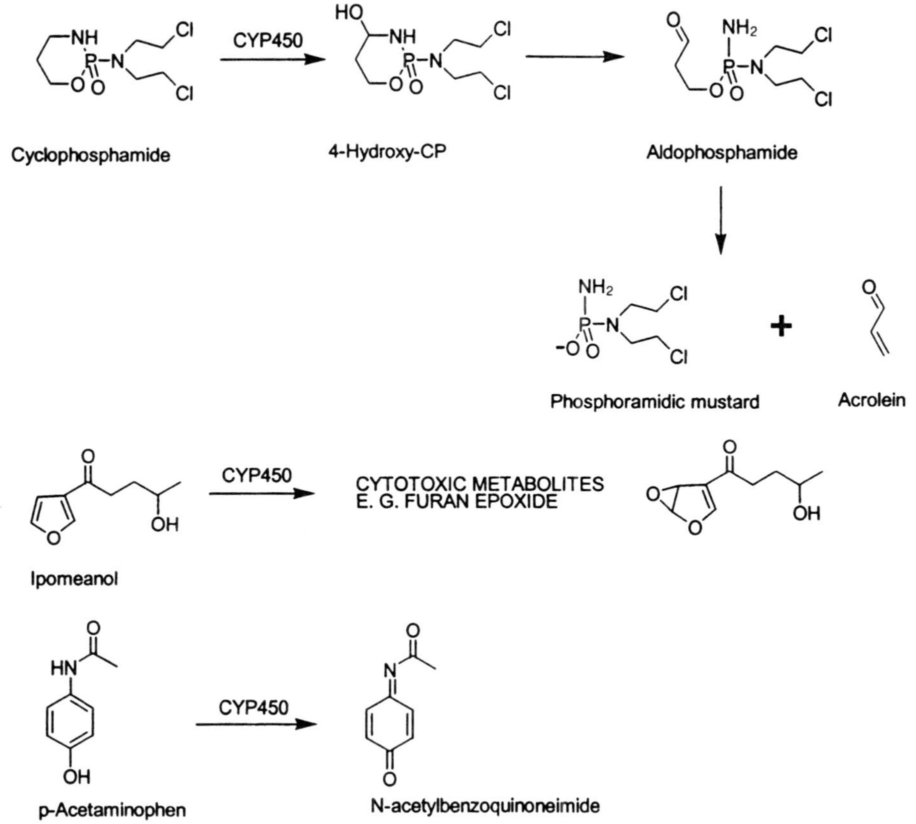

Fig. 10. Prodrugs activated by oxidation by cytochrome P450 isoforms.

specifier. A strategy to expand the range of suitable prodrugs for a given enzyme or to improve the kinetics of activation is to use self-immolative prodrugs.

6.2. Self-Immolative Prodrugs

A self-immolative prodrug can be defined as a compound that following activation by an enzyme, generates an unstable intermediate, which spontaneously extrudes the active drug in a number of subsequent steps. The following elements are important in defining the concept: (1) the activation process is generally of enzymatic nature and is distinct from the drug extrusion step; (2) the drug is generated by an extrusion process (following fragmentation of prodrug); (3) the site of activation is separated from the site of extrusion.

The potential advantages of self-immolative prodrugs vs direct prodrugs include the improvement of unfavorable kinetics of enzymatic activation of a prodrug because of unsuitable electronic or steric features of the drug linked to the specifier moiety, better stability of linkage between drug and specifier (*94*), and a wider range of drugs

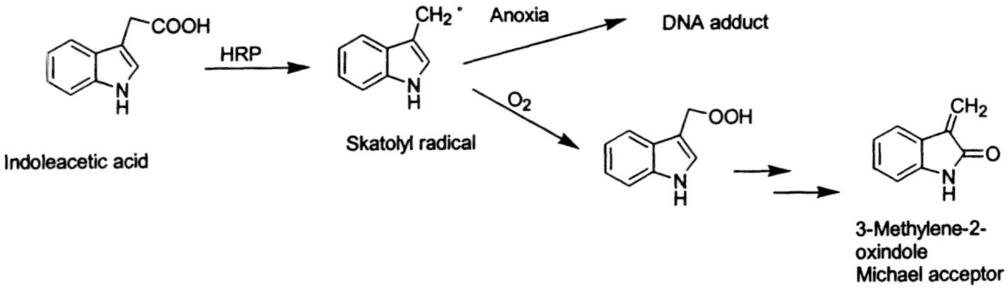

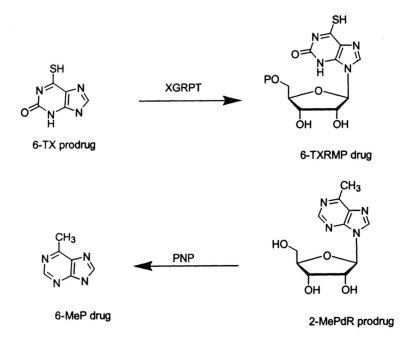

Fig. 11. Activation of indoleacetic acid by peroxidation with horseradish peroxidase.

Fig. 12. Prodrugs activated by ribosyl transfer.

that can be converted into prodrugs for a given activating system unrestricted by the structural substrate requirement of the enzyme.

Several types of self-immolative process can be distinguished based on the extrusion mechanism. The most commonly used in the design of prodrugs for GDEPT are 1,6-elimination, 1,4-elimination, and intramolecular cyclization.

The most used triggering processes for self-immolation are reduction and hydrolytic cleavage.

6.2.1. Prodrugs Fragmenting by 1,6-Elimination

1,6-Eliminaton is characteristic for benzylic systems. It requires an electron-donating substituent in the 4-position with respect to the benzylic methylene bearing a leav-

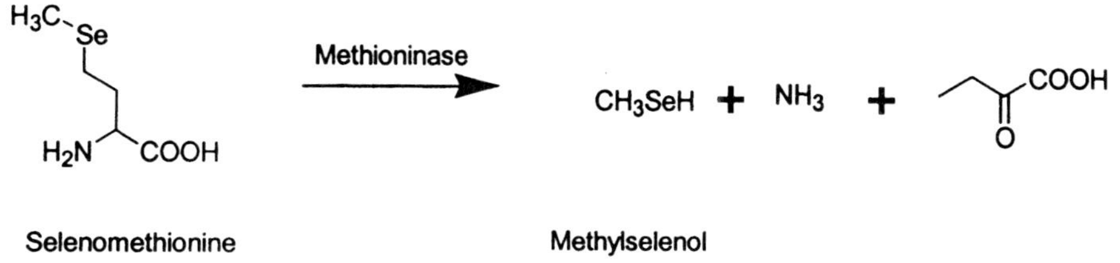

Fig. 13. Activation of selenomethionine by α,β-elimination.

ing group. The high reactivity of the benzylic position, *para*-substituted with hydroxy or amino groups is the result of the strong electron-donating ability of these substituents that trigger a 1,6-elimination with the formation of *para*-quinone methide or iminoquinone methide *(95)*.

Reduction of 4-nitrobenzyl prodrugs to 4-amino or 4-hydroxylaminobenzyl by NR transforms a stabilizing electron-withdrawing group into a electron-donating one, with consequent fragmentation and release of cytotoxic drugs. This system has been used to produce prodrugs from enediynes *(63)*, *seco*-amino-cyclopropylindoles *(64)*, and pyrrolobenzodiazepines *(65)* for GDEPT with NR. The same system for ADEPT with NR was used to release aliphatic and aromatic nitrogen mustards, actinomycin D, mytomycin C *(96)*, and tallimustine *(97)* (*see* **Fig. 14**).

Reduction of azide to amino and disulfide to thiol have also been proposed as reductive triggering processes for self-immolative release of drugs. The finding that CPG2 can cleave ureas and carbamates as well as amides led to the design of self-immolative nitrogen mustard and anthracycline prodrugs *(55,56)*. The nitrogen mustard prodrugs are stabilized by deactivation of the *para* amino or hydroxy of the linker as urea or carbamate. Following cleavage by CPG2 and subsequent spontaneous decomposition of the carbamic or carbonic acid formed with loss of CO_2, the electron density on the para substituent is restored, leading to 1,6-elimination and drug generation (*see* **Fig. 15**).

In self-immolative prodrugs for β-glucuronidase and α- and β-galactosidase, the anthracycline moiety is connected to the glycosyl specifier via an optionally substituted benzylic phenol or aniline. The phenol is masked in the prodrug as a glycosidic ether *(57,98)* and the aniline linker as carbamate *(84,99)*. Cleavage of the glycosidic bond triggers the self-immolative process (*see* **Fig. 16**).

6.2.2. Prodrugs Fragmenting by 1,4-Elimination

Anthracycline prodrugs for β-glucuronidase and β-galactosidase similar to those described earlier, but with a 2-amino- or 2-hydroxybenzylic instead of 4-amino- or 4-hydroxybenzylic linker have been synthesized *(98,99)*. These linkers are fragmenting by 1,4-elimination. However, these prodrugs are poorer substrates for the activating enzymes, probably the result of the closer proximity of the anthracycline to the glycosyl (*see* **Fig. 16**).

Another example is provided by β-lactamase prodrugs. Hydrolysis of the lactam bond releases the electron-donating endocyclic amine, which pushes a pair of elec-

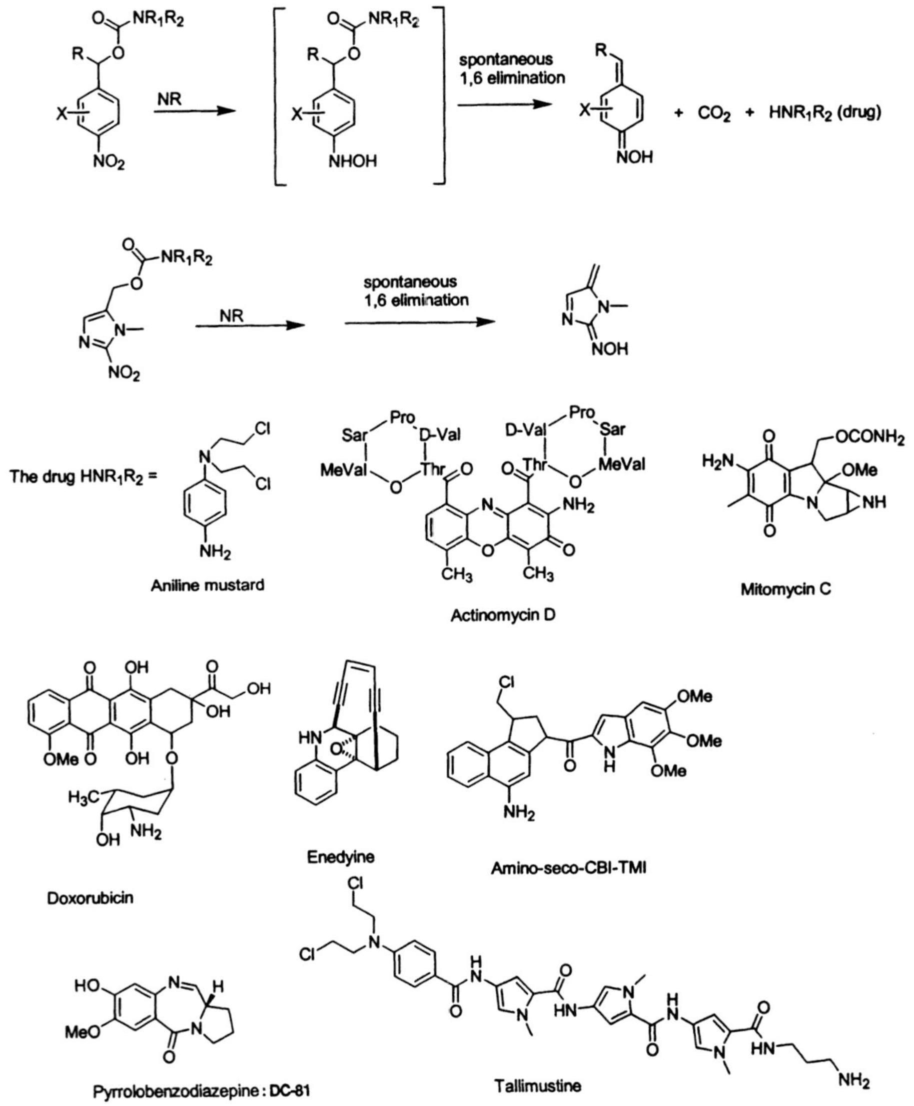

Fig. 14. Self-Immolative prodrugs activated by reduction of a nitro group by NR.

trons through the conjugated bond, leading to expulsion of the exocyclic methylene-bound leaving group (*see* **Fig. 17**).

Several β-lactamase prodrugs have been developed for ADEPT to release aliphatic *(100)* and aromatic nitrogen mustards *(101)*, vinca alkaloids *(102)*, anthracyclines *(103)*, and platinum compounds *(104)*. Recently, this system has been proposed for GDEPT *(105)*.

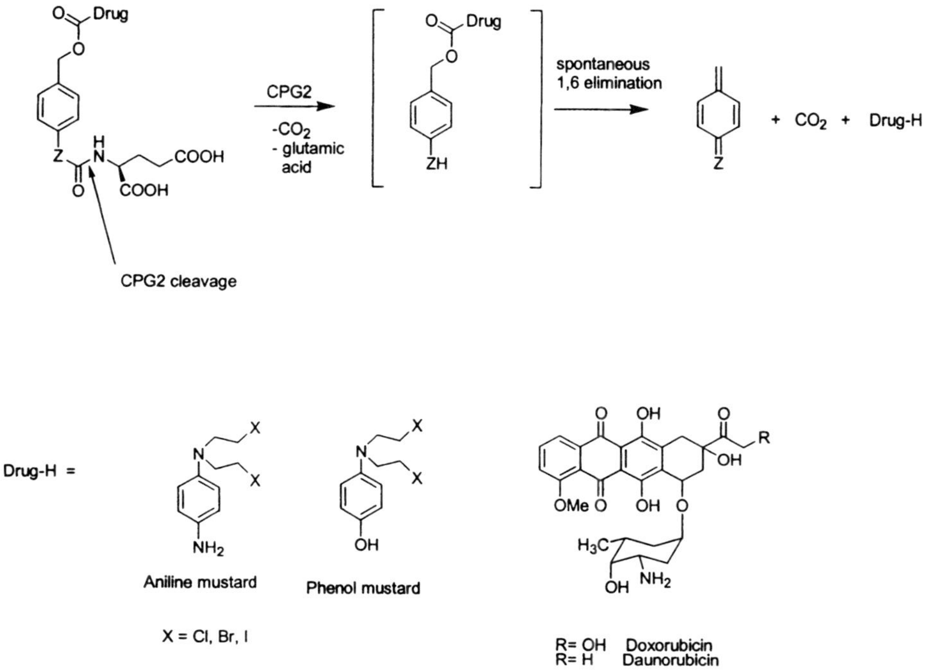

Fig. 15. Self-immolative prodrugs activated by CPG2.

6.2.3. Prodrugs Fragmenting by 1,2-Elimination

The first self-immolative anticancer prodrug, although not described as such when it was introduced into the clinic, is cyclophosphamide. The triggering process for its activation is the 4-hydroxylation by cytochrome P450, generating a hemiacetal. In a first 1,2-elimination step, the cyclic hemiacetal converts to the open aldophosphamide. The α-proton (with respect to the aldehyde) becomes acidic and is removed in a second 1,2-elimination step with generation of toxic phosphoramide mustard (*see* **Fig. 10**).

6.2.4. Prodrugs Fragmenting by Cyclization

There is a wealth of self-immolative prodrugs activated by cyclization. The general principle is the formation of a nucleophilic, electron-rich group (such as amino, hydroxylamino, hydroxy) in a sterically constrained position with respect to an entropically favorable carboxylic or carbonic acid derivative of the drug. The nucleophilic attack of the newly formed nucleophile on the acyl group with elimination of drug moiety would generate a stable five- or six-membered ring in an intramolecular process. A combination of entropic and energetic factors concurs to drive the process toward drug elimination, once the required starting nucleophile is formed. An example proposed for GDEPT is based on the reduction of 2-(2,6-dinitro phenyl)amino-propanamide to a hydroxylamine derivative, followed by cyclization with extrusion of a drug *(106)*. (**Fig. 18D**). The entropic factor here is increased by hydrogen-bonding between the

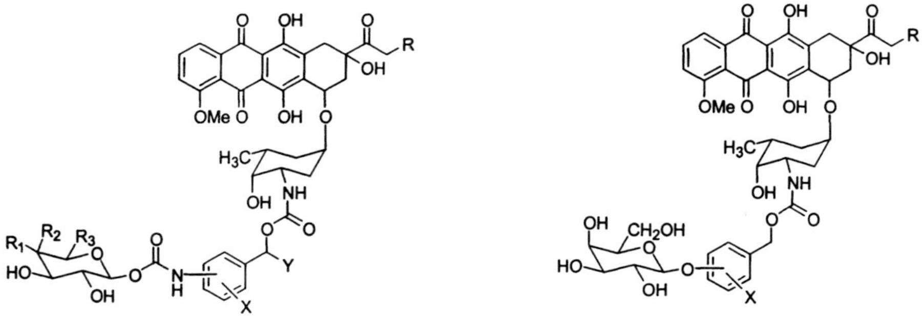

R = H (daunorubicin), OH (doxorubicin)
R₁ = H, R₂ = OH or R₁ = OH, R₂ = H
R₃ = CH₂OH, COOH
X = ortho- or para- Cl, Br
Y = H, C₆H₁₃

X = ortho- or para-Cl, NO₂

Fig. 16. Self-immolative prodrugs activated by glycosidases.

aromatic N-H and the vicinal nitro group, locking the amide in a conformation favorable to cyclization. Aniline mustards and amino-*seco*-cyclopropylindole compounds have been used has drugs. Unfortunately, the prodrugs are poor substrates for NR. Several other self-immolative prodrugs activated via cyclization have been proposed for ADEPT [e.g., taxol prodrugs *(107)*] and can potentially be used for GDEPT. Examples of prodrug structures releasing the drug via cyclization are presented in **Fig. 18**.

6.3. The General Structure of a Self-Immolative Prodrug

An example of self-immolative prodrug activated by CPG2 via 1,6-elimination is presented in **Fig. 19**. Several elements can be distinguished in a self-immolative prodrug, such as: specifier moiety, trigger, linker, linker–drug bond, and drug.

A summary of the component elements of the self-immolative prodrugs proposed for GDEPT is described in **Table 1**.

1. Specifier moiety. The moiety provides the specificity for the expressed enzyme. It is present in both direct and self-immolative prodrugs. The specifier moieties used so far in GDEPT are presented in **Table 1**.

2. Triggers: The triggering processes have been discussed in some detail earlier. The main triggers are glycosyl ether, urea, and carbamate (cleaved by hydrolysis), nitro (activated by reduction), and aromatic or aliphatic carbon (activated by hydroxylation) (*see* **Table 1**).

3. Linkers. The linker separates the specifier moiety from the drug and is responsible for the drug extrusion by different mechanisms during the second step. The linker–drug fragment resulted after enzymatic activation is inherently unstable, breaking down with the release of the drug. However, the kinetics of fragmentation is dependent on the structure of the linker, the substituents, and the type of extrusion process. For linkers that release the drug via 1,6- and 1,4-elimination, the kinetics is usually faster than the first enzymatic step. For linkers based on through-space cyclization, it can be quite slow and become the rate-determining step. Improvement to linkers targeted the kinetics of enzymatic activation, the fine-tuning of fragmentation rate following activation, the stability of the prodrug and the pharmacokinetic properties:

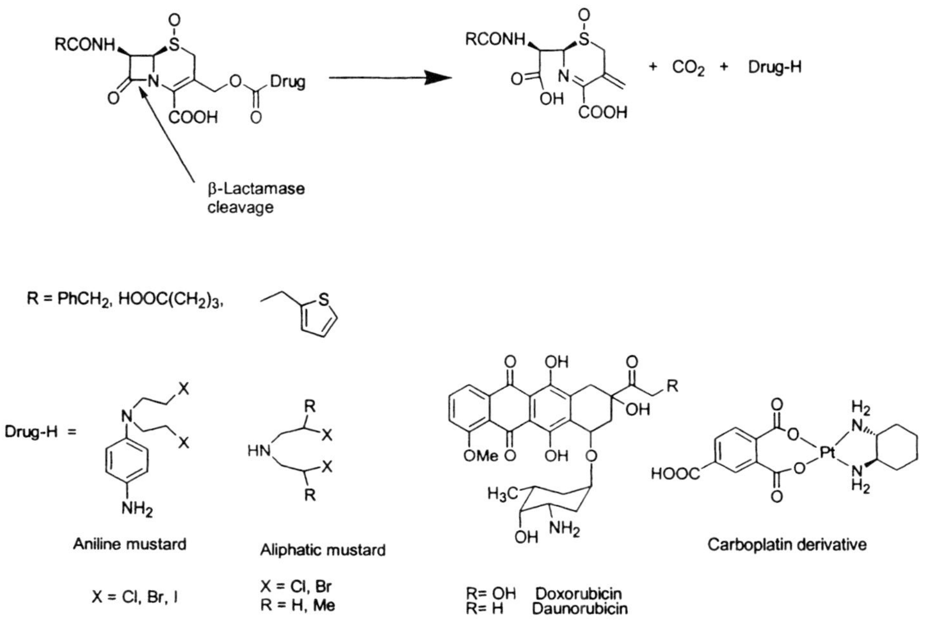

Fig. 17. Self-immolative prodrugs for activation by β-lactamase.

a. The linkers and the kinetics of enzymatic activation. The introduction of a linker has been found in some cases to increase the rate of enzymatic activation. The enzymatic hydrolysis was quite ineffective when galactose was directly bound to the 14-OH of doxorubicin through a classical glycosidic linkage. Introduction of a nitro-substituted linker between galactose and the amino group of doxorubicin greatly improved the kinetics (98). However, this is not always the case. For example, the self-immolative prodrugs of aromatic nitrogen mustard for CPG2 (55) have poorer kinetics of activation than the direct prodrugs (20).

Often, linkers that fragment by 1,4-elimination have slower kinetics of enzymatic activation than those following a 1,6-elimination pathway (98,99).

b. The effect of the substituents. A few systematic studies have been undertaken on the effect of the substitution pattern on the rate of fragmentation of the unstable linker drug intermediate. For anthracycline–spacer–β-glucuronyl prodrugs (see Fig. 16), where the 4-aminobenzyl linker is connected to glucuronyl via a carbamate linkage, the rate of release of prodrug is very similar for unsubstituted or 2-Cl-, 2-Br-, 3-Cl-, or 3-Br-substituted para-benzylic linkers (about 100 min). The ortho-benzylic linker is slower (about 900 min). This difference is most likely because of slower enzymatic activation rather than slower fragmentation (99). However, these values (100 min and 900 min) do not reflect the true rate of fragmentation, which is faster than the rate of enzymatic cleavage. The direct influence of the substituents on the fragmentation rate was measured using the radiolytic reduction of nitrobenzyl carbamates as model prodrugs (108). The real rate of fragmentation, triggered by the conversion of nitro to hydroxylamino was one order of magnitude faster, in the range of 10 min. The release

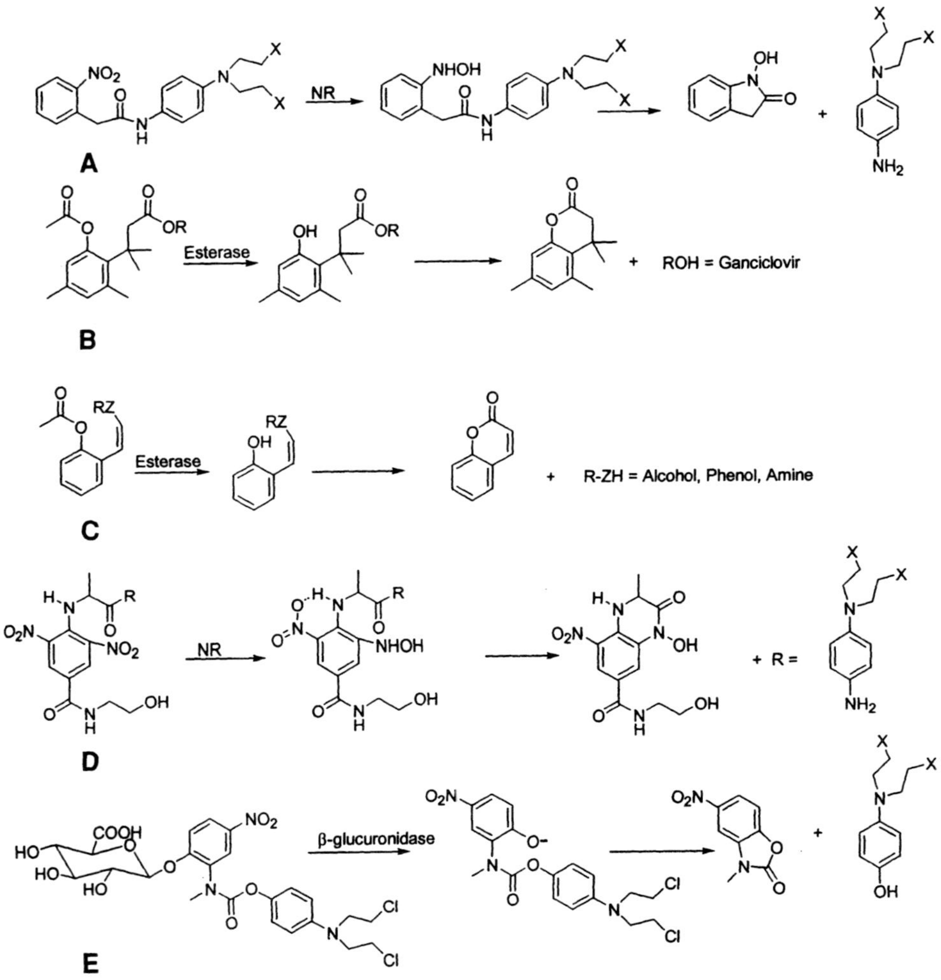

Fig. 18. Self-immolative prodrugs activated by cyclization: (**A**) Nitroarylamide prodrugs; (**B**) trimethyl lock; (**C**) coumarin-based linkers; (**D**) H-bonding conformational lock; (**E**) phenolate-based linker.

of an amino group, which is even more electron-donating than hydroxylamine, is expected to induce an even faster fragmentation. Methylation of the benzylic position and electron-donating subtituents on the aromatic ring increase the rate of fragmentation, presumably by stabilization of the developing positive charge at the benzylic position. Strongly electron-withdrawing substituents like 2-NO_2 or 3-NO_2 slow down the fragmentation to 188 min and 65 min, respectively.

Self-immolative prodrugs using 4-hydroxybenzyl linkers, where the phenolic group is blocked as a galactosyl ether, have been synthesised for α-galactosidase. The insufficient acidity of the unsubstituted phenol prevents the rapid fragmentation of the

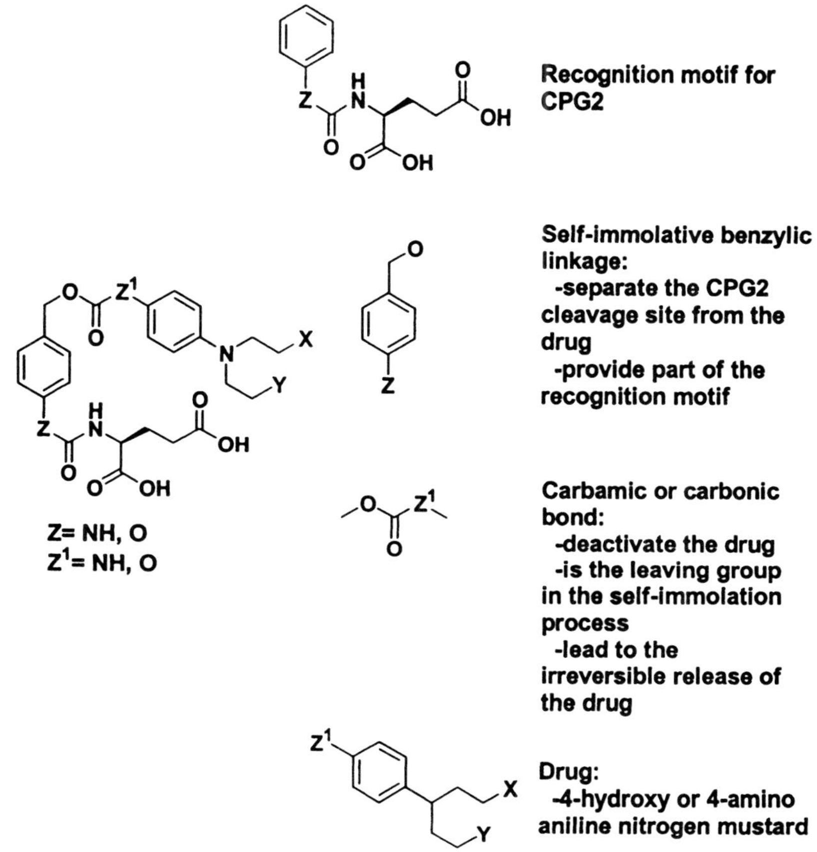

Fig. 19. Structural elements of a self-Immolative prodrug for CPG2.

prodrug *(109)*. Substitution with 3-NO$_2$ or 3-Cl increases the rate of fragmentation considerably. The 2-hydroxy-5-nitro-benzylic linker (activated by 1,4-elimination) decomposes slower, and the intermediate can be detected for 4–5 h. The optimal linker was considered to be the 3-nitro-4-hydroxybenzylic one (as the 3-chloro equivalent afforded somewhat less stable prodrugs) *(57,98)*.

For linkers activated by through space cyclization, this second step can be rate determining. A study on the cyclization of 2-aminoarylamides (compounds A, **Fig. 18**) formed following reduction of 2-nitroarylamides found a variation of more than 50,000-fold in the rate of cyclization, dependent mainly on the geometry of the system *(110)*. Ingenious substitution of the linker to increase the steric strain prior to cyclization (trimethyl lock lactones, compound B, **Fig. 18**) *(111)*, locking the geometry in the cis conformation (coumarin-based linkers, compound C, **Fig. 18**) *(112)*, H-bonding conformational lock (compound D, **Fig. 18**) *(106)*, and phenolate rather than phenol as attacking nucleophile (compound E) *(113)* were all found to increase greatly the rate of cyclisation to a few minutes.

Table 1
Characteristics of Self-immolative Prodrugs for Enzymes Used in GDEPT

Enzyme	Specifier	Trigger	Process of fragmentation	Linker–drug bond	Drugs
Glycosidases	α- and β-glycosyl or glucuronyl	Hydrolysis of glycosyl ether or carbamate	1,6-Elimination, 1,4-Elimination cyclization	Carbamate, phosphoric ester, quaternary ammonium	Anthracyclines, phosphoramide mustards, aromatic mustards, MDR modulators
Nitroreductase	Nitro-aromatics	Reduction of nitro function	1,6-Elimination 1,4-elimination, cyclization	Carbamate, carbonate, quaternary ammonium, amide	Aromatic and aliphatic mustards, mitomycin C, actinomycin D, doxorubicin, enediynes, cyclopropyl-indole, benzodiazepine, tallimustine
Carboxy-peptidase G2	Glutamic acid linked to aromatic nucleus	Hydrolysis of amide, carbamate, or urea	1,6-Elimination	Carbamate, carbonate	Anthracyclines, aromatic mustards
β-Lactamase	β-Lactams	Hydrolysis of lactam amide	1,4-Elimination	Carbamate	Aliphatic and aromatic mustards, vinca alkaloids, anthracyclines, cisplatin
Cytochrome P450		C-hydroxy-lation	Two successive 1,2-eliminations	Phosphoric ester	Phosporamide mustard
Tyrosinase	Dopamine analogs	Oxidation of catechol to ortho-quinone	Cyclization and hydrolysis	Carbamate, carbonate	Anthracyclins, aromatic and aliphatic mustards

182

4. Linker–drug bond. This has a double role: to deactivate the drug and to provide the leaving group in self-immolation. The most common linkage for prodrugs containing an amine functionality is the carbamate. The carbamate lowers the electron density of the amino group, with subsequent ablation or reduction of activity. For example, in 4-aminoaniline nitrogen mustard prodrugs, the high reactivity resulting from the *para* amino group is reduced 32-fold by conversion to carbamate *(55)*. Upon activation, the elimination process extrudes the unstable carbamic acid that loses CO_2, affording the amino drug in an irreversible process. The effect of the basicity of the extruded amine on the fragmentation of carbamates was studied *(114)*. The rate of fragmentation was found to be independent of the pK_a of the leaving amine and of pH. A competing reaction of condensation of the released amine with the reactive iminoquinomethide was found at pH > 5 and concentrations >50 μM. The cytotoxicity of the released amino drug should therefore be below 50 μM to avoid loss because of this competitive reaction.

Amino drugs can also be attached as amides in prodrugs activated by cyclization (*see* **Fig. 18**, compounds A) *(110)*.

Another option for tertiary amino drugs is their conversion to a quaternary ammonium salt, which makes them a good leaving group, the positively charged nitrogen atom effectively becoming an electron-withdrawing functionality. This method has been used for prodrugs of mechloramine activated by one-electron reduction *(115)* and for the MDR modulator verapamil *(116)* (*see* **Fig. 20**).

For phenol drugs, attachment as carbonates could deactivate the phenol mustard and provide the leaving group as carbonic acid. Unfortunately, the carbonates tend to be unstable in physiological conditions *(55)*. A better alternative is the ether linkage, which is more stable, although slower to self-immolate and not deactivating the electronic density of the phenol to the same extent as the carbonate (*see* **Fig. 21**) *(117)*.

Alcohol drugs have been coupled to the linker as reverse carbamate and as esters. Whereas the reversed carbamate failed to regenerate the alcohol by 1,6-elimination, it was useful for prodrugs activated by cyclization *(116)*. The ester linkage regenerates taxol by cyclization *(107)*.

Another leaving group released in a self-immolative prodrug is the phosphoric ester of the phosphoramidic mustard (*see* **Fig. 22**) *(118)*.

5. The drugs. Several drugs have been released from self-immolative prodrugs, such as anthracyclines, aromatic and aliphatic nitrogen mustards, enediynes, cyclopropylindoles, taxol, talimustine, etoposide, combretastatin, tallimustine, mytomycin C, and actinomycin D.

7. Optimization of Prodrugs

In order to obtain the best results from a GDEPT enzyme/prodrug system, the prodrug should be optimized. Issues that have to be addressed include the following:

• Cytotoxicity differential
• Cytotoxicity of released drug
• Bystander effect (BE)
• Stability of prodrug and drug
• Kinetics of activation
• Pharmacological properties

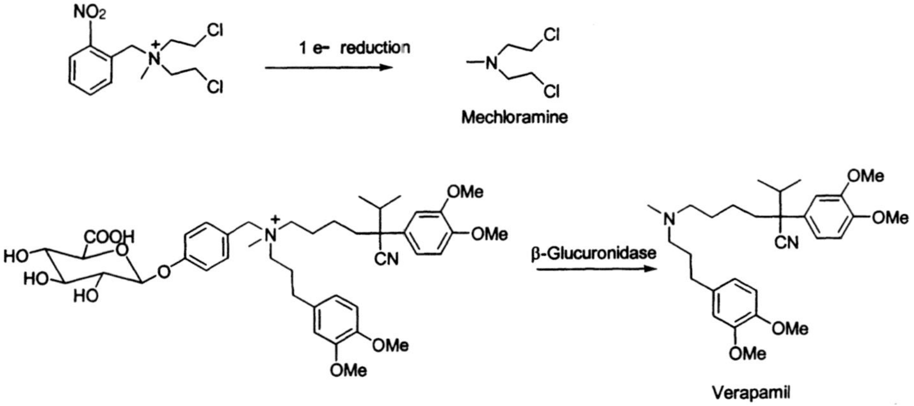

Fig. 20. Self-immolative prodrugs with quaternary ammonium as the leaving group.

7.1. Improving the Cytotoxicity Differential

The cytotoxicity differential can be described by the potential of activation (the ratio between drug and prodrug in a nonexpressing cell line) or by the degree of activation (the ratio of cytotoxicity of prodrug between expressing and nonexpressing cell line). The potential of activation represents the maximum differential achievable with a prodrug, whereas the degree of activation measures the actual differential *(7)*. Theoretically, the degree of activation can at best be equal to the potential of activation. Usually, complete activation is not achieved because of limitations in enzymatic kinetics or side reactions.

There are several general strategies to generate cytotoxicity differentials between drugs and their corresponding prodrugs. The main strategies employed for both direct and self-immolative prodrugs design are as follows:

1. Electronic switches: reversing or altering the electronic effect of a key functional group, with consequent increase in the reactivity of the prodrug. This is the mechanism of activation of nitrogen mustard prodrugs whereby the conversion of electron-withdrawing nitro (*see* **Fig. 20**), weakly electron-donating urea (*see* **Fig. 2**), or amide (*see* **Fig. 18**) to strongly electron-donating amine or hydroxylamine increases the reactivity of the aromatic mustard and subsequently the rate of DNA alkylation. Other enzymatic conversions with the same effect in aromatic systems are amide to carboxylate (*see* **Fig. 1**) and carbamate (*see* **Fig. 2**) or phosphate (*see* **Fig. 3**) to hydroxy. The same applies to cyclopropylindoles (*see* **Fig.14**), where the release of the amino or hydroxy stabilizes the key alkylating cyclopropyl ring. In enediyne carbamate prodrugs (*see* **Fig. 14**), liberation of the free amine increases electron density, promoting opening of the epoxide with the change of conformation of the enediyne macrocycle. This triggers the Bergman cyclization, forming diradicalic specia, which induces DNA double-strand breaks *(16)*.
   As a rule, the magnitude of the shift in electronic effect parallels the cytotoxicity differential. This holds true, especially for nitrogen mustards. Differentials of up to 200-fold have been obtained with 4-aminoaniline mustards deactivated as carbamates or ureas (the differences in Hammett constants $\Delta\sigma_p=0.42$ for urea and 0.49 for carbamates) *(20,119)*.

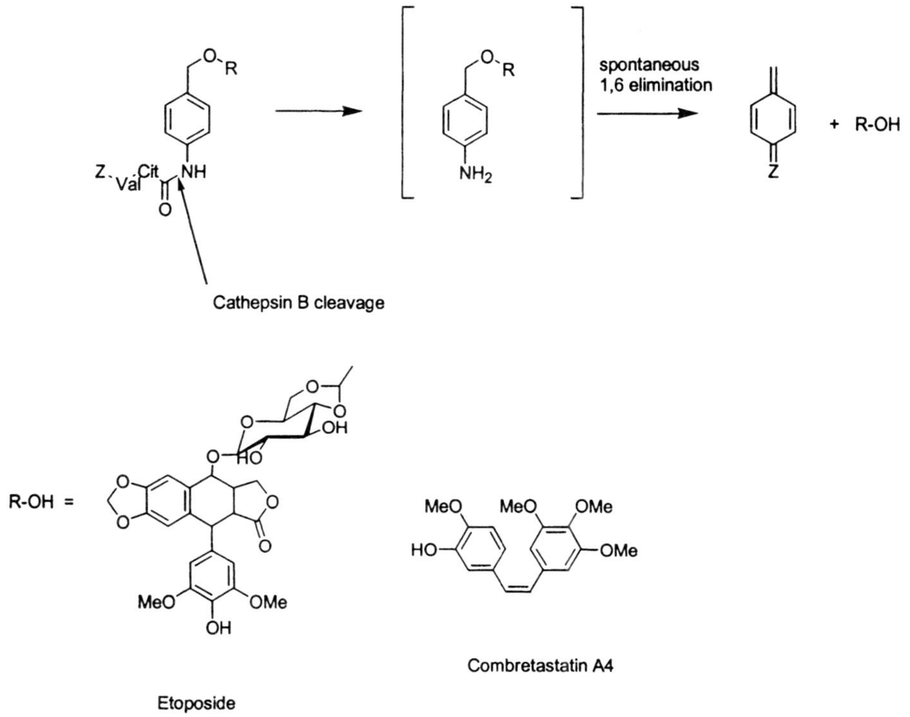

Fig. 21. Self-immolative ether prodrugs.

For aromatic mustard prodrugs activated by reduction of nitro group to hydroxylamine ($\Delta\sigma_p=1.12$), differentials of 100 to 2500 have been achieved *(54)*. Although not directly comparable because it is deactivated directly rather than via an aromatic ring, for quaternary ammonium prodrugs of mechloramine (that would correspond to $\Delta\sigma_p=1.64$), a 3000-fold differential was observed *(115)*. In the aromatic nitrogen mustard class, differentials can be manipulated by substitutions on the aromatic ring (e.g., *ortho* substituents with respect to the mustard tend to increase toxicity of the drug by steric effects) *(120)* and by varying the leaving groups on the mustard (usually using Br, I, or mixed Cl-mesyl mustards tends to achieve higher differentials than Cl) *(54)*.

2. Prodrugs acting by cell exclusion. In this case, the prodrug is charged or very hydrophilic and cannot penetrate the cell membrane to reach its cellular target. Upon activation and cleavage of the charged/hydrophobic moiety, it becomes more lipophilic and cell permeable. Examples of this class are etoposide phosphate (activated by phosphatases; *see* **Fig. 3**) *(58)* and β-glucuronide anthracycline prodrugs (activated by β-glucuronidase; *see* **Figs. 4** and **16**) *(82)*.

3. Hindrance or blocking of key interaction with active sites. Thus, the prodrug is unable to interact with its target. An example is the dipeptide MTX prodrugs for CPA (*see* **Fig. 1**), where the key α-carboxylate of the glutamic acid is blocked as amide, preventing interaction with the reduced folate carrier (RFC) and cellular uptake, as well as polyglutamation with conversion to a more active drug against thymidylate synthetase *(28)*. Conjugation

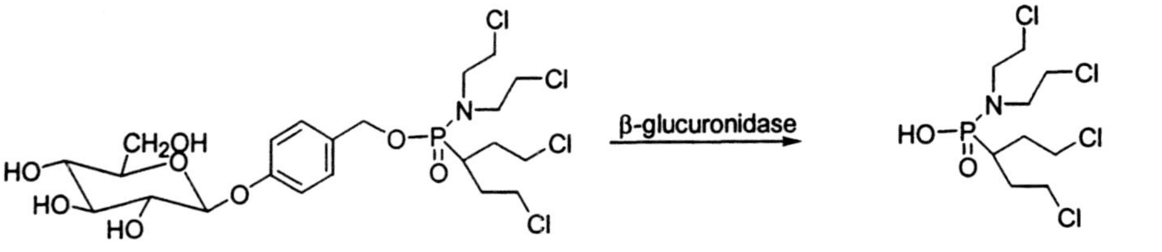

Fig. 22. Self-immolative prodrugs with phosphate ester as the leaving group.

of taxol at the critical 2'-OH with a β-glucuronyl-linker moiety decreases the cytotoxicity by two orders of magnitude, and in the presence of β-glucuronidase, a 30-fold activation occurs *(107)*. In a cephalosporin–vinblastine prodrug, the bulky side chain deactivates the prodrug, presumably by hindering the binding to tubulin *(19)*. The same mechanism probably applies for the CPT11 prodrug, where, following activation by rabbit carboxylesterase, the released OH group has an important role in the interaction with topoisomerase 1 (*see* Fig. 2) *(80)*.

4. Conversion of the prodrug to a substrate for endogenous enzymes. Phosphorylation of nucleoside-like prodrugs to nucleotides by various kinases (HSV-TK, varicella zoster virus thymidine kinase [VZV-TK], deoxycytidine kinase [dCK]) generate monophosphate precursors that are phosphorylated further to triphosphates by endogenous enzymes and then used as polymerase substrates to generate stunted DNA (*see* **Fig. 6**). The prodrug itself is poor or not a substrate for endogenous enzymes prior to conversion to the monophosphate. A similar principle is used for cytosine deaminase, which converts 5-FC to 5-FU (*see* **Fig. 5**), a substrate for uracil phosphoribosyl transferase to generate a TS inhibitor, and for XGPRT, transferring a deoxyribosyl phosphate to 6-TG or 6-TX (*see* **Fig. 12**). Huge differentials have been achieved by this method [e.g., 44,000-fold for GCV in TK-transfected osteosarcoma *(121)*].

5. Formation of a reactive functional group. This strategy is based on the conversion of an inert functional group (in a compound containing no reactive functionality) to a reactive moiety that can react nonspecifically with cellular components. Examples are conversion of the double bond in the furan ring of ipomeanol to a reactive epoxide by Cyt P450 *(90,122)* or transformation by the same enzyme of the benign N-acylated 4-aminophenol (acetaminophen) to *N*-acetylbezoquinoneimine capable of a Michael addition reaction with cellular nucleophiles (*see* **Fig. 10**) *(123)*. Conversion of selenoether (in selenomethionine) to the cellular poison methylselenol (*see* **Fig. 13**) *(93)* and formation of H_2O_2, as a source of hydroxyl radicals, from D-amino acids by D-amino acids oxidase (DAAO) *(91)*, are other examples. An activation of 400-fold has been obtained with the methioninase/selenomethionine system.

6. Formation or activation of a second interactive group. Activation of CB1954 by NR transforms a weak DNA monoalkylator into a bifunctional DNA crosslinking compound. The second alkylating group is generated from the conversion of nitro to hydroxylamine, and acetylation of the latter by CoA transferases, generating a reactive intermediate. This intermediate eliminates acetate, with formation of NH+, a very reactive group for nucleophiles (*see* **Fig. 7**) *(66)*.

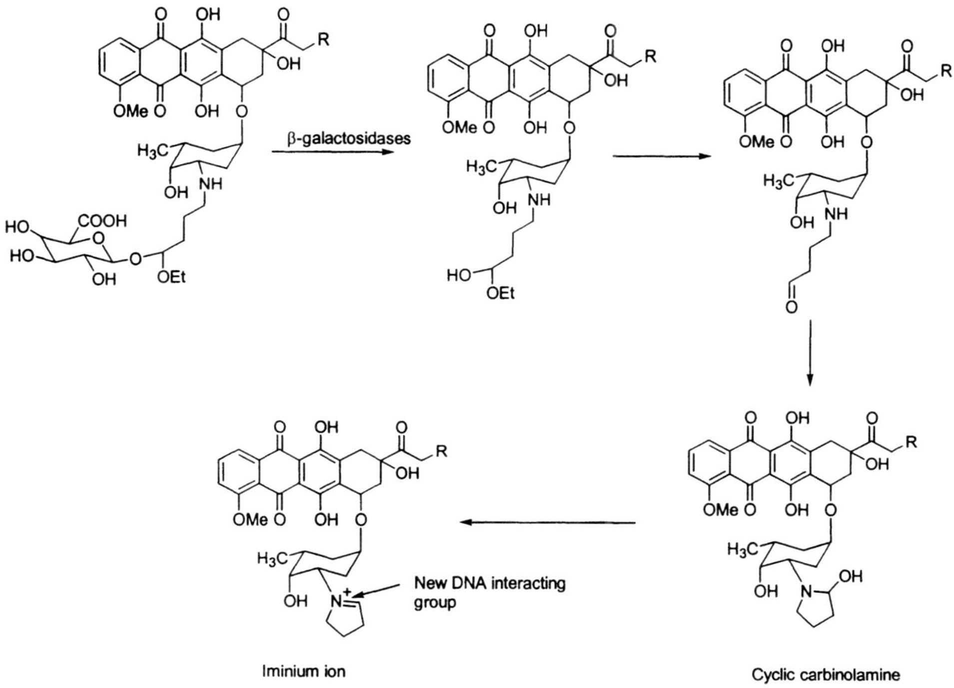

Fig. 23. Prodrug activated by formatin of a second reactive group.

N-(4-Ethoxy-4-β-glucuronyl)butyl-anthracyclines are prodrugs for β-glucuronidase *(124)*. The linkage between the glucuronyl and doxorubicin is simply an N-alkyl chain, which preserves the electron density on the nitrogen and only mildly hinders the DNA interaction of anthracyclins (IC_{50}=0.1 μM, similar to that of unsubstituted doxorubicin; IC_{50}=inhibitory concentration that achieves 50% cell death). Upon activation, the N-alkyl group is converted spontaneously to a cyclic carbinolamine, that ultimately generates a very reactive iminium ion, capable of covalent DNA bonding (*see* **Fig. 23**). Doxorubicin has two elements that contribute to DNA complexation, the aglycon and the daunosamine moiety. Both interact with DNA by hydrogen or electrostatic bonds. Conversion of one of the DNA interaction sites (the amino group in daunosamine) from a weak non-covalent ligand to a very reactive iminium ion generating covalent bonds with DNA can increase the cytotoxicity 10,000 fold.

7.2. Cytotoxicity of Released Drugs

The released drug needs to be as cytotoxic as possible because of the limitations of the activation mechanism and of cell penetration *(19)*. For self-immolative carbamate prodrugs, it was found that competing side reactions occur at concentrations higher than 50 μM *(114)*. The less cytotoxic drugs also tend not to achieve total cell killing at their solubility limit.

In order to improve the cytotoxicity of the released drug, the range of prodrugs that can be activated by a certain enzyme should be expanded, so that very cytotoxic compounds can be converted into relatively noncytotoxic efficient substrates for the respective enzyme. The CMDA prodrug, consisting of a benzoic mustard drug conjugated to glutamic acid, releases the benzoic acid mustard with an IC_{50} of 130 μM following CPG2 activation *(177)*. In order to obtain prodrugs for CPG2 releasing more cytotoxic drugs, phenol and aniline mustards were coupled to glutamic acid. The drugs formed from these latter prodrugs attained an IC_{50} of 0.2 μM *(20)*.

Another possibility for expanding the range of drugs released from prodrugs for a certain enzyme is the self-immolative approach. Anthracycline prodrugs have been obtained for CPG2 *(56)*, and enedyin *(63)* and amino-*seco*-cyclopropylindol prodrugs *(64)* for NR using this approach.

7.3. Bystander Effect

Improvement of the BE *(see* Chapter 1) is very important for GDEPT, as the vectors in use so far very rarely achieve more than 10–15% efficacy of transfection in vivo, and usually less than this. Two mechanisms for the BE can be encountered, depending on the type of prodrugs used. For prodrugs releasing drugs unable to cross cell membranes, cell-to-cell contact is required. HSV-TK with ganciclovir is an example where gap junctions seem to be required for a BE. For prodrugs generating diffusible drugs based on passive diffusion or active transport, no such conditions are required. Activation by secreted or surface-tethered enzymes tends to increase the BE for diffusible drugs.

For prodrugs requiring cell–cell contact for BE, both cellular and prodrug factors influence the magnitude of the effect. GDEPT in the MDA-MB-35 breast cancer cell line produce a smaller BE than 9L glioma with HSV-TK and VZV-TK and pyrimidine nucleoside prodrugs BVDU and BVaraU, consistent with the level of gap junctions *(125)*. Purine nucleoside prodrugs consistently produced a better BE than pyrimidine nucleoside prodrugs with HSV-TK and VZV-TK and the effect is less dependent on cell line *(121,125)*.

Prodrugs generating diffusible drugs usually achieve a better BE, at least in vitro. A comparison of several prodrug systems *(126,127)* demonstrated a higher bystander effect for CD/5-FC and NR/CB1954 (generating diffusible metabolites) than for HSV-TK and dCK/araC, whose metabolites are phosphorylated and cannot cross the cell membrane.

A systematic study on structural modifications of the dinitrobenzamide mustard prodrug SN 23862 *(see* **Fig.** 7) for NR brought about improvements in cytotoxicity differentials, BE, and solubility of prodrugs. In this study, the prodrugs generating more active drugs (mustard moiety containing bromo and iodo as leaving group) mounted a better BE and better cytotoxicity differentials *(54)*. However, in studying three novel prodrugs for CPG2, the prodrugs generating more stable benzoic acid mustard drugs produced a better BE in vivo (at 10% and 50% cells expressing surface-tethered CPG2). The prodrug generating a more reactive phenol mustard afforded the best cytotoxicity differential at 100% cells expressing CPG2, but the bystander effect was poorer *(61)*. This can be explained by the fact that the most reactive drug (the phenol mustard) reacts at the site of generation, becoming inactivated before diffusing to bystander cells. The benzoic mustard drugs are more stable and have time to diffuse to neighboring cells. Clearly, one factor influencing the BE is the stability of the released drug, and an optimum is required for a good BE.

7.4. Stability of Prodrugs and Drugs

The chemical and biological half-lives of released drugs should be optimised. If they are too short, they can generate a high log kill locally, but they do not have time to reach their molecular target and also to reach neighboring cells to achieve a good BE. Too long a half-life engenders the risk of leakage of drug out of the tumor into the systemic circulation and damage to normal tissues. There are suggestions that the optimal half-life should be between seconds and a few minutes *(21)*. Based on a diffusion range in the tumor of 100–200 μm, the optimum half-life can be calculated to be about 1 min *(128)*. Therefore, a compromise between the maximum local efficacy and the maximum BE should be reached. It is possible that a combination of prodrugs releasing drugs with different $t_{1/2}$ would be more efficient.

For aromatic nitrogen mustard prodrugs and drugs, the chemical half-life and the ratio of reactivities between drug and prodrug can be fine-tuned by the pattern of substitution on the aromatic ring. The reactivity varies linearly with the Hammett sigma parameter for *para* substituents (σ_p) and to a lesser extent with the Hammett sigma parameter for *meta* substituents (σ_m). The effect of the *ortho* substituents is more difficult to predict. Apart from the electronic effects, the *ortho* substituents produce steric hindrance of resonance, twisting the nitrogen mustard moiety and disrupting the conjugation with the aromatic nucleus, with consequent increase in reactivity of the mustard. This effect increases with the bulkiness of the *ortho* substituent. Another factor that drastically affects the half-life of the mustard is the leaving group, with reactivities increasing in the order F<<Cl<Br<I<MesO (MesO= mesyloxy) *(120)*. Based on this analysis, prodrugs generating drugs with shorter half-lives and higher ratio of reactivity prodrugs: drugshave been obtained by using 4-hydroxy- and 4-amino-aniline instead of the benzoic nitrogen mustards, testing various substituents in the 2- and 3-positions, and replacing bis-chloro mustard with bis-iodo or bis-bromo *(20)*.

The stability of prodrugs in physiological conditions is important to prevent premature release of drug and general toxicity. Especially when the released drugs are alcohols or phenols and the attachment of the specifier moiety is in the hydroxy group, instability in serum can occur. The carbonate linkage between drug and specifier is not very stable chemically and even less stable to serum esterases. Self-immolative prodrugs of phenol nitrogen mustard for NR and CPG2 connected to the linker via a carbonate bond are as toxic as the drug, presumably because of fast unspecific hydrolysis with release of phenol drug *(55,96)*. Ester prodrugs are also hydrolyzed in human serum, but sterically hindered ones tend to be more stable *(107,129)*. More stable prodrugs of phenol drugs can be obtained using carbamate linkers activated by cyclization *(113)* or the stable ether bond instead of carbonate, which still undergo 1,6-elimination from the 4-aminobenzyl linker *(117)*. The prodrugs where the drug contains an amino group, connected as a carbamate, by contrast are quite stable. The amide linkage in prodrugs is usually stable in vivo; however, surprising instability can occur if the amide is substrate for endogenous peptidases *(28)*. The effect of the aromatic linker substitution on the stability of self-immolative prodrugs is quite minor *(98,99)*.

7.5. Kinetic Factors

The kinetics of activation of a prodrug is described by the parameters K_M and k_{cat} or V_{max}. K_M is a measure of the affinity of the substrate for the enzyme and k_{cat} or V_{max} describe the rate of substrate conversion. These parameters are important in determining the rate of drug release from prodrug at the site of activation, the local concentration of released drug, and the amount of prodrug required to achieve a significant concentration of drug. A prodrug with high affinity for the enzyme (low K_M) and high rate of activation (high k_{cat}) is likely to be more efficient. Although the comparison of kinetics between different enzyme/prodrug systems is difficult, because of the inconsistent way the data are determined and expressed in literature, it appears that systems with better kinetics have better activity *(7)*. However, a rapid release of drug can be more effective for proliferating cells, whereas a slow constant release might be more efficient against quiescent cells.

The differences in kinetics are reflected in cytotoxicity differentials in experiments in vitro when the incubation time is varied. When comparing 2-aminoanthracene (2-AA) and 4-ipomeanol (4-IM) prodrugs for cyt P450 4B1 at 48 h continuous exposure, the cytotoxic effect was similar. However, if the exposure was short (30–60 min), a much weaker effect was obtained with 4-IM than 2-AA. 2-AA produced maximal cell killing upon 5 h exposure, whereas 4-IM achieved the same effect only after 48 h incubation. These results can be explained by kinetic differences between the activation of prodrugs, but the interplay between the prodrug mode of action and the cell cycle has also been offered as an explanation *(130)*. The same effect was observed in the activation of the prodrug CB1954 by two forms of NR expressed at different cellular locations. The wild-type cytosolic/nuclear enzyme had better activity than mitochondrial expression. No obvious difference in cytotoxicity was observed at long exposure times. However, the difference becomes obvious (in favor of the wild-type NR), when short exposures were used, which are likely to reflect more accurately the situation in vivo *(31)*.

Attempts to improve the kinetics of activation have focused on two directions: improving the enzyme and improving the prodrug.

7.5.1. Improving the Enzyme

In several cases, it has been found that orthologous enzymes or enzymes with similar profiles of activity from different species can have very different kinetics for a substrate. For example, the rat DT-diaphorase is a better activating enzyme than the human DT-diaphorase for CB-1954, with a K_M slightly lower and a k_{cat} sevenfold better. The *E. coli* NR has a similar K_M, but the k_{cat} is much higher (360 min^{-1} compared to 4.1 for rat and 0.64 min^{-1} for the human enzyme). This enzyme is the enzyme of choice for GDEPT based on the reduction of the nitro group *(66)*. The rabbit carboxylesterase is 100-1000-fold more efficient in activating the prodrug CPT-11 than the human homologue *(80)*. The yeast cytosine deaminase (CD) has better kinetics for the 5-FC prodrug than the bacterial CD and was also shown to be a more effective system*(131)*. Another way of modifying the enzyme is by protein engineering and mutagenesis. An example is the engineering of HSV-TK, which produced mutants with increased sensitivity to both GCV and ACV. This enhancement can be explained by kinetic factors. Compared to wild type, the K_M was slightly higher for GCV and ACV in the mutant, but much higher (35-fold) for the endogenous thymidine substrate. The k_{cat} was reduced for GCV and ACV (6-fold and 8-fold, respectively) but much more reduced for thymidine (88-fold). As a consequence, the specificity constant (k_{cat}/K_M) for thymidine was 3000-fold lower in mutant than in wild type, whereas the reduction of the same constant for GCV was only 40-fold. The mutant displayed greatly reduced competition for the active site and better selectivity for the prodrug substrates than for endogenous thymidine *(132)*.

7.5.2. Improving the Prodrug

Scanning various substrate prodrugs for an enzyme, altering the linkage between drug and specifier, structure–activity correlations between substitution patterns and kinetics, and increasing the spatial separation between specifier and drug using self-immolative linkers have been instrumental in obtaining substrates with a favorable kinetic profile for GDEPT.

Sixty compounds were assessed as substrates for *E. coli* purine nucleoside phosphorylase, and the prodrugs with the best kinetics that also fulfill several other criteria were chosen for further evaluation *(18)*. Several bioreductive prodrugs were assessed for NR for GDEPT. Apart from CB1954, nitrofurazone was found to have reasonable cytotoxicity differentials, and the rate of reduction was 10 times faster than CB1954 *(133)*.

In some cases, obtaining the optimal kinetic profile does not mean increasing the rate of activation. A drop in the kinetic performance of prodrugs for an enzyme is acceptable if the advantages obtained by modifying the structure more than compensate the loss in enzyme activity. In these cases, the stress shifts from enhancing the kinetics to minimizing the loss in the rate of activation while still preserving the benefits of the new structure. The best substrates for CPG2 were based on benzoic acid derivatives, coupled to glutamic acid as amides *(120)*. Benzoic acid mustards, as exemplified by CMDA, release less potent drugs. More potent aniline and phenol mustards can be released from prodrugs where the drug is coupled to glutamic acid as urea or carbamates rather than amide *(79)*. However, the rate of cleavage is reduced in these prodrugs with respect to CMDA. The lead compound in a series of phenol nustard prodrugs had a similar K_M to CMDA, but the k_{cat} was 20 times lower *(20)*. Despite this, the prodrug had a better cytotoxicity differential and performed better than CMDA in vivo *(61)*.

Structure–activity studies have been performed in order to determine the optimal structure of a prodrug for an enzyme. One of the criteria of assessment is the kinetics of activation. The effect of the substitution on the aromatic ring of the prodrugs for CPG2 on the kinetics has been investigated. It was found that both steric and electronic effects play a role in the kinetics *(20,120)*. The substituents on the aromatic ring also influence the fragmentation of the self-immolative prodrugs, as discussed earlier *(98,99,108)*.

An additional approach to improving the kinetics of activation is to use self-immolative linkers. Whereas the direct carbamate linker between the α-galactosyl and doxorubicin was poorly cleaved by α-galactosidase, the insertion of an 4-aminobenzyl linker afforded good substrates for the enzyme *(84)*. The rationale for the effect is probably the increased distance between the specifier and the drug, releasing the steric hindrance around the site of activation. Increasing the distance between drug and specifier even further by using multiple cascade linkers improved the kinetics even more, as demonstrated for a series of self-immolative prodrugs for plasmin *(134)*. However, in some cases, introduction of a linker can actually worsen the kinetics *(55)*. This can be explained by the fact that the direct prodrug sat comfortably in the catalytic pocket of the enzyme, whereas the larger self-immolative one is oversized for the pocket and clashed sterically with other residues of the protein.

For self-immolative prodrugs, the kinetics of activation is complicated by the fact that there are two steps: enzymatic reaction and fragmentation. The rate-determining step is usually the first; however, there are exceptions.

7.6. Physicochemical and Pharmacological Properties

The properties of prodrugs determined in vitro do not always correlate with in vivo results, because of the complexity of living systems and factors such as biodistribution, metabolism, retention time, excretion, and so forth that can be grouped under the heading of pharmacological properties. Also of importance are the physicochemical properties such as water solubility and lipophilicity, which also influence cellular uptake and metabolism.

The biodistribution of prodrugs of clinical use was determined for several systems. Uptake of cyclophoshamide in lung tumors was very variable *(135)*. An option to improve the tumor concentration of prodrug and achieve a more sustained concentration was to use a polymer based implant containing cyclophosphamide, which was demonstrated to be activated by virally trasfected CYP2B1 *(136)*.

The prodrug should be reasonably stable to metabolism to avoid premature drug release or deactivation. Plasma instability of some self-immolative prodrugs containing a carbonate or ester linkage was discussed previously. Inhibition of liver cyclophosphamide-metabolizing enzymes has been found to have a beneficial effect in GDEPT with CYP450 *(137)*.

Substitution of the linker part of self-immolative prodrugs with halogens and aliphatic chains was undertaken in order to increase serum albumin binding and, therefore, retention time *(99)*. Binding to serum proteins stabilizes the nitrogen mustard prodrugs for CPG2, without apparent adverse effect on activation.

The lipophilicity of prodrugs and released drugs is an important consideration in their design. The optimal lipophilicity enables drugs to permeate cells efficiently but not become sequestered in the lipid membrane so they cannot mount a BE *(61)*. Fluorinated analogs of CMDA were designed to improve the lipophilicity of prodrugs for CPG2 and increase cell uptake *(61,138)*. A lipophilic ester of the prodrug GCV with elaidic acid (E-GCV) was synthesized and was found to have better cytotoxicity than the parent prodrug. The increased cytotoxicity seems to be the result of the longer retention of GCV mono-, di-, and triphosphates in cells treated with E-GCV than with GCV *(139)*. The lipophilicity of 4-ipomeanol, a small-molecule substrate for CYP4B1, allows it to cross the blood–brain barrier, and therefore it is used for GDEPT treatment of glioma following systemic administration *(140)*.

For drugs that are too lipophilic, increasing the water solubility would increase the bioavailability of the prodrug. For example, nitrogen mustard prodrugs for NR containing solubilizing groups, such as diethylamino-ethyl or 2, 3-dihydroxypropyl, increased the water solubility of the prodrug but also decreased their cytotoxicity compared to the unsubstituted ones. Nevertheless, one of these new prodrugs had a better differential and BE than the bis-chloro mustard lead *(54)*.

It should be noted that pharmacological requirements, and especially lipophilicity of prodrugs, are very different according to the site of expression of the enzyme. Intracellularly expressed enzymes require lipophilic prodrugs, whereas prodrugs for surface-tethered or secreted enzymes should be hydrophilic and potentially excluded form the cells, whereas the released drugs have to be up taken in tumor cells.

8. Conclusion

The development of tailored prodrugs is a promising approach to achieve success in GDEPT. Currently, the main problem of any gene therapy method is the lack of an efficient safe vector for gene delivery. As progress is made in the area of vector development, there is a need for better prodrugs that will compensate the shortcomings of the actual vectors (by mounting a BE) and will take advantage of the future generations of improved vectors. Also, no prodrug at the moment is optimal, and various prodrugs can work better in selective tumors.

Several improved prodrugs have been obtained by design and synthesis. This is a trend likely to continue in the future, as there is much potential to optimize the prodrugs. Prodrugs tailored for a specific enzyme system are addressing the specific issues raised such as poor kinetics, small cytotoxicity differentials, and inadequate lipophilicity.

As more enzymes are developed to be expressed tethered on the surface of the cells or secreted, prodrugs developed for ADEPT can be now used in GDEPT. Several examples have been presented in this chapter. The borderline between ADEPT and GDEPT tends to disappear for prodrugs, although there are still very different approaches in terms of enzyme targeting (*see* Chapter 26).

The expansion of the range of drugs that can be released from prodrugs is set to continue, including very cytotoxic drugs and self-immolative prodrugs.

Engineering of the enzyme in order to accommodate new more selective prodrugs, rational design of new structure of optimal prodrugs based on crystallographic data, and QSAR studies are new exciting developments in the field of prodrug development for GDEPT. Use of cocktails of prodrugs released by the same enzyme or coexpression of several enzymes activating prodrugs with different mechanism of action might also result in improvements in efficacy.

References

1. Greco, O., Folkes, L. K., Wardman, P., Tozer, G. M., and Dachs, G. U. (2000) Development of a novel enzyme/prodrug combination for gene therapy of cancer: horseradish peroxidase/indole-3-acetic acid. *Cancer Gene Ther.* **7,** 1414–1420.

2. Prospective, open-label, parallel-group, randomized multicenter trial comparing the efficiency of surgery, radiation, and injection of murine cells producing herpes simplex virus thymidine kinase vector followed by intravenous ganciclovir against the efficacy of surgery and radiation in the treatment of newly diagnosed, previously untreated glioblastoma, *NIH OBA Human Gene Transfer Clinical Trials Database/***NIH protocol number: 157-(1996–08)** Available at www4.od.nih.gov/oba/rac/clinicaltrial.

3. Connors, T. A. (1995) The choice of prodrugs for gene directed enzyme prodrug therapy of cancer. *Gene Ther.* **2,** 702–709.

4. Springer, C. J. and Niculescu-Duvaz, I. (1996) Gene directed enzyme prodrug therapy (GDEPT): choice of prodrugs. *Adv. Drug Deliv. Rev.* **22,** 351–364.

5. Niculescu-Duvaz, I., Spooner, R. A., Marais, R., and Springer, C. J. S. (1998) Gene-directed enzyme prodrug therapy. *Bioconjug. Chem.* **9,** 4–22.

6. Melton, R., Connors, T., and Knox, R. J. (1999) The use of prodrugs in targeted anticancer therapies. *S. T. P. Pharm. Sci.* **9,** 13–33.

7. Springer, C. J. and Niculescu-Duvaz, I. (2000) Prodrug-activating systems in suicide gene therapy. *J. Clin. Investig.* **105,** 1161–1167.

8. Xu, G. and McLeod, H. L. (2001) Strategies for enzyme/prodrug cancer therapy. *Clin. Cancer Res.* **7,** 3314–3324.

9. Denny, W. A. (2001) Prodrug strategies in cancer therapy. *Eur. J. Med. Chem.* **36,** 577–595.

10. Greco, O. and Dachs, G. U. (2001) Gene directed enzyme/prodrug therapy of cancer: Hystorical appraisal and future prospectives. *J. Cell. Physiol.* **187,** 22–36.

11. Chen, L., Waxman, D. J., Chen, D., and Kufe, D. C. (1996) Sensitization of human breast cancer cells to cyclophosphamide and ifosfamide by transfer of a liver cytochrome P450 gene. *Cancer Res.* **56,** 1331–1340.

12. Marais, R., Spooner, R. A., Stribbling, S. M., Light, Y., Martin, J., and Springer, C. J. S. (1997) A cell surface tethered enzyme improves efficiency in gene-directed enzyme prodrug therapy. *Nature Biotechnol.* **15,** 1373–1377.

13. Kojima, A., Hackett, N. R., Ohwada, A., and Crystal, R. G. (1998) In vivo human carboxylesterase cDNA gene transfer to activate the prodrug CPT-11 for local treatment of solid tumors. *J. Clin. Investig.* **101,** 1789–1796.

14. McCart, J. A., Puhlmann, M., Lee, J., et al. (2000) Complex interaction between the replicating oncolytic effect and the enzyme/prodrug effect of vaccinia-mediated tumor regression. *Gene Ther.* **7,** 1217–1223.

15. Griffiths, L., Binley, K., Iqball, S., et al. (2000) The macrophage—a novel system to deliver gene therapy to pathological hypoxia. *Gene Ther.* **7,** 255–262.

16. Denny, W. A. and Wilson, W. R. (1998) The design of selectively-activated anti-cancer prodrugs for use in antibody-directed and gene-directed enzyme-prodrug therapies. *J. Pharm. Pharmacol.* **50,** 387–394.

17. Niculescu-Duvaz, I., Baracu, I., and Balaban, A. T. (1990) Alkylating agents, in Chemistry of Antitumour Agents. Wilman, D. E. V., ed., Blackie & Son: London, pp. 63–130.

18. Secrist, J. A. III, Parker, W. B., Allan, P. W., et al. (1999) Gene therapy of cancer: activation of nucleoside prodrugs with *E. coli* purine nucleoside phosphorylase. *Nucleosides Nucleotides* **18,** 745–757.

19. Denny, W. A. (1996) The design of selectively-activated prodrugs for cancer chemotherapy. *Curr. Pharm. Des.* **2**, 281–294.
20. Springer, C. J., Dowell, R. L., Burke, P. J., et al. (1995) Optimization of alkylating prodrugs derived from phenol and aniline mustards: a new clinical candidate prodrug (ZD2767) for ADEPT. *J. Med. Chem.* **38**, 5051–5065.
21. Denny, W. and Wilson, W. R. (1993) Bioreducible mustards: a paradigm for hypoxia-selective prodrugs of diffusible cytotoxins (HPDCs). *Cancer Metastases Rev.* **12**, 135–151.
22. Siim, B. G., Denny, W. A., and Wilson, W. R. (1997) Nitro reduction as an electronic switch for bioreductive drug activation. *Oncol. Res.* **9**, 357–369.
23. Patterson, L. H. and Raleigh, S. M. (1998) Reductive Metabolism: Its Application in Prodrug Activation, IOS, 1998.
24. Jaffar, M., Williams, K. J., and Stratford, I. J. (2001) Bioreductive and gene therapy approaches to hypoxic diseases. *Adv. Drug Deliv. Rev.* **53**, 217–228.
25. Bagshawe, K. D., Springer, C. J., Searle, F., et al. (1988) A cytotoxic agent can be generated selectively at cancer sites. *Br. J. Cancer* **58**, 700–703.
26. Niculescu-Duvaz, I. and Springer, C. J. (1995) Antibody-directed enzyme prodrug therapy (ADEPT): a targeting strategy in cancer chemotherapy. *Curr. Med. Chem.* **2**, 687–706.
27. Satchi, R., Connors, T. A., and Duncan, R. (2001) PDEPT: polymer-directed enzyme prodrug therapy I. HPMA copolymer-cathepsin B and PK1 as a model combination. *Br. J. Cancer* **85**, 1070–1076.
28. Hamstra, D. A., Page, M., Maybaum, J., and Rehemtulla, A. (2000) Expression of endogenously activated secreted or cell surface carboxypeptidase A sensitizes tumor cells to methotrexate-α-peptide prodrugs. *Cancer Res.* **60**, 657–665.
29. Heine, D., Muller, R., and Brusselbach, S. (2001) Cell surface display of a lysosomal enzyme for extracellular gene-directed enzyme prodrug therapy. *Gene Ther.* **8**, 1005–1010.
30. Weyel, D., Sedlacek, H.-H., Muller, R., and Brusselbach, S. (2000) Secreted human β-glucuronidase: a novel tool for gene-directed enzyme prodrug therapy. *Gene Ther.* **7**, 224–231.
31. Spooner, R. A., Maycroft, K. A., Paterson, H., Friedlos, F., Springer, C. J., and Marais, R. (2001) Appropriate subcellular localisation of prodrug-activating enzymes has important consequences for suicide gene therapy. *Int. J. Cancer* **93**, 123–130.
32. Alrabiah, F. A. and Sacks, S. L. (1996) New antiherpesvirus agents—their targets and therapeutic potential. *Drugs* **52**, 17–32.
33. Marley, J. (1997) Antiviral therapy in herpes zoster: a review. *Antiviral Chem. Chemoth.* **8** (**Suppl. 1**), 37–42.
34. Maudgal, P. C. and Declerq, E. (1991) Bromovinyldeoxyuridine treatment of herpetic-keratitis clinically resistant to other antiviral agents. *Curr. Eye Res.* **10 (Suppl. S)**, 193–199.
35. Averett, D. R., Koszalka, G. W., Fyfe, J. A., Roberts, G. B., Purifoy, D. J. M., and Krenitsky, T. A. (1991) 6-Methoxypurine arabinoside as a selective and potent inhibitor of Varicella–Zoster virus. *Antimicrob. Agents Chemother.* **35**, 851–857.
36. Ishiguro, K., Taira, S., Sasaki, T., and Nariuchi, H. (1988) Depletion of Mycoplasma from infected cell lines by limiting dilution in 6-methylpurine deoxyriboside. *J. Immunol. Methods* **108**, 39–43.
37. Besnard, C., Monthioux, E., and Jami, J. (1987) Selection against expression of the *Escherichia Coli* gene gpt in hrpt+ mouse teratocarcinoma and hybrid cells. *Mol. Cell Biol.* **7**, 4139–4141.
38. Marr, J. J. (1991) Purine analogs as chemotherapeutic agents in leishmaniasis and American trypanosomiasis. *J. Lab. Clin. Med.* **118**, 111–119.

39. Ghannoum, M. A. and Rice, L. B. (1999) Antifungal agents: mode of action, mechanism of resistance, and correlation of these mechanisms with bacterial resistance. *Clin. Microbiol. Rev.* **12,** 501.

40. Kondo, K., Sakamoto, J., Nakazato, H., et al. (2000) A phase III randomized study comparing doxifluridine and 5-fluorouracil as supportive chemotherapy in advanced and recurrent gastric cancer. *Oncol. Rep.* **7,** 485–490.

41. Cheson, B. D. and Simon, R. (1987) Low-dose Ara-C in acute nonlymphocytic leukemia and myelodysplastic syndromes—a review of 20 years experience. *Semin. Oncol.* **14 (Suppl. 1),** 126–133.

42. Colvin, O. M. (1999) An overview of cyclophosphamide development and clinical applications. *Curr. Pharm. Des.* **5,** 555–560.

43. Franck, R. W. and Tomasz, M. (1990) The chemistry of mitomycins, in Wilman, D. E. W., ed., *Chemistry of Antitumor Agents,* Blackie & Son Ltd., London and Glasgow, pp. 379–394.

44. Vanhoefer, U., Harstrick, A., Achterrath, W., Cao, S. S., Seeber, S., and Rustum, Y. M. (2001) Irinotecan in the treatment of colorectal cancer: clinical overview. *J. Clin. Oncol.* **19,** 1501–1518.

45. Grant, S. C., Kris, M. G., Young, C. W., and Sirotnak, F. M. (1993) Edatrexate, an antifolate with antitumor activity—a review. *Cancer Invest.* **11,** 36–45.

46. Lee, D. J., Trotti, A., Spencer, S., et al. (1998) Concurrent tirapazamine and radiotherapy for advanced head and neck carcinomas: a phase II study. *Int. J. Radiat. Oncol. Biol. Phys.* **42,** 811–815.

47. Nakamuro, K., Okuno, T., and Hasegawa, T. (2000) Metabolism of selenoamino acids and contribution of selenium methylation to their toxicity. *J. Health Sci.* **46,** 418–421.

48. Wolf, C. R., Statham, C. N., McMenamin, M. G., et al. (1982) The relationship between the catalytic activities of rabbit pulmonary cytochrome P-450 isozymes and the lung-specific toxicity of the furan derivative, 4-ipomeanol. *Mol. Pharmacol.* **22,** 738–744.

49. Ellard, S. and Parry, J. M. (1993) A comparative study of the use of primary chinese-hamster liver cultures and genetically-engineered immortal V79 chinese-hamster cell-lines expressing rat liver CYP1A1, 1A2 and 2B1 cDNAs in micronucleus assays. *Toxicology* **82,** 131–149.

50. Roberts, J. J., Friedlos, F., and Knox, R. J. (1986) CB 1954 (2,4-dinitro-5-aziridinyl benzamide) becomes a DNA interstrand crosslinking agent in Walker tumour cells. *Biochem. Biophys. Res. Commun.* **140,** 1073–1078.

51. Folkes, L. K. and Wardman, P. (2001) Oxidative activation of indole-3-acetic acids to cytotoxic species—a potential new role for plant auxins in cancer therapy. *Biochem. Pharmacol.* **61,** 129–136.

52. Miner, D. J. and Kissinger, P. T. (1979) Evidence for the involvement of *N*-acetyl-*p*-quinoneimine in acetaminophen metabolism. *Biochem. Pharmacol.* **28,** 3285–3290.

53. De Clercq, E., Andrei G., De Bolle, L., et al. (2001) Acyclic/carbocyclic guanosine analogues as anti-herpesvirus agents. *Nucleosides Nucleotides Nucleic Acids* **20,** 271–285.

54. Friedlos, F., Denny, W. A., Palmer, B. D.,and Springer, C. J. (1997) Mustard prodrug for activation by *Escherichia coli* nitroreductase in gene-directed enzyme prodrug therapy. *J. Med. Chem.* **40,** 1270–1275.

55. Niculescu-Duvaz, D., Niculescu-Duvaz, I., Friedlos, F. F., et al. (1998) Self-immolative mustard prodrugs for suicide gene therapy. *J. Med. Chem.* **41,** 5297–5309.

56. Niculescu-Duvaz, I., Niculescu-Duvaz, D., Friedlos, F., et al. (1999) Self-immolative anthracycline prodrugs for suicide gene therapy. *J. Med. Chem.* **42**, 2485–2489.
57. Ghosh, A. K., Khan, S., Marini, F., Nelson, J. A., and Farquhar, D. (2000) A daunorubicin β-galactoside prodrug for use in conjunction with gene-directed enzyme prodrug therapy. *Tetrahedron Lett.* **41**, 4871–4874.
58. Hayes, G. M., Carpenito, C., Davis, P. D., Dougherty, S. T., Dirks, J. F., and Dougherty, G. J. (2002) Alternative splicing as a novel means of regulating the expression of therapeutic genes. *Cancer Gene Ther.* **9**, 133–141.
59. Simonova, M., Wall, A., Weissleder, R., and Bogdanov, A. J. (2000) Tyrosinase mutants are capable of prodrug activation in transfected nonmelanomic cells. *Cancer Res.* **60**, 6656–6662.
60. Marais, R., Spooner, R. A., Light, Y., Martin, J., and Springer, C. J. (1996) Gene-directed enzyme prodrug therapy with a mustard prodrug/carboxypeptidase G2 combination. *Cancer Res.* **56**, 4735–4742.
61. Friedlos, F., Davies, L., Scanlon, S., et al. (2002) Three new prodrugs for suicide gene therapy using carboxypeptidase G2 elicit bystander efficacy in two xenograft models. *Cancer Res.* **62**, 1724–1729.
62. Hamstra, D. A. and Rehemtulla, A. (1999) Toward an enzyme/prodrug strategy for cancer gene therapy: endogenous activation of carboxypeptidase A mutants by the PACE/Furin family of propeptidases. *Hum. Gene Ther.* **10**, 235–248.
63. Hay, M. P., Wilson, W. R., and Denny, W. A. (1999) Nitrobenzyl carbamate prodrugs of enediynes for nitroreductase gene-directed enzyme prodrug therapy (GDEPT). *Bioorg. Med. Chem. Lett.* **9**, 3417–3422.
64. Hay, M. P., Sykes, B. M., Denny, W. A., and Wilson, W. R. (1999) A 2-nitroimidazole carbamate prodrug of 5-amino-1-(chloromethyl)-3-[(5,6,7-trimethoxyindol-2-yl)carbonyl]-1,2-dihydro-3*H*-benz[e]indole (amino-*seco*-CBI-TMI) for use with ADEPT and GDEPT. *Bioorg. Med. Chem. Lett.* **9**, 2237–2242.
65. Sagnou, M. J., Howard, P. W., Gregson, S. J., Eno-Amooquaye, E., Burke, P. J., and Thurston, D. E. (2000) Design and synthesis of novel pyrrolobenzodiazepine (PBD) prodrugs for ADEPT and GDEPT. *Bioorg. Med. Chem. Lett.* **10**, 2083–2086.
66. Grove, J. I., Searle, P. F., Weedon, S. J., Green, N. K., McNeish, I. A., and Kerr, D. J. (1999) Virus-directed enzyme prodrug therapy using CB1954. *Anti-Cancer Drug Des.* **14**, 461–472.
67. Alena, F., Jimbow, K., and Ito, S. (1990) Melanocytotoxicity and antimelanoma effects of phenolic amine compounds in mice in vivo. *Cancer Res.* **50**, 3743–3747.
68. Riley, P. A., Cooksey, C. J., Johnson, C. I., Land, E. J., Latter, A. M., and Ramsden, C. A. (1997) Melanogenesis-targeted anti-melanoma pro-drug development: effect of side chain variations on the cytotoxicity of tyrosinase-generated ortho-quinones in a model screening system. *Eur. J. Cancer* **33**, 135–143.
69. Tando, M., Thomas, P. D., Shokravi, M., et al. (1998) Synthesis and antitumor effect of the melanogenesis-based antimelanoma agent *N*-propionyl-4-*S*-cysteaminylphenol. *Biochem. Pharmacol.* **55**, 2023–2029.
70. Jordan, A. M., Khan, T. H., Osborn, H. M. I., Photiou, A., and Riley, P. A. (1999) Melanocyte-directed enzyme prodrug therapy (MDEPT): development of a targeted treatment for malignant melanoma. *Bioorg. Med. Chem.* **7**, 1775–1780.
71. Jordan, A. M., Khan, T. H., Malkin, H., Osborn, H. M. I., Photiou, A., and Riley, P. A. (2001) Melanocyte-directed enzyme prodrug therapy (MDEPT): development of second generation prodrugs for targeted treatment of malignant melanoma. *Bioorg. Med. Chem.* **9**, 1549–1558.

72. Rauth, A. M., Melo, T., and Misra, V. (1998) Bioreductive therapies: an overview of drugs and their mechanisms of action. *Int. J. Radiat. Oncol. Biol. Phys.* **42,** 755–762.

73. Springer, C. J. and Niculescu-Duvaz, I. (2002) Gene-directed enzyme prodrug therapy, in *Anticancer Drug Development* (Baguley, B. C. and Kerr, D. J., eds.), Academic, San Diego, CA.

74. Cortes, M. L., de Felipe, P., Martin, V., Hughes, M. A., and Izquierdo, M. (1998) Succesful use of a plant gene in the treatment of cancer in vivo. *Gene Ther.* **5,** 1499–1507.

75. Aghi, M., Kramm, C. M., and Breakefield, X. O. (1999) Folylpolyglutamyl synthetase gene transfer and glioma antifolate sensitivity in culture and in vivo. *J. Natl. Cancer Inst.* **91,** 1233–1241.

76. Aghi, M., Hochberg, F., and Breakfield, X. O. (2000) Prodrug activation enzymes in cancer gene therapy. *J. Gene Med.* **2,** 148–164.

77. Springer, C. J., Antoniw, P., Bagshave, K. D., Searle, F., Bisset, G. M., and Jarman, M. (1990) Novel prodrugs which are activated to cytotoxic alkylating agents by carboxypeptidase G2. *J. Med. Chem.* **33,** 677–681.

78. Smith, G. K., Banks, S., Blumenkopf, T. A., et al. (1997) Towards antibody directed enzyme prodrug therapy with the T268G mutant of human carboxypeptidase A1 and novel in vivo stable prodrugs of methotrexate. *J. Biol. Chem.* **272,** 15,804–15,816.

79. Dowell, R., Springer, C. J., Davies, D. H., et al. (1996) New mustard prodrugs for antibody-directed enzyme prodrug therapy: alternative to the amide link. *J. Med. Chem.* **39,** 1100–1105.

80. Wierdl, M., Morton, C. L., Weeks, J. K., Danks, M. K., Harris, L. C., and Potter, P. M. (2001) Sensitization of human tumor cells to CPT-11 via adenoviral-mediated delivery of a rabbit liver carboxylesterase. *Cancer Res.* **61,** 5078–5082.

81. Senter, P. D., Saulnier, M. G., Schreiber, G. J., et al. (1988) Antitumor effects of antibody alkaline-phosphatase conjugates in combination with etoposide phosphate. *Proc. Natl. Acad. Sci. USA* **85,** 4842–4846.

82. Haisma, H. J., Boven, E., Vanmuijen, M., Dejong, J., Vandervijgh, W. J. F., and Pinedo, H. M. (1992) A monoclonal antibody-β-glucuronidase conjugate as activator of the prodrug epirubicin-glucuronide for specific treatment of cancer. *Br. J. Cancer* **66,** 474–478.

83. Roffler, S. R., Wang, S. M., Chern, J. W., Yeh, M. Y., and Tung, E. (1991) Antineoplastic glucuronide prodrug treatment of human tumor-cells targeted with a monoclonal-antibody enzyme conjugate. *Biochem. Pharmacol.* **42,** 2062–2065.

84. Azoulay, M., Florent, J.-C., Monneret, C., et al. (1995) Prodrugs of anthracycline antibiotics suited for tumor-specific activation. *Anti-Cancer Drug Des.* **10,** 441–450.

85. Huber, B. E., Austin, E. A., Richards, C. A., Davis, S. T., and Good, S. S. (1994) Metabolism of 5-fluorocytidine to 5-fluorouracil in human colorectal tumor cells transduced with the cytosine deaminase gene: significant antitumor effects when only a small percentage of tumor cells express cytosine deaminase. *Proc. Natl. Acad. Sci. USA* **91,** 8302–8306.

86. Whartenby, K. A., Darnowski, J. W., Scott, M. F., and Calabresi, P. (2002) A role for MAP kinase in the antitumor activity of a nucleoside analog. *Cancer Gene Ther.* **9,** 37–43.

87. Krohne, T. U., Shankara, S., Geissler, M., et al. (2001) Mechanism of cell death induced by suicide genes encoding purine nucleoside phosphorylase in human hepatocellular carcinoma cells in vitro. *Hepatology* **34,** 511–518.

88. Akyurek, L. M., Nallamshetty, S., Aoki, K., Yang, Z.-Y., Nabel, G. J., and Nabel, E. G. (2001) Coexpression of guanylate kinase with thymidine kinase enhances prodrug cell killing in vitro and suppresses vascular cell proliferation in vivo. *Mol. Ther.* **3,** 779–786.

89. Jounaidi, Y. and Waxman, D. J. (2000) Combination of the bioreductive drug tirapazamine with the therapeutic prodrug cyclophosphamide for P450/P450-reductase based cancer gene therapy. *Cancer Res.* **60,** 3761–3769.

90. Lakhanpal, S., Donehower, R. C., and Rowinsky, E. K. (2001) Phase II study of 4-ipomeanol, a naturally occuring alkylating furan, in patients with advanced hepatocellular carcinoma. *Invest. New Drugs* **19,** 69–76.

91. Stegman, L. D., Zheng, H., Neal, E. R., et al. (1998) Induction of cytotoxic oxidative stress by D-alanine in brain tumor cells expressing Rhodotorula Gracilis D-amino acids: a cancer gene therapy strategy. *Hum. Gene Ther.* **9,** 185–193.

92. Tamiya, T., Ono, Y., Wei, M. X., Mroz, P. J., Moolten., F. L., and Chiocca, E. A. (1996) *Escherichia coli* gpt gene sensitizes rat glioma cells to killing by 6-thioxanthine or 6-thioguanine. *Cancer Gene Ther.* **3,** 155–162.

93. Miki, K., Xu, M., Gupta, A., et al. (2001) Methioninase cancer gene therapy with selenomethionine as suicide prodrug substrate. *Cancer Res.* **61,** 6805–6810.

94. Carl, P. L., Chakravaty, P. K., and Katzenellenbogen, J. A. (1981) A novel connector linkage applicable in prodrug design. *J. Med. Chem.* **24,** 479–480.

95. Wakselman, M. (1983) 1, 4 - and 1, 6-elimination from hydroxy- and amino-substituted benzyl systems: chemical and biochemical applications. *Nouv. J. Chim.* **7,** 439–447.

96. Mauger, A. B., Burke, P. J., Somani, H. H., Friedlos, F., and Knox, R. J. (1994) Self-immolative prodrugs: candidates for antibody-directed enzyme prodrug therapy in conjunction with a nitroreductase enzyme. *J. Med. Chem.* **37,** 3452–3458.

97. Lee, M., Simpson, J. E., Woo, S., et al. (1997) Synthesis of an aminopropyl analog of the experimental anticancer drug tallimustine, and activation of its 4-nitrobenzylcarbamoyl prodrug by nitroreductase and NADH. *Bioorg. Med. Chem. Lett.* **7,** 1065–1070.

98. Gesson, J.-P., Jacquesy, J.-C., Mondon, M., et al. (1994) Prodrugs of anthracyclines for chemotherapy via enzyme-monoclonal antibody conjugates. *Anti-Cancer Drug Des.* **9,** 409–423.

99. Leenders, R. C. G., Damen, E. W. P., Bijsterveld, E. J. A., et al. (1999) Novel anthracycline–spacer–β-glucuronide, –β-glucoside, and –β-galactoside prodrugs for application in selective chemotherapy. *Bioorg. Med. Chem.* **7,** 1597–1610.

100. Alexander, R. P., Beeley, N. R. A., O'Driscott, M., et al. (1991) Cephalosporin nitrogen mustard carbamate prodrugs for ADEPT. *Tetrahedron Lett.* **32,** 3269–3272.

101. Svensson, H. P., Kadow, J. F., Vrudhula, V. M., Wallace, P. M., and Senter, P. D. (1992) Monoclonal antibody–β-lactamase conjugates for the activation of a cephalosporin mustard prodrug. *Bioconjug. Chem.* **3,** 176–181.

102. Meyer, D. L., Jungheim, L. N., Law, K. L., et al. (1993) Site-specific prodrug activation by antibody–β-lactamase conjugates: regression and long term growth inhibition of human colon carcinoma xenograft models. *Cancer Res.* **53,** 3956–3963.

103. Jungheim, L. N., Sheperd, T. A., and Kling, J. K. (1993) Synthesis of a cephalosporin–doxorubicin antitumor prodrug: a substrate for an antibody-targeted enzyme. *Heterocycles* **35,** 339–348.

104. Hanessian, S. and Wang, J. (1993) Design and synthesis of a cephalosporin carboplatinum prodrug activatable by a beta-lactamase.*Canadian J. Chem.* **71,** 896–906.

105. Moore, J., Ohmstede, C., Dickerson, S., et al. (1997) Gene therapy utilizing enzymes capable of extracellular conversion of multiple prodrugs. *Proc. Am. Assoc. Cancer Res.* **38,** 379.

106. Sykes, B. M., Atwell, G. J., Hogg, A., Wilson, W. R., O'Connor, C. J., and Denny, W. R. (1999) N-Substituted 2-(2,6-dinitrophenylamino)propanamides: novel prodrugs that release a primary aminevia nitroreduction and intramolecular cyclization. *J. Med. Chem.***42,** 346–355.

107. de Bont, D. B. A., Leenderens, R. G. G., Haisma, H. J., van der Meulen-Muileman, I., and Scheeren, H. W. (1997) Synthesis and biological activity of β-glucuronyl carbamate-based prodrugs of paclitaxel as potential candidates for ADEPT. *Bioorg. Med. Chem.* **5**, 405–414.

108. Hay, M. P., Sykes, B. M., Denny, W. A., and O'Connor, C. J. (1999) Substituent effects on the kinetics of reductively-initiated fragmentation of nitrobenzyl carbamates designed as triggers for prodrugs. *J. Chem. Soc. Perkin Transactions 1* **19**, 2759–2770.

109. Andrianomenjanahary, S., Dong, X., Florent, J.-C., et al. (1992) Synthesis of novel targeted pro-prodrugs of anthracyclins potentially activated by a monoclonal antibody galactosidase conjugate. *Bioorg. Med. Chem. Lett.* **9**, 1093.

110. Atwell, G. J., Sykes, B. M., O'Connor, C. J., and Denny, W. A. (1994) Relationships between structure and kinetics of cyclisation of 2-aminoaryl amides: potential prodrugs of cyclisation-activated aromatic mustards. *J. Med. Chem.* **37**, 371–380.

111. Dillon, M. P., Cai, H., and Maag, H. (1996) Application of the "trimethyl lock" to ganciclovir, a pro-prodrug with increased oral bioavailability. *Bioorg. Med. Chem. Lett.* **6**, 1653–1656.

112. Wang, B., Zhang, H., and Wang, W. (1996) Chemical feasability studies of a potential coumarin-based prodrug system. *Bioorg. Med. Chem. Lett.* **6**, 945–950.

113. Schmidt, F., Florent, J.-C., Monneret, C., Straub, R., Czech, J., Gerken, M., and Bosslet, K. (1997) Glucuronide prodrugs of hydroxy compounds for antibody directed enzyme prodrug therapy (ADEPT): a phenol nitrogen mustard carbamate. *Bioorg. Med. Chem. Lett.* **7**, 1071–1076.

114. Sykes, B. M., Hay, M. P., Bohing-Herceg, D., Helsby, N. A., O'Connor, C. J., and Denny, W. A. (2000) Leaving group effects in reductively triggered fragmentation of 4-nitrobenzyl carbamates. *J. Chem. Soc. Perkin Trans. 1* **10**, 1601–1608.

115. Tercel, M., Wilson, R. W., Anderson, R. F., and Denny, W. A. (1996) Hypoxia selective antitumor agents. 12. Nitrobenzyl quaternary ammonium salts as bioreductive prodrugs of the alkylating agent mechloramine. *J. Med. Chem.* **39**, 1084–1094.

116. Desbene, S., Dufat-Trinh Van, H., Michel, S., et al. (1999) Application of the ADEPT strategy to the MDR resistance in cancer chemotherapy. *Anti-Cancer Drug Des.* **14**, 93–106.

117. Toki, B. E., Cerveny, C. G., Wahl, A. F., and Senter, P. D. (2002) Protease-mediated fragmentation of p-amidobenzyl ethers: a new strategy for the activation of anticancer prodrugs. *J. Org. Chem.* **67**, 1866–1872.

118. Ghosh, A. K., Khan, S., and Farquhar, D. (1999) A β-galactoside phosphoramide mustard prodrug for use in conjunction with gene-directed enzyme prodrug therapy. *Chem. Commun.* **24**, 2527–2528.

119. Hansch, C., Leo, A., and Hoekman, D. (1995) *Exploring QSAR. Hydrophobic, Electronic and Steric Constants*, American Chemical Society, Washington, DC.

120. Springer, C. J. and Niculescu-Duvaz, I. (1995) Antibody-directed enzyme prodrug therapy (ADEPT) with mustard prodrugs. *Anti-Cancer Drug Des.* **10**, 361–372.

121. Degreve, B., DeClerq, E., and Balzarini, J. (1999) Bystander effect of purine nucleoside analogues in HSV-tk suicide gene therapy is superior to that of pyrimidine nucleoside analogues. *Gene Ther.* **6**, 162–170.

122. Rainov, N. G., Dobberstein, K. U., Sena-Esteves, M., et al. (1998) New prodrug activation gene therapy for cancer using cytochrome P450 4B1 and 2-aminoanthracene/4-ipomeanol. *Hum. Gene Ther.* **9**, 1261–1273.

123. Thatcher, N. J., Edwards, R. J., Lemoine, N. R., Doehmer, J., and Davies, D. S. (2000) The potential of acetaminophen as a prodrug in gene-directed enzyme prodrug therapy. *Cancer Gene Ther.* **7**, 521–525.

124. Bakina, E., Wu, Z., Rosenblum, M., and Farquhar, D. (1997) Intensely cytotoxic anthracycline prodrugs: glucuronides. *J. Med. Chem.* **40**, 4013–4018.
125. Grignet-Debrus, C., Cool, V., Baudson, N., Velu, T., and Calberg-Bacq, C.-M. (2000) The role of cellular- and prodrug-associated factors in the bystander effect induced by the varicella zoster and herpes simplex viral thymidine kinases in suicide gene therapy. *Cancer Gene Ther.* **7**, 1456–1468.
126. Hoganson, D. A., Batra, R. K., Olsen, J. C., and Boucher, R. C. (1996) Comparison of the effects of three different toxin genes and their level of expression on cell growth and bystander effect in lung adenocarcinoma. *Cancer Res.* **56**, 1315–1323.
127. Nishihara, E., Nagayama, Y., Narimatsu, M., et al. (1998) Treatment of thyroid carcinoma cells with four different suicide gene/prodrug combinations in vitro. *Anticancer Res.* **18**, 1521–1526.
128. Patterson, A. V. and Harris, A. L. (1999) Molecular chemotherapy for breast cancer. *Drugs Aging* **14**, 75–90.
129. Hu, L., Liu, B., and Hacking, D. R. (2000) 5'-[2-(2-Nitrophenyl)-2-methylpropionyl]-2'-deoxy-5-fluorouridine as a potential bioreductively activated prodrug of FUDR: synthesis, stability and reductive activation. *Bioorg. Med. Chem. Lett.* **10**, 797–800.
130. Frank, S., Steffens, S., Fischer, U., Tlolko, A., Rainov, N. G., and Kramm, C. M. (2002) Differential cytotoxicity and bystander effect of the rabbit cytochrome P450 4B1 enzyme gene by two different prodrugs: Implications for pharmacogene therapy. *Cancer Gene Ther.* **9**, 178–188.
131. Kievit, E., Bershad, E., Ng, E., et al. (1999) Superiority of yeast over bacterial cytosine deaminase for enzyme/prodrug gene therapy in colon cancer. *Cancer Res.* **59**, 1417–1421.
132. Kokoris, M. S., Sabo, P., Adman, E. T., and Black, M. E. (1999) Enhancement of tumor ablation by a selected HSV-1 thymidine kinase mutant. *Gene Ther.* **6**, 1415–1426.
133. Bailey, S. M., Knox, R. J., Hobbs, S. M., et al. (1996) Investigation of alternative prodrugs for use with *E. coli* nitroreductase in "suicide gene" approaches to cancer therapy. *Gene Ther.* **3**, 1143–1150.
134. de Groot, F. M. J., Loos, W. J., Koekkoek, R., et al. (2001) Elongated multiple electronic cascade and cyclization spacer systems in activatable anticancer prodrugs for enhanced drug release. *J. Org. Chem.* **66**, 8815–8830.
135. Bohnenstengel, F., Friedel, G., Ritter, C. A., et al. (2000) Variability of cyclophosphamide uptake into human bronchial carcinoma: consequences for local bioactivation. *Cancer Chemother. Pharmacol.* **45**, 63–68.
136. Ichikawa, T., Petros, W. P., Ludeman, S. M., et al. (2001) Intraneoplastic polymer-based delivery of cyclophosphamide for intratumoral bioconversion by a replicating oncolytic viral vector. *Cancer Res.* **61**, 864–868.
137. Huang, Z., Raychowdhury, M. K., and Waxman, D. J. (2000) Impact of liver P450 reductase suppression on cyclophosphamide activation, pharmacokinetics and antitumoral activity in a cytochrome P450-based cancer gene therapy model. *Cancer Gene Ther.* **7**, 1034–1042.
138. Springer, C. J., Niculescu-Duvaz, I., and Pedley, B. R. (1994) Novel prodrugs of alkylating agents derived from 2-fluoro- and 3-fluorobenzoic acids for antibody-directed enzyme prodrug therapy. *J. Med. Chem.* **37**, 2361–2370.
139. Balzarini, J., Degreve, B., Andrei, G., et al. (1998) Superior cytostatic activity of the ganciclovir elaidic acid ester due to the prolonged intracellular retention of ganciclovir anabolites in herpes simplex virus type 1 thymidine kinase gene-transfected tumor cells. *Gene Ther.* **5**, 419–426.

140. Mohr, L., Rainov, N. G., Mohr, U. G., and Wands, J. R. (2000) Rabbit cytochrome P450 4B1: a novel prodrug activating gene for pharmacogene therapy of hepatocellular canrcinoma. *Cancer Gene Ther.* **7**, 1008–1014.

10

Cytochrome P450-Based Gene Therapies for Cancer

E. Antonio Chiocca and David J. Waxman

1. Introduction: Role of Cytochrome P450s in Anticancer Drug Metabolism and Carcinogen Activation

Cytochrome P450 (CYP) is composed of a family of hemeprotein mono-oxygenases that catalyze reactions as diverse as the biosynthesis of steroid hormones, metabolism of fat-soluble vitamins, oxidation of unsaturated fatty acids, and metabolism of drugs, pollutants, and other xenobiotics (for a review, see **ref. 1**). About 55 *CYP* genes, grouped into 17 gene families, are present in the human genome. *CYPs* belonging to gene families 1, 2, and 3 are particularly active in drug and xenobiotic metabolism and are most abundantly expressed in the liver and other tissues that come in contact with foreign chemicals. Large interindividual variations in *CYP* expression and, consequently, CYP-dependent drug metabolism are seen in humans, as a result of both genetic and environmental factors.

In the context of cancer, a large number of investigative studies on *CYPs* have focused on their role as bioactivators of procarcinogens. For instance, CYP1A1 catalyzes the activation of airborne polycyclic aromatic hydrocarbons, such as benzo(*a*)pyrene, in the lung to yield DNA-alkylating carcinogenic metabolites. The finding of functionally important single-nucleotide polymorphisms (SNPs) in *CYP1A1* and in other carcinogen-activating *CYPs* raises the possibility that these SNPs may be linked to interindividual differences in susceptibility to environmental carcinogens in the human population. For example, an A to G polymorphism in exon 7 of *CYP1A1* leads to an Ile to Val substitution that is found more commonly in patients afflicted with lung cancer in a Japanese population (*2*).

Cytochrome P450s play an important role in the metabolism of several widely used anticancer drugs (for a review, see **ref. 1**). Typically, CYP-catalyzed drug metabolism (including anticancer drug metabolism) leads to drug inactivation. However, in the case of several cancer chemotherapeutic drugs, including cyclophosphamide (CPA) and its isomer ifosfamide (IFA), CYP metabolism converts an inactive prodrug to an

From: *Methods in Molecular Medicine, Vol. 90, Suicide Gene Therapy: Methods and Reviews*
Edited by: C. J. Springer © Humana Press Inc., Totowa, NJ

active chemotherapeutic metabolite *(3)*. Individual variation in *CYP* expression profiles may thus be associated with individual differences in anticancer drug metabolism and pharmacokinetics and, potentially, individual differences in drug toxicity and clinical response. The potential impact of pharmacogenetics—in particular, allelic variations in *CYP* genes—on the metabolism of anti-cancer drugs such as CPA or IFA is suggested by the finding that two allelic variants of *CYP2C18*, one with a Met(385) and the other with a Thr(385) allele *(4)*, exhibit up to a sixfold difference in catalytic efficiency in IFA activation *(5)*. Cancer patients with this SNP who are treated with IFA might exhibit an altered therapeutic index compared to the remainder of the population. Several other anticancer drugs, such as taxol, tamoxifen, and flutamide, are converted into inactive metabolites by *CYPs (6–8)*. Accordingly, SNPs in the *CYPs* that inactivate these drugs may potentially contribute to individual differences in therapeutic indices and anticancer responses encountered in the clinic.

Studies of *CYP*-dependent pharmacogenomics and anticancer pharmacology are thus important to cancer therapeutics and may lead to important advances in our understanding of cancer epidemiology and cancer biology. As will be discussed, the detailed understanding of the role of CYPs in the conversion of anticancer prodrugs into active drug metabolites can be exploited to enhance the responsiveness of tumor cells using a novel gene therapy for cancer treatment. Studies initially reported in 1994 demonstrate that CYPs have the potential to enhance chemotherapeutic responses when incorporated into an anticancer regimen in a gene-based treatment strategy *(9)*. In this chapter, we review recent studies demonstrating the efficacy of CYP-based cancer gene therapy and discuss how these studies have established a firm preclinical basis for clinical trials that have recently been initiated.

2. Clinical Uses of CPA

Cyclophosphamide is an oxazaphosphorine alkylating agent prodrug used in two distinct clinical settings (*see* **Fig. 1**). CPA is a widely used anticancer agent, and it is a pleiotropic immunosuppressive drug that can rapidly decrease lymphocyte counts, affecting B-cell maturation and antibody production and decreasing macrophage/monocyte, natural killer (NK) cells, and cytokine generation *(10,12)*. CPA can affect multiple arms of the immune system, but it is more effective in its inhibition of the innate responses as well as of the adaptive humoral responses. Accordingly, CPA is effective in treating autoimmune disorders and as a countermeasure against organ rejection in transplant recipients.

As an anticancer drug, CPA and its chemical isomer IFA are typically used in combination with other chemotherapeutic agents. CPA is a cell-cycle-phase-nonspecific anticancer agent *(10)*. It is an important component of chemotherapeutic regimens currently employed in the treatment of breast, lung, and ovarian cancers, sarcomas, and a variety of childhood cancers *(10)*. CPA is also employed in the treatment of other cancers, including certain brain tumors. CPA diffuses rapidly across cell membranes, including in the liver, where it is subject to CYP-catalyzed activation to yield the polar metabolite 4-hydroxy-CPA (*see* **Fig. 2** and **Subheading 3.**) *(13)*. Like many anticancer drugs, CPA has a relatively narrow therapeutic index, and careful dosing and schedules must be

CPA 4-hydroxyCPA PM

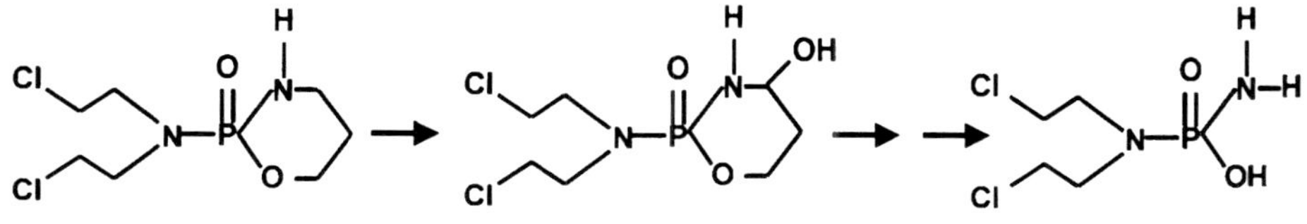

Fig. 1. A summary of the pathway of CPA activation. CPA is activated by members of the cytochrome P450 family into 4-hydroxycyclophosphamide, which spontaneously decomposes into the active metabolite, phosphoramide mustard.

employed to minimize harmful side effects. Chemically activated forms of CPA have been synthesized (e.g., 4-hydroperoxy-CPA and mafosfamide), but these are of limited clinical utility because of dose-limiting toxicities *(14,15)*.

3. Activation of CPA and IFA by CYP2B Enzymes

Cyclophosphamide is inactive until it is converted into its active metabolites in a reaction mediated by a CYP-catalyzed hydroxylation reaction at C-4 (*see* **Fig. 1**). The resulting metabolite, 4-hydroxy-CPA (4-OH-CPA), equilibrates with the ring-opened aldophosphamide, which spontaneously decomposes in a β-elimination reaction to yield equimolar amounts of acrolein and phosphoramide mustard. The latter metabolite is the therapeutically active anticancer agent responsible for DNA alkylation and tumor cell toxicity, whereas the former contributes to some of the host toxicities of CPA, including hemorrhagic cystitis and other side effects *(10)*. CPA metabolism primarily occurs in the liver and is catalyzed by CYP enzymes. The finding that the rate of hepatic CPA activation can be induced by the liver CYP inducer phenobarbital provided the first clue that this metabolism was catalyzed by a phenobarbital-inducible liver CYP enzyme. In studies of CPA 4-hydroxylation using liver microsomes isolated from rats treated with phenobarbital, reconstituted enzyme systems, enzyme CYP2B1 was shown to be the most active of 11 rat CYPs examined (2B1, 2B2, 2C11, 2A2, 2C6, 1A1, 2C12, 2A1, 2C13, 3A1, 1A2) *(11)*. Activation of CPA was established using a variety of enzymatic assays, including measuring the binding to bovine serum albumin (BSA) of [^{14}C]acrolein, formed from [^{14}C]CPA, and the alkylation of calf thymus DNA by [^{3}H]phosphoramide mustard derived from [*chloroethyl*-^{3}H]CPA. CYP2B1 activation of CPA (turnover rate of approx 26 nmol metabolite/min/nmol P-450) proceeded at a ≥ 10-fold higher rate than that catalyzed by the other CYPs.

Subsequent studies of human CYP enzymes demonstrated that CYP2B6, together with several CYP2C enzymes, plays a key role in the activation of CPA in human liver tissue *(16,17)*. By contrast, IFA activation in human liver was found to be primarily carried out by CYP3A4 *(16)*. Therefore, species-specific differences in the metabolism of these prodrugs are readily apparent and need to be taken into account in considering CYPs for therapeutic exploitation.

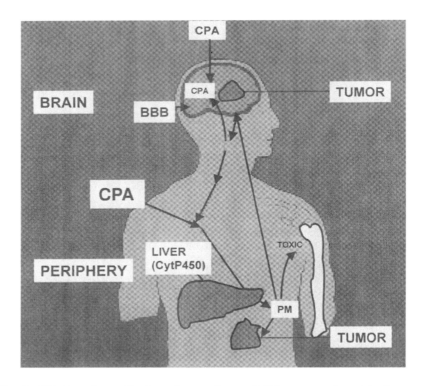

Fig. 2. CPA is activated by hepatic cytochrome P450 enzymes into 4-hydroxycyclo-phosphamide. The latter gives rise to phosphoramide mustard, which acts as an anticancer agent. However, transport of this metabolite across the blood brain barrier is not very efficient. In this case, the gene therapy paradigm includes: (1) endogenous tumor cells in the brain that are transduced to express one of the cytochrome P450 enzymes, responsible for CPA bioconversion (such as CYP2B1), and (2) local CPA administration. This may provide a means for more effective chemotherapy of the brain tumor.

4. *CYP* Gene Transfer Confers on Tumor Cells a Novel Chemosensitivity to CPA

In the late 1980s, a novel prodrug activation gene therapy strategy for cancer treatment was introduced *(18–20)*. The thymidine kinase enzyme encoded by herpes simplex virus type 1, HSV-TK, phosphorylates and thereby activates nucleoside analogs such as acyclovir and ganciclovir (GCV). This phosphorylation enables the nucleoside to ultimately be metabolized to a triphosphate, which can be incorporated into replicating viral DNA, thus terminating the growing DNA chain, leading to an effective antiviral therapy. This same strategy can be applied to kill human tumor cells: In tumor cells that are stably transfected with *HSV-TK* and then treated with a nucleoside analog, phosphorylated acyclovir (or phosphorylated GCV) becomes incorporated into the replicating tumor cell's DNA, leading to tumor cell death. The emerging field of cancer gene therapy became enamored with this strategy: Viral and nonviral vectors could be genetically engineered to deliver the *HSV-TK* gene into tumors, thereby rendering these neoplasms chemosensitive to GCV. The preclinical and clinical application of this treatment strategy to a variety of cancers and proliferative disorders has now been tested *(21,22)*. Although the basic concept has been verified and validated, the poor delivery of *HSV-TK* into tumors has proven to be a major limitation and has led to the failure of such trials *(23)*.

Investigation of other possible prodrug-activation gene therapy strategies for treatment of brain tumors led to the consideration of the CYP-activated prodrug CPA. CPA can be used to treat brain tumors, but its use is hampered by the requirement that CPA be activated in the liver, followed by transport to the tumor of the activated metabolite 4-OH-CPA and/or its ring-opened derivative aldophosphamide. Furthermore, to be effective, 4-OH-CPA needs to diffuse across cell membranes and then decompose intracellularly to yield phosphoramide mustard, a hydrophilic compound with poor capacity for diffusion across lipid membranes. In particular, the blood–brain barrier (BBB) can effectively hamper CPA's anticancer effects in treating brain tumors. In fact, the level of phosphoramide mustard assayed in brain tissue when CPA is activated in the liver is quite low (*see* **Fig. 2**) *(13)*. One solution to this problem would be to provide for delivery and activation of CPA within the brain, directly within the tumor itself.

The finding that CYP2B1 is an active catalyst of CPA activation *(11)* provided the opportunity to evaluate whether the use of CYP2B1 to activate CPA within tumor cells might serve as an effective prodrug-activation gene therapy strategy. To test this proposal, rat *CYP2B1* cDNA was transfected into rat glioma cells, which thereby acquired chemosensitivity to CPA. CYP2B1 was then cloned into a retroviral vector and retroviral producer cells were generated. Treatment of subcutaneous and brain tumors by vector producer cell injection resulted in an enhanced therapeutic effect compared to control treatment *(3)*. These experiments demonstrated that a strategy coupling *CYP2B1* gene transfer into tumors with CPA treatment had the potential for exploitation as an alternative to *HSV-TK*/GCV.

Further exploitation of this strategy against rat 9L gliosarcoma and human MCF7 breast carcinoma cells, stably transfected with *CYP2B1* and grown in vivo as subcutaneous tumors, was also demonstrated *(24,25)*. Thus, *CYP*-based gene therapy not only has the potential for applications in the treatment of brain tumors but could also be used to enhance the chemosensitivity of systemic tumors. The large extent of chemosensitization of the systemic tumors was somewhat unexpected, given that these tumors are already exposed to high levels of circulating 4-OH-CPA generated by hepatic CYP enzymes. In other studies, an adenoviral vector expressing *CYP2B1* was developed and shown to sensitize a variety of rodent and human tumor cells to both CPA and IFA *(25)*. Intratumoral CYP-dependent CPA activation led to an initial accumulation of tumor cells in the S-phase of the cell cycle, followed by an even more substantial accretion of cells at the G2-M-phase at later time-points. This finding is consistent with CPA-metabolite-induced damage to cellular DNA, which is manifest as G2-M cell cycle arrest. It is not known if this arrest is mediated by p21 and/or by proteins involved in the repair of DNA damage. However, recent studies have established that CYP-activated CPA induces a caspase 9-dependent apoptotic pathway *(70)*.

Together, these initial findings established the feasibility of pursuing a *CYP*-based gene therapy that utilizes established anticancer prodrugs. Several important details remained to be determined, including the optimal method for delivery of the *CYP* transgene into tumors, the route, vehicle, and schedule for delivery of the prodrug to achieve optimal efficacy and minimal toxicity, and whether the therapeutic effect could be further enhanced by combination with other treatment strategies.

5. The Bystander Effect

The original reports describing GCV/*HSV-TK*-based cancer gene therapy included an in vitro experiment that described a "bystander" cytotoxic effect. In this experiment, HSV-TK-expressing tumor cells and nonexpressing tumor cells were cocultivated in the presence of the prodrug GCV. As expected, HSV-TK-expressing cells died following GCV treatment, but, unexpectedly, the cocultivated HSV-TK nonexpressing cells were also susceptible to GCV cytotoxicity. This effect was not mediated by conditioned medium from the HSV-TK-expressing cells; rather, it required direct contact between the two cell populations *(26,27)*. There was a dose–effect relationship whereby greater toxicity was imparted to naïve cells in proportion to the fraction of HSV-TK-expressing cells found in the coculture. Further in vitro characterization of this effect suggested that it was mediated by passage of phosphorylated GCV metabolites across cellular gap junctions, although endocytosis of HSV-TK-expressing apoptotic bodies by naïve tumor cells was also invoked as a mechanism for the bystander toxicity. To further complicate matters, in vivo bystander toxicity was also shown to be the result of immunologic crossreactive responses *(28–30)*. Similar bystander responses have been described for other prodrug-activating gene therapies *(31,32)*. Such bystander responses are highly significant because they may greatly amplify the cytotoxic response to include cells well beyond the cells that are initially transduced with the therapeutic, prodrug-activating gene. This is an important feature, given that an effective, anticancer strategy must kill every tumor cell within the population, and for the forseeable future, gene transfer paradigms are unlikely to reach every cell within a neoplasm.

Characterization of the CPA/*CYP2B1* gene transfer strategy with regard to its potential for bystander cytotoxicity revealed an important difference in comparison to HSV-TK: Conditioned medium from CPA-treated cells that stably expressed CYP2B1 was cytotoxic to naive tumor cells, consistent with the presence in the medium of a diffusible, activated CPA metabolite, such as 4-OH-CPA *(24,33)*. This was shown to occur both with rat C6 and 9L glioma cell lines as well as human U87 and Gli36 glioma cells. The presence of 4-OH-CPA in conditioned medium was confirmed by a semicarbazide trapping fluorometric method *(4,58)* and, more recently, by a gas chromatographic–mass spectrometric technique (GC-MS) *(34)*. The production of diffusible metabolites with CPA/*CYP2B1* gene therapy is a feature that is intrinsic to 4-OH-CPA and results in a bystander effect that, unlike that of activated GCV, is independent of gap-junctional communication or apoptotic cell body endocytosis (*see* **Fig. 3**). More recently, other prodrug-activating gene therapies have been described whose bystander effect can be mediated by conditioned medium and are thus similar to the CPA/*CYP2B1* gene therapy paradigm *(35,36)*.

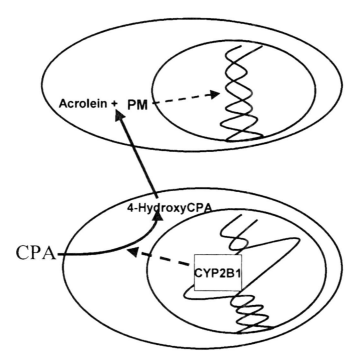

Fig. 3. The "bystander" effect with CPA/*CYP2B1* gene therapy is attributable to the diffusion of active CPA metabolites (presumably 4-hydroxycyclophosphamide) from the "converting" tumor cell into other tumor cells. In the latter, decomposition of 4-hydroxyCPA gives rise to the active metabolites (acrolein and PM). The latter possesses DNA alkylating properties that lead to observed cytotoxic effects.

6. *CYP* Gene Delivery: The Replicating Virus Strategy

Clinical trials of cancer gene therapy most commonly involve inoculation of a replication-defective vector (viral or nonviral) into the neoplastic mass. Typically, analysis of the inoculated tumor tissue reveals a pattern of gene expression that is localized along the needle tract, with little evidence for diffusion of the vector from the site of injection *(23,37)*. For example, stereotactic injection of either a lacZ-expressing adenoviral vector or a retroviral vector into a malignant human glioma resulted in infection of a minority of tumor cells located less than 1 cm from the needle tract *(38)*. Extremely low tumor transduction rates in cells primarily located around the needle injection tract have also been observed in a clinical trial involving stereotactic injection of HSV-TK-expressing retroviral vector producer cells into recurrent human malignant gliomas *(23)*. These findings prompted the development of methods to improve the anatomic extent of tumor transduction by a gene therapy vector.

One approach to accomplish this objective involves the use of a replication conditional, oncolytic virus (OV) to deliver the therapeutic gene into the tumor. OVs are genetically altered viruses with deletions that restrict viral replication in normal cells but permit replication in tumor cells *(39,71)*. Additional approaches that can provide for tumor-selective replication include the use of tumor-specific promoters to drive viral replication *(40)* and alteration of the viral tropism to infect only desired target cells *(41)*. The process of viral replication and expression of viral genes is toxic to the host cell and leads to its rapid demise. Additional inflammatory changes within the tumor can also contribute to the virus' anticancer action.

Oncolytic viruses can be engineered to deliver therapeutic genes, including prodrug-activating genes, thus providing for multimodal mechanisms of tumor cytotoxicity *(42)*. Because the time frame of viral replication can typically last from 12 to 24 h (depending on the virus employed), expression of the therapeutic gene within an infected tumor cell may be of short duration. However, the continuous process of viral replication and subsequent propagation within the tumor can render this expression temporally and anatomically extensive within the tumor mass *(43)*. In addition, if expression of the therapeutic gene expressed by an OV leads to formation of a diffusible factor or cytotoxic metabolite, such as 4-OH-CPA, then even a brief period of production within the infected cell could confer a significant antitumor effect.

A large number of OVs have been developed, based on herpes simple virus (HSV), adenovirus, vaccinia virus, reovirus, and others *(39,71)*. HSV-based OVs have been engineered to possess genetic alterations in the viral gene locus *(UL39)* that encodes the viral ICP6 protein and/or the ICP34.5 protein. The former alteration restricts viral replication to cells with elevated levels of deoxynucleoside triphosphate pools, a product of cellular ribonucleotide reductase (RR) function *(44,45)*. Because *RR* gene transcription is strictly regulated by the p16/pRB tumor suppressor pathway, replication of HSV OVs with defective ICP6 function is likely to target defects in this particular tumor suppressor pathway. In contrast, it remains unclear how viral defects in ICP34.5 function are associated with selective replication in tumors. At least two different HSV OVs have entered into clinical trials and several more are likely to begin clinical testing *(46,47)*.

To test the utility of OVs for delivering a therapeutic *CYP* gene, a HSV-based OV that expresses *CYP2B1* was engineered. *CYP2B1* cDNA was subcloned into the UL39 (ICP6) locus of HSV under transcriptional control of the endogenous ICP6 promoter *(48)*. Expression of *CYP2B1* in cell lines infected with this novel OV, designated as rRp450, was confirmed by Western blot analysis and by GC-MS assays of 4-hydroxy-CPA production in infected cell supernatants *(34)*. A schedule of four inoculations of rRp450, given every other day for 1 wk with a single injection of CPA between the first two doses, was employed and shown to be more effective in controlling ectopic growth of human tumor xenografts than either therapy applied alone.

One interesting and important finding relates to the effects of the activated CPA metabolite 4-OH-CPA. When rRp450 titers were determined in infected cells exposed to CPA, minimal effects on viral titers were found both in vitro and in vivo *(48)*. This indicates that activated CPA displays anticancer activity but minimal antiviral effects. In contrast, activated GCV exhibits both antiviral and anticancer effects. Thus, in the presence of GCV, replication of rRp450 is completely inhibited. This reflects the fact that rRp450, like all other HSVs, expresses the *HSV-TK* gene and is an important point to be considered in the context of cancer therapies utilizing OVs. The combination of rRp450 with CPA for tumor therapy is expected to provide for continuous viral replication within the tumor mass, with anticancer effects resulting not only from the OV's direct cytotoxic effects but also from the tumor cytotoxicity of activated CPA. By contrast, when rRp450 and GCV are used in combination, viral replication in strongly inhibited, such that the observed anticancer effects are provided primarily mediated by the activated GCV *(42)*.

An additional and relevant consideration concerns the immunosuppressive properties of CPA. In the context of a replicating OV and of the humoral and cellular immune responses against it, transient immunosuppression provided by activated CPA favors continuous viral replication and anticancer effects in vivo, particularly when the OV is delivered intravascularly *(49)*. Suppression of innate antiviral responses, such as the classical and lectin pathways of complement activation as well as the production of antiviral cytokines, is a likely mechanism responsible for the observed effects of CPA on OV treatment *(50,72,73)*.

In summary, CPA/*CYP2B1* gene delivery to tumors can be carried out in an effective manner by combination with OV therapy of tumors. The combination of 4-OH-CPA-mediated toxicity toward tumor cells with minimal effects on viral replication and the suppression of antiviral immune responses results in enhanced anticancer responses associsted with intratumoral OV replication.

7. Synergy With Other Gene Therapies

Other improvements in CPA/*CYP2B1* gene therapy may derive from combinations of prodrug activation strategies *(51)*. Application of traditional parameters of drug-interaction studies to prodrug-activation gene therapies has recently been investigated. Ganciclovir/HSV-TK can be combined with CPA/*CYP2B1* gene therapy and the occurence of pharmacologic synergy or antagonism has been ascertained *(42)*. Using stably transfected 9L rat gliosarcoma cells, the method of Chou–Talalay *(52)* as well as the classical isobologram method can be applied to exclude the possibility of antagonism that may be deleterious to anticancer effects and to demonstrate pharmacologic synergy between the two gene therapies. The observed synergy can be further validated by mechanistic proposals and studies. GCV's metabolites are nucleoside analogs, whereas CPA's metabolites are alkylating agents. Reports that other nucleoside analogs are pharmacologically synergistic in their anticancer action with other alkylating agents *(53,54)* leads to the hypothesis that the observed synergy arises at the level of DNA repair: After DNA chain alkylation by the CPA metabolite phosphoramide mustard, single nucleotide excision repair mediated by DNA polymerases δ and ε ensues. Activated GCV is thought to primarily affect these polymerases *(55)*. Therefore, inhibition of alkylated DNA nucleotide excision repair by GCV may represent the mechanism of observed synergy. To test this hypothesis, tumor cells were treated with CPA/*CYP2B1* gene therapy and the amount of alkylated DNA then assayed as a function of time in the presence or absence of GCV/HSV-TK gene therapy. Following CPA/*CYP2B1* gene therapy, there was a time-dependent decrease in alkylated DNA, suggesting a fairly rapid nucleotide excision repair. However, in the presence of GCV/HSV-TK gene therapy, this repair was significantly retarded, suggesting a mechanistic explanation for the observed pharmacologic synergy (*see* **Fig. 4**).

This combined gene therapy regimen has been applied in the context of rRp450, the tumor-selective HSV oncolytic virus discussed earlier. Antitumor effects both in vivo and in vitro were significantly enhanced by the combination of GCV/*HSV-TK* with CPA/*CYP2B1*, as evaluated in rat 9L gliosarcoma cells infected with the replicating rRp450. However, one note of caution must be provided. Activated GCV will destroy rRp450 and its ability to replicate; thus, the beneficial effects of combining GCV/ HSV-TK, the replicating virus, and CPA/*CYP2B1* may not be seen in all tumors and in all tumor cell lines. The interplay between replicating HSV and GCV activation will depend on the extent of gap-junction formation between tumor cells and the replicative ability of the virus. When virus replicates well and/or gap-junction formation is low, GCV will primarily antagonize the oncolytic effect. However, when conditions do not favor viral replication and/or when gap-junction formation is prominent, GCV activation combined with OV treatment will result in a more prominent anticancer effect than either treatment alone.

Further confirmation of the potentially beneficial interactions between prodrug-activation strategies involving alkylating agents and nucleoside analogs has been provided in studies using encapsulated cells engineered to express both *CYP2B1* and cytosine deaminase *(CD) (56)*. The latter enzyme converts the prodrug 5-fluorocytosine (5-FC) into the anti-cancer drug 5-fluorouracil (5-FU). After cell encapsulation and implantation into TS/A murine adenocarcinoma or GR murine mammary carcinoma tumors, treatment with IFA in combination with 5-FC resulted in more potent anticancer effects than treatment with either prodrug alone. By contrast, when parental, nontransduced cells were used, the combination of prodrugs was not as effective as either prodrug used alone. Independent confirmation of the enhanced anticancer effect of these two forms of prodrug-activating gene therapy was thus obtained.

8. Delivery of CPA Via Polymers

In order to maximize local cytotoxicity and minimize systemic side effects, local tumoral activation of CPA by transferred *CYP* cDNAs might also benefit from local delivery of the prodrug. Recently, intratumoral application of a polymer impregnated with the chemotherapeutic agent BCNU was approved by the U.S. Food and Drug Administration (FDA) for local treatment of malignant gliomas *(57)*. Based on the same concept, local application of a polymeric formulation of CPA was tested to ascertain whether increased intraneoplastic concentrations of the prodrug's active metabolites when compared to controls could be observed after tumor inoculation with rRp450 *(34)*. The results obtained demonstrated that there was a 10-fold increase in peak levels of activated CPA metabolites in rRp450-inoculated tumors treated with polymeric CPA compared to rRp450-inoculated tumors treated with systemic CPA. This translated to AUC (area under the curve) values of approx 800 µg/mg/h for the former compared to only approx 3 µg/mg/h for the latter. When systemic blood levels of CPA metabolites were measured for each method of prodrug delivery, no differences in AUC values were seen (approx 3 µg/mL/h). Thus, when compared to systemic CPA delivery, polymer-based local delivery of CPA into a tumor that expresses

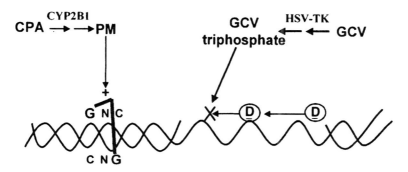

Fig. 4. Mechanism postulated to be responsible for the observed synergy between CPA/ *CYP2B1* and GCV/*HSV-TK* gene therapies. The active metabolite of CPA (PM) produces inter- and intrastrand crosslinks between guanine residues within the sequence 5'-GNC-3'. Such crosslinks can be excised and repaired by DNA repair enzymes, such as DNA polymerase delta (D). However, the active metabolite of GCV (GCV triphosphate) functions as an inhibitor of DNA polymerase delta activity, thus potentiating the effects of PM.

CYP2B1 substantially increases the concentration of CPA's cytotoxic metabolites within the neoplastic mass without increasing their systemic concentration.

9. Coexpression of P450 Reductase Enhances CPA/CYP-Based Gene Therapy

The P450 system is actually comprised of two polypeptide components, the heme-containing cytochrome P450 and the flavoprotein P450 reductase (P450R). These two proteins are localized in the endoplasmic reticulum. P450R is a flavin adenine dinucleotide (FAD)- and flavin mononucleotide (FMN)-containing flavoenzyme that catalyzes the transfer of electrons required for all microsomal P450-dependent mono-oxygenase reactions. A total of two electrons are transferred from NADPH to P450R, first to FAD, then to FMN, and then on to the P450 hemeprotein, which utilizes these reducing equivalents to hydroxylate its substrates. Therefore, P450R and P450 need to be coexpressed for CYP2B1 or CYP2B6 to be catalytically active in the context of cancer gene therapy. Although tumor cells have been reported to express sufficient P450R to allow for expression of the transduced CYP gene's intrinsic capability to activate CPA, supplementation of cellular P450R levels by P450R gene transfer substantially enhances the cytotoxic potency of CPA/*CYP2B1* gene therapy in vitro and in vivo *(58)*. For example, in studies of rat 9L gliosarcoma cells that were stably transfected with *CYP2B1*, *P450R*, or both cDNAs in combination, up to a 4- to 10-fold increase in P450R enzyme activity could be achieved by delivery of the P450R gene. This resulted in increased CPA conversion, as measured by formation of CPA's activated metabolites, when compared to control cells. Tumor excision studies demonstrated up to a 10-fold increase in CPA's cytotoxicity toward 9L gliosarcoma cells stably transfected with *CYP2B1* and *P450R* when compared to 9L tumor cells transfected with CYP2B1 alone.

The incorporation of P450R into the P450-based gene therapy strategy not only increases CYP2B1-mediated conversion of CPA to alkylating metabolites but also provides for the ability to convert other prodrugs into active anticancer agents *(59)*. One such agent is tirapazamine (TPZ), a bioreductive prodrug that is particularly active against hypoxic cells. TPZ is activated by P450R, via a one-electron reduction, into a nitroxide radical that causes single- and double-strand DNA breaks. This TPZ radical can be further converted into an inactive product by a second one-electron reduction. Under normoxic conditions, the TPZ radical can be rapidly reoxidized, concomitantly producing reactive oxygen species and superoxide radicals. Because both prodrugs are metabolized by the same *CYP/P450R* gene combination, concern might exist about antagonism from CPA and TPZ competition for the same enzymatic sites. However, the addition of TPZ to CPA was found to augment the cytotoxic effects against 9L cells retrovirally transduced with both *CYP2B6* and *P450R* when treated under either normoxic or hypoxic conditions. Moreover, the in vivo anticancer effects of this prodrug combination were significant, increasing tumor growth delay from 23 d in CPA-treated mice to 35 d in mice treated with CPA plus TPZ. This benefit was partially offset by some increase in host toxicity, manifested by body weight loss, which may have been the result of drug-induced nausea. These findings demonstrate the important principle that transduction of tumor cells with *P450R* not only increases CYP-catalyzed CPA activation but also provides an additional capability for activation of bioreductive prodrugs.

10. Suppression of Liver P450 Prodrug Activation

Another pharmacologic approach to increasing the therapeutic index of CPA/CYP gene therapy involves the selective inhibition of hepatic metabolism of the prodrug *(60)*. This could have the desirable effect of decreasing the systemic toxicity of activated CPA metabolites while increasing the availability of systemically delivered prodrug to tumor cells that express CYP. One approach to inhibition of hepatic but not tumor-cell-catalyzed CPA activation takes advantage of the fact that, in rat liver, the P450R gene is regulated by thyroid hormone, which is required for enzyme expression. This thyroid hormone dependence provides a means to downregulate P450R expression and enzyme activity by using antithyroid drugs such as methimazole (MMI). MMI treatment of rats significantly inhibits liver P450R expression, thereby reducing hepatic *CYP*-mediated prodrug activation. P450R expression and P450R activity in transfected rat 9L tumors is not inhibited by MMI, as expected from the fact that the *P450R* transgene is under control of a heterologous, non-thyroid-hormone-dependent promoter. This selective inhibition of hepatic CPA activation resulted in a 30% decrease in peak plasma concentration and a twofold increase in half-life of the activated CPA metabolite. Correspondingly, MMI treatment improved the anticancer effect of CPA (75 mg/kg) against subcutaneous 9L tumors transfected with *CYP2B1* and *P450R*, although this improvement was not apparent at a higher dose of CPA (100 mg/kg). An advantage of using MMI in this context is that it decreases the incidence of CPA side effects, such as body weight loss and hematuria. Inhibition of weight loss may be a consequence of the hypothyroid state induced by MMI, whereas the decrease in hematuria may be the result of the reduction in urinary excretion of acrolein, one of CPA's metabolites, associated with MMI's inhibition of hepatic and kidney CPA metabolism.

A second pharmacologic approach to improve the balance between tumor vs hepatic CPA activation uses liver CYP enzyme-specific chemical inhibitors (61). In rats, the hepatic enzymes CYP2C6 and CYP2C11 make major contributions to the activation of CPA into its cytotoxic metabolites. Five inhibitors of CYPs were tested: metyrapone and chloramphenicol, both known inhibitors of CYP2B subfamily of P450 enzymes; DDEP (3,5-dicarbethoxy-2,6-dimethyl-4-ethyl-1,4-dihydropyridine) and 1-aminobenzotriazole, which inhibit CYP2C P450 enzymes; and SKF-525A, a general P450 inhibitor. In vitro, significant reductions in liver microsomal activation of CPA were observed with all 5 P450 inhibitors. Pharmacokinetic studies in rats confirmed the inhibitory action of these compounds, with 1-aminobenzotriazole causing a sevenfold increase in the half-life of the activated CPA metabolite 4-OH-CPA. However, only modest effects of these inhibitors on CPA's anticancer activity against 9L/*2B1-P450R* tumors were obtained, and no amelioration of CPA's toxic side effects were observed. Unlike the relatively selective inhibitory action of MMI against liver P450R, the chemical CYP inhibitors studied lack sufficient hepatic CYP inhibitory potency and selectivity to achieve the desired liver-specific inhibitory effect. The testing and evaluation of more specific and more potent liver CYP inhibitors could lead to improved therapeutic results, if differences between the transduced tumor CYP and the hepatic CYP catalysts of CPA activation can be exploited based on differences in P450 enzyme structure or transcriptional regulation.

11. Antiangiogenic Scheduling of CPA

One of the critical and essential steps in tumorigenesis is the active recruitment of a neovascular supply by the growing neoplastic mass. The balance between angiogenic and antiangiogenic factors dictates the establishment not only of a tumor mass but also that of metastatic foci. Recently, Browder et al. reported a significant antiangiogenic effect associated with a novel schedule of CPA administration, involving a repeated, 6-d cycle of CPA at a dose that is lower that the commonly used intermittent high-dose CPA schedule (62). Investigation of the therapeutic effectiveness of this antiangiogenic CPA schedule in combination with CYP gene therapy revealed that 9L tumors expressing CYP2B6 and P450R, established in the flank of scid mice, could be erradicated by a 6-d repeated course of CPA (140 mg/kg) given over 11 cycles (63). The conventional CPA schedule in this tumor model, 150 mg/kg CPA given twice over a period of 24 h, did not produce tumor eradication although it did produce significant tumor growth delay. The change in schedule also ameliorated toxicity in the animals, as indicated by the minimization of body weight loss. Several weeks after cessation of CPA treatment, regrowth of four of eight 9L/2B1-P450R tumors was observed. Three of the four tumors responded to a second course of CPA treatment. This novel CPA schedule was then applied to very large tumors (8–19% of animal's body weight). Substantial regression of the large tumors was achieved, although some resistance to CPA was encountered toward the end of the schedule. Analysis of the mechanism of resistance revealed that the 9L/2B6-P450R tumors had lost the transduced *P450R* gene and *P450R* enzyme activity as well as reduced expression of the CYP2B6 and, hence, the ability to activate CPA efficiently. Importantly, the resistant tumor cells did not acquire intrinsic cellular resistance to CPA (e.g., by overexpression of aldehyde dehydrogenase). This finding underscores the importance of continuous expression of the prodrug-activating CYP transgene, a feat that might be achievable by repeated treatment with the gene therapy vector or by use of replicating agents or self-perpetuating vector systems.

12. CYP2B1 Delivery Using Encapsulated Cells or Macrophages

In addition to the use of viral vectors for transduction of CYP cDNAs, described earlier, several cellular and other nonviral CYP delivery methods have been investigated. In one approach, feline kidney cells were transfected with a CYP2B1 cDNA expression plasmid and then encapsulated into cellulose–sulfate capsules in order to protect the cells from the host immune system (*64*). Capsules contained up to 10^4 cells and cell viability studies in mice showed that approx 50% of the cells were alive 4 wk after encapsulation. In vivo efficacy studies were then performed using human pancreatic tumors established in the flank of nude mice. When the tumors reached a size of 1 cm^3, 20–40 capsulates containing CYP2B1-expressing cells were implanted directly into the tumor followed by treatment with IFA. Four of 12 tumors regressed completely, and the remaining tumors showed evidence of partial responses. These encouraging results have provided a basis for a clinical trial of IFA with CYP2B1 gene therapy in pancreatic cancer patients (*see* **Subheading 15.**).

Macrophages, which can infiltrate tumors and may predominate in hypoxic regions of a tumor, could serve as a useful delivery vehicle for prodrug-activating genes, such as CYPs. In a recent study, adenoviral vectors expressing human *CYP2B6* were used to infect primary human macrophages (*65*). Treatment of these cells with CPA did not affect the viability of the macrophages, as assessed by mitochondrial function. The *CYP*-expressing macrophages were then incubated with tumor cells growing in culture as spheroids, which they were able to infiltrate. Subsequent treatment with CPA resulted in a decrease in spheroid tumor volume as well as a decrease in spheroid clonogenic efficiency. Similar results were obtained when a hypoxia-responsive DNA enhancer was used to regulate expression of CYP2B6 in the macrophages. Therefore, the use of intact cells to deliver CYP enzyme activity into tumors, allowing for CPA chemosensitization, provides an exciting alternative to direct injection of viral vectors. Both the extent of prodrug activation catalyzed by these cells and the distribution of these cells within tumors require further investigation and will be a critical factor in the success of this approach.

13. Activation of 4-Ipomeanol by CYP4B1

The rabbit CYP enzyme CYP4B1 has been shown to activate the prodrugs 4-ipomeanol (4IM) and 4-aminoanthracene (4-AA) into their respective anticancer alkylating metabolites (*66*). In fact, 4IM was originally synthesized as a potential cancer chemotheraputic agent, but human clinical trials revealed a lack of efficacy as well as host toxicity. This is most likely the result of inefficient activation of the prodrug by the endogenous human CYP4B enzyme, whose catalytic activity with the prodrug substrate is only 1% that of the corresponding rabbit enzyme CYP4B1. Therefore, transfer of the rabbit *CYP4B1* might provide a means to achieve increased activation of 4IM in tumors. To test this hypothesis, cultured rat 9L gliosarcoma or human U87 glioma cells were stably transfected with *CYP4B1* and then treated with 4-AA. A significant drug-dependent antiproliferative effect was observed, and fluorescence-activated cell sorter (FACS) analysis revealed that this effect was the result of apoptotic cell death. Crosslinking assays showed that DNA from treated cells was alkylated and in vivo studies confirmed a significant anticancer action for this gene therapy strategy. Similar results were observed with hepatocellular carcinoma cell lines. Therefore, 4IM or 2-AA in combination with CYP4B1 gene transfer provides a second example of CYP-mediated activation of prodrugs into their alkylating agents.

14. Prodrug Activation by Other CYPs

Recently, exploitation of other CYPs and their abilities to activate anticancer prodrugs has been reported. For instance, several human CYP2C enzymes has been shown to activate CPA *(4)* and CYP3A has been shown to activate IFA *(4)* as well as the prodrug AQ4N *(67)*. CYP1A2 can metabolize acetaminophen into the toxic metabolite NABQI *(68)*. This exploits a minor pathway of acetaminophen activation. Generally, the drug is eliminated in the liver by conjugation, forming sulfate or glucuronide derivatives. A minor pathway consists of drug oxidization into NABQI by CYP1A2, CYP3A4, and CYP2E1, with CYP1A2 carrying out the majority of hepatic activity. NABQI is cytotoxic presumably because of its oxidation and arylation of protein thiol groups. In fact, when Chinese hamster ovary cells, stably transfected with a CYP1A2 cDNA, were exposed to acetaminophen, decreases in cell viability were evident. A bystander effect was also observed, although it remained unclear if this effect was mediated by diffusible metabolites.

15. Clinical Trials

The preclinical studies summarized in the chapter indicate that further evaluation of the potential of CYP-based gene therapies leading to human clinical trials are warranted. In the United Kingdom, clinical trials for breast cancer, using a human *CYP2B6* cDNA delivered by intratumoral injections of a retroviral vector followed by systemic CPA treatment, are being pursued in a phase I setting. Preliminary findings in a group of 12 patients have shown a good safety record and encouraging evidence regarding efficacy (Kingsman, Oxford Biomedica, personal communication). In Germany, a separate trial of patients with pancreatic cancer treated using encapsulated cells that express rat *CYP2B1* followed by treatment with IFA has also shown evidence of safety and encouraging results regarding efficacy *(69)*. Clearly, more conclusive proof of efficacy will have to await results from phase II/III trials.

In conclusion, the available evidence shows the versatility and potential for CYP-based prodrug-activation gene therapies. Multiple CYPs appear to be useful for the activation of different prodrugs and, even in the context of one CYP/prodrug combination, multiple variables can be modified to render treatment more effective. More extensive clinical trials appear warranted and should provide for a more conclusive test of the efficacy and utility of this treatment strategy.

References

1. Hasler, J. A. (1999) Pharmacogenetics of cytochromes P450. *Mol. Aspects Med.* **20,** 12–24, 25–137.
2. Kawajiri, K., Eguchi, H., Nakachi, K., Sekiya, T., and Yamamoto, M. (1996) Association of CYP1A1 germ line polymorphisms with mutations of the p53 gene in lung cancer. *Cancer Res.* **56,** 72–76.
3. Sladek, N. E. (1988) Metabolism of oxazaphosphorines. *Pharmacol. Ther.* **37,** 301–355.
4. Jounaidi, Y., Hecht, J. E., and Waxman, D. J. (1998) Retroviral transfer of human cytochrome P450 genes for oxazaphosphorine-based cancer gene therapy. *Cancer Res.* **58,** 4391–4401.
5. Chang, T. K., Yu, L., Goldstein, J. A., and Waxman, D. J. (1997) Identification of the polymorphically expressed CYP2C19 and the wild-type CYP2C9-ILE359 allele as low-K_m catalysts of cyclophosphamide and ifosfamide activation. *Pharmacogenetics* **7,** 211–221.
6. Harris, J. W., Rahman, A., Kim, B. R., Guengerich, F. P., and Collins, J. M. (1994) Metabolism of taxol by human hepatic microsomes and liver slices: participation of cytochrome P450 3A4 and an unknown P450 enzyme. *Cancer Res.* **54,** 4026–4035.
7. Crewe, H. K., Ellis, S. W., Lennard, M. S., and Tucker, G. T. (1997) Variable contribution of cytochromes P450 2D6, 2C9 and 3A4 to the 4-hydroxylation of tamoxifen by human liver microsomes. *Biochem. Pharmacol.* **53,** 171–178.
8. Shet, M. S., McPhaul, M., Fisher, C. W., Stallings, N. R., and Estabrook, R. W. (1997) Metabolism of the antiandrogenic drug (Flutamide) by human CYP1A2. *Drug Metab. Dispos.* **25,** 1298–1303.
9. Wei, M. X., Tamiya, T., Chase, M., et al. (1994) Experimental tumor therapy in mice using the cyclophosphamide-activating cytochrome P450 2B1 gene. *Hum. Gene Ther.* **5,** 969–978.
10. Colvin, O. M. (1999) An overview of cyclophosphamide development and clinical applications. *Curr. Pharm. Des.* **5,** 555–560.
11. Clarke, L. and Waxman, D. J. (1989) Oxidative metabolism of cyclophosphamide: identification of the hepatic monooxygenase catalysts of drug activation. *Cancer Res.* **49,** 2344–2350.
12. Bryant, J., Clegg, A., and Milne, R. (2001) Systematic review of immunomodulatory drugs for the treatment of people with multiple sclerosis: is there good quality evidence on effectiveness and cost? *J. Neurol. Neurosurg. Psychiatry* **70,** 574–579.
13. Genka, S., Deutsch, J., Stahle, P. L., et al. (1990) Brain and plasma pharmacokinetics and anticancer activities of cyclophosphamide and phosphoramide mustard in the rat. *Cancer Chemother. Pharmacol.* **27,** 1–7.
14. Levine, E. S., Friedman, H. S., Griffith, O. W., Colvin, O. M., Raynor, J. H., and Lieberman, M. (1993) Cardiac cell toxicity induced by 4-hydroperoxycyclophosphamide is modulated by glutathione. *Cardiovasc. Res.* **27,** 1248–1253.
15. Schuster, J. M., Friedman, H. S., Archer, G. E., et al. (1993) Intraarterial therapy of human glioma xenografts in athymic rats using 4-hydroperoxycyclophosphamide. *Cancer Res.* **53,** 2338–2343.
16. Huang, Z., Roy, P., and Waxman, D. J. (2000) Role of human liver microsomal CYP3A4 and CYP2B6 in catalyzing N-dechloroethylation of cyclophosphamide and ifosfamide. *Biochem. Pharmacol.* **59,** 961–972.

17. Chang, T. K., Weber, G. F., Crespi, C. L., Waxman, D. J., (1993) Differential activation of cyclophosphamide and ifosphamide by cytochromes P-450 2B and 3A in human liver microsomes. *Cancer Res.* **53,** 5629–5637.

18. Moolten, F. L., Wells, J. M., Heyman, R. A., and Evans, R. M. (1990) Lymphoma regression induced by ganciclovir in mice bearing a herpes thymidine kinase transgene. *Hum. Gene Ther.* **1,** 125–134.

19. Takamiya, Y., Short, M. P., Ezzeddine, Z. D., Moolten, F. L., Breakefield, X. O., and Martuza, R. L. (1992) Gene therapy of malignant brain tumors: a rat glioma line bearing the herpes simplex virus type 1-thymidine kinase gene and wild type retrovirus kills other tumor cells. *J. Neurosci. Res.* **33,** 493–503.

20. Moolten, F. L. and Wells, J. M. (1990) Curability of tumors bearing herpes thymidine kinase genes transferred by retroviral vectors. *J. Natl. Cancer Inst.* **82,** 297–300.

21. Chung, R. Y. and Chiocca, E. A. (1998) Gene therapy for tumors of the central nervous system. *Surg. Oncol. Clin. North Am.* **7,** 589–602.

22. Wildner, O. (1999) In situ use of suicide genes for therapy of brain tumours. *Ann. Med.* **31,** 421–429.

23. Harsh, G. R., Deisboeck, T. S., Louis, D. N., et al. (2000) Thymidine kinase activation of ganciclovir in recurrent malignant gliomas: a gene-marking and neuropathological study. *J. Neurosurg.* **92,** 804–811.

24. Chen, L. and Waxman, D. J. (1995) Intratumoral activation and enhanced chemotherapeutic effect of oxazaphosphorines following cytochrome P-450 gene transfer: development of a combined chemotherapy/cancer gene therapy strategy. *Cancer Res.* **55,** 581–589.

25. Chen, L., Waxman, D. J., Chen, D., and Kufe, D. W. (1996) Sensitization of human breast cancer cells to cyclophosphamide and ifosfamide by transfer of a liver cytochrome P450 gene. *Cancer Res.* **56,** 1331–1340.

26. Freeman, S. M., Abboud, C. N., Whartenby, K. A., et al. (1993) The "bystander effect" tumor regression when a fraction of the tumor mass is genetically modified. *Cancer Res.* **53,** 5274–5283.

27. Culver, K. W., Ram, Z., Wallbridge, S., Ishii, H., Oldfield, E. H., and Blaese, R. M. (1992) In vivo gene transfer with retroviral vector-producer cells for treatment of experimental brain tumors. *Science* **256,** 1550–1502.

28. Tapscott, S. J., Miller, A. D., Olson, J. M., Berger, M. S., Groudine, M., and Spence, A. M. (1994) Gene therapy of rat 9L gliosarcoma tumors by transduction with selectable genes does not require drug selection. *Proc. Natl. Acad. Sci. USA* **91,** 8185–8189.

29. Barba, D., Hardin, J., Sadelain, M., and Gage, F. H. (1994) Development of anti-tumor immunity following thymidine kinase-mediated killing of experimental brain tumors. *Proc. Natl. Acad. Sci. USA* **91,** 4348–4352.

30. Felzmann, T., Ramsey, W. J., and Blaese, R. M. (1997) Characterization of the antitumor immune response generated by treatment of murine tumors with recombinant adenoviruses expressing HSVtk, IL-2, IL-6 or B7-1. *Gene Ther.* **4,** 1322–1329.

31. Mullen, C. A., Coale, M. M., Lowe, R., and Blaese, R. M. (1994) Tumors expressing the cytosine deaminase suicide gene can be eliminated in vivo with 5-fluorocytosine and induce protective immunity to wild type tumor. *Cancer Res.* **54,** 1503–1506.

32. Mullen, C. A., Kilstrup, M., and Blaese, R. M. (1992) Transfer of the bacterial gene for cytosine deaminase to mammalian cells confers lethal sensitivity to 5-fluorocytosine: a negative selection system. *Proc. Natl. Acad. Sci. USA* **89,** 33–37.

33. Wei, M. X., Tamiya, T., Rhee, R. J., Breakefield, X. O., and Chiocca, E. A. (1995) Diffusible cytotoxic metabolites contribute to the in vitro bystander effect associated with the

cyclophosphamide/cytochrome P450 2B1 cancer gene therapy paradigm. *Clin Cancer Res.* **1,** 1171–1177.

34. Ichikawa, T., Petros, W. P., Ludeman, S. M., et al. (2001) Intraneoplastic polymer-based delivery of cyclophosphamide for intratumoral bioconversion by a replicating oncolytic viral vector. *Cancer Res.* **61,** 864–868.

35. Kuriyama, S., Masui, K., Sakamoto, T., et al. (1998) Bystander effect caused by cytosine deaminase gene and 5-fluorocytosine in vitro is substantially mediated by generated 5-fluorouracil. *Anticancer Res.* **18,** 3399–3406.

36. Connors, T. A. (1995) The choice of prodrugs for gene directed enzyme prodrug therapy of cancer. *Gene Ther.* **2,** 702–709.

37. Ram, Z., Culver, K. W., Oshiro, E. M., et al. (1997) Therapy of malignant brain tumors by intratumoral implantation of retroviral vector-producing cells. *Nature Med.* **3,** 1354–1361.

38. Puumalainen, A. M., Vapalahti, M., Agrawal, R. S., et al. (1998) Beta-galactosidase gene transfer to human malignant glioma in vivo using replication-deficient retroviruses and adenoviruses. *Hum. Gene Ther.* **9,** 1769–1774.

39. Smith, E. R. and Chiocca, E. A. (2000) Oncolytic viruses as novel anticancer agents: turning one scourge against another. *Expert Opin. Invest. Drugs* **9,** 311–327.

40. Chung, R. Y., Saeki, Y., and Chiocca, E. A. (1999) B-myb promoter retargeting of herpes simplex virus gamma34.5 gene-mediated virulence toward tumor and cycling cells. *J. Virol.* **73,** 7556–7564.

41. Suzuki, K., Fueyo, J., Krasnykh, V., Reynolds, P. N., Curiel, D. T., and Alemany, R. (2001) A conditionally replicative adenovirus with enhanced infectivity shows improved oncolytic potency. *Clin. Cancer Res.* **7,** 120–126.

42. Aghi, M., Chou, T. C., Suling, K., Breakefield, X. O., and Chiocca, E. A. (1999) Multimodal cancer treatment mediated by a replicating oncolytic virus that delivers the oxazaphosphorine/rat cytochrome P450 2B1 and ganciclovir/herpes simplex virus thymidine kinase gene therapies. *Cancer Res.* **59,** 3861–3865.

43. Ichikawa, T. and Chiocca, E. A. (2001) Comparative analyses of transgene expression mediated by a replication-conditional vs. defective viral vector. *Cancer Res.* **61,** 5336–5339.

44. Jacobson, J. G., Leib, D. A., Goldstein, D. J., et al. (1989) A herpes simplex virus ribonucleotide reductase deletion mutant is defective for productive acute and reactivatable latent infections of mice and for replication in mouse cells. *Virology* **173,** 276–283.

45. Coen, D. M., Goldstein, D. J., and Weller, S. K. (1989) Herpes simplex virus ribonucleotide reductase mutants are hypersensitive to acyclovir. *Antimicrob. Agents Chemother.* **33,** 1395–1399.

46. Rampling, R., Cruickshank, G., Papanastassiou, V., et al. (2000) Toxicity evaluation of replication-competent herpes simplex virus (ICP 34.5 null mutant 1716) in patients with recurrent malignant glioma. *Gene Ther.* **7,** 859–866.

47. Markert, J. M., Medlock, M. D., Rabkin, S. D., et al. (2000) Conditionally replicating herpes simplex virus mutant, G207 for the treatment of malignant glioma: results of a phase I trial. *Gene Ther.* **7,** 867–874.

48. Chase, M., Chung, R. Y., and Chiocca, E. A. (1998) An oncolytic viral mutant that delivers the CYP2B1 transgene and augments cyclophosphamide chemotherapy. *Nature Biotechnol.* **16,** 444–448.

49. Ikeda, K., Ichikawa, T., Wakimoto, H., et al. (1999) Oncolytic virus therapy of multiple tumors in the brain requires suppression of innate and elicited antiviral responses. *Nature Med.* **5,** 881–887.

50. Ikeda, K., Wakimoto, H., Ichikawa, T., et al. (2000) Complement depletion facilitates the infection of multiple brain tumors by an intravascular, replication-conditional herpes simplex virus mutant. *J. Virol.* **74,** 4765–4775.

51. Aghi, M., Kramm, C. M., Chou, T. C., Breakefield, X. O., and Chiocca, E. A. (1998) Synergistic anticancer effects of ganciclovir/thymidine kinase and 5-fluorocytosine/cytosine deaminase gene therapies. *J. Natl. Cancer Inst.* **90**, 370–380.

52. Chou, T. C., Motzer, R. J., Tong, Y., and Bosl, G. J. (1994) Computerized quantitation of synergism and antagonism of taxol, topotecan, and cisplatin against human teratocarcinoma cell growth: a rational approach to clinical protocol design. *J. Natl. Cancer Inst.* **86**, 1517–1524.

53. Andersson, B. S., Sadeghi, T., Siciliano, M. J., Legerski, R., and Murray, D. (1996) Nucleotide excision repair genes as determinants of cellular sensitivity to cyclophosphamide analogs. *Cancer Chemother. Pharmacol.* **38**, 406–416.

54. Li, L., Keating, M. J., Plunkett, W., and Yang, L. Y. (1997) Fludarabine-mediated repair inhibition of cisplatin-induced DNA lesions in human chronic myelogenous leukemia-blast crisis K562 cells: induction of synergistic cytotoxicity independent of reversal of apoptosis resistance. *Mol. Pharmacol.* **52**, 798–806.

55. Ilsley, D. D., Lee, S. H., Miller, W. H., and Kuchta, R. D. (1995) Acyclic guanosine analogs inhibit DNA polymerases alpha, delta, and epsilon with very different potencies and have unique mechanisms of action. *Biochemistry* **34**, 2504–2510.

56. Kammertoens, T., Gelbmann, W., Karle, P., et al. (2000) Combined chemotherapy of murine mammary tumors by local activation of the prodrugs ifosfamide and 5-fluorocytosine. *Cancer Gene Ther.* **7**, 629–636.

57. Anon. (1998) Gliadel wafers for treatment of brain tumors. *Med. Lett. Drugs Ther.* **40**, 92.

58. Chen, L., Yu, L. J., and Waxman, D. J. (1997) Potentiation of cytochrome P450/cyclophosphamide-based cancer gene therapy by coexpression of the P450 reductase gene. *Cancer Res.* **57**, 4830–4837.

59. Jounaidi, Y. and Waxman, D. J. (2000) Combination of the bioreductive drug tirapazamine with the chemotherapeutic prodrug cyclophosphamide for P450/P450-reductase-based cancer gene therapy. *Cancer Res.* **60**, 3761–3769.

60. Huang, Z., Raychowdhury, M. K., and Waxman, D. J. (2000) Impact of liver P450 reductase suppression on cyclophosphamide activation, pharmacokinetics and antitumoral activity in a cytochrome P450-based cancer gene therapy model. *Cancer Gene Ther.* **7**, 1034–1042.

61. Huang, Z. and Waxman, D. J. (2001) Modulation of cyclophosphamide-based cytochrome P450-based gene therapy using liver P450 inhibitors. *Cancer Gene Ther.* **8**, 450–458.

62. Browder, T., Butterfield, C. E., Kraling, B. M., et al. (2000) Antiangiogenic scheduling of chemotherapy improves efficacy against experimental drug-resistant cancer. *Cancer Res.* **60**, 1878–1886.

63. Jounaidi, Y. and Waxman, D. J. (2001) Frequent, moderate-dose cyclophosphamide administration improves the efficacy of cytochrome P-450/cytochrome P-450 reductase-based cancer gene therapy. *Cancer Res.* **61**, 4437–4444.

64. Lohr, M., Muller, P., Karle, P., et al. (1998) Targeted chemotherapy by intratumour injection of encapsulated cells engineered to produce CYP2B1, an ifosfamide activating cytochrome P450. *Gene Ther.* **5**, 1070–1078.

65. Griffiths, L., Binley, K., Iqball, S., et al. (2000) The macrophage—a novel system to deliver gene therapy to pathological hypoxia. *Gene Ther.* **7**, 255–2562.

66. Rainov, N. G., Dobberstein, K. U., Sena-Esteves, M., et al. (1998) New prodrug activation gene therapy for cancer using cytochrome P450 4B1 and 2-aminoanthracene/4-ipomeanol. *Hum Gene Ther.* **9**, 1261–1273.

67. McCarthy, H. O., Yakkundi, A., McErlane, V., et al. (2003) Bioreductive GDEPT using cytochrome P450 3A4 in combination with AQ4N. *Cancer Gene Ther.* **10**, 40–48.

68. Thatcher, N. J., Edwards, R. J., Lemoine, N. R., Doehmer, J., and Davies, D. S. (2000) The potential of acetaminophen as a prodrug in gene-directed enzyme prodrug therapy. *Cancer Gene Ther.* **7,** 521–525.

69. Lohr, M., Hoffmeyer, A., Kroger, J., et al. (2001) Microencapsulated cell-mediated treatment of inoperable pancreatic carcinoma. *Lancet* **357,** 1591–1592.

70. Schwartz, P. S. and Waxman, D. J. (2001) Cyclophosphamide induces caspase 9-dependent apoptosis in 9L tumor cells. *Mol. Pharmacol.* **60,** 1268–1279.

71. Antonio Chiocca, E. (2002) Oncolytic viruses. *Nat. Rev. Cancer* **2,** 938–950.

72. Wakimoto, H., Ikeda, K., Abe T., et al. (2002) The complement response against an oncolytic virus is species-specific in its activation pathways. *Mol. Ther.* **5,** 275–282.

73. Wakimoto, H., Johnson, P. R., Knipe, D. M., Chiocca, E. A. (2003) Effects of innate immunity on herpes simplex virus and its ability to kill tumor cells. *Gene Ther.* **10,** 983–990.

11

Tumor Sensitization to Purine Analogs by *E. coli* PNP

Kimberly V. Curlee, William B. Parker, and Eric J. Sorscher

1. Introduction

This chapter describes an approach to destroying malignant cells by effectively changing the tumor phenotype through the delivery of *Escherichia coli* purine nucleoside phosphorylase (PNP). In the presence of nucleoside prodrugs, this nonhuman enzyme in purine metabolism causes the death of the transfected (transduced) cells through the release of a highly potent antitumor agent. Importantly, the properties of the liberated compounds kill not only the transfected (transduced) cells but cause the efficient destruction of tumor cells that do not express the gene (i.e., bystander cells). In addition, the cytotoxic agents are active against both proliferating and nonproliferating tumor cells and, therefore, unlike other antitumor agents, this system can target the nonproliferating component of solid tumors. Many common cancers (including prostate, breast, colon, lung, brain, melanoma, pancreas, ovarian, kidney) progress to become untreatable and eventually cause death. Compounds are available that could abolish these tumors, but they are too toxic to systematically administer safely to cancer patients. We have shown that some of these compounds are remarkably potent and can abolish otherwise refractory human cancers when produced within the tumor mass by virtue of expression of *E. coli* PNP.

2. Overview Concerning Unique Properties of the *E. coli* PNP System

The *E. coli* PNP system has several characteristics that distinguish it from other suicide gene therapy strategies. The most important characteristics for killing cancer cells are summarized in this section and elaborated upon in the body of this chapter.

2.1. High Bystander Activity

Entire cell populations can be killed when as few as 0.1–1% of the cells in the culture express the *E. coli* PNP gene. In addition, the mechanism of bystander activity for *E. coli* PNP is not dependent on gap junctions (connexins) and does not require

From: *Methods in Molecular Medicine, Vol. 90, Suicide Gene Therapy: Methods and Reviews*
Edited by: C. J. Springer © Humana Press Inc., Totowa, NJ

cell-to-cell contact, such as the herpes simplex virus–thymidine kinase (*HSV-TK*) system. The cellular mechanisms governing nucleoside and nucleobase transport are well understood and form the basis of effective antitumor and antiviral therapy using nucleoside analogs; that is, purine analogs can quickly and readily cross membranes to get to their intracellular targets.

2.2. Novel Cell Killing Mechanism

A second important characteristic underscores the mechanism of cell killing for the two toxins generated by *E. coli* PNP: methyl purine (6-MeP) and 2-fluoro-adenine (2-F-Ade). These two agents are converted to ATP analogs, which inhibit RNA and/or protein synthesis. This mechanism of cell killing is therefore different from that of all other anticancer agents, including ganciclovir nucleotides (generated by *HSV-TK*) and 5-fluorouracil (5-FU) (produced by cytosine deaminase). Because RNA and protein synthesis are important to all cells regardless of their proliferative status, these two compounds kill both nonproliferating and proliferating cells.

2.3. Targets Nonproliferating Cells

Activity against nonproliferating cells is of particular importance to the treatment of solid tumors, which often have a very low growth fraction (*see* **Subheading 5.**). The in vivo effectiveness of PNP substrates such as 6-MeP-dR (6-methyl purine-deoxyribose), F-dAdo (fluoro-deoxyadenosine), and F-araAMP (flouro-arabinosyl adenosine monophosphate) against slow growing tumors provides in vivo evidence of the activity of 6-MeP and 2-F-Ade against nonproliferating cells.

2.4. High Potency

2-Flouro-adenine is 1000 times more potent (and 6-MeP is 10 times more potent) than 5-FU, the toxin produced by the cytosine deaminase suicide gene therapy system. It is possible that 2-F-Ade and 6-MeP could cause tumor regressions in animals under conditions (equal expression of activating enzymes) where 5-FU or ganciclovir–monophosphate would have little effect. Given the difficulty of selectively delivering genes to tumor cells in an intact animal, the potency of these agents (particularly 2-F-Ade) may allow the *E. coli* PNP suicide gene to work when only a small amount of gene expression is achieved.

2.5. Short Treatment Period

Another important characteristic embodies effectiveness of prodrugs against cells expressing *E. coli* PNP after only a short treatment period. Excellent in vivo antitumor activity has been demonstrated with 6-MeP-dR after only a single dose of the compound. This characteristic has particular importance in the context of gene therapy, because when only a small percentage of cells are transduced, it is important that the toxin be immediately toxic to the whole tumor. Otherwise, if prolonged therapy was necessary to kill the tumor (as with many current suicide gene therapies), cells that express the activating gene could be eliminated prior to obtaining a significant antitumor effect. Furthermore, the duration of gene expression with many of the current vectors is limited to only a few days. Obviously, it is necessary to treat with prodrug when the suicide gene is being expressed.

2.6. Effective Against Large Tumors

Finally, we have shown that 6-MeP-dR is effective in vivo against large tumors (700 mg) that express *E. coli* PNP, which is a very stringent test for antitumor activity.

3. Considerations Regarding *E. coli* PNP Biochemistry

The *E.coli* purine nucleoside phosphorylase gene product cleaves nucleoside prodrugs, including 6-MeP-dR (which is cleaved to 6-MeP) and 2-F-dAdo (which is cleaved to 2-F-Ade), to highly toxic purine bases (*see* **Fig. 1**). 2-F-araA, a clinically approved chemotherapeutic, is also metabolized to 2-F-Ade. **Table 1** shows the kinetic constants underlying these enzymatic reactions. Although reversible phosphorolysis of (2'-deoxy) purine ribonucleosides to free base and (2'-deoxy) ribose-1-phosphate is a shared property of prokaryotic and eukaryotic PNPs, the mammalian enzymes (e.g., taken from human or bovine red blood cells) differ fundamentally in sequence, structure and function from their bacterial counterparts *(1–4)*. Prokaryotic PNPs are hexameric (believed to act as a set of functional dimers), whereas the mammalian enzymes exist as trimers. Moreover, mammalian enzymes accept only guanosine and inosine as substrates, whereas bacterial enzymes such as *E. coli* PNP also accept adenosine and are permissive for several ribose modifications. The structural and functional dichotomy is also reflected in the activity of enzymatic blockers. Formycin A, for example, abrogates *E. coli* PNP activity with a $k_1 = 5$ μM, but is completely inactive against the human enzyme. An extensive literature regarding the high-resolution crystal structure of prokaryotic and mammalian PNP, substrate, and inhibitor activities and details regarding of oligomerization and active site conformation are available for both enzymatic families. Modifying the prokaryotic enzyme, prodrug, or both has recently become a realistic possibility for further improving this general approach to cancer gene therapy.

4. *E.coli* PNP as a Prodrug Activation Strategy

The limitations that exist in gene delivery vehicles make it likely that robust bystander activity will be required to treat human tumors by "suicide" gene therapy *(5)*. It is reasonable to imagine that bystander cell killing with compounds that do not readily partition across the plasma membrane will not be adequate to overcome a low efficiency of gene delivery. The strategy to transfect cells with *E. coli* PNP and subsequently treat with nontoxic deoxyadenosine analogs utilizes membrane-permeant prodrugs and liberates membrane-permeant chemotherapeutic toxins *(6,7)*. Nucleoside monophosphates (such as those derived from *HSV-TK*) are trapped inside the cell in which they are formed. Even if a nucleoside monophosphate such as ganciclovir monophosphate were released following cell lysis, the metabolite would not be capable of entering neighboring cells and would be degraded (inactivated) to the nucleoside by phosphatases. However, a toxic adenine analog formed after conversion by *E. coli* PNP would be converted by adenine phosphoribosyl transferase to toxic nucleotides and kill all transfected cells and would diffuse out of the cell and kill surrounding cells that were not transfected. These enzymatic features distinguish *E. coli* PNP from other prodrug activation strategies, such as *HSV-TK*.

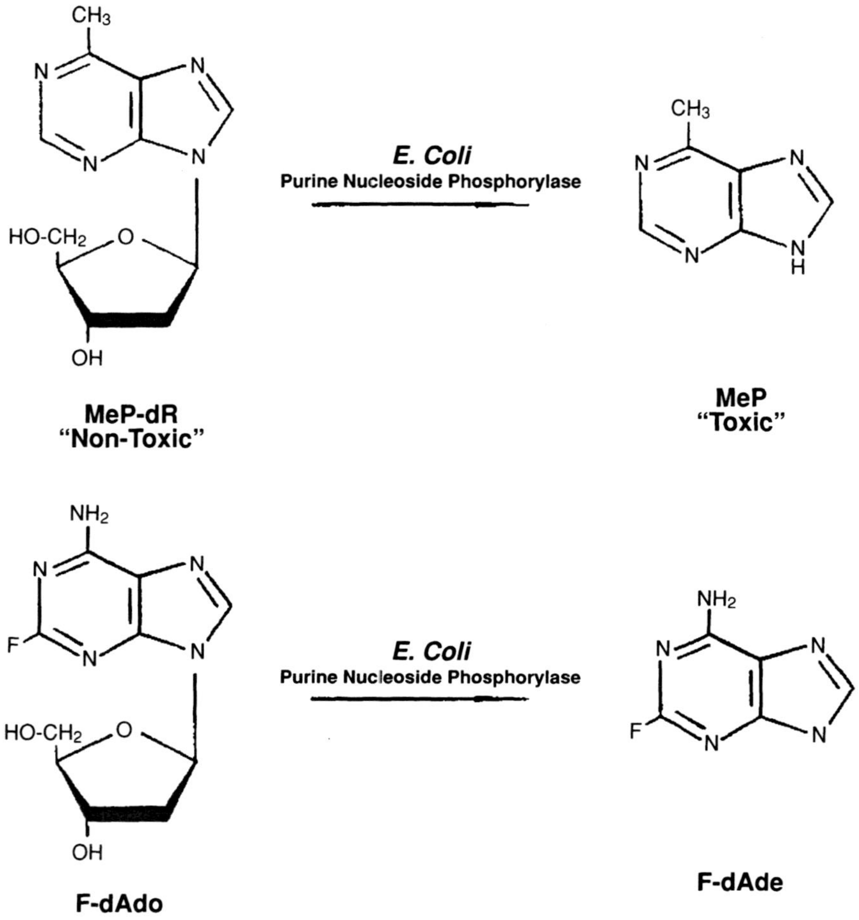

Fig. 1. Conversion of nucleosides by *E. coli* PNP.

5. Rationale for Developing Methods for Killing Refractory Tumors With a Low Growth Fraction

Most conventional chemotherapeutic drugs derive antitumor specificity from the ability to kill dividing (as opposed to nondividing) cells. Many chemotherapies are suitable for systemic administration specifically because they are most toxic to cells that are dividing. This leads to an acceptable level of damage in other, rapidly proliferating tissues (cellular compartments such as the bone marrow, intestinal tract, hair follicles, etc.). However, many refractory tumors are refractory precisely because they have a very low growth fraction (i.e., a relatively small percentage of tumor cells are dividing at any particular point in time). For example, it has been estimated in hormone refractory prostate cancer that approx 5% of the cells are dividing and that the low growth fraction explains the poor response to therapy (*8–10*). In refractory colon,

Table 1
Kinetic Constants for Nucleosides as Substrates for *E. coli* PNP

Analog	K_m (μM)	V_{max} (nmol/h/mg)	V_m/K_m
MeP-dR	126	1,500,000	11,000
F-dAdo	22	430,000	20,000
F-araA	960	6,000	6

breast, glioma, melanoma, and non-small-cell lung cancers, the growth fractions are estimated at 0.4%, 4%, 10–30%, 10–40%, and approx 40%, respectively *(11–16)*. Even if 75% of the cells in an otherwise refractory tumor were proliferating during a cumulative exposure to chemotherapy and even if all of these cells were completely eradicated by treatment, the tumor would remain at two doubling times away from regaining pretreatment dimensions. As a consequence, it may be unrealistic to expect drugs that kill mainly nondividing cells to cure large tumors of these types. This explanation is generally acknowledged as a reason for the failure of conventional chemotherapy against many tumors.

6. Features of 6-MeP and 2-F-Ade Related to Therapy of Refractory, Slow-Growing Tumor Cells

Several points may be considered regarding use of 6-MeP and 2-F-Ade as novel forms of chemotherapy. First, as described earlier, toxins such as 6-MeP and 2-F-Ade are extremely potent antitumor cell agents (IC_{50}'s of 100 n*M* and 10 μM, respectively) *(17)*. Once compounds such as 6-MeP are generated within a solid tumor, they appear to have a very long half-life within the tumor tissue itself and are only very slowly released from solid tumor masses (e.g., half-life of greater than 24 h) *(18)*. This long tumor half-life may be part of the explanation for the ability of these drugs to ablate tumors without profound systemic toxicity (i.e., by virtue of very slow release to nontarget tissues). Second, drugs such as 6-MeP and 2-F-Ade are known to be too toxic for systemic administration. In previous studies, no therapeutic margin exists for systemic administration of these compounds (i.e., animals die at drug doses below those that could safely cause tumor regressions) *(19,20)*. However, when these compounds are generated within a tumor mass, the slow release and substantial dilution throughout the remainder of the body limits overall toxicity. Third, it has been shown that toxins such as 6-MeP kill both dividing and nondividing cells *(17)*. This was demonstrated using several independent protocols. In one series of experiments, CEM (T-cell derived) cells were serum starved to arrest growth. Subsequent addition of 6-MeP or 2-F-Ade led to killing of these nonproliferating cells, whereas agents such as flurouracil did not (*see* **Fig. 2**). Nonproliferating Balb-3T3 cells were also studied as an in vitro model. 6-MeP and 2-F-Ade blocked uridine and leucine incorporation into acid-precipitable material in those cells that were in a well-characterized quiescent state and led to cell death (*see* **Fig. 3**) *(17)*. In another study, MRC-5 cells, which do not proliferate once confluent, were killed well after confluency by 6-MeP or 2-F-

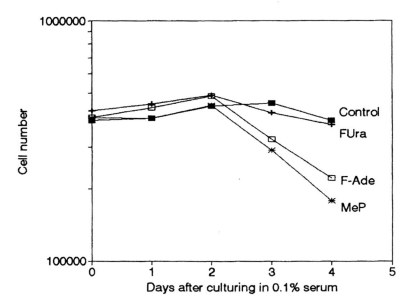

Fig. 2. Effects of FUra, MeP, or F-Ade on cytotoxicity of nonproliferating CEM cells. CEM cells were cultured in medium containing 0.1% serum to induce a nonproliferative state. Forty-eight hours after initiation of the cell cultures in 0.1% serum medium, MeP (10 μg/mL), F-Ade (1 μg/mL), or FUra (10 μg/mL) was added to separate cell cultures. Cell numbers were counted with a Coulter Counter at 24-h intervals from the time the cells were cultured in the 0.1% serum. This experiment was repeated one time with similar results.

Ade. Malignant glioma tumor cells transduced with an inducible *p53* gene exhibited the anticipated, complete arrest of cell growth, as judged by both tetrazonium incorporation and direct counting of trypan blue-excluding cells, after p53 induction. Low micromolar concentrations of 6-MeP killed these cells in culture, even after p53 induction and complete proliferation arrest in vivo. Three doses of 6-MeP-dR in tumors transduced with PNP led to strong antitumor effects and cures without deaths or limiting weight loss because of treatment *(21)*. Because the half-life of 6-MeP-dR in the circulation is less than 30 min *(see* **Fig. 4**), these observations further establish that generation of methyl purine within tumors is capable of safely eliminating both the dividing and nondividing compartments of well-characterized, slow-growing, low-growth-fraction cancer models *(see also* **Subheading 9.5.**).

Both 6-MeP and 2-F-Ade are converted to ATP analogs and block reaction(s) involving ATP so as to result in cell death. These two agents therefore act quite differently from ganciclovir monophosphate or 5-FU, in that they impair one or more enzymes unrelated to DNA synthesis and kill cells that are not actively proliferating. The mechanism of action of these two agents is also quite different from all of the drugs currently used in the treatment of cancer and thus represents a novel way to kill tumor cells. The specific mechanism of these two compounds is not known and may

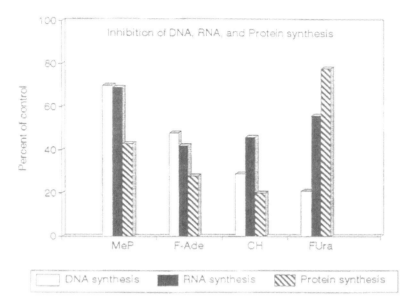

Fig. 3. Inhibition of DNA, RNA, and protein synthesis. Effects of MeP, F-Ade, cyclohexim-ide, and FUra on macromolecular synthesis. CEM cells (approx 300,000 cells/mL) were incu-bated with 100 μM of MeP, 2 μM of F-Ade, 1 μM of cycloheximide, or 1000 μM of FUra. Radiolabeled precursors of DNA ([*methyl*-^{3}H]dThd), RNA ([5-^{3}H]Urd), or protein ([4,5-^{3}H]leucine) were added at 2 μCi/mL 4 h after the addition of the compounds. Samples were taken 1, 2, 3, and 4 h after the addition of radiolabel to determine their incorporation into RNA, DNA, or protein. Because treatment with FUra inhibits thymidylate synthetase, the effect of FUra on DNA and RNA syntheses was determined by measuring the incorporation of [8-^{14}C]Ade into the alkali-stable/acid-insoluble fraction and the total acid-insoluble fraction. The amount of incorporation of [^{3}H]leucine into protein, [^{3}H]dThd into DNA, [^{3}H]Urd into RNA, or [^{14}C]Ade into DNA in a 4-h period was 8, 444, 229, or 1.1 disintegrations per minute (dpm)/ 10^3 cells, respectively. This experiment was repeated, and similar results were obtained.

be difficult to elucidate, because of the many enzymatic reactions that require ATP. It is possible that the incorporation of these agents into RNA results in the disruption of secondary structure (possibly by inhibiting dsRNA deaminase; *see* **ref. 22**), which could explain the inhibition of both RNA and protein synthesis observed previously.

7. Implications of Clinical Trials With *HSV-TK* or Cytosine Deaminase and Ways to Improve the Usefulness of Prodrug Activation

Although early clinical studies have led to encouraging initial results in some cases, in other trials the antitumor effects elicited by the *HSV-TK* or cytosine deaminase gene have been difficult to establish. There is a strong belief that significant improvements will be required if prodrug activation is to become a useful part of cancer therapy. The magnitude and scope of existing clinical studies is large and continuing to expand

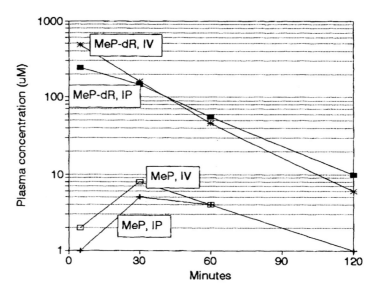

Fig. 4. MeP-dR and MeP plasma concentrations in mice after injection of MeP-dR. Twelve nude mice (*nu/nu*) were injected intraperitoneally with 67 mg/kg of MeP-dR. Three mice were sacrificed 5, 30, 60, and 120 min after injection of MeP-dR, and the mouse plasma was obtained for analysis. Particulate matter was removed from each plasma sample by centrifugation (Centrifree centrifugal filter device, Millipore Corp, Bedford MA). Reverse-phase high-performance liquid chromatography (5 μm BDS Hypersil C-18 column, 150 × 4.6 mm; Keystone Scientific Inc., State College, PA) was used to separate products from substrates, which were detected as they eluted from the column by their absorbance at 254 nm. The mobile phase was 5% acetonitrile in 50 mM ammonium dihydrogen phosphate buffer (pH 4.5) at a flow rate of 1 mL/min. The experiment has been repeated six times with similar results.

(23). The need for improvements in prodrug activation that will augment the clinical efficacy of these trials is evident.

At least two distinct areas have been identified that might improve the usefulness of prodrug activation. First, improved methods for bystander killing have been suggested as a way to augment the overall strategy. It is often recognized that *HSV-TK* is relatively inefficient as a mechanism for bystander killing. When *HSV-TK* phosphorylates ganciclovir to form ganciclovir monophosphate, cellular kinases next generate ganciclovir triphosphate (TP), which elicits DNA chain termination specifically in dividing cells. Bystander killing with *HSV-TK* has been a limitation in vivo and in vitro. When fewer than 10% of cells express *HSV-TK*, efficient killing has been variable and is not consistently obtained in many cell types *(24,25)*. Unlike 6-MeP, ganciclovir nucleotides are not membrane permeant and require direct cell-to-cell contact and/or gap junctions to mediate killing of neighboring cells *(25–31)*. The apparent reliance on gap junctions to transmit an activated toxin that is not membrane permeable precludes many cell types from *HSV-TK* bystander killing *(26–28)*. Vile et al. *(32)* and Caruso et al. *(33)* have shown that the bystander effect of *HSV-TK* in vivo may be largely attributable to immune-mediated clearance of the tumor cells. Tapscott et al. *(34)* have further demonstrated that tumor formation in rats was retarded even without ganciclovir treatment. The requirements of a large number of transduced cells within the tumor, gap junctions, and the immune system for *HSV-TK*/ganciclovir-mediated cell killing may limit the effectiveness of *HSV-TK* in human trials of cancer treatment.

A second area that has been identified as a way to improve prodrug activation is the use of toxins that kill nondividing tumor cells. Because ganciclovir–TP primarily inhibits DNA synthesis, it is less effective than 6-MeP at killing a quiescent (nondividing) compartment of cells in a tumor *(17,35)*. Drugs such as 5-FU also kill primarily nondividing tumor cells and are not likely to ablate otherwise refractory tumors. Even in regional administration, or following direct intratumoral injection, 5-FU may not lead to potent antitumor effects (e.g., hepatic metastasis from colon cancer may not be effectively treated when this compound is infused directly into the portal circulation as part of regional chemotherapy) *(36)*. Important strategies for improving the effectiveness of *HSV-TK* and cytosine deaminase (e.g., augmenting apoptosis, testing combinations of conventional and suicide gene therapies, and improving cell-to-cell communication) are being tested to overcome this barrier *(37–41)*. In either case, it is reasonable to imagine that prodrug activation strategies could be improved if (1) bystander killing and (2) the ability to destroy the nondividing compartment within growing tumors could be better optimized. The *E. coli* PNP gene strategy addresses these two limiting boundaries of prodrug activation in vivo.

8. Studies of *E. coli* PNP Prodrug Activation

Subsequent to the original description of *E. coli* PNP as a way to augment bystander killing *(6,42)*, Vogelstein's laboratory *(43)* confirmed that the approach led to pronounced tumor cell destruction in an H1299 cell model of lung cancer. A novel (chimeric) protein was formed in tumor cells between a mutant p53 and a transcriptional activator. In this way, PNP was expressed only in cells that had undergone a tumorigenic p53 mutation. These experiments indicated a 1000-fold greater killing effect of tumor cells as a result of *E. coli* PNP expression, even when <3% of the cells expressed the PNP gene *(43)*. In another study, a direct comparison of the usefulness of *HSV-TK*, cytosine deaminase, and *E. coli* PNP was made in vitro. Nestler and colleagues *(44)* used a novel foamy virus vector to test these three sensitization genes in hamster kidney fibroblasts (BHK-21), fibrosarcoma (HT 1080 and CMS5), glioblastoma (A172), and hepatoma (HepG2) cell lines. Green fluorescent protein transduction into target cells, and parental cells were examined as controls. The PNP gene killed each cell type in a rapid dose-dependent fashion that was faster than *HSV-TK*- or cytosine deaminase-induced cytotoxicity and was found to be more effective as a suicide gene across several cancer cell types in vitro *(44)*. Lockett and colleagues *(35)* showed that expression of *E. coli* PNP led to profound killing of human prostate (PC-3) and breast cancer (MCF-7, T47-D2) cells in vitro. Otherwise identical adenoviral vectors encoding *HSV-TK* or *E. coli* PNP were directly compared. The prostate cells were refractory to killing by *HSV-TK*, (multiplicity of infections [MOIs] of 10, 20, 50, or 100 led to no more than 50% inhibition of growth because of ganciclovir), whereas the PNP gene abolished 100% of these cells at every viral MOI tested. Breast cancer cells in vitro were completely resistent to *HSV- TK*/ganciclovir at all MOIs tested but were completely ablated by PNP/6-MeP-dR. More recently, it was shown that when adenovirus encoding either the *E. coli* PNP or the *HSV-TK* gene were compared for their ability to mediate regressions of a PC-3 prostate tumor model in nude mice, PNP led to stronger antitumor effects and cures than *HSV-TK* and 20% long-term survivors (>450 d, compared with no long-term survivors in the *HSV-TK*/ganciclovir group) *(45)*. A high degree of melanoma specificity (with profound bystander killing) has been demonstrated by situating the *E. coli* PNP gene downstream of a murine or human tyrosinase promoter *(42,46)*. Moreover, *E. coli* PNP can also be incorporated into an attenuated vaccinia vector *(47)*. This vector exhibits a strong tropism toward dividing cancer cells, and in combination with 6-MeP-dR, it was shown to kill entire populations of melanoma (pMel1), colon (MC-38), hepatoma (Hepa 16), and adenocarcinoma (Wi Dr, HT-29) cancer cell types in vitro. Direct targeting of metastatic colon tumors in vivo and complete regressions and cures of these cancers were achieved with *E. coli* PNP. In the same study, direct comparisons were also made with cytosine deaminase/5-FC and cytotoxicity by *E. coli* PNP was found to be more rapid and complete. Strong in vivo antitumor effects in mouse models of liver carcinoma have also been shown recently *(48,49)*.

9. Selected Examples of In Vitro and In Vivo Bystander Killing Using *E. coli* PNP

9.1. Summary

The use of *E. coli* PNP as a suicide gene is fundamentally different from *HSV-TK* or other suicide genes because it (1) provides a toxin that kills tumors with a low growth fraction, (2) generates a toxin that readily diffuses between and among tumor cells with potent bystander activity even when 1 in 1000 cells express the gene in vivo, and (3) does not require gap junctions to mediate bystander killing (a requirement for *HSV-TK*) *(6,7,17,21,43,50,51)*. Moreover, intermediate biochemical end-points (e.g., levels of recombinant *E. coli* PNP enzyme within a tumor or amounts of a 6-MeP liberated by tumor cells) can be used to characterize this system and its requirements. Examples of tumor cell killing by this approach in vitro and in vivo are summarized in the following subsections.

9.2. Gap Junctions and Cell-to-Cell Contact Are Not Required for Tumor Cell Killing by E. coli *PNP*

The mechanism of cell killing by *E. coli* PNP can be explained by the level of toxin that is produced. For example, in bystander killing experiments, the amount of 6-MeP released into the medium by *E. coli* PNP is directly measurable. When this same concentration of purified 6-MeP is added to the medium of non-PNP-expressing cells, all cells are killed. Thus, 6-MeP in the medium (whether released by *E. coli* PNP cleavage of 6-MeP-dR or by direct addition of 6-MeP) accounts for all of the cell killing that is observed *(7,21,42)*. Tumor cell killing also exhibits dose and time dependence on both the level of *E. coli* PNP expressed and the amount of 6-MeP generated *(7,42)*. These results indicate a simple and straightforward mechanism of bystander killing by *E. coli* PNP that differs fundamentally from *HSV-TK*. Because both prodrug and toxin are freely membrane permeant, gap junctions or cell-to-cell contact are not required for bystander killing mediated by *E. coli* PNP (*see* **Fig. 5A–C**).

9.3. In Vitro Tumor Cell Killing Mediated by E. coli PNP

Multiple tumor cell types have been assayed for the ability of *E. coli* PNP to mediate sensitization to prodrugs such as 6-MeP-dR in vitro, including human and mouse, melanoma (B-16, Mel 1, Mel 21), human, mouse, and rat glioma (D54, MT-539, RT-2), human lung (A549), cervical (HeLa), colon (T84, HT29), hepatic (Hep-2), lymphoid (H-9), prostate (DU154, LNCap), murine breast (16/c), ovarian (SKOV3), and primate kidney (293). In all cases, strong bystander cell killing and/or destruction of entire tumor cell populations was observed when a very small fraction of the cells (e.g., 1–5%) expressed the *E. coli* PNP gene. Cytotoxicity was correlated to the formation of 6-MeP in tumor cells expressing PNP (an example is shown in **Figs. 6** and **7**).

Experiments using retrovirus, adenovirus, or lipid transfection methods have demonstrated the protocol independence of cell killing with *E. coli* PNP. In one study of MuLV-transduced B-16 (melanoma), 16/c (breast) carcinoma, and MT539 (glioma) cells, 100% cell killing was observed when 2–4% of cells expressed *E. coli* PNP *(42)*. In studies of MT539 cells, treatment with 100 μM 6-MeP-dR was found to kill 100% of cells when as few as 1% expressed PNP. Further, the conversion of 6-MeP-dR to 6-MeP was found to continue after all of the cells were dead, confirming the stability of the PNP enzyme in the medium *(7)*. In studies using cationic liposomes for transient transfection of human colonic carcinoma (T84) cells, 100% of cells were killed when 0.1–0.2% of cells expressed PNP and a similar result was found in human melanoma (Mel 1) cells *(6,42)*. Similar results have been observed in vitro using an adenoviral vector to transfer *E. coli* PNP to target cells.

9.4. In Vivo Tumor Cell Killing Mediated by E. coli PNP Using Retroviral Cell Lines

In the D54 (human glioma) cell line developed for studies of *E. coli* PNP (*see* **Figs. 8–12**), expression is driven by a relatively weak (SV40 early) promoter in pLNSX *(21)*. When glioma tumors expressed the *E. coli* PNP gene in 100% of the cells, rapid tumor regressions and cures were observed after three doses of prodrug therapy with 6-MeP-dR (*see* **Fig. 8**); similar antitumor effects were observed after a single dose of 6-MeP-dR *(18)*. Strong antitumor effects were also noted with 2-F-araA (fludarabine, a clinically approved agent) (*see* **Fig. 9**). In all of these studies, antitumor effects and cures were observed specifically in the tumors which expressed *E. coli* PNP and were treated with a prodrug. Experiments in D54 glioma cells showed that F-dAdo was also capable of mediating potent antitumor effects (*see* **Fig. 10**). Once again, no antitumor activity was noted in control tumors treated with a prodrug but lacking *E. coli* PNP, or in tumors expressing *E. coli* PNP, in the absence of a prodrug.

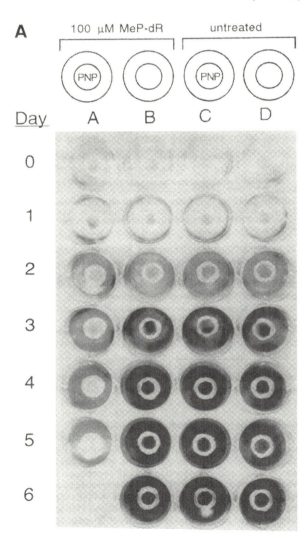

Fig. 5. (**A**) Bystander activity of 6-MeP-dR in D54 cells expressing *E. coli* PNP. D54 cells seeded inside or outside a cloning ring (removed) are separated by a thin ring of vacuum grease. All surrounding cells (outside the ring) are D54 parental cells. In columns A and C, cells inside the ring are D54-PNP cells, and in columns B and D, the inside cells are D54 parental cells. Columns A and B were treated with 100 μ*M* 6-MeP-dR for 6 d. On each day, a row of cells was fixed and stained with crystal violet. (**B**) Effect of exposure to 6-MeP-dR for 24 and 48 h on bystander cell killing. D54 cells were situated as in Column A of (**A**). Magnification of D54 parental cells outside of the rings is ×100 (reduced from original magnification). (**C**) The rate of MeP-dR conversion correlates with an increased rate of cell death. MT539 (murine glioma) and MT539-PNP cells were mixed together from 1% PNP cells to 100% PNP cells and treated with 100 μ*M* MeP-dR. The amount of PNP activity in the medium of treated cells was determined by measuring the proportion of MeP-dR converted to MeP.

B

D54 Parental Cells Outside Rings, Exposed to 100 µM MePdR

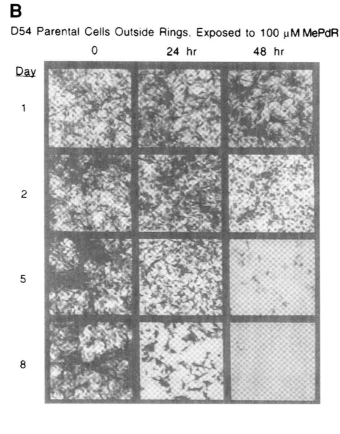

Fig. 5(B)

9.5. Significance of In Vivo Tumor Regressions Mediated by E. coli PNP

The results shown in **Figs. 8–10** apply to tumors in which 100% of cells express *E. coli* PNP and therefore do not test bystander killing in vivo. Nevertheless, these experiments remain important for three reasons. First, they indicate that the general approach (to cleave 6-MeP-dR or other prodrugs) can be safely accomplished in vivo without undue toxicity to the host. At the doses studied in these experiments, animal weights were acceptable and none developed lethargy or had other evidence of systemic toxicity despite generation of highly toxic compounds (which kill both dividing and nondividing cells) within tumor tissues. Cured animals lived normal life expectancies for mice following the regressions of their tumors.

Importantly, the maximum tolerated dose (MTD) of 6-MeP-dR (and other prodrugs) is lower (by approx 35%) in animals that carry PNP-expressing tumors. As one might predict, intratumoral expression of the PNP gene reset the MTD, and an otherwise safe dose of prodrug led to weight loss and death in test animals if their tumors expressed

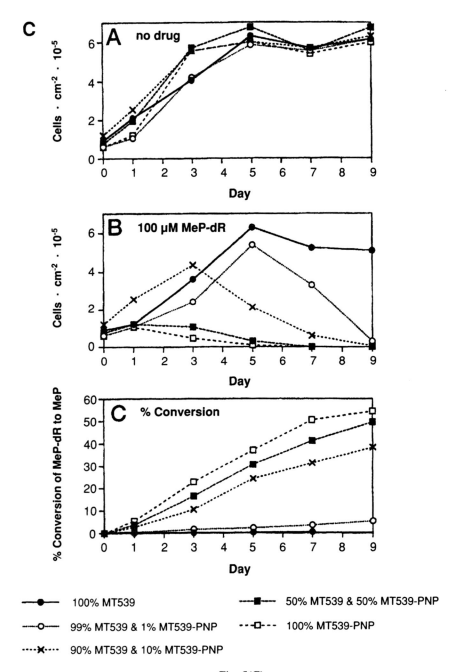

Fig. 5(C)

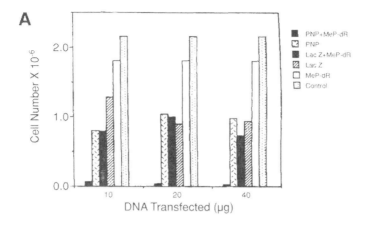

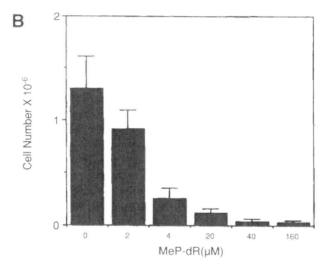

Fig. 6. Enhanced toxicity of MeP-dR mediated by *E. coli* PNP expression. **(A)** Nontransfected T84 (human colonic carcinoma) cells or cells transfected with 10, 20, or 40 μg of cDNA containing either the *E. coli* PNP or *LacZ* genes under control of the SV-40 early promoter (in otherwise comparable vector contexts) were transfected into $(1–2) \times 10^5$ colonic carcinoma cells using a 1 : 1 molar mixture of the cationic lipid DOTMA/DOPE. Two days after transfection, MeP-dR was added to wells as shown to a concentration of 160 μm. After 5 d, the cells were removed from each well and the number of trypan blue-excluding cells were determined with a hemocytometer. **(B)** Approximately 2×10^5 cells per well were transfected with 6 μg of the *E. coli* PNP cDNA as described in **(A)**. Two days after transfection, increasing concentrations of MeP-dR were added to the wells as shown, and after 5 d, the dye-excluding cells were counted. Bars represent mean ± SD from three measurements. These experiments have been repeated five times with essentially identical results. DOTMA, 2,3-dioleoyloxypropyl-1-trimethyl ammonium bromide; DOPE, dioleoylphosphatidylethanolamine.

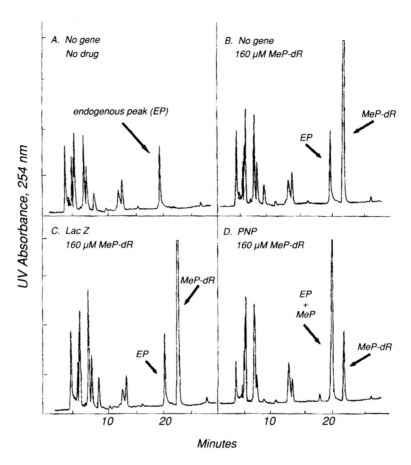

Fig. 7. Detection of MeP in medium of T84 cells transfected with *E. coli* PNP. The medium from T84 cells treated as in **Fig. 6** was collected 5 d after the addition of 160 μ*M* MeP-dR and analyzed by high-performance liquid chromatography for the appearance of MeP. Repeat experiments in HEp-2 cells gave similar results.

E. coli PNP. However, by reducing the administered dose of prodrug in the setting of PNP tumors, tumor regressions and cures were observed despite the generation of 6-MeP or 2-F-Ade. This result has significance, because it indicates that the toxicity of the overall approach can be controlled if prodrug concentration is carefully titrated and shows that although the anticipated toxicity was observed, it can be overcome by adjusting the prodrug dosing scheme.

Second, these results differ from other prodrugs (such as *HSV-TK* or cytosine deaminase) where longer prodrug schedules (generally one to several weeks) are required to establish antitumor effects. The activity of a foreshortened schedule (one to three doses of 6-MeP dR; *see* **Fig. 8**) may be explained in part by the stability of toxic compounds (>24 h) specifically within tumors expressing *E. coli* PNP *(18)*.

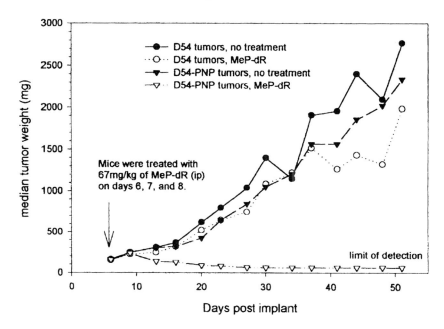

Fig. 8. Effect of MeP-dR on D54 tumors that express *E. coli* PNP (all cells express *E. coli* PNP).

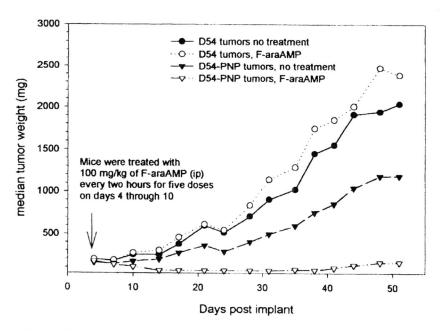

Fig. 9. Effect of F-araAMP on D54 tumors that express *E. coli* PNP (all cells express *E. coli* PNP).

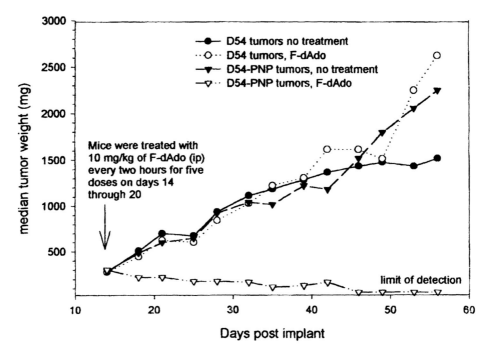

Fig. 10. Effect of F-dAdo on D54 tumors that express *E. coli* PNP (all cells express *E. coli* PNP).

Moreover, the ability to cure tumors after very short courses of therapy may be desirable from the standpoint of prodrug activation. One can argue that the need for repeat or long-term prodrug dosing could otherwise lead to progressive destruction of the very cells expressing the tumor sensitization (or "suicide") gene and lessen the efficacy of subsequent cycles of prodrug.

Third, the results help define a threshold (target) level for intratumoral expression of *E. coli* PNP, above which antitumor effects might be anticipated. **Figures 11** and **12** show the result of mixing experiments with lower percentages of cells expressing the *E. coli* PNP gene and the antitumor effects that were observed. Although a dose dependence has been shown in vivo *(21)*, significant antitumor effects were only observed when 20% or greater of cells expressed the gene (under the control of the relatively weak SV40 promoter).

10. Boundaries to Bystander Killing by *E. coli* PNP

Using recent, state-of-the-art expression vectors (e.g., lentivirus and adenovirus), it should be possible to generate much higher levels of *E. coli* PNP expression (on a per cell basis) than in experiments such as those shown in this chapter. Both the prodrug and the toxin generated as part of *E. coli* PNP prodrug activation are freely membrane permeant. Therefore, it is possible that the number of cells expressing *E. coli* PNP

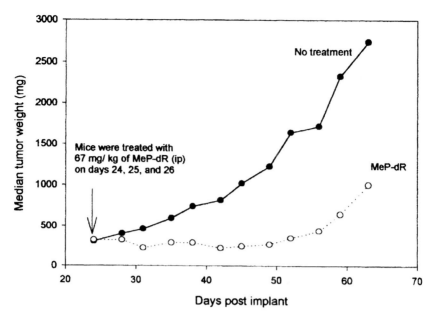

Fig. 11. Effect of MeP-dR on D54 tumors in which 20% of the tumor cells express *E. coli* PNP.

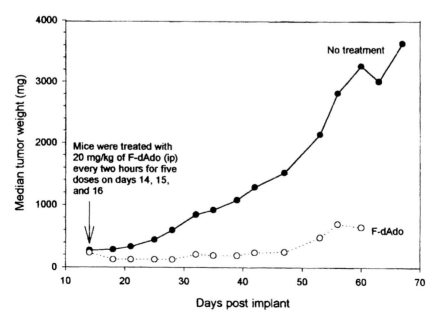

Fig. 12. Effect of F-dAdo on D54 tumors in which 20% of the tumor cells express *E. coli* PNP.

might be a less important determinant of overall bystander killing than the absolute level of PNP enzyme within a tumor cell population or a growing tumor mass. In other words, if 10-fold fewer cells in a tumor express 10-fold higher enzyme on a per cell basis, the magnitude of bystander killing might remain constant despite a much lower number of cells expressing the gene. This predication has been borne out in vitro *(7,42)*, but it will require rigorous testing in vivo.

11. Summary and Conclusions

Prodrug activation is an important strategy for the development of new cancer therapies. From both the practical and conceptual points of view, development of prodrug activation genes in the past has been limited by factors such as inadequate bystander killing, the failure to kill both dividing and nondividing cells, and the inability to target tumors with a low growth fraction. Many untreatable human malignancies are refractory to conventional chemotherapy specifically because antitumor compounds are directed against dividing cells, whereas these same tumors have a comparatively low growth fraction. Toxins such as ganciclovir triphosphate (generated by the action of the *HSV-TK* on ganciclovir) and 5-FU (generated by the action of *E. coli* cytosine deaminase on 5-florocytosine) are, in most cases, ineffective against the nondividing compartment within growing tumors, based on the mechanism of action of these drugs (DNA chain termination and inhibition of thymidylate synthetase, respectively). Part of the rationale underlying the development of an *E. coli* PNP gene therapy strategy is to study drugs that can kill both dividing and nondividing cells and to develop ways to safely administer these specifically within growing tumors.

References

1. Mao, C., Cook, W. J., Zhou, M., Koszalka, G. W., Krenitsky, T. A., and Ealick, S. E. (1997) The crystal structure of *Escherichia coli* purine nucleoside phosphorylase: a comparison with the human enzyme reveals a conserved topology. *Structure* **5(10)**, 1373–1383.
2. Ealick, S. E., Rule, S. A., Carter, D. C., et al. (1990) Three-dimensional structure of human erythrocytic purine nucleoside phosphorylase at 3.2 A resolution. *J. Biol. Chem.* **265(3)**, 1812–1820.
3. Zimmerman, T. P., Gersten, N., Ross, A. F., and Meich, R. P. (1971) Adenine as substrate for purine nucleoside phosphorlase. *Can. J. Biochem.* **49**, 1050–1054.
4. Jensen, K. F. and Nygaard, P. (1975) Purine nucleoside phosphorylase from *Escherichia coli* and *Salmonella typhimurium*. Purification and some properties. *Eur. J. Biochem.* **51**, 253–265.
5. Springer, C. J. and Niculescu-Duvaz, I. (2000) Prodrug-activating systems in suicide gene therapy. *J. Clin. Invest.* **105(9)**, 1161–1167.
6. Sorscher, E. J., Peng, S., Bebok, Z., Allan, P. W., Bennett, L. L., Jr., and Parker, W. B. (1994) Tumor cell bystander killing in colonic carcinoma utilizing the *E. coli* Deo D gene and generation toxic purines. *Gene Ther.* **1**, 233–238.
7. Hughes, B. W., King, S. A., Allan, P. W., Parker, W. B., and Sorscher, E. J. (1998) Cell to cell contact is not required for bystander cell killing by *E. coli* purine nucleoside phosphorylase. *J. Biol. Chem.* **273**, 2322–2328.

8. Dionne, C. A., Camoratto, A. M., Jani, J. P., et al. (1998) Cell cycle-independent death of prostate adenocarcinoma is induced by the trk tyrosine kinase inhibitor CEP-751 (KT6587). *Clin. Cancer Res.* **4(8)**, 1887–1898.
9. Sai, S., Takashi, M., Miyake, K., and Koshikawa, T. (1991) Study of growth fraction on fine needle aspirated prostatic tissue smear using monoclonal antibody Ki-67. *Hinyokika Kiyo—Acta Urol. Japon.* **37**, 881–886.
10. Sadi, M. V. and Barrack, E. R. (1991) Determination of growth fraction in advanced prostate cancer by Ki-67immunostaining and its relationship to the time to tumor progression after hormonal therapy. *Cancer* **67**, 3065–3071.
11. Tay, D. L., Bhathal, P. S., and Fox, R. M. (1991) Quantitation of G0 and G1 phase cells in primary carcinomas. Antibody to M1 subunit of ribonucleotide reductase shows F1 phase restriction point block. *J. Clin. Invest.* **87**, 519–527.
12. Giangaspero, F., Doglioni, C., Rivano, M. T., Pileri, S., Gerdes, J., and Stein, H. (1987) Growth fraction in human brain tumors defined by the monoclonal antibody Ki-67. *Acta Neuropathol.* **74**, 179–182.
13. Pierard, G. E. and Pierd-Franchimont, C. (1997) Stochastic relationship between the growth fraction and vascularity of thin malignant melanomas. *Eur. J. Cancer* **33**, 1888–1892.
14. Crafts, D. C., Hoshino, T., and Wilson, C. B. (1977) Current status of population kinetics in gliomas. *Bull. Cancer* **64**, 115–124.
15. Fontanini, G., Pingitore, R., Bigini, D., et al. (1992) Growth fraction in non-small cell lung cancer estimated by proliferating cell nuclear antigen and comparison with Ki-67 labeling and DNA flow cytometry data. *Am. J. Pathol.* **141**, 1285–1290.
16. Vescio, R. A., Connors, K. M., Bordin, G. M., et al. (1990) The distinction of small cell and non-small cell lung cancer by growth in native-state histoculture. *Cancer Res.* **50**, 6095–6099.
17. Parker, W. B., Allan, P. W., Shaddix, S. C., et al. (1998) Metabolism and metabolic actions of 6-methylpurine and 2-fluoroadenine in human cells. *Biochem. Pharmacol.* **55**, 1673–1681.
18. Gadi, V. K., Alexander, S. D., Waud, W. R., Alan, P., Parker, W. B., and Sorscher, E. J. (2002) A long acting suicide gene toxin, 6-methyl purine, inhibits slow growing tumors after a single administration. *J. Pharmacol. Exp. Ther.* **304**, 1280–1284.
19. Skipper, M. E., Montgomery, J. A., Tomson, J. R., and Schabel, F. M., Jr. (1959) Structure–activity relationship and cross resistance observed on a series of purine analogues against experimental neoplasm. *Cancer Res.* **19**, 425–437.
20. Philips, F. S., Sternberg, S. S, Hamilton, L., and Clarke, D. A. (1954) The toxic effects of 6-mercaptopurine and related compounds. *Ann. NY Acad. Sci.* 283.
21. Parker, W. B., King, S. A., Allan, P. W., et al. (1997) In vivo gene therapy of cancer with *E. coli* purine nucleoside phosphorylase. *Hum. Gene Ther.* **8**, 1637–1644.
22. Bass, B. L. (1992) The dsRNA unwinding/modifying activity: Fact and fiction. *Semin. Dev. Biol.* **3**, 425–433.
23. Clinical Gene Therapy Trial Data base. Available from www.wiley.com/wileychi/genm...er+Therapy&subcategory=.*&start=40.
24. Sacco, M. G., Benedetti, S., Duflotdancer, A., et al. (1996) Partial regression, yet incomplete eradication of mammary tumors in transgenic mice by retrovirally mediated HSV-TK transfer in vivo. *Gene Ther.* **3**, 1151–1156.
25. Beck, C., Cayeux, S., Lupton, S. D., Dorken, B., and Blankenstein, T. (1995) The thymidine kinase/ganciclovir-mediated "suicide" effect is variable in different tumor cells. *Hum. Gene Ther.* **6**, 1525–1530.

26. Dilber, M. S., Abedi, M. R., Christensson, B., et al. (1997) Gap junctions promote the bystander effect of herpes simplex virus thymidine kinase in vivo. *Cancer Res.* **57,** 1523–1528.
27. Elshami A. A., Saavedra, A., Zhang, H., et al. (1996) Gap junctions play a role in the "bystander effect" of the herpes simplex virus thymidine kinase/ganciclovir system in vitro. *Gene Ther.* **3,** 85–92.
28. Fick, J., Barker, F. N., Dazin, P., Westphale, E. M., Beyer, E. C., and Israel, M. A. (1995) The extent of heterocellular communication mediated by gap junctions is predictive of bystander tumor cytotoxicity in vitro. *Proc. Natl. Acad. Sci. USA* **92,** 11,071–11,075.
29. Imaizumi, K., Hasegawa, Y., Kawabe, T., et al. (1998) Bystander tumoricidal effect and gap junctional communication in lung cancer cell lines. *Am. J. Respir. Cell Mol. Biol.* **18,** 205–212.
30. Freeman, S. M., Abboud, C. N., Whartenby, K. A., et al. (1993) The "bystander effect": tumor regression when a fraction of the tumor mass is genetically modified. *Cancer Res.* **53,** 5274–5283.
31. Marini, III., F.C., Nelson J. A., and Lapeyre, J. N. (1995) Assessment of bystander effect potency produced by intratumoral implantation of HSVtk-expressing cells using surrogate marker secretion to monitor tumor growth kinetics. *Gene Ther.* **2,** 655–659.
32. Vile, R. G., Nelson, J. A., Castleden, S., Chong, H, and Hart, I. R. (1994) Systemic gene therapy of murine melanoma using tissue specific expression of the HSVtk gene involves an immune component. *Cancer Res.* **54,** 6228–6234.
33. Caruso, M., Pham-Nguyen, K., Kwong, Y. L., et al. (1996) Adenovirus-mediated interleukin-12 gene therapy for metastatic colon carcinoma. *Proc. Natl. Acad. Sci. USA* **93,** 11,302–11,306.
34. Tapscott, S. J., Miller, A. D., Olson, J. M., Berger, M. S., Groudine, M., and Spence, A. M. (1994) Gene therapy of rat 9L gliosarcoma tumors by transduction with selectable genes does not require drug selection. *Proc. Natl. Acad. Sci. USA* **91,** 8185–8189.
35. Lockett, L. J., Molloy, P. L., Russell, P. J., and Both, G. W. (1997) Relative efficiency of tumor cell killing in vitro by two enzyme-prodrug systems delivered by identical adenovirus vectors. *Clin. Cancer Res.* **3,** 2075–2080.
36. DeVita, V. T., Hellman, S., and Rosenberg, S. A. (1997) Cancer: Principles & Practice of Oncology, 5th ed., Lippincott–Raven, Philadelphia, Vol. 2, p. 1176.
37. Moriuchi, S., Oligino, T., Krisky, D., et al. (1998) Enhanced tumor cell killing in the presence of ganciclovir by herpes simplex virus type 1 vector-directed coexpression of human tumor necrosis factor-alpha and herpes simplex virus thymidine kinase. *Cancer Res.* **58,** 5731–5737.
38. Freytag, S. O., Pogulski, K. R., Paielli, D. L., Gilbert, J. D., and Kim, J. H. (1998) A novel three-pronged approach to kill cancer cells selectively: concomitant viral, double suicide gene, and radiotherapy. *Hum. Gene Ther.* **9,** 1323–1333.
39. Beltinger, C., Fulda, S., Kammertoens, T., Meyer, E., Uckert, W., and Debatin, K. M. (1999) Herpes simplex virus thymidine kinase/ganciclovir-induced apoptosis involves ligand-independent death receptor aggregation and activation of caspases. *Proc. Natl. Acad. Sci. USA* **69,** 8699–8704.
40. Chen, S. H., Kosai, K., Xu, B., et al. (1996) Combination suicide and cytokine gene therapy for hepatic metastases of colon carcinoma: sustained antitumor immunity prolongs animal survival. *Cancer Res.* **56,** 3758–3762.
41. Heise, C., Sampson-Johannes, A., Williams, A., McCormick, F., Von Hoff, D. D., and Kirn, D. H. (1997) ONYX-015, and E1B gene-attenuated adenovirus, causes tumor-specific cytolysis and antitumoral efficacy that can be augmented by standard chemotherapeutic agents. *Nature Med.* **3,** 639–645.

42. Hughes, B. W., Wells, A. H., Bebok, Z., et al. (1995) Bystander killing of melanoma cells using the human tyrosinase promoter to express the *Escherichia coli* purine nucleoside phosphorylase gene. *Cancer Res.* **55,** 3339–3345.

43. Da Costa, L. T., Jen, J., Tong-Chuan, H., Chan, T. A., Kinzler, K. W., and Vogelstein, B. (1996) Converting cancer genes into killer genes. *Proc. Natl. Acad. Sci. USA* **93,** 4192–4196.

44. Nestler, U., Heinkelein, M., Lucke, M., et al. (1997) Foamy virus vectors for suicide gene therapy. *Gene Ther.* **4,** 1270–1277.

45. Martiniello-Wilks, R., Garcia-aragon, J., Daja, M. M., et al. (1998) In vivo gene therapy for prostate cancer: preclinical evaluation of two different enzyme-directed prodrug therapy systems delivered by identical adenovirus vectors. *Hum. Gene Ther.* **9,** 1617–1626.

46. Park, B. J., Brown, C. K., Hu, Y., et al. (1999) Augmentation of melanoma-specific gene expression using a tandem melanocyte-specific enhancer results in increased cytotoxicity of the purine nucleoside phosphorylase gene in melanoma. *Hum. Gene Ther.* **10,** 889–898.

47. Puhlmann, M., Gnant, M., Brown, C. K., Alexander, H. R., and Bartlett, D. L. (1999) Thymidine kinase-deleted vaccinia virus expressing purine nucleoside phosphorylase as a vector for tumor-directed gene therapy. *Hum. Gene Ther.* **10,** 649–657.

48. Krohne, T. U., Shankara, S., Geissler, M., et al. (2001) Mechanisms of cell death induced by suicide genes encoding purine nucleoside phosphorylase and thymidine kinase in human hepatocellular carcinoma cells in vitro. *Hepatology* **34(3),** 511–518.

49. Mohr. L., Shankara, S., Yoon, S. K., et al. (2000) Gene therapy of hepatocellular carcinoma *in vitro* and *in vivo* in nude mice by adenoviral transfer of the *Escherichia coli* purine nucleoside phosphorylase gene. *Hepatology* **31(3),** 606–614.

50. Gadi, V. K., Alexander, S. D., Kudlow, J. E., Allan, P., Parker, W. B., and Sorscher, E. J. (2000) In vivo sensitization of ovarian tumors to chemotherapy by expression of *E. coli* purine nucleoside phosphorylase in a small fraction of tumor cells. *Gene Ther.* **7,** 1738–1743.

51. Secrist, J. A., Parker, W. B., Allan, P. W., et al. (1999) Gene therapy of cancer: activation of nucleoside prodrugs with *E. coli* purine nucleoside phosphorylase. *Nucleosides Nucleotides* **18,** 745–757.

12

Enzyme–Prodrug Systems

Carboxylesterase/CPT-11

Mary K. Danks and Philip M. Potter

1. Introduction

The development of enzyme–prodrug approaches for targeted treatment of human tumors has gained momentum in the last decade, especially with the advent of antibodies, viral vectors, and nonviral delivery systems that might be suitable for use in vivo. However, relatively few novel enzyme–prodrug combinations have been developed for use with these vectors. Because tumors differ in their intrinsic sensitivity to specific classes of chemotherapeutic agents, it is unlikely that any single enzyme–prodrug combination will be effective for all types of cancer. The design of additional vectors, enzymes, and prodrugs needs to be pursued. This section discusses the use of carboxylesterases (CEs) to activate the prodrug CPT-11 {irinotecan, 7-ethyl-10-[4-(1-piperidino)-1-piperidino]carbonyloxycamptothecin}.

1.1. Enzyme–Prodrug Combinations

The most well-characterized enzyme–prodrug combinations to date are herpes simplex virus thymidine kinase/ganciclovir and *Escherichia coli* cytosine deaminase/5-fluorocytosine (5-FC). These combinations illustrate the concept of introducing a viral or bacterial enzyme to provide an activity that is absent in mammalian cells. Expression of the appropriate enzyme activates the respective prodrug preferentially in cells engineered to express each enzyme. Theoretically, tumor-specific cytotoxicity can be achieved by this approach. However, in vivo, when host cells are manipulated to express foreign proteins, the potential exists for induction of an immune response that may limit the utility of the approach. To minimize these problems and to provide an additional useful enzyme–prodrug combination that has a molecular mechanism of cytotoxicity distinct from those of ganciclovir and 5-FC, we have developed and characterized a system that uses a mammalian CE to convert the anticancer camptothecin

From: *Methods in Molecular Medicine, Vol. 90, Suicide Gene Therapy: Methods and Reviews*
Edited by: C. J. Springer © Humana Press Inc., Totowa, NJ

prodrug CPT-11 to its active moiety, SN-38 (7-ethyl-10-hydroxycamptothecin; *see* **Fig. 1**). Most of the work discussed here focuses on the use of this combination in a viral-directed enzyme prodrug therapy (VDEPT) approach, but investigation for potential applications using other delivery systems is ongoing.

1.2. Carboxylesterase/CPT-11

1.2.1. CPT-11

CPT-11 (*see* **Fig. 1**) is a water-soluble camptothecin derivative and an inhibitor of topoisomerase I *(1)*. CPT-11 has demonstrated remarkable antitumor activity both in animal models and in phase II/III trials and is commonly used in the treatment of colon cancer *(1–10)*. CPT-11 is also being tested currently for its efficacy in a wide range of malignancies, including non-small-cell lung cancer, rhabdomyosarcoma, and neuro-blastoma.

Following administration of a range of doses of the drug to humans, low concentrations of SN-38 are observed in the plasma of patients. One study further documented that the percentage of CPT-11 converted to SN-38 decreased as the drug dose increased *(11)*, suggesting that the enzymes responsible for drug activation became saturated and that increasing the amount of CPT-11 administered past a critical level likely provided no additional therapeutic benefit. However, the encouraging results of early clinical trials also indicate that tumor-selective expression of an efficient CPT-11-activating enzyme might well increase both antitumor response and the therapeutic index of the drug.

1.2.2. Activation and Toxicity of CPT-11 in Patients

The activation of CPT-11 in humans has been thought to be mediated by the hepatic CEs *(12,13)* even though extensive studies had failed to identify a single enzyme responsible for catalysis of this drug. However, in the last year, both a human liver CE (hCE2) and a human intestinal CE (hiCE) have been identified that efficiently activate CPT-11 *(14,15)*. Butyrylcholinesterases can also convert CPT-11 to SN-38, although the exact contribution that these enzymes play in drug metabolism remains unclear *(16)*. It now appears that, in vivo, CPT-11 is metabolized both in the liver and in the small intestine. Interestingly, these results suggest that the secretory diarrhea observed in some patients to whom CPT-11 is administered may result, at least in part, from local activation of CPT-11 in the intestine by hiCE. Additionally, a cholinergic syndrome very likely the result of direct inhibition of acetylcholinesterase by CPT-11 has also been observed *(16,17)*.

Evidence of in vivo activation of CPT-11 by endogenous human enzymes notwithstanding, the percent of prodrug converted to its active analog ranges from <1% to only about 5% for most schedules of administration. In light of the curative potential of CPT-11 when sufficient plasma levels of SN-38 can be achieved *(7)*, the potential for tissue-specific expression of active CEs to increase levels of SN-38 in tumor cells and dramatically increase the therapeutic index of CPT-11 merits further investigation.

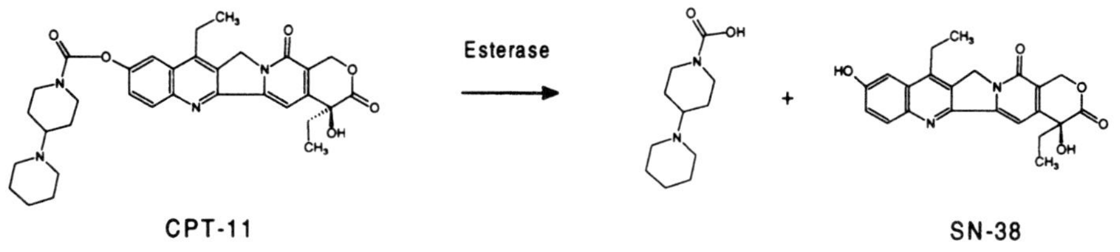

CPT-11   SN-38

Fig. 1. Metabolic activation of CPT-11 to SN-38 by esterases.

1.2.3. Metabolites of CPT-11

Many articles describing in vivo metabolites of CPT-11 have been published and a comprehensive review of these studies and the physiological importance of each metabolite is beyond the scope of this chapter. Suffice it to say that the major metabolites of CPT-11 that appear to be clinically relevant include CPT-11, SN-38, a glucuronide-conjugated form of SN-38 (SN-38G), and APC. A procedure to extract these metabolites from biological samples and an high-performance liquid chromatography (HPLC) method to separate and quantitate their concentration is described in **Subheadings 3.1., 3.2., and 3.3.**

1.2.4. Isolation of a Carboxylesterase That Activates CPT-11

For most schedules of administration, less than 5% of CPT-11 administered to patients is converted to SN-38, suggesting that in vivo CEs are expressed at low levels or that human enzymes activate this prodrug inefficiently. Therefore, more efficient esterases needed to be identified for VDEPT approaches with CPT-11. To screen carboxylesterases from mammalian sources for drug activation, a simple fluorometric assay was designed to quantitate CPT-11 and SN-38 (*see* **Subheading 3.4.**). Using this method, rat and mouse serum CEs and rabbit and pig liver CEs were demonstrated to catalyze CPT-11 efficiently *(18)*. The N-terminus of the rabbit liver CE (rCE) was sequenced and degenerate oligonucleotides were designed to amplify a partial cDNA by polymerase chain reaction (PCR). Following amplification, sequence analysis confirmed that the DNA fragment demonstrated homology to cDNAs encoding previously described CEs. 5' and 3' RACE were then performed to isolate the complete cDNA for rCE *(18)*.

1.2.5. Rabbit Liver Carboxylesterase (rCE)

The rCE is a 565-amino-acid protein with a predicted molecular weight of 62,287 Da *(18)*. The N-terminus of the nascent protein contains a 19-residue signal peptide that directs the enzyme to the endoplasmic reticulum *(19,20)*; however, these amino acids are not present in the mature protein (*see* **Fig. 2**). The four C-terminal amino acids HIEL anchor the protein within the endoplasmic reticulum, and deletion of these residues results in secretion of the CE from the cell *(19,20)*. The secreted enzyme is functional, catalyzing the metabolism of both simple and complex CE substrates *(21)*.

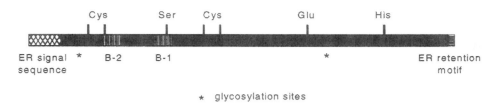

Fig. 2. Schematic representation of the rCE. The active-site residues (Ser221, Glu353, His467), two cysteine disulfide bonds (Cys), and two glycosylation sites (*) are marked. In addition, the B-1 and B-2 esterase motifs and the endoplasmic reticulum signal peptide and retention sequences are indicated.

Extracts of mammalian cells expressing rCE metabolize simple esters such as o-nitrophenyl acetate (o-NPA) and o-nitrophenyl butyrate (o-NPB) as well as more complex substrates such as naphthyl acetate and CPT-11 *(21)*. Metabolism of the classic esterase substrate o-NPA to nitrophenol is readily monitored spectrophotometrically and this assay is useful as a screening technique for CE activity (*see* **Subheading 3.5.**).

However, although many esterases metabolize o-NPA, for example, fewer enzymes of this family activate CPT-11. Therefore, although the o-NPA assay is rapid and useful for preliminary assessment of overall CE activity in biological samples, it is essential to confirm results obtained by determining activation of CPT-11 itself (*see* **Subheading 3.3.** or **3.4.**).

1.2.6. Human Carboxylesterases

As mentioned earlier, one of the potential problems with VDEPT approaches is induction of an immune response when transgenes are of nonhuman origin. Although rCE is highly homologous to several human CEs and unlikely to initiate a clinically significant immune response, identification of a human CE that efficiently activates CPT-11 may be better tolerated than rCE. To this end, computer searches of protein databases with the rCE amino acid sequence identified over 100 homologous enzymes. Of these, a human alveolar macrophage CE (hCE1) *(22)* had the greatest homology to the rabbit protein: Human macrophage CE is greater than 81% identical and 86% similar to the rabbit sequence (*see* **Fig. 3**). Unexpectedly, whereas hCE1 and rCE metabolized small esters such as o-NPA and o-NPB with similar efficiency *(21)*, hCE1 activated CPT-11 approx 650-fold less efficiently than rCE *(23)*.

More recently, a human intestinal CE (hiCE) (*see* **Fig. 3**) has been identified that efficiently converts CPT-11 to SN-38 *(15)*, and a similar activity has been identified in the small intestine of normal mice and in mice deficient in plasma esterase *(24)*. Database searches for DNA sequences encoding human CEs did identify a cDNA encoding a human intestinal CE; however, the investigators who isolated and described this cDNA sequence did not demonstrate the function of the encoded protein *(25)*. When the cDNA of hiCE was expressed in COS-7 cells, analysis of cell sonicates confirmed that the encoded CE efficiently metabolized both o-NPA and CPT-11.

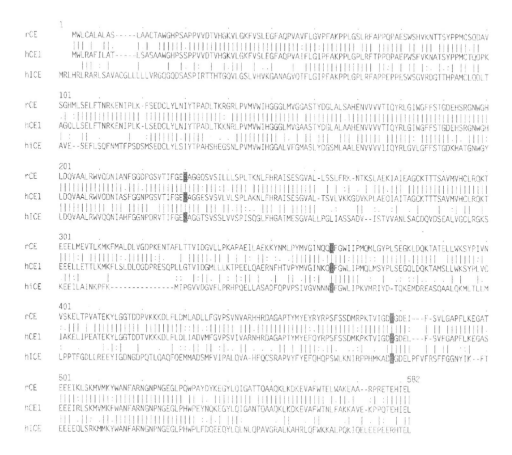

Fig. 3. Alignments of the rabbit (rCE), human liver 1 (hCE1), and human intestinal carboxylesterase (hiCE) amino acid sequences. The active-site residues are shaded.

Analysis of the protein sequences indicated that hiCE was very similar (>99% identical) to a previously reported liver CE, hCE2, with the exception that hiCE contained 10 amino acids at the N-terminus that were not present in hCE2. It is likely that this leader sequence is crucial for routing of the protein to the endoplasmic reticulum and for correct intracellular processing and enzymatic function, because expression of the hCE2 cDNA in mammalian cells results in little *o*-NPA or CPT-11 metabolism in comparison to hiCE cDNA (Khanna and Potter, unpublished results).

1.2.7. Computer Predictive Analysis of the Substrate Specificity of Human and Rabbit Carboxylesterases

In an attempt to understand the inability of hCE1, compared to hiCE and rCE, to metabolize CPT-11, we performed computer-predictive modeling of the three pro-

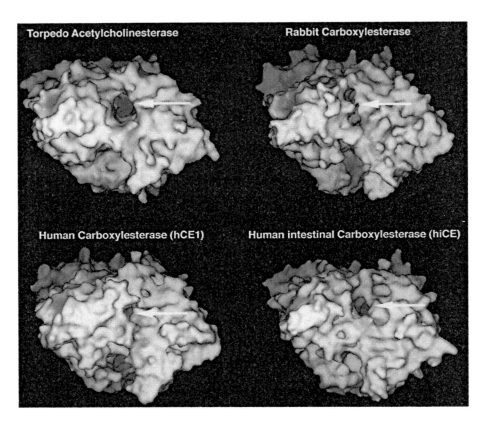

Fig. 4. Computer-predicted models of the rabbit, human liver 1, and human intestinal carboxylesterase. Models were generated using the electric eel (Torpedo) acetylcholinesterase X-ray crystal structure as a template with the computer programs, MODELLER 4 *(27)* and *spock*. Molecular surfaces generated from van der Waals radii of the atoms are colored red for negative charge, blue for positive charge, and white for neutral. The entrance to the active-site gorge, indicated by the yellow arrow, is considerabley smaller in hCE1 compared to rCE and hiCE, accounting for its reduced ability to activate CPT-11.

teins. Because the three-dimensional (3D) structure of mammalian CEs is not known, we modeled hCE1, hiCE, and rCE based on the coordinates of the electric eel acetylcholinesterase *(26)*. The eel acetylcholinesterase demonstrates approx 35% amino acid identity and approx 45% similarity with rCE, hCE1 and hiCE. Importantly, the critical catalytic amino acids residues, a triad of serine, histidine, and glutamic acid, are conserved among the four proteins.

Modeling studies demonstrated that the amino acid residues that interact directly with substrates lie at the distal end of a long narrow gorge and that substrate specificity is restricted by steric constraints dictated by amino acid residues at the entrance of this gorge (*see* **Fig. 4**) *(21)*. Computer-docking analyses of each protein with CPT-11 indicated that the entrance to the catalytic gorge of hCE1 was too narrow to permit entry of the drug into this cleft. In contrast, CPT-11 readily enters the gorge and has access to the catalytic amino acids of both hiCE and rCE. Kinetic studies with substrates containing large bulky ester substituents yielded results that were consistent with the modeling studies *(21)*. Very recently, rCE has been crystallized and the structure is being determined (Potter and Redinbo, unpublished results). Additional studies are ongoing to compare the suitability of rCE and hiCE for use in VDEPT approaches and also to compare the relative utility of intracellular vs secreted rCE and hiCE for specific VDEPT applications.

1.2.8. Expression of rCE Sensitizes Human Tumor Cells to CPT-11

Several approaches were taken to evaluate the extent to which expression of rCE and, more recently, hiCE sensitizes human tumor cells to CPT-11. First, human tumor cell lines were transfected transiently or stably with plasmids encoding rCE, and the concentration of CPT-11 required to inhibit growth or eradicate the clonogenic potential of CE-expressing and vector-transfected controls was determined. The effect of rCE/CPT-11 was assessed both in cell lines grown in culture and as xenografts in severe combined immunodeficient (SCID) mice. Second, adenoviral vectors encoding rCE were constructed and cell lines were transduced with various amounts of virus to produce different levels of expression of the rCE to evaluate the effect of incremental increases in rCE activity on conversion of CPT-11 to SN-38 intracellularly. Growth-inhibition assays, clonogenic assays, and adenoviral construction were performed by standard methods and these methods are not included in this chapter.

In in vitro assays, the IC_{50} values for CPT-11 in human tumor cell lines expressing rCE were 8- to 80-fold lower than for plasmid-transfected control cells *(18,20,23,28)*. A typical example of a survival curve of cells transfected with rCE is shown in **Fig. 5**. This degree of sensitization is particularly impressive, as it has been demonstrated that as little as a two-fold increase in the dose of CPT-11 can effect complete regressions of human tumor xenografts compared to a minimal transient response at the original dose (2.5 vs 1.25 mg/kg/d; *(7)*. Similar to results with cell lines, rCE expression sensitized human tumor xenografts to CPT-11, and complete, long-term "tumor" regressions with no regrowth were observed following administration of CPT-11 to xenograft-bearing mice (*see* **Fig. 6**) *(23)*.

Further, as suggested from in vitro enzyme analysis studies, more recent experiments show that hiCE metabolizes CPT-11 relatively efficiently and, as expected, also sensitizes human tumor cells to CPT-11 *(15)*. In contrast, as alluded to earlier, cell lines expressing hCE1 were not sensitized to CPT-11 *(23)*. Experiments are ongoing to compare the efficacy of hiCE and rCE for specific VDEPT applications.

1.2.9. VDEPT With Carboxylesterases and CPT-11; Comparison With Other Enzyme–Prodrug Combinations

Virus-directed enzyme prodrug therapy with CPT-11 has several advantages not offered by other model systems. First, CPT-11 demonstrates considerable antitumor activity as a single agent, indicating an intrinsic sensitivity of several types of solid

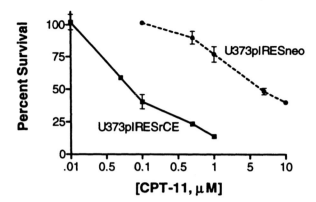

Fig. 5. Expression of rCE sensitizes the U373 glioblastoma cell line to CPT-11. U373 cells were transfected with control pIRESneo plasmid or pIRESrCE plasmid-encoding rCE. Expression of rCE was verified using *o*-NPA as a substrate. U373 cells expressing rCE were approx 80-fold more sensitive to CPT-11 than were cells transfected with the control plasmid.

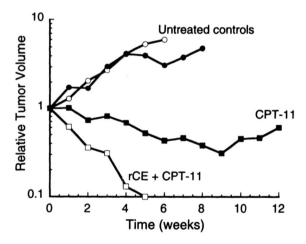

Fig. 6. Expression of rCE sensitizes U373 xenografts in SCID mice to CPT-11. U373 cells stably transfected with pIRESneo or pIRESrCE plasmid were established as subcutaneous xenografts in SCID mice. When the xenografts reached a volume of approx 0.5 cm^3, the mice were treated with three courses of CPT-11 at 5 mg/kg/d, daily for 5 d, for two wk. Xenografts that did not express rCE (as indicated by the CPT-11 curve) showed stable disease, but did not regress. Xenografts that expressed rCE (as indicated by the rCE + CPT-11 curve) regressed completely and did not regrow.

tumors to this drug. Second, xenograft experiments show that CPT-11 has a steep dose–response curve, suggesting that even relatively modest increases in drug activation in tumor cells might produce remarkable increases in antitumor activity. Third, the molecular cytotoxic target of SN-38, topoisomerase I, is an essential enzyme; and, as yet, no resistance-conferring mutations have been identified in this gene from tumors of patients undergoing treatment with camptothecins. Fourth, because the basis for substrate specificity of most human CEs vs rCE and hiCE is now known, novel prodrugs based on existing or new classes of antitumor agents could be designed to be activated by these enzymes. VDEPT combination chemotherapy would almost certainly be more efficacious than single-agent therapy. Fifth, SN-38 freely passes through cell membranes, thereby increasing the likelihood that a bystander effect might be seen in tumor cells adjacent to those engineered to express rCE or hiCE. Additionally, rCE and hiCE are functional when they are localized either intracellularly in the endoplasmic reticulum or secreted from the cell, also providing the opportunity for inducing apoptosis in neighboring cells that do not express the transgene. All of the above considerations, in addition to extensive information regarding most effective and least toxic schedules of administration of CPT-11, are regarded as potential advantages of this novel enzyme–prodrug system.

1.2.10. VDEPT With rCE and CPT-11; Application to Cancer Therapy

Our initial studies to assess the potential of this enzyme–prodrug combination in the treatment of human cancer have concentrated on two specific applications. The first is the selective eradication, or purging, of neuroblastoma cells from bone marrow or peripheral stem cells to be used for autologous stem cell rescue. The second approach involves the use of tumor-specific expression vectors to specifically express rCE in tumor cells. The current status of each of these approaches is summarized briefly.

The rationale for investigating the use of rCE/CPT-11 in purging is twofold: Purging is accomplished ex vivo and therefore provides a simple system with which to test the efficacy of any given prodrug enzyme–prodrug combination. More importantly, gene-marking studies have demonstrated that tumor cells contaminate autologous stem cell grafts and that these tumor cells contribute to the relapse of children with neuroblastoma *(29)*. Hence, if autologous "transplants" are to be used for therapy of high-risk neuroblastoma, tumor cells must be purged prior to reinfusion. To effect this purging, adenoviral vectors encoding rCE are used at a concentration that selectively transduces tumor cells but not human CD34$^+$ marrow repopulating cells. Mixtures of hematopoietic cells/neuroblastoma cells are exposed sequentially to adenovirus and CPT-11 to induce apoptosis specifically in the tumor cells. Conditions that result in complete eradication of neuroblastoma cells but are not toxic to hematopoietic progenitor cells or nonobese diabetic (NOD)/SCID mouse repopulating cells have been identified *(30,31*, and Wagner et al., unpublished data). This method is likely applicable to purging any type of solid tumor cell having an intrinsic sensitivity to CPT-11 similar to that of neuroblastoma cells.

The second approach toward application of the rCE/CPT-11 system involves the use of tumor-specific expression vectors to deliver the rCE cDNA using adenoviral vectors, but to express rCE specifically in tumor cells that overexpress N-MYC or c-MYC. We have modified the ornithine decarboxylase (ODC) promoter to be a potent and specific regulator of transcription of rCE in tumor cells that overexpress the oncogene c-*myc (32)*. Because the MYC family of proteins are transcription factors *(33–35)* and ODC is a target gene regulated by these factors *(36,37)*, selective upregulation of rCE in a tumor cell-specific fashion appears achievable *(31)*.

1.2.11. Future Directions

Whether a drug-activating enzyme is delivered to a tumor by antibody, viral vector, or nonviral delivery systems, each component of enzyme–prodrug approaches must be optimized to maximize antitumor effects and minimize toxicities. Depending on the individual application, specific characteristics may or may not be desirable. For purging, for example, a bystander effect might result in toxicity to hematopoietic stem cells, which would prevent reconstitution of the patient's marrow. In this instance, a bystander effect or collateral cell death would be harmful. In contrast, a bystander effect might be highly desirable when attempting to treat residual disease of a partially resected solid tumor. The potential benefits/toxicities of many aspects of each approach must be evaluated. Essential components of each approach include the intrinsic sensitivity of a particular tumor type to the activated prodrug, the subcellular localization of the enzyme (intracellular or extracellular), the ability of each prodrug/ active drug to traverse the cell membrane, the tumor specificity of antibodies used to deliver drug-activating enzymes, the strength of putative tumor-specific promoters used to regulate specific transgenes, and so forth. Our own current studies focus on comparing the efficacy and toxicity of rCE and hiCE with various viral constructs, including adenoviruses and retroviruses in which expression of intracellular or secreted forms of each enzyme are regulated by different tumor-cell-specific promoters. It will be essential to determine the length of time for which transgenes are expressed in vivo. The most effective viral vectors are being combined with schedules of administration of CPT-11 designed to produce transient, high levels of CPT-11 compared to sustained, lower levels of CPT-11. This comparison is being performed because it is unknown which approach will produce the most tumor-cell-selective toxicity in xenografts that express high levels of CE. Further, additional classes of chemotherapeutic agents are being developed that will also be activated preferentially by rCE and hiCE to achieve combination, tumor-selective chemotherapy.

2. Materials

2.1. Source of Enzyme Activity

Rabbit liver carboxylesterase (Sigma Chemicals, St. Louis, MO).

2.2. Extraction of CPT-11, SN-38, and Other Metabolites from Biological Samples

Methanol (Sigma Chemicals).

2.3. HPLC Detection of Metabolites of CPT-11

1. HPLC-grade acetonitrile (Aldrich Chemical Co., Milwaukee, WI).
2. A 3.9 × 300-mm Nova-Pak C18 60A 4-µm column (Waters Corp., Milford, MA).
3. A high-performance FP920 fluorescence detector (Jasco Corp.).
4. Acidified methanol is prepared by adding 5 µL of 1 *M* HCl to 1 mL of methanol, and the reagent is stored at –20°C.

2.4. Fluorometric Detection of the Conversion of CPT-11 to SN-38

Spectrophotometric-grade methanol (Aldrich Chemical Co.).

2.5. Spectrophotometric Detection of CE
Activity Using o-NPA as a Substrate

HEPES and *o*-nitrophenyl acetate (Sigma Chemicals).

3. Methods
3.1. Source of Enzyme Activity

If a liquid sample such as serum is to be analyzed for CE activity, no preparation or special precautions are necessary prior to analysis, as CEs are stable enzymes. If cell pellets or tissue preparations are to be used as the source of the enzyme, sonicate the cells or tissue in a small volume of 50 m*M* HEPES, pH 7.4, and use the protein suspension for enzyme assays. Do not centrifuge the cell sonicates prior to analysis, because a majority of CE activity is in the particulate fraction.

3.2. Extraction of CPT-11, SN-38, and Other
Metabolites from Biological Samples

1. To each sample, an equal volume of cold acidic methanol is added, and the mixture is vortexed for 10 s and placed on dry ice for 10 min. The sample is then stored at –70°C for a minimum of 1 h.
2. Prior to analysis, the sample is centrifuged at 100,000*g* for 30 min at 4°C. The supernatant is then used for HPLC or fluorometric analysis (*see* **Subheadings 3.3.** or **3.4.**). (*See* **Notes 1** and **2**.)

3.3. HPLC Detection of Metabolites of CPT-11

1. The supernatant from **Subheading 3.2.** is applied to a 300 × 3.9-mm 4-μ*m* Nova-Pak C_{18} column equilibrated in 75 m*M* ammonium acetate, 25% acetonitrile, pH 4.0, at a flow rate of 1 mL/min. Under these conditions, SN-38G, APC, CPT-11, and SN-38 (all lactones) elute at 2.6, 4.1, 5.8, and 7.5 min, respectively (*see* **Fig. 7**).
2. All compounds are detected with a Jasco FP-920 fluorescence detector using an excitation wavelength of 375 nm and an emission wavelength of 550 nm.
3. Detection limits are 10, 20, 20, and 2 pg/μL for SN-38G, APC, CPT-11, and SN-38, respectively.

3.4. Fluorometric Detection of the Conversion of CPT-11 to SN-38

1. As a positive control for samples to be analyzed, incubate 20 units of rabbit liver carboxylesterase (*see* **Note 3**) with 1 μ*M* CPT-11, in a total volume of 1 mL of 50 m*M* HEPES, pH 7.4, at 37°C, for 1–18 ho. (*See* **Note 4**.)
2. Add an equal volume of cold acidified methanol (5 μL of 1 *M* HCl per milliliter of metha-nol) to each sample, vortex, and centrifuge at approx 20,000*g* for 2 min at 4°C. Remove and save supernatant.
3. Place supernatant in a Hitachi F2000 fluorimeter with an excitation wavelength of 377 nm and record the emission profile between 300 and 600 nm.
4. Under these conditions, CPT-11 and SN-38 emission maxima occur at 427 and 549 nm, respectively (*see* **Fig. 8**). (*See* **Notes 5** and **6**.)

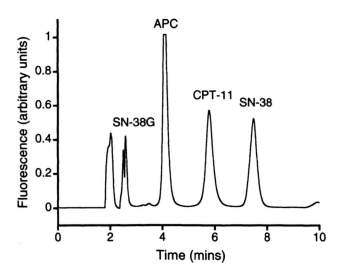

Fig. 7. HPLC chromatogram of CPT-11 and its metabolites. SN-38G, APC, CPT-11′, and SN-38 elute at 2.6, 4.1, 5.8, and 7.5 min, respectively. The SN-38G signal occasionally occurs as a doublet and this may represent the lactone and hydroxyacid forms of the molecule.

3.5. Spectrophotometric Detection of CE
Activity Using o-NPA as a Substrate

This assay monitors the conversion of o-nitrophenyl acetate to o-nitrophenol spectrophotometrically. The rate of product formation is dependent on the amount of CE activity in the sample and can be calculated using the molar extinction coefficient (εm) for o-nitrophenol ($13.6 \times 10^3 \ M^{-1} \ cm^{-1}$).

1. Keep all samples and substrate on ice.
2. Prepare extracts by sonicating cells in minimal volumes (30–300 μL) of 50 mM HEPES, pH 7.4, on ice for 5 s. Do not centrifuge sample because many carboxylesterases are attached to endoplasmic reticulum (ER) membranes.
3. Samples are assayed in quadruplicate and compared to a blank that contains only HEPES buffer. Aliquot 83 μL of sample into the bottom of a plastic cuvet. Typically, 20–80 μL of tissue culture media, 0.5–10 μL for human or animal sera, or 0.1–10 μL of cell extracts will be required.
4. In a 15-mL tube, mix together 900 μL of 50 mM HEPES, pH 7.4, and 17 μL of substrate (32.6 mg/mL of o-NPA in methanol) for each cuvet; that is, for 5 samples, use 5400 μL of assay buffer + 102 μL of substrate. Vortex briefly.
5. As quickly as possible, dispense 917 μL into each cuvet and start a timer halfway through.
6. Place cuvets in spectrophotometer and blank at 420 nm. After 1 min from the addition of the substrate, start the spectrophotometer so that 10 readings will be taken at 1-min intervals.
7. Compare with a no extract control or boiled extract.
8. Plot absorbance values vs time and determine slope of linear regression. Typically, R^2 values should exceed 0.99. The slope will represent ΔA_{420}/min.
9. If the sample is a cell extract, determine the protein concentration of the samples.

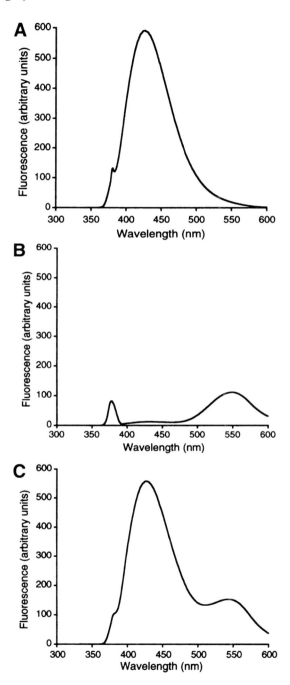

Fig. 8. Fluorometric scans of 5 μ*M* CPT-11 (**A**), 5 μ*M* SN-38 (**B**), and 5 μ*M* of both (**C**), using an excitation wavelength of 375 nm and emission wavelengths from 300 to 600 nm.

3.6. Calculations

Because the extinction coefficient of *o*-nitrophenol is 13,600 at 420 nm, we can calculate μmoles/min/mg as follows:

$$\frac{\text{Slope of curve} \times [1000/\text{sample vol }(\mu L)]}{\text{Protein Conc. (mg/mL)}} = \text{OD/min/mg}$$

$$\text{To convert to } \mu\text{moles/min/mg:} \frac{\text{OD/min/mg}}{0.0136}$$

where OD = optical density.

4. Notes

1. To allow efficient detection and quantitation of CPT-11 and its metabolites in biological samples, removal of protein, DNA, and other particulate matter is achieved by methanol precipitation. In addition, because both CPT-11 and SN-38 can exist as isomers (hydroxyacid and lactone forms), samples are acidified prior to analysis. Below pH 4.0, the equilibrium between the two isoforms shifts so that only the lactone form is present, facilitating quantitation of the total amount of drug.

2. A more extensive sample preparation is needed prior to injecting samples onto an HPLC column than is needed for simple fluorometric analysis. The method in **Subheading 3.1.** is suitable for both HPLC and fluorometry. However, for samples to be analyzed by fluorometry, it is necessary only to (1) add an equal volume of cold, acidified methanol, (2) vortex, (3) centrifuge at approx 20,000*g* for 2 min, and (4) place the supernatant in a cuvet for analysis.

3. Sigma sells rabbit liver carboxylesterase both as a suspension in ammonium sulfate and as a powder in Tris buffer. The activity of the enzyme in the ammonium sulfate suspension is stable for up to 6 mo at 4°C. After reconstitution, the enzyme in Tris buffer is stable only for a very short time and should be used immediately after reconstitution.

4. Concentrations of CPT-11, the amount of enzyme, and the incubation time can be tailored to accommodate prodrug concentrations from 0.5 to 100 μ*M*. Reaction conditions of 20 units of enzyme activity, 1 μ*M* CPT-11, and an 18-h incubation results in >50% conversion of CPT-11 to SN-38.

5. A methanol peak will be visible at approx 300 nm; the size of this peak varies with the temperature of the solution.

6. The lactone and hydroxyacid forms of each compound (CPT-11 and SN-38) have similar excitation/emission spectra; therefore, this assay does not differentiate between active (lactone) and inactive (hydroxyacid) forms of the compounds, as is possible by some of the more sophisticated HPLC methods.

References

1. Tanizawa, A., Fujimori, A., Fujimori, Y., and Pommier, Y. (1994) Comparison of topoisomerase I inhibition, DNA damage, and cytotoxicity of camptothecin derivatives presently in clinical trials. *J. Natl. Cancer Inst.* **86,** 836–842.
2. Houghton, P. J., Cheshire, P. J., Hallman, J. D., 2nd, et al. (1995) Efficacy of topoisomerase I inhibitors, topotecan and irinotecan, administered at low dose levels in protracted schedules to mice bearing xenografts of human tumors. *Cancer Chemother. Pharmacol.* **36,** 393–403.

3. Houghton, J. A., Cheshire, P. J., Hallman, J. A., et al. (1996) Evaluation of irinotecan in combination with 5-fluorouracil or etoposide in xenograft models of colon adenocarcinoma and rhabdomyosarcoma. *Clin. Cancer Res.* **2,** 107–118.

4. Bissery, M. C., Vrignaud, P., Lavelle, F., and Chabot, G. G. (1996) Preclinical antitumor activity and pharmacokinetics of irinotecan (CPT-11) in tumor-bearing mice. *Ann. NY Acad. Sci.* **803,** 173–180.

5. Bissery, M. C., Vrignaud, P., Lavelle, F., and Chabot, G. G. (1996) Experimental antitumor activity and pharmacokinetics of the camptothecin analog irinotecan (CPT-11) in mice. *Anticancer Drugs* **7,** 437–460.

6. Thompson, J., Zamboni, W. C., Cheshire, P. J., et al. (1997) Efficacy of oral irinotecan against neuroblastoma xenografts. *Anticancer Drugs* **8,** 313–322.

7. Thompson, J., Zamboni, W. C., Cheshire, P. J., et al. (1997) Efficacy of systemic administration of irinotecan against neuroblastoma xenografts. *Clin. Cancer Res.* **3,** 423–431.

8. Baker, L., Khan, R., Lynch, T., et al. (1997) Phase II study of irinotecan (CPT-11) in advanced non-small cell lung cancer (NSCLC). *Proc. Annu. Meet. Am. Soc. Clin. Oncol.* **16,** A1658 (abstract).

9. Escudier, B., Fizazi, K., Rolland, F., et al. (1997) Phase II study of irinotecan (CPT 11) in pretreated (A) or not pretreated (B) patients (pts) with advanced renal cell carcinoma. *Proc. Annu. Meet. Am. Soc. Clin. Oncol.* **16,** A1188 (abstract).

10. Furman, W. L., Stewart, C. F., Poquette, C. A., et al. (1999) Direct translation of a protracted irinotecan schedule from a xenograft model to a Phase I trial in children. *J. Clin. Oncol.* **17,** 1815–1824.

11. Rivory, L. P., Haaz, M.-C., Canal, P., Lokiec, F., Armand, J.-P., and Robert, J. (1997) Pharmacokinetic interrelationships of irinotecan (CPT-11) and its three major plasma metabolites in patients enrolled in Phase I/II trials. *Clin. Cancer Res.* **3,** 1261–1266.

12. Rivory, L. P., Bowles, M. R., Robert, J., and Pond, S. M. (1996) Conversion of irinotecan (CPT-11) to its active metabolite, 7-ethyl-10-hydroxycamptothecin (SN-38), by human liver carboxylesterase. *Biochem. Pharmacol.* **52,** 1103–1111.

13. Slatter, J. G., Su, P., Sams, J. P., Schaaf, L. J., and Wienkers, L. C. (1997) Bioactivation of the anticancer agent CPT-11 to SN-38 by human hepatic microsomal carboxylesterases and the in vitro assessment of potential drug interactions. *Drug Metab. Dispos.* **25,** 1157–1164.

14. Humerickhouse, R., Lohrbach, K., Li, L., Bosron, W., and Dolan, M. (2000) Characterization of CPT-11 hydrolysis by human liver carboxylesterase isoforms hCE-1 and hCE-2. *Cancer Res.* **60,** 1189–1192.

15. Khanna, R., Morton, C. L., Danks, M. K., and Potter, P. M. (2000) Proficient metabolism of CPT-11 by a human intestinal carboxylesterase. *Cancer Res.* **60,** 4725–4728.

16. Morton, C. L., Wadkins, R. M., Danks, M. K., and Potter, P. M. (1999) CPT-11 is a potent inhibitor of acetylcholinesterase but is rapidly catalyzed to SN-38 by butyrylcholinesterase. *Cancer Res.* **59,** 1458–1463.

17. Petit, R. G., Rothenberg, M. L., Mitchell, E. P., Compton, L. D., and Miller, L. L. (1997) Cholinergic symptoms following CPT-11 infusion in a phase II multicenter trial of 250 mg/m^2 irinotecan (CRT-11) given every two weeks. *Proc. Annu. Meet. Am. Soc. Clin. Oncol.* **16,** A953 (abstract).

18. Potter, P. M., Pawlik, C. A., Morton, C. L., Naeve, C. W., and Danks, M. K. (1998) Isolation and partial characterization of a cDNA encoding a rabbit liver carboxylesterase that activates the prodrug Irinotecan (CPT-11). *Cancer Res.* **52,** 2646–2651.

19. Potter, P. M., Wolverton, J. S., Morton, C. L., Whipple, D. O., and Danks, M. K. (1998) In situ subcellular localization of epitope tagged human and rabbit carboxylesterases. *Cytometry* **32,** 223–232.

20. Potter, P. M., Wolverton, J. S., Morton, C. L., Wierdl, M., and Danks, M. K. (1998) Cellular localization domains of a rabbit and a human carboxylesterase: influence on irinotecan (CPT-11) metabolism by the rabbit enzyme. *Cancer Res.* **58**, 3627–3632.

21. Wadkins, R. M., Morton, C. L., Weeks, J. K., et al. (2001) Structural constraints affect the metabolism of CPT-11 by esterases. *Mol. Pharmacol.* **60**, 355–362.

22. Munger, J. S., Shi, G. P., Mark, E. A., Chin, D. T., Gerard, C., and Chapman, H. A. (1991) A serine esterase released by human alveolar macrophages is closely related to liver microsomal carboxylesterases. *J. Biol. Chem.* **266**, 18,832–18,838.

23. Danks, M. K., Morton, C. L., Krull, E. J., et al. (1999) Comparison of activation of CPT-11 by rabbit and human carboxylesterases for use in enzyme/prodrug therapy. *Clin. Cancer Res.* **5**, 917–924.

24. Morton, C. L., Wierdl, M., Oliver, L., et al. (2000) Activation of CPT-11 in mice: Identification and analysis of a highly effective plasma esterase. *Cancer Res.* **60**, 4206–4210.

25. Schwer, H., Langmann, T., Daig, R., Becker, A., Aslanidis, C., and Schmitz, G. (1997) Molecular cloning and characterization of a novel putative carboxylesterase, present in human intestine and liver. *Biochem. Biophys. Res. Commun.* **233**, 117–120.

26. Sussman, J. L., Harel, M., Frolow, F., et al. (1991) Atomic structure of acetylcholinesterase from Torpedo californica: a prototypic acetylcholine-binding protein. *Science* **253**, 872–879.

27. Sali, A. and Blundell, T. J. (1993) Comparative protein modelling by satisfaction of spatial restraints. *J. Mol. Biol.* **234**, 779–815.

28. Danks, M. K., Morton, C. L., Pawlik, C. A., and Potter, P. M. (1998) Overexpression of a rabbit liver carboxylesterase sensitizes human tumor cells to CPT-11. *Cancer Res.* **58**, 20–22.

29. Rill, D., Santana, V., Roberts, W., et al. (1994) Direct demonstration that autologous bone marrow transplantation for solid tumors can return a multiplicity of tumorigenic cells. *Blood* **84**, 380–383.

30. Wagner, L. M., Guichard S. M., Burger, R. Z., et al. (2002) Efficacy and toxicity of a virus-directed enzyme prodrug therapy purging method: practical assessment and application to bone marrow samples from neuroblastoma patients. *Cancer Res.* **62**, 5001–5007.

31. Meck, M., Wierdl, M., Wagner, L., et al. (2001) A VDEPT approach to purging neuroblastoma cells from hematopoeitic cells using adenovirus encoding rabbit carboxylesterase and CPT-11. *Cancer Res.*, **61**, 5083–5089.

32. Iyengar, R. V., Pawlik, C. A., Krull, E. J., et al. (2001) Use of a modified ornithine decarboxylase promoter to achieve efficient c-MYC or N-MYC-regulated protein expression. *Cancer Res.* **61**, 3045–3052.

33. Blackwell, T. K., Kretzner, L., Blackwood, E. M., Eisenman, R. N., and Weintraub, H. (1990) Sequence-specific DNA binding by the c-Myc protein. *Science* **250**, 1149–1151.

34. Blackwood, E. M. and Eisenman, R. N. (1991) Max: a helix–loop–helix zipper protein that forms a sequence-specific DNA-binding complex with Myc. *Science* **251**, 1211–1217.

35. Kretzner, L., Blackwood, E. M., and Eisenman, R. N. (1992) Myc and Max proteins possess distinct transcriptional activities. *Nature* **359**, 426–429.

36. Bello-Fernandez, C. and Cleveland, J. L. (1992) c-myc transactivates the ornithine decarboxylase gene. *Curr. Topics Microbiol. Immunol.* **182**, 445–452.

37. Bello-Fernandez, C., Packham, G., and Cleveland, J. L. (1993) The ornithine decarboxylase gene is a transcriptional target of c-Myc. *Proc. Natl. Acad. Sci. USA* **90**, 7804–7808.

13

Enzyme–Prodrug Systems

Thymidine Phosphorylase/5'-Deoxy-5-Fluorouridine

Alexandre Evrard, Joseph Ciccolini, Pierre Cuq, and Jean-Paul Cano

1. Introduction

Thymidine phosphorylase (E.C. 2.4.2.4) (TP), also described as the angiogenic platelet-derived endothelial cell growth factor (PD-ECGF) *(1–4)*, is a homodimeric enzyme with a monomeric molecular mass of about 55 kDa *(5,6)* that phosphorolytically cleaves thymidine to yield thymine and deoxyribose-1-phosphate (dR-1-P) *(7,8)*. TP is expressed in various human cells and tissues and plays a role in plasma thymidine homeostasis *(9–11)*. The levels of expression in different human tissues can vary up to 15-fold *(12)*. Moreover, TP levels are increased in several types of malignant tumors when compared to the non-neoplastic regions of these tissues *(13)* and also in the plasma from tumor-bearing animals and cancer patients *(14)*.

Thymidine phosphorylase is also a key enzyme in the metabolic activation of fluoropyrimidines that share the physiological pathway of pyrimidines (*see* **Fig. 1**). TP is responsible for the conversion of 5'-deoxy-5-fluorouridine (5'dFUrd, Doxifluridine) to 5-fluorouracil (5-FU), and because of its reversible phosphorolytic activity, assumes also the conversion of 5FU to its anabolite 5-fluoro-2'-deoxyuridine (5FdUrd) if sufficient dR-1-P co-factor is available *(15,16)*. 5-FU has been reported to be activated through two distinct pathways *(17,18)*. The first, initiated by 5-FU conversion to 5-fluorouridine (FUrd) by uridine phosphorylase, leads to fluororibonucleotides incorporation into RNA. The second, initiated by 5-FU conversion to 5-fluoro-2'-deoxyuridine (FdUrd) by thymidine phosphorylase (TP), leads to thymidylate synthase inhibition by 5-fluoro-2'-deoxyuridine monophosphate (FdUMP) and to fluorodeoxyribonucleotides incorporation into DNA.

Transfection experiments have provided evidence that overexpression of TP confers sensitivity of various cancer cells to 5'dFUrd and enhances 5-FU cytotoxicity

From: *Methods in Molecular Medicine, Vol. 90, Suicide Gene Therapy: Methods and Reviews*
Edited by: C. J. Springer © Humana Press Inc., Totowa, NJ

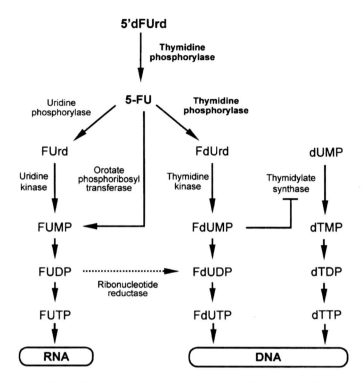

Fig. 1. Metabolic activation pathways of fluoropyrimidines.

(19–22). Furthermore, several authors have described a neighboring cytotoxicity on adjacent, untransfected cells (23–25). Unlike the HSV-TK/ganciclovir system, which requires gap junctions between adjacent tumor cells (26,27), the bystander effect observed with TP and fluoropyrimidines does not require cell–cell contact. The mechanism by which this diffusible bystander effect occurs is unclear. A first hypothesis is diffusion of toxic anabolites of 5'dFUrd toward untransfected cells (i.e., 5-FU itself as a freely diffusible molecule or its anabolite 5-fluoro-2'-deoxyuridine, which is able to cross the cell membrane through a in and out nucleoside transport system) (28,29). Alternatively, this bystander effect could be explained by the extracellular depletion of thymidine by transfected cells. This depletion would lead to a thymidineless death of untransfected cells insofar as thymidine would not be available for the salvage pathway (16). Whatever it is, the exact mechanism of bystander effect in the TP/5'dFUrd system remains to be elucidated.

We describe here a strategy to obtain stable transfectants of cancer cells expressing high TP expression. The presented TP activity assay is useful, on the one hand, to assess TP expression in transfected cells and, on the other hand, to check basal TP activity of target cells. High-performance liquid chromatographic (HPLC) analysis of tritiated fluopyrimidines metabolism is carried out to evaluate the relative importance of the metabolic activation pathways. Finally, we describe cytotoxicity assays to assess the sensitivity of transfected cells compared to wild-type cells and to evidence a bystander effect.

2. Materials
2.1. Stable Transfection

1. Petri dishes, 5 and 10 cm in diameter.
2. 24-Well plates.
3. Growth medium.
4. OptiMEM™ (Life Technologies) (*see* **Note 1**).
5. Dulbecco's phosphate-buffered saline (PBS).
6. Lipofectamine™ reagent (Life Technologies).
7. Geneticin™ (Life Technologies).
8. Mammalian expression vector containing TP cDNA (*see* **Fig. 2** and **Note 2**).
9. Cloning rings (*see* **Note 3**).
10. Sterilized silicone.
11. Incubator 37°C, 5% CO_2.

2.2. TP Activity

1. Sterilized cell scrapers (for adherent cells).
2. 1 *M* Tris-HCl, pH 8.0
3. 5 *M* NaCl.
4. Phenylmethylsulfonyl fluoride (PMSF) (*see* **Note 4**).
5. Aprotinin (*see* **Note 4**).
6. Triton X-100.
7. Bradford reagent (Sigma or Bio-Rad) *(30)*.
8. Bovine serum albumin (BSA).
9. PBS.
10. Thymidine.
11. Thymine (for calibration curve).
12. KH_2PO_4.
13. 0.2 *N* NaOH.

2.3. Determination of [³H]-Fluorinated Metabolites

1. 100 μCi [³H]-5'dFUrd or [³H]-5-FU (Dupont NEN).
2. High-performance liquid chromatographic (HLPC)-grade methanol.
3. K_2HPO_4.
4. Tetrabutylammonium nitrate.
5. Orthophosphoric acid.
6. 0.45-μm Membrane filter.
7. HPLC system coupled to ultraviolet (UV) and radiometric detectors.
8. Lichrospher 100 RP8, 5-μm column.
9. Ultima-Flow scintillation liquid (Packard).
10. Standards (Sigma) : 5-FU, 5'dFUrd, 5FUrd, 5FdUrd, 5FdUMP, 5-fluoro-2'-uridine monophosphate (5FUMP), and 5-fluoro-2'-uridine diphosphate (5FUDP) (*see* **Note 5**).
11. Speed-Vac.

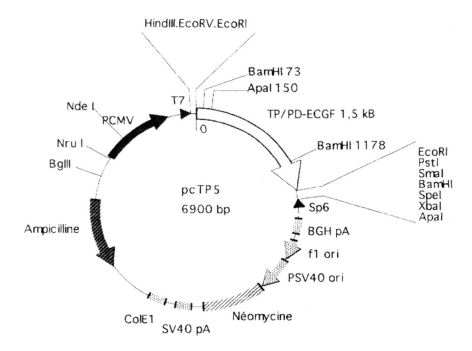

Fig. 2. Schematic diagramm of the mammalian expression vector pcTP5 used for stable transfection of thymidine phosphorylase cDNA in tumor cells (*see* **Note 2**). Mains features are a strong promoter derived from cytomegalovirus and a neomycine-resistance gene allowing selection of recombinant clones with geneticin (G418).

2.4. Cell-Sensitivity Assays

1. 96-Well microtiter plates.
2. Multichannel pipet and tips.
3. Syringe (10 or 20 mL) and syringe filter (0.2–0.8 μm).
4. Neutral red solution at 3.3 g/L (Sigma N2889).
5. Dimethyl sulfoxyde (DMSO).
6. Acetic acid (glacial).
7. Ethanol absolute.
8. PBS.
9. Growth medium adapted to the cell type of interest.
10. Microtiter plate reader with 540-nm filter.
11. Membrane culture inserts for 96-well plates (Anopore, pore size=0.02 μm; Nunc) for assessment of bystander effect in noncontact conditions.

3. Methods

3.1. Stable Transfection

This is a lightly modified version of the manufacturer's (Life Technologies) procedure that gave the best results on several mammalian cell lines.

1. Seed $(1-5) \times 10^6$ target cells in a 5-cm-diameter $(20\text{-}cm^2)$ Petri dish in appropriate serum containing growth medium. Incubate overnight at 37°C in a fully humidified atmosphere of 5% CO_2 in air. On the day of transfection, cells shoud be approx 80% confluent.

2. Prepare two sterile tubes with 220 µL optiMEM and dilute 4 µg plasmid DNA (solution A) in one tube and 25 µL Lipofectamine™ (solution B) in the other tube (*see* **Note 1**). Mix solutions A and B by gently pipetting and incubate at room temperature for 30 min to allow the liposomes–DNA complexes to form.

3. During incubation, rinse cells twice with optiMEM or another serum-free medium. At the end of incubation, add 1.7 mL optiMEM to the liposomes–DNA complexes, mix by gently pipetting, and pour the solution on rinsed cells; be careful to overlay all the cells' monolayer. Incubate for 5 h at 37°C in a fully humidified atmosphere of 5% CO_2 in air (*see* **Note 6**).

4. Remove the transfection mixture, rinse twice, and replace with serum containing the growth medium. Incubate cells at 37°C, 5% CO_2 for 48–72 h; do not allow the cells to pass beyond the confluence state.

5. Harvest cells using trypsin and replate in three 10-cm-diameter Petri dishes (i.e., an approx 1/12 passage; *see* **Note 7**) in selective growth medium containing 1 mg/mL geneticin (*see* **Note 8**). Incubate cells at 37°C, 5% CO_2 for 2–3 wk. Medium should be replaced every day during the first week to remove efficiently untransfected dead cells and cellular debris. Afterward, the medium could be changed only every 2 or 3 d. Check the appearance of colonies. Mark individualized clones well with an indelible marker by surrounding them on the dishes' bottom.

6. When clones reach a size of approx 5 mm, they can be isolated as follows. Fill a 24-well plate with selective growth medium (approx 1 mL per well). Remove growth medium from the Petri dishes, rinse the cells twice with PBS, and remove all of the remaining liquid by aspiration. With sterilized tongs, steep the rim of cloning rings in sterilized silicone and place them around selected clones (*see* **Note 3**). Add 20 µL trypsin in each cloning ring and harvest the cells by a gently and pipetting in and out (change tip for each new clone) and transfer in the 24-well plate.

7. Grow isolated clones by replacing medium every 2 d. At this time, geneticin concentration can be reduced to 500 µg/mL. When cells are subconfluent, harvest using trypsin and expand to large quantities for TP activity and liquid nitrogen storage.

3.2. TP Activity

Samples must be stored on ice throughout the procedure to conserve thymidine phosphorylase activity.

3.2.1. Cell Lysis

1. Seed approx 5×10^6 cells in a 5-cm-diameter $(20\text{-}cm^2)$ Petri dish in appropriate serum containing growth medium. Incubate overnight at 37°C in a fully humidified atmosphere of 5% CO_2 in air. On the day of lysis, cells shoud be approx 80% confluent.

2. Prepare a lysis buffer containing 50 mM Tris-HCl (pH 8.0), 150 mM NaCl, 100 µg/mL PMSF, 1 µg/mL aprotinin and 1% Triton X-100 (*see* **Note 4**).

3. Wash cells monolayers twice on a flat aluminum tray on ice with cold PBS, carefully remove all remaining PBS by pipetting, and add 100 µL of lysis buffer for the 20-cm² culture dishes (*see* **Note 9**). Incubate on ice for 5 min.

4. Harvest the lysates with sterilized cell scrapers (change for each cell type) and transfer into microtubes with a micropipetting device. For the case of cells growing in a suspen-

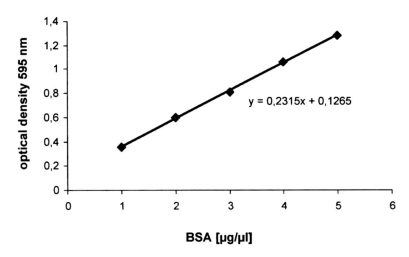

Fig. 3. Protein standard curve obtained by mixing 20 µL of BSA dilutions with 5 ml of diluted (1/5) Bradford reagent. The curve is linear up to 5 µg/µL; sample concentration is calculated from the linear regression curve equation.

    sion, pellet cells by gently centrifugation, add lysis buffer, and mix by pipetting lysate into and out of a disposable pipette.

5. Centrifuge lysates at 20,000g for 30 min at 4°C. TP, as a cytosolic protein, is located in the supernatant. Transfer supernatants into clean microtubes. Depending on cell type, the obtained volume is approx 200–300 µL (*see* **Note 10**).

6. To assess protein contents of cleared lysates, prepare a 1/5 dilution of Bradford reagent in sterile ultrapure water; dispense the diluted solution into aliquots of 5 mL in appropriate plastic tubes. For each lysate, add 20 µL of supernatant to 5 mL of diluted Bradford reagent. An additional tube with 20 µL of lysis buffer is used as a blank. Gently mix tubes by inversion and incubate at room temperature for 5 min. Check the appearance of a blue coloration, except for the blank.

7. Measure the optical density of samples at 595 nm using the blank tube as a zero. Calculate the protein concentration (µg/µL) of lysates by reference to a standard curve obtained with BSA (*see* **Fig. 3**). Subconfluent 20-cm^2 culture dishes usually yield 2–5 µg/µL protein. In any case, adjust protein concentration to 2 µg/µL by adding lysis buffer.

3.2.2. TP Activity Assay

    This assay is a modified version of a previously described procedure *(12)* based on the spectrophotometric monitoring at 300 nm of the conversion of thymidine to thymine.

1. Prepare a reaction mixture (substrate) consisting of 10 mM thymidine and 10 mM KH$_2$PO$_4$ in ultrapure water and adjust pH to 8.4. This solution can be dispensed into aliquots and kept for long-term storage at –20°C.

2. For each sample, prepare two microtubes with 50 µL of cells lysate (corresponding to 100 µg of total protein). Prepare two additional microtubes with 50 µL of lysis buffer for blank reactions. The first serie of microtubes is for t_0 (i.e., without incubation) and the second one is for t_f (i.e., after incubation).

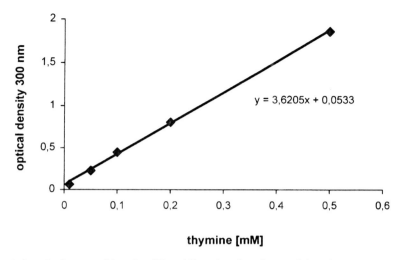

Fig. 4. Standard curve of thymine. Thymidine phosphorylase activity of samples is expressed as pmol of thymine formed/μg protein/h as described (*see* **Note 12**).

3. Add 150 μL of reaction mixture in each tube by using a multidispense pipet. Immediatly add 800 μL of 0.2 *N* NaOH in the t_0 series of microtubes, mix gently by inversion, and keep at –4°C. Incubate the t_f series of microtubes for 4 h at 37°C (*see* **Note 11**). After incubation, stop the reaction by adding 800 μL of 0.2 *N* NaOH and keep at 4°C.

4. Measure the optical density of samples at 300 nm using blank reactions as a zero for the corresponding series (there is usually no difference between the t_0 and the t_f blank). The final volume of sample (1 mL) is suitable for the use of quartz microcuvets.

5. Calculate the amount of thymine in the reaction mixture using a calibration curve (*see* **Note 12**). TP activity is expressed as pmol thymine formed/μg protein/h (*see* **Fig. 4**).

3.3. Determination of [³H]-Fluorinated Metabolites

Monitoring of fluoropyrimidines tumoral activation into nucleosides and/or nucleotides is performed by reverse-phase HPLC analysis with flow radiometric detection. Briefly, after exposing the cells to radiolabelled drugs, cytosols are isolated and subjected to HPLC analysis.

3.3.1. Cell Treatment and Cytosol Isolation

1. Seed approx 1×10^6 cells in 25-cm² culture flasks and allow attachment to proceed overnight.

2. Expose the cells to 100 μCi of [³H]-FUra or [³H]-5'dFURd (about 2 μ*M* final concentration) for time intervals ranging from 0.5 up to 72 h (*see* **Note 13**).

3. Wash the cells twice with standard PBS solution and harvest the culture by trypsin. Isolate the cells by gentle centrifugation (200*g*) and wash the pellet twice with PBS.

4. Resuspend the pellet in 600 μL of 60% methanol and vortex at room temperature for at least 30 min. Using an ultrasonic probe may improve the lysis process. Store the suspension at –20°C overnight and centrifuge at 18,000*g* for 30 min. Supernatant can be stored at –20°C until analysis. Before HPLC injection, methanol evaporation is carried out by using a Speed-Vac, and a mobil phase (100 μL) was added to the residue.

3.3.2. HPLC Analysis

1. Mobile-phase preparation: Dissolve 0.3 g of K_2HPO_4 (final concentration: 50 mM) and 1.7 g of tetrabutylammonium nitrate (final concentration: 5 mM) in 1000 mL of distilled water. Adjust the pH to 6.8 using diluted orthophosphoric acid. The solution is then filtered through a 0.45-μm membrane and degassed under a stream of helium.

2. Chromatographic conditions: Our HPLC consists of a HP1090 system (Hewlett-Packard) coupled to an A200 radioactive flow detector (Packard). Separation is achieved using a Lichrospher 100 RP8 5-μm column (Hewlett-Packard). The mobile phase pumped at a rate of 1 mL/min consist of a mix between the phosphate buffer solution and 12% (0–9 min) to 16% (10–50 min) gradient of methanol. A high-flash-point Ultima-Flow scintillation liquid (Packard) is pumped at a flow rate of 0.8 mL/min to ensure proper detection within the detector cell. In our laboratory, data acquision and signal processing are carried out using the built-in A200 acquisition software (Packard).

3. The different peaks were identified by comparing retention times with standards (*see* **Note 5**). Typical retention times are (for example) as follows: 5FU, 4 min; 5FUrd, 6 min; 5FUMP, 31 min; 5FdUMP, 34 min; 5FUDP, 41 min; 5FUTP, 44 min (*see* **Fig. 5**).

3.4. Cell Sensitivity Assay

3.4.1. Neutral Red Assay

1. Seed approx 5×10^3 cells/well in a microtiter plate in a final volume of 150 μL/well of appropriate growth medium. Do not feel the outer wells (i.e., columns 1 and 12 and lines A and H) to avoid an edge effect. Furthermore, column 1 must be kept free of cells for the use as a blank for the microtiter plate reader. The optimal cellular density depends on the doubling time and should be determined for each cell line (*see* **Note 14**). Incubate for 24 h at 37°C in a fully humidified atmosphere of 5% CO_2 in air.

2. Prepare serial dilutions of fluoropyrimidines up to nine concentrations in growth medium. We usually use concentrations ranging from 0.01 to 100 μM prepared as shown in **Fig. 6**. The higher concentration is obtained by a $1/1000^e$ dilution of 0.1 M stock solutions of 5FU or 5'dFUrd (aliquots at −20°C in DMSO). Prepare an aditionnal tube of growth medium with $1/1000^e$ DMSO for control cells (*see* **Note 15**).

3. Remove the growth medium from the plates by gentle inversion in a tray and absorption of the remaining liquid on absorbent paper. Add 150 μL/well of increasing concentrations of toxicity by using a plastic tank and a mutichannel pipet. First, add the growth medium with DMSO in column 2 as a control for untreated cells. Thereafter, add the nine dilutions of toxicity from columns 3 to 11. Incubate for 72 h at 37°C in a fully humidified atmosphere of 5% CO_2 in air.

4. Prepare a 1/100 neutral red dilution in medium (final concentration 33 mg/L) (*see* **Note 16**) and filter by using a syringe with an adaptable 0.2-μm filter to remove possible crystals. Remove the growth medium from the plates as describe in **step 3** and refill wells with 150 μL of neutral red solution, including column 1 as a blank. Incubate for 4 h at 37°C to allow the neutral red uptake into living cells.

5. Remove the neutral red solution and rinse twice carefully with PBS (including blank column). Add 150 μL of a solution consisting of glacial acetic acid (1%)–ethanol (50%) (v/v) in each well (including the blank column). Incubate for 15 min at room temperature on a plate shaker.

6. Read absorbance at 540 nm (A_{540}) with a plate reader using the blank column as a zero. Calculate the mean of six wells for each column. Results are expressed as the percentage

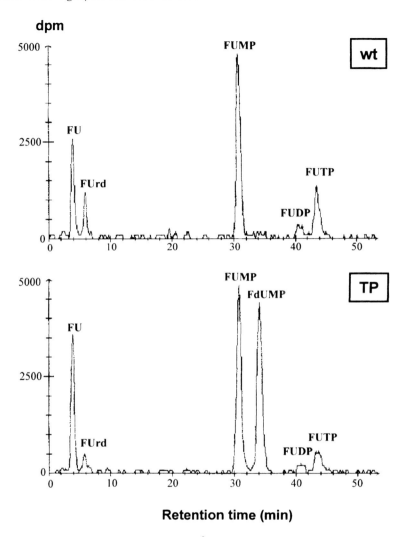

Fig. 5. Metabolic activation patterns of [³H]5FU in human colorectal adenocarcinoma LS174T cells. Wild-type **(upper)** or TP-transfected **(lower)** cells were incubated for 4 h in the presence of 100 µCi [³H]5FU and resulting metabolites were identified by HPLC coupled to a radiometric detection. TP transfection leads to a significant accumulation of 5FdUMP, which is considered the main active metabolite of 5'dFUrd and 5FU.

of cell viability obtained as follows: % cell viability = (A_{540} drug treated/A_{540} control) × 100. Experiments are usually carried out in triplicate and the final result is the mean ± SEM of the three separate assays.

7. A conventional cytotoxicity graph is obtained by plotting the percentage of cell viability (y-axis) against the drug concentration (x-axis, log scale). Characteristic points such IC_{50} or IC_{90} can be calculated graphically or with a suitable curve-fitting software (*see* **Fig. 7**).

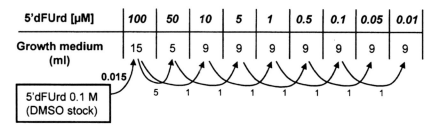

5'dFUrd [µM]	100	50	10	5	1	0.5	0.1	0.05	0.01
Growth medium (ml)	15	5	9	9	9	9	9	9	9

Fig. 6. Schematic diagram for the preparation of fluoropyrimidines serial dilution used in the neutral red cytotoxicity assay. The indicated volumes are suitable for the setup of eight microtiter plates.

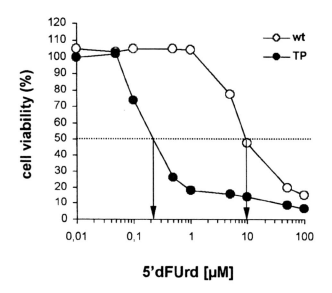

5'dFUrd [µM]

Fig. 7. Cell viability of wild-type (wt) and TP-transfected human colorectal adenocarcinoma LS174T cells obtained with the neutral red assay. IC_{50} values are determined graphically or with a suitable curve-fitting software.

3.4.2. Assessment of Bystander Effect

The aim of these assays is to assess the neighboring cytotoxicity of transfected cells toward untransfected cells after fluoropyrimidines treatment. In the first assay, both cell types are mixed and cell viability is assessed on the whole population. The second assay is useful for studying the requirement of direct cell–cell contact for the bystander effect. In this experiment, wild-type and transfected cells are grown separately in the same medium using membrane culture inserts and cell viability is assessed only on wild-type cells.

3.4.2.1. COCULTURE WITH CELL CONTACT

1. Harvest cells using trypsin, and after counting, mix wild-type and transfected cells in various ratios (from 0% up to 100% of transfected cells; 10% of transfected cells is defined as a ratio of 0.1). Growth medium should not contain selective agent such G418 (geneticin). We usually prepare a range of 11 ratios as follows: 0, 0.1, 0.2, 0.3, 0.4, 0.5, 0.6, 0.7, 0.8, 0.9, and 1.
2. Seed mixed cells in two microtiter plates (approx 5×10^3 cells/well; *see* **Note 14**); each column should correspond to one ratio (column 2 for ratio 0, column 3 for ratio 0.1, etc.). In this case, the entire plate can be used insofar as the viability of treated cells from a plate will be compared column to column with the untreated cells from another plate. Column 1 must be kept free of cells for the use as a blank. Incubate for 24 h at 37°C in a fully humidified atmosphere of 5% CO_2 in air.
3. Remove growth medium from plates as described in **Subheading 3.4.1.**, **step 3** and add fresh medium containing a predetermined concentration of fluoropyrimidine in a treated plate (*see* **Note 17**) or fresh medium alone in the control plate. Incubate for 72 h at 37°C in a fully humidified atmosphere of 5% CO_2 in air.
4. Proceed to the neutral red assay as described **Subheading 3.4.1.** The percentage of cell viability is calculated for each ratio by comparing, column to column, the mean A_{540} from the treated plate to the drug-free plate. This experimental cell viability is to be compared to the theoretical cell viability that would be observed in absence of the bystander effect (*see* **Fig. 8**). The theoretical cell viability for each transfected cells ratio could be calculated as follows:

   Theoretical cell viability (%) = $[(CV_{wt})(1-r)] + [(CV_t)r]$
   where CV_{wt} is the cellular viability (%) of wild-type cells alone (column 2),
   CV_t is the cellular viability (%) of transfected cells alone (column 12), and,
   r is the ratio of transfected cells.

3.4.2.2. COCULTURE IN NONCONTACT CONDITIONS

1. Seed wild-type (untransfected) cells in two microtiter plates as described in **Subheading 3.4.1.**
2. Set the strip of membrane culture inserts on plates, avoiding air bubbles under the membrane. Seed wild-type (on one plate) and transfected cells (on the other plate) in culture inserts in a final volume of 50 µL. We usually use the same amount of cells in inserts as in the bottom chamber (i.e., 5×10^3 cells/well) in order to obtain a TP-transfected cells ratio of 0.5, which usually leads to a strong bystander effect. Incubate for 24 h at 37°C in a fully humidified atmosphere of 5 % CO_2 in air.
3. Remove membrane culture inserts and put them temporarily on new empty plates (take care to respect column position). Remove growth medium from the plates by inversion and refill with serial dilutions of fluoropyrimidine of interest prepared as described in **Subheading 3.4.1.**, **step 2** (150 µL/well).
4. Carefully, remove the growth medium from culture inserts by aspiration (this can be done with a tip and a suction line or with a multichannel pipette) and put the inserts back in their initial positions on the wild-type cells plates (the growth medium including toxicity will diffuse through the membrane). Incubate for 72 h at 37°C in a fully humidified atmosphere of 5% CO_2 in air.
5. After the incubation period, discard the culture inserts and proceed to the standard neutral red assay as described in **Subheading 3.4.1.** Plot the percentage of cell viability against

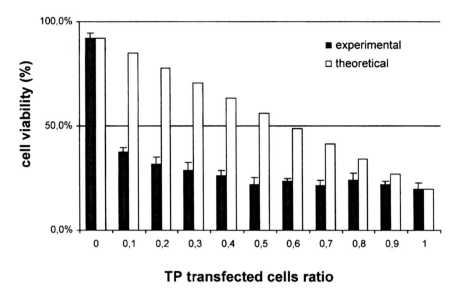

TP transfected cells ratio

Fig. 8. Cell viability of wild-type and TP-transfected LS174T cells mixed at various ratio, incubated with 5 μ*M* 5'dFUrd and assessed with the neutral red assay. The difference between experimental and theoretical viabilities displays a bystander effect. A TP-transfected cell ratio of 0.1 is sufficient to obtain approx 60% cell death and a ratio of 0.3 is sufficient for a maximal effect on the whole cell population.

drug concentration (log scale) for the two plates. The diffusibility of the bystander effect is evidenced by the fact that wild-type cells cocultured with transfected cells are more sensitive to the toxic effect of fluoropyrimidines than wild-type cells cocultured with others wild-type cells (*see* **Fig. 9**).

4. Notes

1. OptiMEM™ is a medium designed for transfection, but it could be replaced by standard serum-free medium without a substantial decrease of transfection efficacy. Optimal quantities of Lipofectamine and DNA should be determined for each cell lines, however, indicated amounts (i.e., 25 μL Lipofectamine and 4 μg DNA for 5-cm-diameter dishes) gave the best transfection efficacy for a wide variety of cell lines.
2. The pcTP5 vector was obtained by cloning the human TP cDNA (Genbank accession number M63193) into the *Xba*I/*Hin*dIII cloning sites of the mammalian expression vector pcDNA3 (Invitrogen).
3. Plastic or glass cloning rings are available in different sizes; the diameter of the cloning ring should fit the size of the clone that is to be isolated.
4. Phenylmethylsulfonyl fluoride (PMSF) is extremely toxic to the mucous membrane, eyes, and skin and should be handled with care. Stock solutions can be prepared at 10 mg/mL in isopropanol and stored at –20°C. Aprotinin and PMSF are protease inhibitors rapidly inactivated in aqueous solution; lysis buffer must be prepared on ice just before cell lysis.
5. For cost reasons and because all of the radiolabeled standards are not commercially available, a preliminary identification of the retention times can be performed with a UV detector set at 264 nm *(31)*.

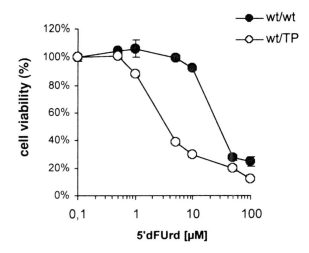

Fig. 9. Cell viability of wild-type LS174T cells cocultured in noncontact conditions either with TP-transfected cells or with others wild-type cells and assessed with the neutral red assay. The increase cytotoxicity observed on wild-type cells cocultured with TP-transfected cells evidences the diffusibility of the bystander effect.

6. A 5-h incubation period with liposomes–DNA complexes is usually sufficient. We often noted a decreased in cell viability with longer incubations because of Lipofectamine toxicity and serum starvation.
7. Transfected cells must imperatively be dilute to respect a 1/10 passage at least; otherwise, clones would not be separated enough for isolation with cloning rings.
8. Geneticin sensitivity varies among cell type and the manufacturer recommends assessing wild-type cell sensitivity using a range from 100 to 1200 µg/mL. The neutral red assay described in this chapter could be used to determine the optimal geneticin concentration (i.e., the lowest concentration that leads to a maximal toxicity).
9. A volume of buffer as low as 100 µL is sufficient to ensure cell lysis and permits obtaining a protein concentration >2 µg/µL, suitable for TP activity assay but also for direct loading in sodium dodecyl sulfate–polyacrylamide gel electrophoresis gel for Western blot analysis.
10. At this step, lysates can be stored at –80°C. However, we noted a significant decrease in TP activity after long-term storage and we recommend, when possible, working on fresh samples.
11. Kinetic experiments carried out in our laboratory determined that the amont of thymine formed is maximal after a 4 h incubation time.
12. For the standard curve of thymine, dissolve 12.6 mg thymine in 10 mL of a dilution buffer (= 10 mM) containing 0.5 mL lysis buffer, 1.5 mL substrate (10 mM thymidine, 10 mM KH_2PO_4), and 8 mL of 0.2 N NaOH (note that the dilution buffer has the same composition as the reaction mixture at the time of spectrophotometric measure). Prepare serial dilution from 0.01 to 10 mM in the same buffer, read the optical density (OD) at 300 nm, and plot OD_{300} (*y*-axis) against thymine concentration (*x*-axis) (*see* **Fig. 4**).

13. Because of rate-limiting steps, metabolism kinetic of fluoropyrimidines varies among cell type and the apparition of tritiated metabolites should be monitored during at least three different incubation periods.
14. The optimal cellular density for neutral red assay is the one that leads to confluent state in untreated (control) cells at the end of the assay. Depending on cell type, the optimal density usually ranges from 3×10^3 to 10×10^3 cells/well.
15. Although dimethyl sulfoxyde diluted to $1/1000^e$ is normally nontoxic for cells, it is necessary to grow the control cells in the same conditions than the treated cells.
16. Phenol red, used as a pH indicator in most growth media, does not interfere with neutral red.
17. The fluoropyrimidine concentration is critical and should be chosen after cellular viability determination of wild-type and transfected cells in a standard neutral red assay. The optimal concentration is the one that involves a maximal cytotoxicity on transfected cells with a minimal cytotoxicity on wild-type cells.

References

1. Ishikawa, F, Miyazono, K., Hellman, U., et al. (1989) Identification of angiogenic activity and the cloning and expression of platelet derived endothelial cell growth factor. *Nature* **338**, 557–562.
2. Moghaddam, A. and Bicknell, R. (1992) Expression of platelet-derived endothelial cell growth factor in *Escherichia coli* and confirmation of its thymidine phosphorylase activity. *Biochemistry* **31**, 12,141–12,146.
3. Sumizawa, T., Furukawa, T., Haraguchi, M., et al. (1993) Thymidine phosphorylase activity associated with platelet-derived endothelial cell growth factor. *J. Biochem.* **114**, 9–14.
4. Miyadera, K., Sumizawa, T., Haraguchi, M., et al. (1995) Role of thymidine phosphorylase activity in the angiogenic effect of platelet derived endothelial cell growth factor/ thymidine phosphorylase. *Cancer Res.* **55**, 1687–1690.
5. Desgranges, C., Razaka, G., and Rabaud, H. (1981) Catabolism of thymidine in human blood platelets—purification and properties of thymidine phosphorylase. *Biochim. Biophys. Acta* **654**, 211–218.
6. Miyazono, K., Okabe, T., Urabe, A., Takaku, F., and Heldin, C.H. (1987) Purification and properties of an endothelial cell growth factor from human platelets. *J. Biol. Chem.* **262**, 4098–4103.
7. Friedkin, M. and Roberts, D. (1953) The enzymatic synthesis of nucleosides. Thymidine phosphorylase in mammalian tissue. *J. Biol. Chem.* **207**, 245–256.
8. Krenitsky T. A. (1968) Pentosyl transfer mechanisms of the mammalian nucleoside phosphorylase. *J. Biol. Chem.* **243**, 2871–2875.
9. Zimmerman, M. and Seidenberg, J. (1964) Deoxyribosyl transfer. Thymidine phosphorylase and nucleoside deoxyribosyltransferase in normal and malignant tissue. *J. Biol. Chem.* **230**, 2618–2621.
10. Shaw, J., Smillie, R. H., Miller, A. E., and MacPhee, D. G. (1988) The role of blood platelets in nucleoside metabolism: regulation of thymidine phosphorylase. *Mutat. Res.* **200**, 117–131.
11. Fox, S. B., Moghaddam, A., Westwood, M., et al. (1995) Platelet-derived endothelial cell growth factor thymidine phosphorylase expression in normal tissues-an immunohistochemical study. *J. Pathol.* **176**, 183–190.
12. Yoshimura, A., Kuwazuru, Y., Furukawa, T., Yoshida, H., Yamada, K., and Akiyama, S. (1990) Purification and tissue distribution of human thymidine phosphorylase; high expression in lymphocytes, reticulocytes and tumors. *Biochim. Biophys. Acta* **1034**, 107–113.

13. Obrien, T. S., Fox, S. B., Dickinson, A. J., et al. (1996) Expression of the angiogenic factor thymidine phosphorylase/platelet-derived endothelial cell growth factor in primary bladder cancers. *Cancer Res.* **56,** 4799–4804.

14. Luccioni, C., Beaumatin, J., Bardot, V., and Lefrancois, D. (1994) Pyrimidine nucleotide metabolism in human colon carcinomas: comparison of normal tissues, primary tumors and xenografts. *Int. J. Cancer* **58,** 517–522.

15. Ciccolini, J., Peillard, L., Evrard, A., et al. (2000) Enhanced antitumor activity of 5-fluorouracil in combination with 2'-deoxyinosine in human colorectal cell lines and human colon tumor xenografts. *Clin. Cancer Res.* **6,** 1529–1535.

16. Ackland, S. P. and Peters, G. J. (1999) Thymidine phosphorylase: its role in sensitivity and resistance to anticancer drugs. *Drug Resist. Updates* **2,** 205–214.

17. Rustum, Y. M., Harstrick, A., Cao, S., et al. (1997) Thymidylate synthase inhibitors in cancer therapy: direct and indirect inhibitors. *J. Clin. Oncol.* **15,** 389–400.

18. Sobrero, A. F., Aschele, C., and Bertino, J. R. (1997) Fluorouracil in colorectal cancer—A tale of two drugs: implications for biochemical modulation. *J. Clin. Oncol.* **15,** 368–381.

19. Schwartz, E. L., Baptiste, N., Wadler, S., and Makower, D. (1995) Thymidine phosphorylase mediates the sensitivity of human colon carcinoma cells to 5-fluorouracil. *J. Biol. Chem.* **270,** 19,073–19,077.

20. Haraguchi, M., Furukawa, T., Sumizawa, T., and Akiyama, S. (1993) Sensitivity of human KB cells expressing platelet-derived endothelial cell growth factor factor to pyrimidine antimetabolites. *Cancer Res.* **53,** 5680–5682.

21. Patterson, A.V., Zhang, H., Moghaddam, A., et al. (1995) Increased sensitivity to the prodrug 5'-deoxy-5-fluorouridine and modulation of 5-fluoro-2'-desoxyuridine sensitivity in MCF-7 cells transfected with thymidine phosphorylase. *Br. J. Cancer* **72,** 669–675.

22. Evrard, A., Cuq, P., Robert, B., Vian, L., Pèlegrin, A., and Cano, J. P. (1999) Enhancement of 5-fluorouracil cytotoxicity by human thymidine phosphorylase expression in cancer cells: in vitro and in vivo study. *Int. J. Cancer* **80,** 465–470.

23. Kato, Y., Matsukawa, S., Muraoka, R., and Tanigawa, N. (1997) Enhancement of drug sensitivity and a bystander effect in PC-9 cells transfected with a platelet-derived endothelial cell growth factor thymidine phosphorylase cDNA. *Br. J. Cancer* **75,** 506–511.

24. Evrard, A., Cuq, P., Ciccolini, J., Vian, L., and Cano, J.P. (1999) Increased cytotoxicity and bystander effect of 5-fluorouracil and 5-deoxy-5-fluorouridine in human colorectal cancer cells transfected with thymidine phosphorylase. *Br. J. Cancer* **80,** 1726–1733.

25. Morita, T., Matsuzaki, A. and Tokue, A. (2001) Enhancement of sensitivity to capecitabine in human renal carcinoma cells transfected with thymidine phosphorylase cDNA. *Int. J. Cancer* **92,** 451–456.

26. Fick, J., Barker, F. G. II, Dazin, P., Westphale, E. M., Beyer, E. C., and Israel, M. A. (1995) The extent of heterocellular communication mediated by gap junctions is predictive of bystander tumor cytotoxicity in vitro. *Proc. Natl. Acad. Sci. USA* **92,** 11,071–11,075.

27. Denning, C. and Pitts, J. D. (1997) Bystander effect of different enzyme–prodrug systems for cancer gene therapy depend on different pathways for intercellular transfer of toxic metabolites, a factor that will govern clinical choice of appropriate regimes. *Hum. Gene Ther.* **8,** 1825–1835.

28. Lonn, U., Lonn, S., Nylen, U., and Winblad, G. (1989) 5-Fluoropyrimidine-induced DNA damage in human colonadenocarcinoma and its augmentation by the nucleoside transport inhibitor dipyridamole. *Cancer Res.* **49,** 1085–1089.

29. Grem, J. L. and Fischer, P. H. (1986) Alteration of fluorouracil metabolism in human colon cancer cells by dipyridamole with a selective increase in fluorodeoxyuridine monophosphate levels. *Cancer Res.* **46,** 6191–6199.

30. Bradford, M. M. (1976) A rapid and sensitive method for the quantitation of microgram quantities of protein utilizing the principle of protein-dye binding. Anal. Biochem. **72,** 248–254.
31. Ciccolini, J., Peillard, L., Aubert, C., Formento, P., Milano, G., and Catalin, J. (2000) Monitoring of the intracellular activation of 5-fluorouracil to deoxyribonucleotides in HT29 human colon cell line: application to modulation of metabolism and cytotoxicity study. Fundam. Clin. Pharmacol. 14, 147–154.

14

Methods to Improve Efficacy in Suicide Gene Therapy Approaches

Targeting Prodrug-Activating Enzymes Carboxypeptidase G2 and Nitroreductase to Different Subcellular Compartments

Silke Schepelmann, Robert Spooner, Frank Friedlos, and Richard Marais

1. Introduction

Current cancer chemotherapy strategies are often hampered by the lack of tumor selectivity, resulting in unwanted damage to healthy tissue. Gene-directed enzyme–prodrug therapy (GDEPT) *(1)* and virus-directed enzyme–prodrug therapy (VDEPT) *(2)* are suicide gene therapy approaches that aim to deliver cytotoxic agents to tumor cells in a specific manner, thus improving the selectivity of chemotherapy and protecting normal cells from adverse side effects. In the first step, a gene encoding a foreign enzyme is delivered to tumor cells (*see* **Fig. 1**). The aim is to express the enzyme only in the tumor cells and then administer a prodrug. Prodrugs are small molecules that are nontoxic to normal cells, but are converted to potent cytotoxic agents in tumors. In GDEPT, the foreign enzyme performs this conversion, so if the enzyme is successfully targeted, the toxin will only be produced in the tumor, sparing normal tissues from excessive damage.

One of the limitations of GDEPT is that current gene delivery systems cannot target all of the cells within a tumor. Therefore, a so-called "bystander effect" is required, in which cells that express the prodrug-activating enzyme are able to kill nonexpressing, neighboring cells *(3)*. The bystander effect results from the transfer of the toxic drug metabolites from cell to cell either by passive or active mechanisms *(4)*. A number of enzyme/prodrug systems have been described and some of these have now entered the clinic *(4)*. However, there are still a number of hurdles to overcome before GDEPT/VDEPT enters wide clinic use and a number of strategies are currently being explored to improve the efficacy of these approaches.

From: *Methods in Molecular Medicine, Vol. 90, Suicide Gene Therapy: Methods and Reviews*
Edited by: C. J. Springer © Humana Press Inc., Totowa, NJ

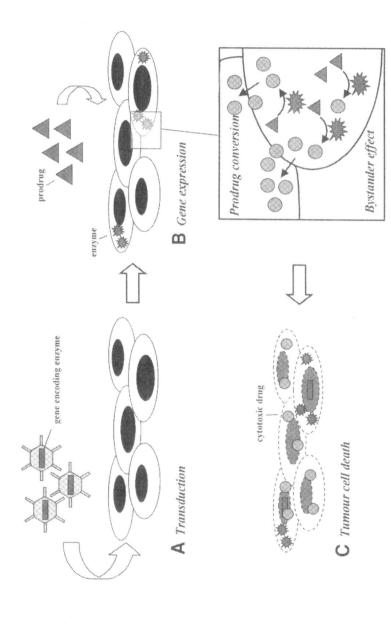

Fig. 1. Schematic diagram of GDEPT. (A) Delivery of the gene encoding the prodrug-activating enzyme by recombinant viruses. (B) Expression of the enzyme by cells that have been transduced. Upon prodrug administration, the enzyme converts the prodrug into the active, cytotoxic drug (magnified square), which spreads to adjacent cells that do not express the enzyme (bystander effect). (C) The cytotoxic drug induces cell death in expressing and nonexpressing cells.

A *Transduction*

B *Gene expression*

Prodrug conversion

Bystander effect

C *Tumour cell death*

gene encoding enzyme

prodrug

enzyme

cytotoxic drug

1.1. Vectors and GDEPT

Substantial effort has been made to develop efficient vectors for tumor-specific gene delivery. A number of delivery systems have been described (naked DNA, bacterial, viral, synthetic delivery vectors), but those based on viral vectors are the most advanced in clinical use *(5–7)*. Viral vectors can be replicating or nonreplicating. Nonreplicating vectors have better safety profiles than replicating vectors, but transduction efficiency is low because they do not spread from the initial site of infection. In contrast, with replicating vectors there are multiple rounds of infection, so the efficiency of gene transduction if far greater *(see also* Chapter 2). For safety reasons, replicating vectors must be restricted to ensure that they do not express foreign genes in normal cells. Viruses such as reovirus appear to be perfectly suited to this application, because they only replicate in cells that have oncogenic RAS *(8)*, so they are naturally selective for tumor cells, 15–30% of which carry activating mutations in RAS *(9)*. However, to date there have been no reports of manipulations of the reovirus genome for expression of foreign proteins.

The choice of gene delivery vector may have an important influence on the efficacy of a specific enzyme and prodrug combination. For example, thymidine kinase (TK) from herpes simplex viruses (HSV) activates the prodrugs acyclovir (ACV) and ganciclovir (GCV) by phosphorylation *(10)*. However, the activated prodrugs are charged and do not partition between cells unless they have gap junctions *(11)*. Because bacteria do not form these structures with mammalian cells, it is unlikely that TK and its prodrugs will be particulary effective if the gene is delivered using bacterial vectors. Similarly, oncolytic viruses such as derivatives of adenovirus and HSV are engineered to kill only tumor cells, leaving normal cells unaffected *(12)*. If these vectors are armed with prodrug-activating enzymes, the cells expressing the enzymes will be killed when the viruses lyse the infected cells to release the new viral progeny. If the bystander effect is dependent on structures such as gap junctions, the vector will effectively destroy the very cells that produce the bystander effect. Thus, the choice of which enzyme/prodrug system should be used to arm a specific vector should be made with great care and improvements can be achieved by manipulating the enzymes that are used in GDEPT protocols to overcome these problems.

1.2. Improved Enzymes for GDEPT Protocols

In selecting enzymes for GDEPT, perhaps the most important consideration is that there should be no endogenous human enzymes to mimic the catalytic activity of the prodrug-activating enzyme. For these reasons, many GDEPT systems use enzymes that are of viral, bacterial, or yeast origin. The most commonly used systems are based on cytosine deaminase (CD) with 5-fluorocytosine (5-FC) and HSV-TK with GCV, both already in clinical trials *(4)*. However, the characteristics of many of the enzymes selected for GDEPT are not optimal for this application and improvements in efficacy can be achieved by manipulating their properties.

One interesting approach has been to use the enzyme, rather than the prodrug, to mediate the bystander effect. The VP22 protein from HSV-1 is able to spread from cell to cell by an unknown mechanism that is independent of the conventional mammalian secretory pathways *(13)*. Importantly, it can carry passenger proteins fused to it and it has been shown to deliver active TK to untransduced cells, mediating a gap-junction-independent bystander effect *(14)*. In vitro, VP22 can spread through cell cultures very efficiently, raising the concern that the enzyme may spread to healthy tissues in patients. However, this does not seem to be a significant problem in vivo because the VP22-TK fusion bystander effect appears to be quite modest in tumor models *(14)*.

Another approach is to improve the kinetics of the enzyme. The two most commonly used prodrugs for TK are acyclovir and ganciclovir. However, therapies with wild-type TK are problematic, because it displays a high K_m toward both prodrugs. The levels of ganciclovir that would be required to achieve a therapeutic effect in humans are immunosuppressive. An enzyme with reduced K_m values for both prodrugs was therefore developed using a random mutagenesis approached targeted to the active site of TK *(15)* (*see also* Chapter 16). Subsequent refinement produced enzymes that could mediate tumor regressions in mice at prodrug concentrations that were ineffective with wild-type TK *(16)*. The substrate specificity of TK has also been altered using a process called DNA family shuffling *(17)*. By fusing random fragments of the TK genes from HSV-1 and HSV-2, novel hybrid proteins were generated that had K_m values for the prodrug zidovudine (AZT) that were threefold to ninefold lower than the values of the parental enzymes *(17)*. Although these hybrids have not been tested against mammalian cells, they were 32- and 16,000-fold more effective at killing *Escherichia coli* expressing HSV-1 TK and HSV-2 TK, respectively.

A slightly different approach is to generate vectors that express two prodrug-activating enzymes as a fusion protein, creating bifunctional chimera that mediate killing by two different prodrugs. Fusion proteins between HSV-1 TK and *E. coli* CD were found to mediate sensitivity to both GCV and 5-FC in vitro and in vivo *(18–20)* (*see also* Chapter 17). Simultaneous treatment with GCV and 5-FC resulted in a synergistic killing, suggesting that the chimera mediates greater cytotoxicity than the individual parental enzymes *(19,20)*. Similarly, a fusion between HSV-1 TK and *E. coli* uracil phosphoribosyltransferase (UP) sensitized tumors to both GCV and 5-fluorouracil (5-FU) *(21)*. The fusion protein was more effective at mediating tumor regression than UP alone in animals treated with both prodrugs (for technical reasons, TK was not tested by itself). Fusion proteins that generate drugs that kill cells through different mechanisms are likely to give enhanced tumor regression and are also likely to provide some protection against resistance to chemotherapy. However, the complexity involved in scheduling two or more prodrugs after vector administration may limit their use in the clinic.

1.3. Improving GDEPT by Targeting the Enzyme to Different Subcellular Compartments

Our own studies on enzyme manipulations have focused on the improvements that can be achieved by expressing prodrug-activating enzymes in different subcellular locations within tumor cells. For these studies, we have used two bacterial enzymes: carboxypeptidase G2 (CPG2) and nitroreductase (NR).

1.3.1. CPG2 and GDEPT

Carboxypeptidase was identified in *Pseudomonas* strain RS-16 as a homodimer composed of subunits with molecular masses of approx 41,800 *(22)*. The monomers are expressed as pro-enzymes with an N-terminal signal peptide that targets them to the periplasm of Gram-negative bacteria. Zinc ions are used as a cofactor and CPG2 cleaves the glutamate moiety from folic acid. It also cleaves glutamated benzoyl nitrogen mustard prodrugs such as CMDA (4-([2-chloroethyl][2-mesyloxyethyl]amino)-benzoyl-L-glutamic acid) to release highly toxic alkylating agents that kill both cycling and noncycling cells (*see* **Fig. 2A**) *(23)*. CPG2 induces prodrug-mediated cell killing when targeted to tumor cells using antibodies in antibody-directed enzyme prodrug therapy (ADEPT) *(24)* and we have demonstrated its potential in GDEPT.

First, we tested whether the enzyme could stimulate prodrug-mediated cell killing when expressed in the cytosol of mammalian cell (*see* **Note 1**). To prevent secretion of wild-type CPG2 in mammalian cells, the first 22 codons of the *cpg2* gene encoding the signal peptide were deleted (*see* **Fig. 3**). This N-terminally deleted CPG2 (called CPG2*) was expressed as an active enzyme in the cytosol of mammalian cells *(25)*, demonstrating that it was correctly folded and dimerized despite the fact that mammalian cytosol and bacterial periplasm are quite different environments. CPG2* sensitized a wide variety of human adenocarcinoma cell lines to CMDA and also mediated a robust bystander effect both in vivo and in vitro *(25)*. This is a somewhat surprising result, because CMDA is charged and thus is unlikely to cross the plasma membrane for intracellular activation. However, CPG2* did not sensitize MDA MB 361 cells to CMDA, because in these cells the plasma membrane was impermeable to the prodrug *(26)*.

The drug that is released from CMDA is more permeable to cells than the prodrug. Therefore, in order to overcome the problem associated with prodrug permeability in MDA MB 361 cells, we tested whether extracellular CPG2 would sensitize these cells to CMDA. However, a fully secreted enzyme could leak from the tumor and mediate prodrug activation in healthy tissues, so in order to prevent this, we tethered the enzyme to the outer surface of the tumor cells. This was achieved using a method borrowed from receptor tyrosine kinases (RTKs). RTKs are integral membrane proteins composed of an extracellular domain that is linked to an intracellular domain via a transmembrane linker *(27)* (*see* **Fig. 3B**). RTKs are synthesized with an N-terminal signal peptide that directs them through the secretory pathway in mammalian cells. However, secretion is stalled by a stop-transfer signal, leaving the transmembrane region to span the membrane and effectively anchoring the extracellular domain to the outer surface of the cell.

Our approach was to replace the extracellular domain of a RTK with CPG2, targeting it for secretion, but anchoring it to the outer surface of mammalian cells with the transmembrane region. The signal peptide of the RTK c-erbB2 was fused to the N-terminus of CPG2* and the transmembrane and stop-transfer region from c-erbB2 was fused to its C-terminus (*see* **Fig. 3A,B**) *(26)*. The intracellular domain was deleted to prevent inappropriate signaling. In mammalian cells, surface tethered CPG2

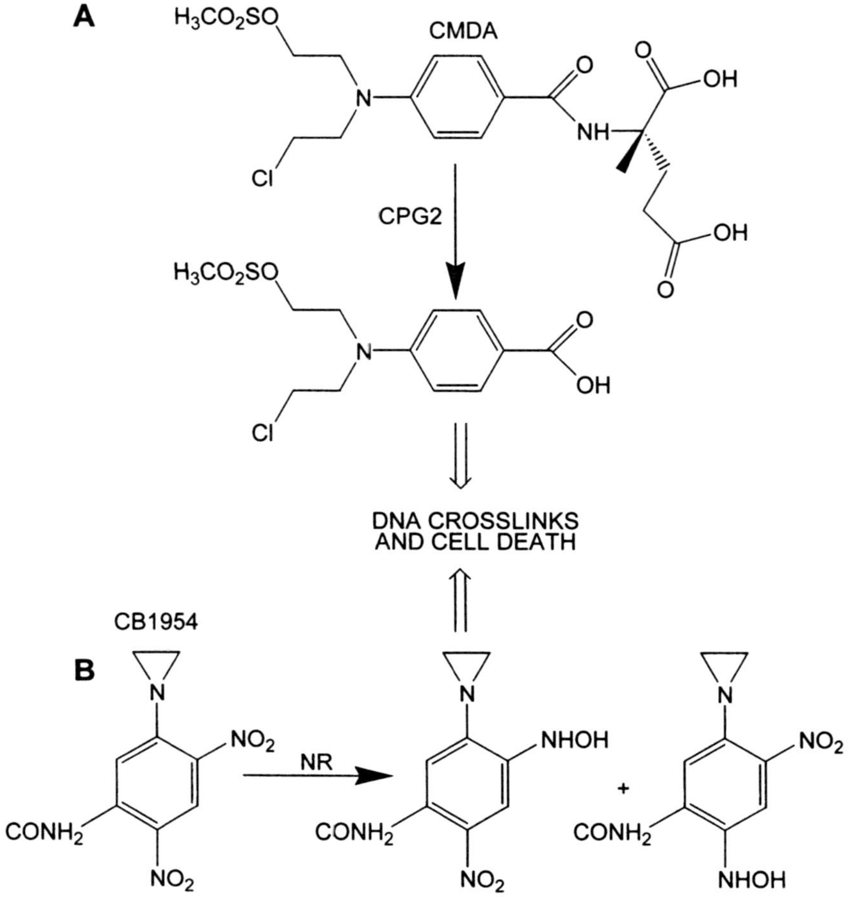

Fig. 2. Activation of prodrugs by CPG2 and NR. (A) Cleavage of CMDA (4-[(2-chloroethyl)(2-mesyloxyethyl)amino] benzoyl-L-glutamic acid) by CPG2 releases the cytotoxic (4-[(2-chloroethyl)(2-mesyloxyethyl)amino] benzoic acid. (B) NR reduces the 2- and 4-nitro groups on CB1954 (5-(aziridin-1-yl)2,4-dinitrobenzamide) to the corresponding hydroxylamine species. A nonenzymatic reaction with thioesters such as acetyl CoA generates the *N*-acetoxy hydroxylamines derivatives and the 4-hydroxylamine is the cytotoxic DNA crosslinking agent.

(stCPG2) was glycosylated on asparagines 222, 264, and 272 (*see* **Notes 2** and **3** and **Fig. 4**), a modification not performed by bacteria. Unfortunately, this glycosylation destroyed the activity of CPG2 *(26)*.

Glycosylation was blocked by mutating these asparagines to glutamines [stCPG2(Q)$_3$] (*see* **Figs. 3A,B** and **4**), and although this recovered activity, it was at some cost because the catalytic activity was substantially reduced (to approx 10% of wild-type) and the K_m toward its substrates significantly increased (by about eightfold for methotrexate) *(26,28)*. We also noted that stCPG2(Q)$_3$ protein expression was con-

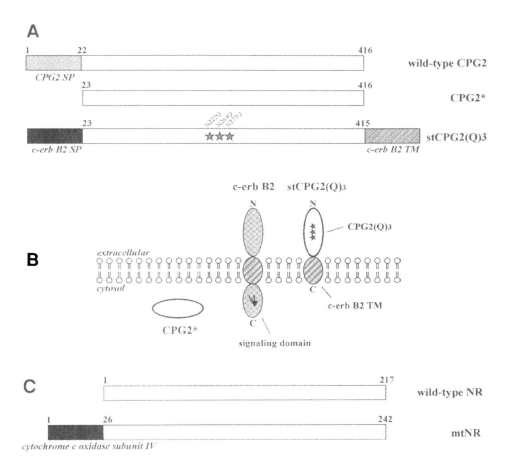

Fig. 3. Schematic representation of the CPG2 and NR constructs. (**A**). Wild-type CPG2 is expressed as a pro-enzyme that encodes a signal peptide (CPG2 SP) at its N-terminus and which is responsible for directing CPG2 to the bacterial periplasm. This peptide was deleted from the gene in CPG2* to force cytosolic expression in mammalian cells. In order to achieve surface-tethered expression of CPG2, the signal peptide from c-erb B2 (c-erb B2 SP) was fused to the N-terminus of CPG2* and the transmembrane region (c-erb B2 TM) was fused to its C-terminus. The glycosylation sites are represented by the star symbols (N222Q, N264Q, N272Q). (**B**) Schematic representation of cellular localization of CPG2 in mammalian cells. See text for details. (**C**) NR was targeted to mitochondria by fusing the enzyme to the signal peptide from mitochondrial cytochrome c oxidase subunit IV, as indicated.

siderably lower in mammalian cells than CPG2* expression (Spooner and Marais, unpublished data). This may be, in part, the result of endoplasmic reticulum (ER)-associated degradation, a process during which misfolded and overexpressed proteins are marked for degradation in the endoplasmic reticulum *(29)*. The combination of these effects was that cells expressing stCPG2(Q)$_3$ had significantly lower levels of

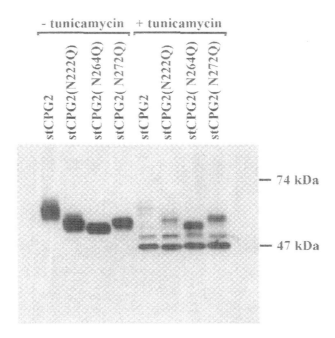

Fig. 4. stCPG2 is glycosylated on three residues. CPG2 Western blot analysis. stCPG2 and variants thereof in which asparagine 222 [stCPG2(N222Q)], asparagine 264 [stCPG2(N264Q)], or asparagine 272 [stCPG2(N272Q)] were mutated to glutamine were expressed in COS cells. The cells were incubated in tunicamycin where indicated and cell extracts were prepared for Western blot analysis.

CPG2 activity associated with them than cells expressing CPG2*. Despite these apparent setbacks, prodrug-dependent killing of tumor cells by stCPG2(Q)$_3$ was more efficient than that mediated by CPG2*. Both enzymes sensitized a wide range of tumor cell lines to CMDA (25,28), but those expressing stCPG2(Q)$_3$ had lower IC$_{50}$ values for CMDA than those expressing CPG2* (25,28) (see **Table 1**). Furthermore, stCPG2(Q)$_3$, but not CPG2*, sensitized MDA MB 361 cells to CMDA and mounted a robust bystander response against these cells both in vitro and in vivo (30). Finally, in a number of other cell lines, both the direct killing of the enzyme-expressing cells and the bystander effect was more rapid in cells expressing stCPG2(Q)$_3$ than in CPG2*-expressing cells (28) (see **Fig 5A**). Thus, despite the apparently unfavorable kinetics and low expression levels, stCPG2(Q)$_3$ offers significant advantages over internal expression, demonstrating the potential for the surface tethering approach. These data also show that CPG2 activity was not the only factor mediating the susceptibility to CMDA.

Table 1
Cytotoxicity of CMDA to Cell Lines Expressing CPG2* or stCPG2(Q)$_3$

Tumor cell line	Clone and protein expressed	IC$_{50}$ (μM CMDA)	Differential cytotoxicity[a] (fold)
WiDr	W1 CPG2*	257 (±15)	12.6
	W2 CPG2*	277 (±38)	11.7
	W3 stCPG2(Q)3	100 (±10)	32.3
	W4 stCPG2(Q)3	147 (±10)	22.0
	β-Gal	3230 (±120)	na[b]
SK-OV-3	S2.34 CPG2*	1289 (±221)	3.2
	S2.4 CPG2*	3196 (±166)	1.3
	S5 stCPG2(Q)3	216 (±31)	19.4
	S6 stCPG2(Q)3	479 (±22)	8.7
	β-Gal	4180 (±452)	na
A2780	A1 CPG2*	23.2 (±2.9)	92.7
	A2 CPG2*	44.4 (±8.1)	48.4
	A3 stCPG2(Q)3	15.6 (±1.5)	138
	A4 stCPG2(Q)3	20.4 (±0.6)	105
	β-Gal	2150 (180)	na

[a]Differential cytotoxicity = IC$_{50}$ β-Gal cell line/IC$_{50}$ CPG2 cell line.
[b]NA = not applicable.

1.3.2. NR and GDEPT

Our studies with the minor flavin mononucleotide (FMN)-dependent nitroreductase from *E. coli* B (NR) have focussed on expressing the enzyme in different intracellular compartments in tumor cells. The functional form of NR is a homodimer of two 24-kDa subunits *(31)* that uses NAD(P)H as a cosubstrate. NR activates the prodrug CB1954 [5-(aziridin-1-yl)2,4-dinitrobenzamide; **Fig. 2B**] and, when expressed in the cytosol of mammalian cells, can mediate CB1954-dependent killing of human mesothelioma *(1)*, colorectal *(32,33)*, pancreatic *(33)*, and ovarian *(32,34)* tumor models. Activation of CB1954 by NR is a two-step process. NR converts CB1954 into a mixture of 2- and 4-hydroxylamines *(35)*, which are thought to react (in an enzyme-independent reaction) with thioesters such as acetyl coenzyme A to generate *N*-acetoxyhydroxylamines (**Fig 2B**). These are potent alkylating agents and the 4-hydroxylamine product is a DNA crosslinking agent *(35)*.

In mammalian cells, the rate-limiting step to prodrug activation is probably the rate at which NAD(P)H is regenerated. In the cytosol, NAD(P)H regeneration depends on glycolysis, whereas in mitochondria, it is regenerated by the more efficient Krebs citric acid cycle. Furthermore, the reducing conditions in bacterial cells are closer to the conditions found in mitochondria than in mammalian cytosol. Therefore, we tested

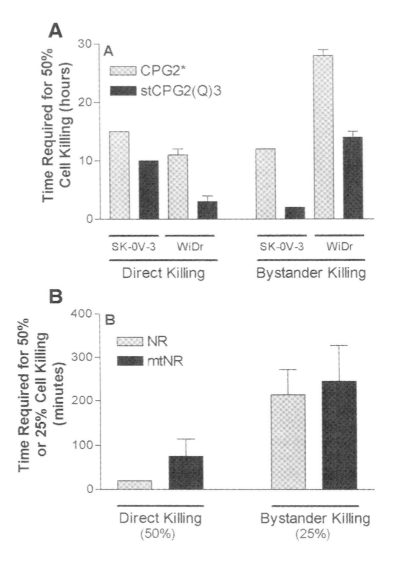

Fig. 5. Enzyme subcellular localization affects the efficiency of prodrug-mediated cell killing. (A) CPG2-mediated cell killing. SK-OV-3 cells (SKOV) or WiDr cells (WiDr) expressing CPG2* or stCPG2(Q)$_3$ were exposed to CMDA (2 mM) for different lengths of time. The length of time required to achieve 50% cell killing was determined using standard regression curves. For bystander analysis, CPG2*- or stCPG2(Q)$_3$-expressing cells (20% of total) were mixed with parental cells expressing β-galactosidase (80% of total). (B) NR-mediated killing. MDA MB 361 cells expressing NR or mtNR were subjected to CB1954 (20 μM) for different lengths of time and the length of time required to kill 50% of the cells was determined. For the bystander analysis, NR or mtNR expressing cells (8%) were mixed with parental cells (92%) and the length of prodrug exposure required to kill 25% of the cells was determined.

whether NR was more active in mitochondria than in mammalian cytosol. NR was targeted to the mitochondrial matrix, by fusing the leader sequence (amino acids 1–25) from mitochondrial cytochrome-c oxidase subunit IV to the N-terminus of NR (creating mtNR) *(36)* (**Fig. 3C**). Whereas NR was evenly distributed between cytosol and nucleus in mammalian cells, mtNR was exclusively expressed in mitochondria *(36)*. Expression of mtNR did not alter the distribution, shape, or number of mitochondria and did not appear to be toxic.

For technical reasons, it was not possible to measure the enzymatic activity of mtNR in vivo to determine if it was actually more active than cytosolic NR. However, mtNR was expressed predominantly as homodimers, whereas NR was a mixture of monomers and dimers *(36)*, suggesting that mitochondrial expression favors the native, active structure, whereas cytosolic NR is only partially in the active conformation. Nevertheless, mtNR was no better than NR at sensitizing cells to CB1954. NR and mtNR produced IC_{50} values with CB1954 in the range of 1.5–3 μM for direct cell killing and of 34 and 40 μM, respectively for bystander-mediated killing *(36)*. However, mtNR-mediated direct cell killing was actually slower than NR-mediated killing, although, curiously, there was little difference in the rate at which bystander killing occurred (*see* **Fig. 5B**) *(36)*.

1.4. Location Location Location!

The bystander effect is an essential aspect of GDEPT approaches. Even with oncolytic viruses, an efficient bystander effect will be required to extend cell killing to uninfected cells, and with armed bacteria, prodrug-mediated cell killing will occur almost entirely by a bystander effect. Improvements in bystander killing can be achieved by manipulating the prodrug-activating enzymes and tailoring their characteristics for specific vector systems.

Manipulating the subcellular location of the enzyme provides a useful approach to achieving improved GDEPT responses. With CPG2, surface-tethered protein had significantly less activity than intracellular CPG2 and yet these proteins were similarly effective in a number of cell types and surface tethering overcame the prodrug permeability problem in MDA MB 361 cells. Similarly, although mtNR appeared to favor the active conformation, it did not provide improved killing over cytosolic/nuclear NR. Thus, maximal enzyme activity does not necessarily translate into maximal cytotoxic efficacy and it may be preferable to induce suboptimal prodrug conversion in a favorable site than to have maximal enzyme activity produce prodrug in a suboptimal site. An alternative interpretation is kinetic. It may be better to have a slow, constant rate of prodrug conversion, provided by a suboptimal enzyme than to have rapid prodrug turnover producing a high but transient level of active drug generated by a highly active enzyme. The optimal rate of prodrug turnover needs to be addressed.

Expressing enzymes in different cellular compartments may also lead to new strategies for prodrug design. Although prodrugs must be able to cross the tumor cell membrane if the prodrug-activating enzyme is expressed intracellularly, membrane translocation becomes unnecessary if activation occurs on the cell surface *(37)*. Thus, cells that are resistant to particular prodrugs because of permeability problems can be rendered sensitive by expressing the activating enzyme on the cell surface. These prodrugs will have to release cell-permeable toxic drugs to reach their target, but because activation will occur in the interstitial spaces of the tumor, all of the local cells (whether or not they express the activating enzyme) will take up the activated drug. Thus, expression of prodrug-activating enzymes on the cell surface may lead to stronger bystander effects in vivo that will not rely on structures such as gap junctions, which are absent in many tumor cells or which are destroyed by the targeting vector.

Other strategies to tether prodrug-activating enzyme to the cell surface have been described. For example, posttranslational addition of glycosylphosphatidylinositol (GPI) has been used as an alternative anchor for CPG2 *(38)*. Similarly, the transmembrane domain of the human PDGF receptor has been fused to a C-terminally truncated version of human β-glucuronidase, an enzyme that activates the prodrug β-glucuronyl-doxorubicin *(39)*. This resulted in the expression of a surface-displayed version of this normally lysosomal enzyme. Fusion of the β-glucuronidase protein with the transmembrane domains of the asialoglycoprotein receptor H1 (ASGPR) and the respiratory syncytial virus (RSV) G-protein were also tested but had undetectable enzymatic activity *(39)*. Surface tethering will not be possible with all proteins. Enzymes that require a cofactor that is not present in the tumor milieu will be inactive if surface tethered. Similarly, enzymes that require a cytosolic cofactor will not be suitable candidates. Thus, the requirement of NR for NAD(P)H excludes this enzyme from surface tethering. In addition, enzymes such as TK that produce a drug that is impermeable to cell membranes will not be effective, as the activated drug will not enter the cells. Furthermore, glycosylation may be a problem if the sites cannot be mutated because they are important for structural integrity or are within the active site of the enzyme. In addition to improved prodrug conversion, surface expression might be expected to stimulate the immune response against infected tumor cells, which may be beneficial. However, a pre-existing immunological memory may make the repeated administration of recombinant viruses unfeasible because cells expressing the activating enzyme may be targeted and destroyed before the prodrug can be administered.

The targeting of NR to the mitochondria produced a somewhat disappointing result. Despite the fact that NR appeared to adopt the active conformation when expressed in the mitochondria, this did not provide a clear advantage over cytosolic expression. It is likely that two opposing processes are responsible for the lack of improved efficiency of mtNR. In mitochondria, the high regenerative potential of NAD(P)H favors high enzyme activity, permitting faster generation of the hydroxylamines. However, the ready availability of acetyl CoA in the mitochondria may also lead to rapid conversion to the *N*-acetoxy alkylating species, trapping most of the cytotoxic agents inside the organelles. Whereas this may poison the mitochondria, it will not lead to an obvious growth delay in vitro, because most cells in culture can survive without mitochondria because of the glycolytic pathway *(40)*.

It is intriguing to note that although mtNR-mediated direct killing of cells was slower than that mediated by cytosolic NR, the magnitude and rate at which the bystander effect occurred were not reduced by mitochondrial expression. This implies that the rate-limiting step in the bystander effect is not the rate at which the active drug is produced, but, rather, is the rate at which it passes to the neighboring cells. This provides another explanation for why mtNR-mediated killing was slower than cytosolic NR-mediated killing. It seems likely that the target of mtNR is nuclear DNA. Therefore, mtNR kills through a pseudobystander effect from mitochondrion to nucleus, which is delayed because the active drug must make this transition.

The potential to target enzymes to different organelles in cells is enormous, because current technology allows us to target proteins to a large number of subcellular locations. It is possible to find peptides in the literature that will allow proteins to be targeted to a number of subcellular organelles, such as the nucleus, the endoplasmic reticulum (inner or outer surface), the plasma membrane, mitochondria (as mentioned earlier), or even the cytoskeleton. As we have shown, appropriate subcellular targeting of enzymes can be very beneficial to GDEPT approaches. Any intracellularly targeted protein will still require cell-permeable prodrugs that release activated drugs that can be transferred to neighboring cells to mediate the bystander effect. Unfortunately, however, it is likely that for each enzyme, the only way to find out whether altering its subcellular localization can improve its efficacy in GDEPT will be to test it.

2. Materials

2.1. CPG2 Activity Assay

1. Phosphate-buffered saline (PBS).
2. Extraction buffer: 250 mM Tris-HCl, 10% (v/v) glycerol, 1% (v/v) Triton X-100, pH 7.5.
3. Assay buffer: 100 mM Tris-HCl, pH 7.3, 260 μM ZnCl$_2$ (store at room temperature).
4. Methotrexate (MTX): 25 mg/mL stock solution. Dissolve in 0.1 N NaOH, then dilute in PBS. The diluted stock is stable for 1 wk refrigerated and for 1 mo frozen at –20°C.
5. Acryl cuvets.

2.2. In Vitro Cytotoxicity Assay

1. CMDA and CB1954: prepare fresh 100X stock solutions in anhydrous dimethyl sulfoxide (DMSO) (*see* **Note 4.**). Use 10 μL/mL for the assay.
2. PBS.
3. [^{3}H]thymidine.
4. Fixing solution: 5% (w/v) trichloroacetic acid in PBS.
5. Solubilization solution: 1% (w/v) sodium dodecyl sulfate (SDS) in 0.2 M NaOH.
6. Scintillation fluid.

2.3. Bystander Cytotoxicity Assay

As for the in vitro cytotoxicity assay (*see* **Subheading 2.2.**).

3. Methods

3.1. Carboxypeptidase G2 Activity Assay on Mammalian Cell Extracts

1. Grow cells in six-well plates to confluence.
2. Wash cells twice with PBS.
3. Add 200 μL extraction buffer per well and lyse cells for 5 min at room temperature (RT). Transfer cell extracts into Eppendorf tubes and spin down cell debris for 5 min at 18,000g (microfuge).
4. The clarified cell extracts can be stored at –70°C.
5. Freshly prepare assay buffer containing 100 μM MTX. For each sample, prepare an acryl cuvet containing 500 μL assay buffer.

6. Dilute each sample (10–100 µL cell extract) in assay buffer. The final volume should be 500 µL.
7. Add 500 µL of the diluted sample to 500 µL assay buffer/100 µM MTX in an acryl cuvet and mix by inverting the cuvet.
   Immediately measure the change in absorbance at 320 nm on a spectrophotometer. As a blank, use cell extract from cells that do not express CPG2. CPG2 activity is detected by the decrease of A_{320} (from A_{320} approx 1 to approx 0.38 within 1–10 min), reflecting the degradation of MTX by CPG2. The molar absorption coefficient of MTX is taken as 8300 L/mol/cm at 320 nm. One unit of enzyme activity is defined as that amount of CPG2 that catalyses the hydrolysis of 1 µmol MTX/min/mL reaction mixture at 37°C.

3.2. In Vitro Cytotoxicity Assay

1. Grow cells in six-well plates until confluent.
2. Dilute the CMDA (CPG2) or CB1954 (NR) stock solutions in complete growth medium immediately prior to use.
3. Aspirate the medium from the cells and replace it with 1.5 mL prodrug-containing medium. Incubate for 24 h. As a control, incubate cells with DMSO-containing medium only.
4. Wash and trypsinise the cells and replate approx 3% of the cells into fresh dishes (*see* **Note 5**). Grow the cells for 4 d.
5. Determine cell viability by incorporation of [³H]thymidine. Add 0.4 mCi/mL growth medium, swirl the plates gently to distribute the [³H]thymidine evenly and incubate for 6 h.
6. Wash cells twice with PBS and fix them for 20 min at 4°C with 5% trichloroacetic acid.
7. Wash the cells twice with methanol and air-dry the cell layer.
8. Solubilize the fixed cells in 1 mL SDS/NaOH per well, transfer the cell extracts into 6 mL of scintillation fluid, shake to form an emulsion, and determine the thymidine incorporation. The results are expressed as percentage of control cells that were treated with DMSO alone.

3.3. Bystander Cytotoxicity Assay

1. Mix cells that express the prodrug-activating enzyme and nonexpressing (parental) cells at varying ratios. Seed cell mixtures into six-well plates and grow them until confluent (*see* **Note 5**). It is important to select cell lines that grow at the same rate to avoid overgrowth of one population of cells at the expense of the other.
2. Treat the cells for 24 h with growth medium containing prodrug as described in **Subheading 3.2.** Use a prodrug concentration that does not affect the growth of the nonexpressing cells (*see* **Note 6**).
3. Trypsinise and replate the cells as earlier and determine the proportion of cells surviving by [³H]thymidine incorporation (*see* **Subheading 3.2.**).

3.3.1. Alternate In Vitro Cytotoxicity Assay Procedure
Optimized for Comparison of Novel Prodrugs

Cell Lines and Culture Conditions: The principal cell lines used for the comparison of prodrugs for CPG2 are WiDr colon carcinoma, LS174T colon carcinoma, and MDA MB 361 breast carcinoma.

Cells are cultured as monolayers in DMEM/10% FBS (fetal bovine serum) in a 5% CO_2 saturation–humidity atmosphere at 37°C using standard tissue culture procedures.

In readiness for the experiment, cells are prepared to be just subconfluent monolayers in 175-cm^2 tissue culture plastic flasks.

DAY 1. PREPARING THE PLATES

The monolayers are trypsinized and the cells pelleted by centrifugation in a conical universal tube at approx 170g for 7 min. After removing the supernatant by aspiration, the pellet is resuspended in 10 mL fresh medium, and the cells thoroughly dispersed into a single-cell suspension by drawing the whole volume 10 times through a blunt-ended 19-gage needle. A dilution of 50X (20 μL + 980 μL) or of 20X (50 μL + 950 μL) is prepared for the colon carcinoma cells or the breast carcinoma cells respectively, and the cell density counted using a hemacytometer. The colon carcinoma cells are then diluted to 5×10^5 cells/mL and the breast carcinoma cells to 2×10^5 cells/mL. For each prodrug to be tested, quadruplicate six-well tissue culture plates are prepared of each cell type and enzyme variety, using 4 mL/well (2×10^6 cells/well) for WiDr and LS174T and 2.5 mL/well (5×10^5 cells/well) for MDA MB 361. These six-well plates are then returned to the incubator for 2 d, after which time they have formed dense monolayers. Greater cell numbers per well and a larger volume of tissue culture medium are used for the colon carcinoma cells compared to the breast carcinoma cells because these cells are smaller and spread out less.

DAY 3. DOSING THE CELLS WITH PRODRUG

The prodrugs are added in two stages. For each prodrug and for each stage, a set of dilution tubes containing tissue culture medium to give 5X 10-fold serial dilutions is prepared in advance. Typically, for each prodrug, these will consist of the following:

> For the first addition: 1 of 5 mL + 4 of 9 mL for transferring 1 mL +9 mL with each dilution.
> For the second addition: 1 of 20 mL + 4 of 18 mL for transferring 2 mL + 18 mL with each dilution.

Two masses of each prodrug are weighed out in small glass vials to provide greater than 50 μL (first addition) and 200 μL (second addition) concentrates at 100X the desired highest dose. The prodrug vials are kept foil-wrapped to protect from light until just before use.

The now-confluent six-well plates for one prodrug treatment are transferred to a tissue culture hood, and the medium is removed by aspiration. The lids are kept on between manipulations to prevent the monolayers from drying out. The first mass of prodrug is dissolved in DMSO, 50 μL of the solution added to the first 5 mL dilution tube, and the 5X 10-fold serial dilutions are performed. A tube containing plain tissue culture medium is used to provide the blank. Immediately after performing the serial dilutions, 225 μL of the blank is added to well 1 of each of the quadruplicates for each cell type/enzyme type, then 225 μL of the most dilute drug solution is added to well 2, and so forth up to the most concentrated prodrug solution in well 6. The plates are agitated to ensure that the small volume of medium flows over the entire cell monolayer, and then returned to the incubator for 1 h. At the half-way stage, the plates are reagitated to disperse the medium.

After 1 h, the second mass of prodrug is dissolved in DMSO, 200 µL added to the first 20-mL dilution tube, and the 5X 10-fold serial dilutions performed as earlier. A larger volume (1.275 mL) is added to the original volume in each well, according to the same pattern as earlier, and the plates returned to the incubator for a further 22 h.

DAY 4. DILUTING THE CELLS

The following are to be prepared in advance:

A capped disposable tube containing 5 mL tissue culture medium for every well of all of the six-well plates used;

A sufficient volume of warmed trypsin/EDTA to provide 1 mL for every well of all of the six-well plates used;

A sufficient volume of fresh tissue culture medium to provide 4 mL for every well of all of the six-well plates used;

An equal number of empty six-well plates to that originally used;

A 96-well plate for each of the original quadruplicate six-well plates.

The cells in each well are harvested by trypsinization. The medium is removed by aspiration, 1 mL trypsin/EDTA added to each well, and the plate returned to the incubator for 5 min. The cell monolayer is then detached and dispersed by repeated pipetting 5X using a 1-mL pipettor, the whole volume transferred to one of the 5-mL dilution tubes, and mixed. A 100-µL volume of this dilution is transferred to a new six-well plate, replicating the pattern of the original, and further diluted by addition of 4 mL fresh tissue culture medium. Using a multichannel pipet, 4X 200 µL of the dilution from the well corresponding to the highest prodrug dose is transferred to wells A1–D1 of a 96-well plate, the second highest to A2–D2, and so on up to A6–D6 for the blank. A single six-well plate will thus fill one quadrant of a 96-well plate. An original quadruplicate set of six-well plates will fill one 96-well plate by repeating the first pattern in the other three quadrants. The 96-well plates are returned to the incubator for 3 d (WiDr and LS174T) or 4 d (MDA MB 361).

This sequence results in a $1/60 \times 1/20 = 1/1200$ dilution, giving a new seeding per well of approximately 2×10^3 cells/well.

DAY 8. STAINING AND SCORING THE PLATES

(**N.B.**: Gloves and eye protection must be worn throughout this procedure): The following solutions are needed:

10% (w/v) trichloroacetic acid (TCA) in tap water;

0.1% sulforhodamine B (SRB) in 1% acetic acid;

a 10-L aspirator of 1% acetic acid;

10 mM Tris-HCL, pH 8.0.

One blank plate is processed along with the experimental plates as follows. The medium in the plates is removed by flicking into a container of bleach, and the plates filled by immersing in a tray of 10% TCA, shaking the plate to ensure that no air bubbles remain and all of the wells are completely filled. The plates are then transferred to a tray filled with a bed of crushed ice for 10 min. The 10% TCA is then removed by flicking into a sink, and the plates extensively washed by five rounds of immersion and draining using a tank of water that is continuously flushed with copious tap water. The plates are then thoroughly blotted onto a pad of tissue and left to air-dry on the bench.

Using a multichannel programmable peristaltic pump, the wells are filled with 50 µL 0.1% SRB in 1% acetic acid and left to stain for 10 min. The dye is then removed by flicking into a sink, and excess dye is rinsed from the wells under a thin stream of 1% acetic acid running from an aspirator. The wells are filled and emptied in this way three to four times until all of the unbound dye has been removed. The plates are then thoroughly blotted again and left to air-dry on the bench.

Using a multichannel programmable peristaltic pump, the wells are filled with 150 µL of 10 mM Tris-HCl, pH 8.0, and agitated for 10 min on a plate shaker, by which time all of the dye has detached from the cell monolayer and completely dispersed into the buffer.

The A_{540} of the wells is then determined using a plate reader. An average blank-well value is derived from the blank plate. The dataset from each quadrant of a 96-well plate, corresponding to the 4 separate prodrug treatments, is used to generate an IC_{50} curve. From each A_{540} value, the blank is subtracted, the quadruplicate values of each set are averaged and expressed as a percentage of the controls, and these percent control growths, are plotted against the log of the dose. The IC_{50} values may then be determined by interpolation or by nonlinear regression.

3.4. Measurement of CPG2 in Tissues

It is frequently desirable to measure levels of CPG2 in the tumors and tissues of experimental mice. Because the enzyme cannot reliably be extracted quantitatively from tissue in such a way as to produce a solution on which absolute determinations can be performed, an externally calibrated method is employed. The digestion of the CPG2 substrate methotrexate (MTX) to generate diaminomethylpteroic acid (DAMPA) and glutamate is followed. A fixed incubation and sample preparation schedule is followed, and the amount of DAMPA formed is quantitated by high-performance liquid chromatography (HPLC).

First, the tissues are excised and may be stored at –70°C until required. The samples are trimmed and weighed to give 50–100 mg. This is homogenized to 10% (w/v) in PBS/1% aprotinin/10% glycerol/260 µM ZnCl$_2$ in a motor-driven Potter homogenizer at 0°C until completely dispersed. For each tissue type, a similar preparation of control material is needed to prepare a standard curve. For assay, the homogenate is diluted by 1/10, and depending on the anticipated concentrations of CPG2, it may need to have been previously diluted with control tissue homogenate. Aliquots of CPG2 assay buffer (250 mM Tris-HCl, pH 7.3/260 µM ZnCl$_2$) plus homogenate to a total volume of 600 µL are placed in a glass 20-mL scintillation vial and equilibrated at 30°C for 30 min in a shaking water bath. Stock 10 mM MTX is prepared by diluting 200 µL pharmaceutical-grade MTX (55 mM) with 900 µL DMSO. The reaction is initiated by addition of 6 µL of this stock to the vials, giving a starting concentration of 100 µM. After 30 min shaking incubation at 30°C, the reaction is stopped by addition of 500 μL methanol/5% TFA. The stopped mixture is then transferred to a micocentrifuge tube and spun for 5 min at 13,000 rpm. The extent to which the DAMPA partitions between the supernatant and the particulate pellet varies with tissue type; hence, a separate standard curve is prepared for each tissue type. Authentic CPG2 solutions are prepared at concentrations of 0.01, 0.02, 0.04, 0.06, 0.08, 0.1, 0.2, 0.4, and 0.6 U/mL. Vials of control tissue are prepared as earlier and spiked with 6 μL (100X dilution) of these solutions and processed as before. The supernatant is then analyzed for DAMPA content by HPLC. Volumes (60 μL) are injected onto a "Hichrom spherisorb" 5-μm SCX column (4.6 × 15 mm) and eluted isocratically with 70% MeOH/20 mM ammonium formate/0.1% TFA, at 1 mL/min at room temperature, and the eluate monitored by absorbance at 307 nm. Under these conditions, the MTX elutes at approx 2.6 min and the DAMPA at 4.6 min. Repeat injections are delayed for 30 min to ensure elution of all material deriving from the tissue. Alternatively, a "Phenomenex Synergi" polar end-capped ether-linked phenyl reverse-phase column is used and eluted with 100 mM ammonium acetate, pH 5.0, and 0–90% methanol gradient over 30 min. Under these conditions, the MTX elutes at approximately 15.5 min and the DAMPA at 20.5 min. The gradient is reset over a further 30 min. A calibration curve is constructed by plotting the area of the DAMPA peak against the concentration of CPG2. This should be a straight line that passes through the origin, which can be used to calculate the CPG2 concentrations in the test tissues. In the event that the concentration of the remaining MTX is seen to be less than 10% of the starting value (dynamic range of the assay exceeded), a repeat is performed, diluting the initial 10% homogenate 10X with its corresponding control homogenate.

3.5. Assessment of the Antitumor Efficacy of Prodrugs for CPG2

Experiments are conducted in accordance with UK Home Office regulations and UKCCCR guidelines. Xenografts are established in nude (nu/nu) female BALB/c mice (20–22 g) by subcutaneous inoculation (0.2 mL) in the right flank of a suspension of MDA MB 361 or WiDr cells (10^7 and $8 × 10^6$ cells, respectively) in PBS. The inocula (5–10 animals per group) consist of cells engineered to express β-galactosidase (control), CPG2* (internally expressed CPG2), or stCPG2(Q)$_3$ (externally expressed CPG2). In order to study in vivo bystander effects, the inocula consist of mixtures of β-galactosidase- and stCPG2(Q)3-expressing cells, comprising 0%, 10%, 50%, or 100% stCPG2(Q)$_3$-expressing cells. After 4 d, mice are divided randomly into control and treated groups, and those in the treated groups are administered prodrugs (d 0). Prodrugs are dissolved in DMSO and diluted 20-fold in 1.26% (w/v) sodium bicarbonate just prior to injection. Each course of prodrug treatment consists of three ip injections over a 2- or 24-h period, to a total preestablished optimal dose. Further courses of prodrug are administered on d 7, 14, 28, and 35, and when palpable tumor remains, on d 42, 56, and 63. When eventual tumor regrowth follows a prolonged tumor-free period, a further course may be administered. Animals are culled if the tumor exceeds 1.5 cm in any dimension. When histology is required, xenografts are established as earlier, and the subjects are treated with similar courses of the prodrugs. Courses are repeated on d 7 and 14. Twenty-four h after the end of the last course, the tumors are excised and fixed in formol–saline. After paraffin mounting, sections (5 μm) are cut, stained with hematoxylin and eosin, and examined microscopically (40× magnification), and representative fields of view are photographed.

4. Notes

1. Generation of stable cell lines. We select our stable cell lines using the antibiotic G418, although other selection protocols can be used. We find that when the Neo® gene and the prodrug-activating enzyme are expressed from the same plasmid, more of the selected colonies express the transgene. Therefore, we use a plasmid called pMCEF—in which the Neo® gene is expressed by a polyoma enhancer and the transgene is expressed off the opposite strand using the elongation factor 1a promoter; in our experience, this promoter is active in a large number of cell types. We use LipofectAMINE (Invitrogen) as our transfection agent of choice. However, the efficiency of transfection depends on the cell type and varies from batch to batch. Therefore, we generally perform a titration for both the DNA concentration and the amount of LipofectAMINE prior to selecting for stable cell lines. We perform our transfections in 35-mm dishes and find that it is more efficient when the cells are relatively (over 90%) confluent. For most cell lines, we use 2–7 μL of lipofectamine with 400–1000 ng of DNA per well. By titrating these reagents against each other using a suitable reporter construct (β-galactosidase, GFP), the best transfection conditions can be established.

   For selecting the cell lines, we transfect cells with high-quality supercoiled plasmid and then replate the cells into G418 48 h later. For each cell line, it is important to establish how sensitive each parental cell line is prior to G418 addition. Generally, the range is from 0.5 to 1.5 mg/mL. The cells from each 35-mm transfected dish are replated into three 100-mm dishes, containing 89%, 10%, and 1% of the cells. The cells are incubated in G418 for up to 2 wk until colonies form. Individual colonies are selected (we simply scrape them off using a 1-μL bacterial innoculation loop) and replated into 24-well plates. Using this plasmid, we have not found it necessary to maintain stock cells in the presence of G418 to ensure that transgene expression is maintained. However, we do revive frozen cells into G418, 48 h after thawing out for 1 wk.

   We screen individual colonies using Western blotting for the transgene. It is therefore often helpful to fuse an antibody tag to the transgene if antibodies are not available. It also allows us to select for a range of levels of transgene expression. Alternatively, transgene expression can be detected using enzyme activity if a convenient assay is available.

2. N- and C-terminal protein tagging. Genes can be modified at their 5' and 3' ends with ease. However, the effects of these modifications to enzyme activity need to be determined. With CPG2, we were able to modify both the N- and the C-termini without affecting enzyme activity. However, with NR, we found that although it was possible to modify the N-terminus, even small modifications to the C-terminus were inactivating *(36)*. Structural data, if available, can provide important information for protein design and may help to predict the consequences of enzyme modifications. The crystal structure of CPG2 reveals that both the N- and C-terminus of the protein are within the catalytic domain of the enzyme, but are positioned on the surface of the molecule and do not contribute to the putative active site *(41)*. By contrast, the crystal structure of NR shows that the C-terminal peptide is important for the activity because it forms part of the catalytic site *(31)*. Therefore, the structural information provides a rational explanation for our experimental observations with these two enzymes. In the absence of structural information, both modifications need to be tested empirically.

3. Posttranslational modification. Expression of nonmammalian enzymes in mammalian cells may result in posttranslational modifications that do not occur in the original organism. Numerous protein modifications have been described, including proteolytic cleavage, glycosylation, phosphorylation, methylation, and acylation. Many of these occur at specific amino acid motifs and can be predicted from the protein sequence using the ExPASy proteomic tools (www.ca.expasy.org). However, the presence of the consensus motifs does not necessarily mean that the modification will occur. Some modifications, such as glycosylation, may be relatively easy to detect, because they induce an increase in apparent molecular mass of the enzyme in denaturing SDS-PAGE (polyacrylamide gel electrophoresis). Furthermore, *N*-linked glycosylation can be blocked using the *Streptomyces* antibiotic tunicamycin which will inhibit this event and restore the expected molecular mass. Prepare tunicamycin as a 1-mg/mL stock in PBS, which can be stored in aliquots at –20°C. Add the antibiotic to the culture medium at a final concentration of 0.1–1 µg/mL. If the concentration is too high, the cells detach from the culture dish. Tunicamycin is toxic and may be carcinogenic, so appropriate safety precautions must be taken.
   N-Linked glycosylation occurs on the asparagine within the consensus motif Asn-Xaa-Ser/Thr (or, in rare cases, Asn-Xaa-Cys) and can be identified using the Prosite program (www.ca.expasy.org/prosite). It is possible to prevent glycosylation by mutating either the asparagine or the serine–threonine. Once again, the consequences of mutating these different amino acids need to be tested empirically. With CPG2, the three glycosylation sites are within the dimerization domain and not all mutants we generated were tolerated *(28)*, although some sites were more flexible than others. It may, therefore, be necessary to test a number of combinations before a suitable combination is discovered.
4. Prodrug stock solutions. The prodrug CMDA is unstable and stock solutions should always be freshly prepared prior to use. Like all nitrogen mustard compounds, CMDA reacts with water molecules. Therefore, it is important to use dry (anhydrous) DMSO as a solvent.
5. Bystander cytotoxicity assays. For bystander studies, cells are grown until confluency prior to prodrug treatment. This allows the cells to form cell–cell contacts, which are necessary for an efficient bystander effect. CPG2 and NR convert their prodrugs into alkylating agents that induce DNA interstrand crosslinks, which prevent the separation of DNA helix strands and thus inhibit DNA replication. Although these events kill both cycling and noncycling cells, the most efficient killing occurs when the cells are growing. Therefore, after exposure to prodrug, we tend to replate the cells to encourage growth and analyze survival after a further 4 d.
6. Prodrug concentration in bystander assays. To assess the prodrug sensitivity of cell lines that do not express prodrug-converting enzymes, treat the cells with varying concentrations and determine the IC_{50} values. These are defined as the prodrug concentration required to kill 50% of the parental cells, compared to DMSO-treated cells. For bystander studies, use the prodrug at concentrations that do not affect the growth of the parental cells (this is usually 10–50% of the IC_{50} of the parental cells; in our experience approx 20 µM CB1954 and 1–2 m*M* CMDA for most cell lines). For some cell lines, it may be necessary to raise the CMDA concentration to 8 m*M*. In this case, it may be beneficial to raise the pH of the medium to prevent precipitation of the compound. This can be done by exposing the medium to air overnight.

References

1. Bridgewater, J. A., Springer, C. J., Knox, R. J., Minton, N. P., Michael, N. P., and Collins, M. K. (1995) Expression of the bacterial nitroreductase enzyme in mammalian cells renders them selectively sensitive to killing by the prodrug CB1954. *Eur. J. Cancer* **31A**, 2362–2370.
2. Huber, B. E., Richards, C. A., and Krenitsky, T. A. (1991) Retroviral-mediated gene therapy for the treatment of hepatocellular carcinoma: an innovative approach for cancer therapy. *Proc. Natl. Acad. Sci. USA* **88**, 8039–8043.
3. Moolten, F. L. (1986) Tumor chemosensitivity conferred by inserted herpes thymidine kinase genes: paradigm for a prospective cancer control strategy. *Cancer Res.* **46**, 5276–5281.
4. Greco, O. and Dachs, G. U. (2001) Gene directed enzyme/prodrug therapy of cancer: historical appraisal and future prospectives. *J. Cell Physiol.* **187**, 22–36.
5. Bermudes, D., Zheng, L. M., and King, I. C. (2002) Live bacteria as anticancer agents and tumor-selective protein delivery vectors. *Curr. Opin. Drug Discovery Dev.* **5**, 194–199.
6. Niculescu-Duvaz, I., Cooper, R. G., Stribbling, S. M., Heyes, J. A., Metcalfe, J. A., and Springer, C. J. (1999) Recent developments in gene-directed enzyme prodrug therapy (GDEPT) for cancer. *Curr. Opin. Mol. Ther.* **1**, 480–486.
7. Xu, G. and McLeod, H. L. (2001). Strategies for enzyme/prodrug cancer therapy. *Clin. Cancer Res.* **7**, 3314–3324.
8. Coffey, M. C., Strong, J. E., Forsyth, P. A., and Lee, P. W. K. (1998) Reovirus therapy for tumors with activated Ras pathway. *Science* **282**, 1332–1334.
9. Bos, J. (1998) All in the family? New insights and questions regarding interconnectivity of Ras, Rap1 and Ral. *EMBO J.* **17**, 6776–6782.
10. Encell, L. P., Landis, D. M., and Loeb, L. A. (1999) Improving enzymes for cancer gene therapy. *Nature Biotechnol.* **17**, 143–147.
11. Vrionis, F. D., Wu, J. K., Qi, P., Waltzman, M., Cherington, V., and Spray, D. C. (1997) The bystander effect exerted by tumor cells expressing the herpes simplex virus thymidine kinase (HSVtk) gene is dependent on connexin expression and cell communication via gap junctions. *Gene Ther.* **4**, 577–585.
12. Wildner, O., Blaese, R. M., and Morris, J. C. (1999) Therapy of colon cancer with oncolytic adenovirus is enhanced by the addition of herpes simplex virus–thymidine kinase. *Cancer Res.* **59**, 410–413.
13. Elliott, G. and O'Hare, P. (1997) Intercellular trafficking and protein delivery by a herpesvirus structural protein. *Cell* **88**, 223–233.
14. Dilber, M. S., Phelan, A., Aints, A., et al. (1999) Intercellular delivery of thymidine kinase prodrug activating enzyme by the herpes simplex virus protein, VP22. *Gene Ther.* **6**, 12–21.
15. Black, M. E., Newcomb, T. G., Wilson, H. M., and Loeb, L. A. (1996) Creation of drug-specific herpes simplex virus type 1 thymidine kinase mutants for gene therapy. *Proc. Natl. Acad. Sci. USA* **93**, 3525–3529.
16. Black, M. E., Kokoris, M. S., and Sabo, P. (2001) Herpes simplex virus-1 thymidine kinase mutants created by semi-random sequence mutagenesis improve prodrug-mediated tumor cell killing. *Cancer Res.* **61**, 3022–3026.
17. Christians, F. C., Scapozza, L., Crameri, A., Folkers, G., and Stemmer, W. P. (1999) Directed evolution of thymidine kinase for AZT phosphorylation using DNA family shuffling. *Nature Biotechnol.* **17**, 259–264.

18. Lee, Y. J., Galoforo, S. S., Battle, P., Lee, H., Corry, P. M., and Jessup, J. M. (2001) Replicating adenoviral vector-mediated transfer of a heat-inducible double suicide gene for gene therapy. *Cancer Gene Ther.* **8,** 397–404.
19. Rogulski, K. R., Kim, J. H., Kim, S. H., and Freytag, S. O. (1997) Glioma cells transduced with an Escherichia coli CD/HSV-1 TK fusion gene exhibit enhanced metabolic suicide and radiosensitivity. *Hum. Gene Ther.* **8,** 73–85.
20. Uckert, W., Kammertons, T., Haack, K., et al. (1998) Double suicide gene (cytosine deaminase and herpes simplex virus thymidine kinase) but not single gene transfer allows reliable elimination of tumor cells in vivo. *Hum. Gene Ther.* **9,** 855–865.
21. Shimizu, T., Shimada, H., Ochiai, T., and Hamada, H. (2001) Enhanced growth suppression in esophageal carcinoma cells using adenovirus-mediated fusion gene transfer (uracil phosphoribosyl transferase and herpes simplex virus thymidine kinase). *Cancer Gene Ther.* **8,** 512–521.
22. Sherwood, R. F., Melton, R. G., Alwan, S. M., and Hughes, P. (1985) Purification and properties of carboxypeptidase G2 from *Pseudomonas* sp. strain RS-16. Use of a novel triazine dye affinity method. *Eur. J. Biochem.* **148,** 447–453.
23. Springer, C. J., Antoniw, P., Bagshawe, K. D., Searle, F., Bisset, G. M., and Jarman, M. (1990). Novel prodrugs which are activated to cytotoxic alkylating agents by carboxypeptidase G2. *J. Med. Chem.* **33,** 677–681.
24. Springer, C. J. and Niculescu-Duvaz, I. I. (1997) Antibody-directed enzyme prodrug therapy (ADEPT): a review. *Adv. Drug Delivery Rev.* **26,** 151–172.
25. Marais, R., Spooner, R. A., Light, Y., Martin, J., and Springer, C. J. (1996) Gene-directed enzyme prodrug therapy with a mustard prodrug/carboxypeptidase G2 combination. *Cancer Res.* **56,** 4735–4742.
26. Marais, R., Spooner, R. A., Stribbling, S. M., Light, Y., Martin, J., and Springer, C. J. (1997) A cell surface tethered enzyme improves efficiency in gene-directed enzyme prodrug therapy. *Nature Biotechnol.* **15,** 1373–1377.
27. Yarden, Y. and Ullrich, A. (1988) Growth factor receptor tyrosine kinases. *Annu. Rev. Biochem.* **57,** 443–478.
28. Spooner, R. A., Martin, J., Friedlos, F., Marais, R., and Springer, C. J. (2000) In suicide gene therapy, the site of subcellular localization of the activating enzyme is more important than the rate at which it activates prodrug. *Cancer Gene Ther.* **7,** 1348–1356.
29. Bonifacino, J. S. and Weissman, A. M. (1998) Ubiquitin and the control of protein fate in the secretory and endocytic pathways. *Annu. Rev. Cell Dev. Biol.* **14,** 19–57.
30. Stribbling, S. M., Friedlos, F., Martin, J., et al. (2000) Regressions of established breast carcinoma xenografts by carboxypeptidase G2 suicide gene therapy and the prodrug CMDA are due to a bystander effect. *Hum. Gene Ther.* **11,** 285–292.
31. Parkinson, G. N., Skelly, J. V., and Neidle, S. (2000) Crystal structure of FMN-dependent nitroreductase from *Escherichia coli* B: a prodrug-activating enzyme. *J. Med. Chem.* **43,** 3624–3631.
32. Friedlos, F., Court, S., Ford, M., Denny, W. A., and Springer, C. (1998) Gene-directed enzyme prodrug therapy: quantitative bystander cytotoxicity and DNA damage induced by CB1954 in cells expressing bacterial nitroreductase. *Gene Ther.* **5,** 105–112.
33. Green, N. K., Youngs, D. J., Neoptolemos, J. P., et al. (1997) Sensitization of colorectal and pancreatic cancer cell lines to the prodrug 5-(aziridin-1-yl)-2,4-dinitrobenzamide (CB1954) by retroviral transduction and expression of the *E. coli* nitroreductase gene. *Cancer Gene Ther.* **4,** 229–238.

34. Searle, P. F., Weedon, S. J., McNeish, I. A., et al. (1998) Sensitisation of human ovarian cancer cells to killing by the prodrug CB1954 following retroviral or adenoviral transfer of the *E. coli* nitroreductase gene. *Adv. Exp. Med. Biol.* **451,** 107–113.
35. Knox, R. J., Friedlos, F., Sherwood, R. F., Melton, R. G., and Anlezark, G. M. (1992) The bioactivation of 5-(aziridin-1-yl)-2,4-dinitrobenzamide (CB1954)—II. A comparison of an *Escherichia coli* nitroreductase and Walker DT diaphorase. *Biochem. Pharmacol.* **44,** 2297–2301.
36. Spooner, R. A., Maycroft, K. A., Paterson, H., Friedlos, F., Springer, C. J., and Marais, R. (2001) Appropriate subcellular localisation of prodrug-activating enzymes has important consequences for suicide gene therapy. *Int. J. Cancer* **93,** 123–130.
37. Springer, C. J. and Niculescu-Duvaz, I. (2000). Prodrug-activating systems in suicide gene therapy. *J. Clin. Invest.* **105,** 1161–1167.
38. Cowen, R. L., Williams, J. C., Emery, S., et al. (2002) Adenovirus-mediated delivery of the prodrug-converting enzyme carboxypeptidase G2 in a secreted or GPI-anchored form: High-level expression of this active conditional cytotoxic enzyme at the plasma membrane. *Cancer Gene Ther.* **9,** 897–907.
39. Heine, D., Muller, R., and Brusselbach, S. (2001) Cell surface display of a lysosomal enzyme for extracellular gene-directed enzyme prodrug therapy. *Gene Ther.* **8,** 1005–1010.
40. Jacobson, M. D., Burne, J. F., King, M. P., Miyashita, T., Reed, J. C., and Raff, M. C. (1993) Bcl-2 blocks apoptosis in cells lacking mitochondrial DNA. *Nature* **361,** 365–369.
41. Rowsell, S., Pauptit, R. A., Tucker, A. D., Melton, R. G., Blow, D. M., and Brick, P. (1997) Crystal structure of carboxypeptidase G2, a bacterial enzyme with applications in cancer therapy. *Structure* **5,** 337–347.

15

Extracellular β-Glucuronidase for Gene-Directed Enzyme–Prodrug Therapy

Sabine Brüsselbach

1. Introduction

Most enzymes used for antibody-directed enzyme–prodrug therapy (ADEPT) and gene-directed enzyme–prodrug therapy (GDEPT) are of bacterial, yeast, or viral origin. These xenogeneic proteins can induce an immune response, which might be a hindrance to their application of these enzymes in humans *(1)*. On the other hand, when choosing a human enzyme for prodrug conversion cleavage by the respective endogenuous enzyme obviously needs to be avoided. Lysosomal enzymes seem to be particularly suitable candidates, because under normal circumstances, the endogenous enzymes are restricted to intracellular vesicles and therefore not available for premature prodrug conversion. In addition, lysosomal enzymes leaking out of cells are rapidly internalized via the mannose-6-phosphate (M6P) receptor expressed on the surface of most cells and at particulary high levels on reticuloendothelial cells *(2,3)*. The human lysosomal enzyme β-glucuronidase has been used for ADEPT *(4–8)* and GDEPT *(9,10)*. This exoglycosidase removes terminal β-glucuronic acids from glycosaminoglycans and other glycoconjugates. The enzyme is highly specific for the glucuronyl residue but has little specificity for the conjugated aglycone. Therefore, different drugs could be developed as prodrugs *(see Table 1)*. Elevated β-glucuronidase levels in tumor tissue have been reported, released from dying tumor cells and invading macrophages and neutrophils *(18,19,36,37)*. β-Glucuronides of different drugs might be exploited for tumor-specific conversion by released endogenous enzymes ("monotherapy") as well as for ADEPT and GDEPT approaches. In the latter cases, the endogenous enzyme released from dying tumor cells after initial prodrug conversion amplifies the effect of the ADEPT/GDEPT system.

From: *Methods in Molecular Medicine, Vol. 90, Suicide Gene Therapy: Methods and Reviews*
Edited by: C. J. Springer © Humana Press Inc., Totowa, NJ

Table 1
Glucuronidated Prodrugs Developed for Monotherapy, ADEPT, and GDEPT

Drug	Prodrug	Application	References
Anthracyclins			
Epirubicin	Epirubicin–glucuronide	ADEPT	*11,12*
Daunorubicin	Daunorubicin–benzyl carbamate spacer–glucuronide (DNR-GA3)	Monotherapy, ADEPT	*13–16*
Doxorubicin	Doxorubicin–benzyl carbamate spacer–glucuronide (Dox-GA3)	Monotherapy, ADEPT	*7,8,16,17*
Doxorubicin	Doxorubicin–nitrophenyl spacer–glucuronide (HMR 1826)	Monotherapy, ADEPT, GDEPT	*5,9,10,18–22*
Daunorubicin and doxorubicin	Daunorubicin and doxorubicin glucuronides		*23*
Doxorubicin	Doxorubicin–nitrophenyl spacer–glucuronide		*24*
Doxorubicin	Doxorubicin–enol ether spacer–glucuronide		*25*
Mustards			
Hydroxyaniline mustard (HAM)	Tetrabutyl HAM glucuronide (BHAMG)	ADEPT	*26,27*
Mustard	Mustard–carbamate spacer–glucuronide		*28*
Nitrogen mustard	Nornitrogen mustard–nitrophenyl–glucuronide		*29*
Other cytotoxic drugs			
diverse	Acetal–glucopyranosiduronates		*30*
Rooperol	Hypoxoside	Monotherapy	*31*
Palitaxel	Palitaxel–carbamate–glucuronide		*32*
9-Aminocamptothecin	9-Aminocamptothecin–aromatic spacer–glucuronide		*33*
5-Fluorouracil	5-Fluorouracil–carbamate spacer–glucuronide	MRS[a]	*34*
MDR inhibitors			
Verapamil, quinine, dipyridamole	MDR inh. glucuronides (for combination with antracyclin prodrugs)		*35*

[a]MRS, magnetic resonance spectroscopy; MDR inh., multiple drug resistance inhibitors.

304

1.1. Cell Biology, Structure, and Properties of Human β-Glucuronidase

The physiological function of β-glucuronidase (β-D-glucuronoside glucurono-sohydrolase; E.C. 3.2.1.31; gene bank accession number M15182) is the turnover of extracellular matrix components. It degrades glucuronic acid-containing glycosami-noglycan, like heparan sulfate, chondroitin sulfate, dermatan sulphate, and hyaluronic acid *(38)*. As a lysosomal enzyme it has an acidic pH optima ranging between 3.8 and 5 *(39)*. The active homotetramer has a Mr of 332,000. There are two active sites located in a large cleft at the interface of two monomers and each cleft has two catalytic centers. Each monomer is arranged as three structural domains as revealed by three–dimensional structure analysis of crystallized human β-glucuronidase *(40)*. The active center is localized in the C-terminal domain with Glu 540 as the catalytic nucleophile and Glu 451 as the acid–base residue *(41,42)*.

Individual subunits of 651 amino acids are synthesized on membrane-bound ribosomes and translocated into the endoplasmic reticulum (ER), where several posttranslational events occur *(43)*. These include signal sequence cleavage (amino acids 1–22), N-linked glycosylation (Asn-173, 272, 420, 631) *(44)*, disulfide bond formation, and homotetramerization. In the Golgi complex, the glycans are modified to expose M6P residues. In the trans-Golgi network, these M6P residues serve as ligands for specific receptors, which transport lysosomal enzymes to a prelysosomal compartment. After pH-dependent dissociation of the receptor–enzyme complex, the receptor relocates to the Golgi, and the enzyme stays in the developing lysosome. β-Glucuronidase undergoes proteolytic C-terminal processing during or after its transport to lysosomes. The C- terminal processing site is the peptide bond between Thr-633 and Arg-634. It has been suggested that the C-terminal fragment influences both the addition and exposure of MGP *(45)*.

The cDNA was first isolated from human placenta *(46)* and the gene has been cloned *(47)*. The human enzyme is 47% similar to Escherichia coli glucuronidase, which has a pH optimum of 7.

In certain pathophysiological conditions, β-glucuronidase is released into the extracellular compartment. In inflammatory joint diseases like rheumatoid arthritis, β-glucuronidase is found in the synovial fluid and contributes to the symptomatology of the disease *(48,49)*. As mentioned earlier, elevated levels of β-glucuronidase have been found in tumors *(18,19,36)*. It has been suggested that the breakdown of the basement membrane, which is necessary for metastasis, is mediated in part by the release of β-glucuronidase *(37)*. Endogenous β-glucuronidase was proposed as a target for prodrug activation by Connors and Whisson in 1966 *(36)*. Thus, mice suffering from advanced plasmacytoma were cured with aniline mustard, which is hydroxylated and glucuronidated in the liver followed by the activation of this endogenously generated prodrug to hydroxyaniline in the tumor tissue, which expresses high amounts of β-glucuronidase. However, clinical trials using aniline mustard have been disappointing, likely the result of insufficient β-glucuronidase activity in tumor areas penetrated by the prodrug. Necrotic areas with high amounts of extracellular β-glucuronidase are less well vascularized, leading to insufficient prodrug supply. Therefore, new strategies are proposed targeting β-glucuronidase to the tumor and especially to those areas where the bloodstream is in contact with the tumor tissue. One possibility of increasing β-glucuronidase concentration at the tumor is the application of tumor-specific antibody–enzyme conjugates (*see* **Subheading 1.2.**). More recently, gene therapeutic approaches are used in order to sensitize the tumor to prodrugs (*see* **Subheading 1.3.**). The inefficacy of conventional cancer chemotherapy is largely the result of dose-limiting, toxic side effects and the generation of multidrug-resistant tumor cells because of insufficient drug concentrations at the tumor site. One aim of enzyme–prodrug therapies is to increase drug concentrations inside the tumor in order to prevent the development of escape mechanisms, but without increasing systemic toxicities.

1.2. Antibody-Directed Enzyme–Prodrug Therapy

The concept of ADEPT was developed by Philpott et al. *(50,51)* and tested by Bagshawe et al. in a pilot clinical trial *(1,52)*. The bacterial enzyme carboxypeptidase G2 (CPG2) conjugated to a monoclonal human carcinoembryonic antigen (CEA)-specific antibody was applied to patients suffering from advanced colorectal cancer. After tumor localization of the antibody–enzyme complex, a mustard glutamate prodrug was applied. All patients studied developed human antimouse antibodies (HAMAs) and anti-CPG2 antibodies emphasizing the need for humanized antibodies and nonimmunogenic proteins. Therefore, an intriguing approach is the use of human enzymes for ADEPT. β-Glucuronidase seems to be an ideal candidate because under nonpathological conditions, the enzyme is localized exclusively intracellularly in lysosomes and not available for cleavage of the systemically applied prodrug. Bosslet et al. fused the cDNA of human β-glucuronidase to the sequence of the humanized Fab fragment of an anti-CEA antibody *(4)*. Therapeutic responses were seen in colon carcinoma xenografts expressing CEA, when the fusion protein was tested in combination with a prodrug of doxorubicin (HMR 1826; *see* **Table 1**). In addition, 4 – to 12-fold higher doxorubicin concentration were found in tumors of mice treated with ADEPT compared to those given drug alone at the maximum tolerable dose (MTD = 12 mg/kg). The prodrug concentration used for these experiments was well below the MTD (> 1600 mg/kg) *(5)*. Haisma´s group developed a conjugate where the human enzyme was crosslinked to a pancarcinoma antigen-specific antibody using stable thioether bonds *(6,8)*. In an ovarian cancer xenograft model, tumor regression was observed in 9 of 10 mice after treatment with the enzyme conjugate and the MTD of a doxorubicin prodrug (DOX-GA3; *see* **Table 1**). In contrast, no regression was seen in mice treated with the MTD of doxorubicin. In addition, the doxorubicin generated by cleavage of HMR 1826 and DOX-GA3 stayed in the tumor because of the high hydrophobicity of the drug. Furthermore, Haisma et al. generated a fusion protein of murine single-chain Fv CD20 antibody and human β-glucuronidase. CD20 is a surface marker specific for B-cell lymphomas. When the fusion protein was specifically bound to Daudi lymphoma cells in cell culture, the prodrug DOX-GA3 induced antiproliferative effects similar to those for doxorubicin *(7)*.

The bacterial enzyme has been used for β-glucuronidase-mediated prodrug activation in vitro *(11,26,27)*. The *E. coli* enzyme has a pH optimum of 7 and therefore seems to be ideal for efficient activation of glucuronidated drugs under physiological conditions. Nevertheless, immunological concerns make the human enzyme a better choice for clinical application, despite the lower enzymatic activity at physiological pH (about 20% of maximal activity at pH 4.5) *(4)*.

1.3. Gene-Directed Enzyme–Prodrug Therapy

In GDEPT, the DNA coding for a prodrug-converting enzyme is delivered to the target tissue by viral or nonviral vectors (see other chapters) or local transduction methods (e.g., electroporation). Most enzymes used at present are of viral and bacterial origin, displaying distinct enzymatic activities and substrate specificities (see other chapters). We have chosen human β-glucuronidase for the development of a new GDEPT approach, where a hydrophilic prodrug is converted to a cell-permeable drug in the extracellular environment. In contrast to established systems using xenogeneic enzymes, the human protein should not elicit an immune response against the prodrug-activating enzyme, which would limit the amount of enzyme available for local prodrug activation and the option to perform multiple cycles of GDEPT.

Targeting and gene transfer efficiency in vivo are other points of concern. Currently available systems are still insufficient for applications in which all cells have to express the transduced gene. For this reason, it is necessary to use an effector mechanism that targets not only the transduced cell itself but also the neighboring cells (bystander effect). Most GDEPT systems available at present function intracellularly and thereby limit the efficacy of the system. In an attempt to improve this situation, prokaryotic carboxypeptidase G2 displayed on the cell surface has been developed for GDEPT *(53)*. We have chosen the human β-glucuronidase to establish a human extracellular cytotoxic effector system for the conversion of a hydrophilic non-cell-permeable prodrug (glucuronide prodrug of doxorubicin, HMR 1826) to the lipophilic, membrane-permeable drug doxorubicin. β-Glucuronidase seems to be a particularly suitable candidate as a prodrug-converting enzyme, because the endogenous enzyme is located in lysosomes and therefore not available for prodrug conversion under normal circumstances. In addition, β-glucuronidase leaking out of cells is rapidly internalized via the M6P receptor on the cell surface as discussed earlier.

Our laboratory has shown that tumor cells transduced to secrete β-glucuronidase can efficiently convert the prodrug HMR 1826 to the toxic drug doxorubicin, and that this GDEPT system can mediate tumor cell killing both in vitro and in vivo *(9)*. The bystander effect is mediated by diffusion of both the secreted β-glucuronidase and the extracellularly activated drug. Nevertheless, a potential problem with this approach lies in the possibility that the secreted enzyme may leak from the tumor with the result of toxic side effects. For this reason, we constructed a cell-membrane-attached form of β-glucuronidase using the platelet-derived growth factor receptor (PDGFR) transmembrane domain (10). Both constructs were tested in a choriocarcinoma xenograft model. Cell lines stably transfected with the secreted form (s-βGluc) or the transmembrane form (TM-βGluc) were injected subcutaneously into nude mice. When tumors had reached a size of approx 40 mm³, prodrug was injected into the tail vein and tumor growth was monitored. As shown in **Fig. 1**, the in vivo growth behavior of s-βGluc- and TM-βGluc-transduced JEG-3 cells in the absence of prodrug treatment resembled that of the nontransduced parental cells, and prodrug treatment had only a slight effect

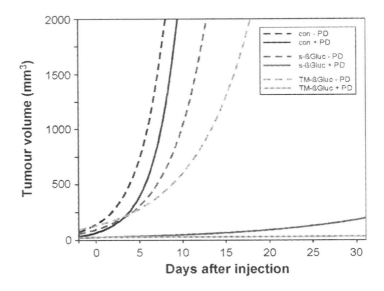

Fig. 1. Effect of the βGluc/β-glucuronyl-doxorubicin system on the growth of JEG-3 choriocarcinoma xenografts in vivo. βGluc expressing cells (s- and TM-βGluc) and nonexpressing
control cells (con) were injected subcutaneously into nude mice. When tumors reached a size
of approx 40 mm^3, the mice were divided into subgroups receiving 100 mg/kg of prodrug HMR
1826 (+PD) or no treatment (–PD). Tumor growth was recorded every 2–3 d. The calculated
tumor volume was plotted against the time after prodrug treatment.

on the nontransduced tumor cells. In contrast, tumors established from βGluc-express-
ing JEG-3 cells regressed after a single prodrug application and in both groups, two
out of six mice remained tumor-free after >6 mo.

1.4. Mucopolysaccharidosis Type VII

Genetic deficiency of β-glucuronidase is the molecular background for the inherited
disorder mucopolysaccharidosis type VII. Several experimental therapies are under
investigation in order to replace the lacking enzyme. Results obtained in these studies
supply useful information about the local and systemic distribution of the enzyme.

Mucopolysaccharidosis type VII (MPS VII) is also called Sly syndrome after the
investigator William S. Sly (54). The disease belongs to a large class of lysosomal
storage disorders that involves central nervous system (CNS) degeneration resulting
in mental retardation and behavioral deficits as the main clinical manifestations
(55,56). Various groups have been delineated according to the affected metabolic pathway and the accumulated substrate: mucopolysaccharidoses, glycoproteinoses,
glycogenosis type II, and lipidoses (57). The lack of β-glucuronidase leads to a progressive accumulation of undegraded glycosaminoglycans within lysosomes, resulting in widespread glycosaminoglycan storage in the brain and visceral organs. In
addition to CNS effects, other symptoms of MPS VII are growth retardation, facial

dysmorphism, joint abnormalities, deafness, corneal clouding, thickening of heart valves, and premature death *(58)*.

Most lysosomal storage diseases are potential candidates for gene therapy because the normal enzyme can be secreted from transduced cells and taken up by adjacent cells to correct the metabolic defect. In order to replace the lacking β-glucuronidase, animal models have been used to explore different therapeutic strategies for the treatment of MPS VII. Most experiments were performed with a spontaneous mouse mutant lacking any detectable β-glucuronidase activity (gus^{mps}/gus^{mps}) *(59–61)*. MPS VII mice suffer from a disorder resembling the human phenotype. This mouse strain has widely been used to test different therapies, including enzyme replacement, cell-based therapies, and gene therapeutic approaches. Special emphasis is put on the reversal of lysosomal storage in the brain to reduce the most severe symptoms (i.e., mental retardation).

1.4.1. Enzyme Replacement Therapy

The systemic application of recombinant protein for the treatment of a lysosomal storage disease is based on the principle of specific internalization of the therapeutic enzyme via M6R and transport to the lysosomes. The first success was achieved in Gaucher's disease, which is the most frequent lysosomal storage disease. The deficiency of β-glucocerebrosidase was corrected by the application of a modified enzyme (Imiglucerase, Cerezyme) *(62)*. In contrast to MPS VII, Gaucher's disease is characterized by the absence of CNS degenerative pathology *(63)*. Enzyme-replacement therapy with recombinant β-glucuronidase in MPS VII mice elicited remarkable improvements in visceral pathology, but had little effect in the brain, because the blood–brain barrier limits the access of the injected protein to the neuronal tissue *(64–69)*.

1.4.2. Cell-Based Therapies

Transplantation of bone marrow from syngeneic wild-type mice into newborn MPS VII mice was shown to prolong life, to improve hearing, retinal function, and bone growth, and to prevent lysosomal storage in many sites, but did not correct the CNS disease *(67,70–74)*. However, bone marrow transplantation (BMT) is still associated with major problems like the high mortality rate, the risk of graft-vs-host disease, and the difficulty of finding a compatible donor.

1.4.3. Gene Therapeutic Approaches

Gene therapeutic approaches for the treatment of MPS VII with ex vivo transduced cells and in vivo gene transfer with recombinant viral vectors have been performed. After transplantation of ex vivo transduced cells, only local effects were observed either in visceral organs after injection into the periphery *(75–78)* or in neurons and glia after injection into the brain *(79–80)*. Promising results were obtained with nonreplicating adenoviral vectors (AVs), adeno-associated virus (AAV)-based vectors, and lentiviral vectors. After intravenous administration of β-glucuronidase-expressing AVs, a transient reduction of lysosomal storage granules in visceral organs was observed, especially in the liver, where up to 88% of wild-type β-glucuronidase activity was measured *(81,82)*. In other visceral, organs less enzymatic activity was detected as a result of the preferential uptake of viral particles in the liver. In contrast, systemic application of recombinant AAVs did not result in any significant benefit *(83)*. Promising results were obtained after intracranial injections of recombinant adenovirus leading to marked reductions of lysosomal storage granules in neurons and glia, even in the noninjected hemisphere *(82,84)*. However, the induction of an immune response limits the application of adenoviral vectors for long-term expression of the transgene and multiple applications of the vector. On the other hand, sustained and stable expression of β-glucuronidase was achieved with AAVs *(85–87)* and lentiviral vectors *(88)*, which enabled a nearly complete correction of the pathology in the injected hemisphere.

The requirements for correction of MPS by gene therapy differ substantially from those that need to be fulfilled for an application to cancer therapy. First, in contrast to cancer gene therapy where transient expression of β-glucuronidase is sufficient, stable or long term expression is needed for the correction of MPS VII pathology. Second, in GDEPT approaches enzyme expression must be restricted to the tumor, whereas for MPS VII treatment, the enzyme can be expressed ubiquitously. Finally, in MPS VII, the replaced β-glucuronidase is needed in its natural surroundings, the lysosome, whereas in GDEPT, extracellular activity is needed for prodrug cleavage.

2. Materials

2.1. Subcellular Localization of s-βGluc and TM-βGluc: Saponin Extraction and Immunoprecipitation

1. ^{35}S-Methionine
2. Optional: Methionine-free cell culture medium and dialysed serum
3. Granular charcoal (Merck 1.02518.)
4. Phosphate buffered saline (PBS).
5. 0.1% Saponin in PBS.
6. Radioimmunoprecipitation assay buffer (RIPA buffer): 10 mM Tris-HCl, pH 7.5, 150 mM NaCl, 0.25% sodium dodecyl sulfate (SDS), 1% Sodium deoxycholate, 1% Nonidet P40, 1 mM dithiothreitol (DTT; add just before usage from 1 M stock solution), protease inhibitors (optional, see Note 1), 0.5 mM phenylmethylsulfonyl fluoride (PMSF; e.g., Sigma P 7626), 50 µg/mL aprotinin (e.g., Sigma A 4529), and 50 µg/mL leupeptin (e.g. Sigma L 2023).
7. Human β-glucuronidase-specific antibody (*see* Note 2).
8. Protein A–sepharose (Amersham Pharmacia Biotech 17-0974).
9. Equipment and buffers for SDS–gel electrophoresis and autoradiography.

2.2. 5-Bromo-4-Chloro-3-Indolyl β-D-Glucuronic Acid (X-gluc) Staining

1. General cell culture equipment.
2. General equipment for the preparation of frozen tissue sections.
3. 25% Glutaraldehyde, histological grade (prepare aliquots and keep at –20°C) for fixation of tissue culture cells.
4. 37% Formaldehyde.
5. PBS.
6. 2% X-gluc dissolved in dimethyl formamide (DMF), store at –20°C.
7. 0.3 M Potassium ferricyanide and 0.3 M potassium ferrocyanide (cyanide solutions should be stored at 4°C in the dark).
8. 0.2 M Sodium acetate buffer, pH 5. Mix seven parts of 0.2 M sodium acetate with three parts of 0.2 M acetic acid.

9. Mowiol:
   a. Add 5 g Mowiol (Calbiochem 475904) to 20 ml PBS.
   b. Stir overnight.
   c. Add 10 ml glycerol.
   d. Stir overnight.
   e. Centrifuge for 1 h at 25,000g.
   f. Remove pellet.
   g. Add 0.02% NaN$_3$;
   h. Store at 4°C.

2.3. Naphthol AS-BI β-D-Glucuronide Staining

1. General cell culture equipment.
2. General equipment for the preparation of frozen tissue sections.
3. Acetone.
4. 37% Formaldehyde solution.
5. PBS.
6. 0.2 M sodium acetate buffer, pH 5. Mix seven parts of 0.2 M sodium acetate with three parts of 0.2 M acetic acid.
7. 2 N HCl.
8. New fuchsin (Serva 30293, Sigma N 0638).
9. Sodium nitrite.
10. Naphthol-AS-BI β-D-glucuronide acid (Sigma N 1857).
11. D-Saccharic acid 1,4-lactone monohydrate (Aldrich 22,293-3).
12. Hematoxylin dye: Mayer's hemalum solution (Merck 1.09249).
13. Mounting medium (e.g., Mowiol; *see* **Subheading 2.2., item 9**).

2.4. ELF-97 β-D-Glucuronide Staining

1. General equipment for the preparation of frozen tissue sections.
2. Fluorescence microscope with a Hoechst/DAPI long-pass optical filter.
3. 37% Formaldehyde solution.
4. PBS.
5. 0.2 M Sodium acetate buffer, pH 5. Mix seven parts of 0.2 M sodium acetate with three parts of 0.2 M acetic acid.
6. ELF-97 β-D-glucuronide (Molecular Probes E-6587).
7. bisBenzimide Hoechst 33258 (*carcinogenic*, Sigma B 2883), stock solution: 2 mM in H$_2$O (can be stored at 4°C in the dark for at least 1 y).
8. Bovine serum albumin (BSA), fraction V (e.g., Sigma A 3912).
9. Mowiol (*see* **Subheading 2.2.**).

2.5. 4-Methylumbelliferyl β-D-Glucuronic Acid (4-MUG) Staining

1. Fluorometer with filter set to measure excitation at 350 nm and emission at 455 nm.
2. PBS.
3. 0.5% Sodium deoxycholate in PBS for extraction of tissue culture cells
4. 1% Bovine Serum Albumin BSA (Fraction V; e.g., Sigma A 3912) in PBS for preparation of organ extracts.
5. 0.1 N NaOH.
6. β-Glucuronidase-specific antibody (*see* **Note 2**).
7. 0.2 M Sodium acetate buffer, pH 5. Mix seven parts of 0.2 M sodium acetate with thee parts of 0.2 M acetic acid.

8. 4-Methylumbelliferyl β-D-glucuronic acid (4-MUG, Sigma M 5664, Molecular Probes M-1490).
9. 4-Methylumbelliferone (4-MU) (Sigma M 1381).
10. D-Saccharic acid 1,4-lactone monohydrate (Aldrich 22,293-3).
11. Stop solution: 0.2 *M* glycin, 0.2% sodium dodecyl sulfate, (SDS), pH 11.1 (freshly made).

2.6. N-(4-β-Glucuronyl-3-Nitrobenzyloxycarbonyl)-Doxorubicin (HMR 1826)

1. General cell culture equipment.
2. Fluorescence microscope with filters to detect the following:
   Doxorubicin: rhodamine filter; β-Glucuronidase (indirect immunofluorescence with green fluorochrome): FITC filter (*optional*); nuclei stained with DNA dye: Hoechst/DAPI long-pass optical filter (*optional*).
3. Dulbecco's modified Eagle's medium (DMEM) with 1.2 g/L NaHCO$_3$ (*see* **Notes 3** and **4**). Prepare DMEM medium from powder (e.g., Invitrogen 52100), but do not add NaHCO$_3$ as recommended. Use tissue culture grade water. Add 1.6 mL of 7.5% NaHCO$_3$ solution (tissue culture grade) to 100 mL DMEM. The pH of the medium should be 7.0 at 37°C and 7% CO$_2$.
4. β-Glucuronyl-doxorubicin (or other prodrug with autofluorescent drug).
5. 37% Formaldehyde.
6. PBS.
7. Mowiol (*see* **Subheading 2.2.**, item 9).
   Optional:
8. 10% Tween-20 in PBS.
9. 10% BSA (Fraction V, e.g., Sigma A 3912) in PBS.
10. β-Glucuronidase-specific antibody (*see* **Note 2**).
11. Secondary antibody conjugated to a green fluorochrome [e.g., DTAF(green)-labeled secondary antimouse antibody, F(ab')$_2$-fragments from Dianova].
12. bisBenzimide Hoechst 33258 (*carcinogenic*; Sigma B 2883), stock solution: 2 m*M* in H$_2$O (can be stored at 4°C in the dark).

3. Methods
3.1. Subcellular Localization of s-β Gluc and TM-β Gluc: Saponin Extraction and Immunoprecipitation

Saponin is a detergent that extracts soluble proteins from cells, but not membrane-integrated proteins. Cells are first radioactive labeled with ^{35}S-methionine and then extracted with saponin. The remaining insoluble fraction is dissolved in a high-detergent buffer. Both fractions, saponin extract and RIPA extract, are immunoprecipitated with a β-glucuronidase-specific antibody. Soluble and membrane integrated forms can be visualized by autoradiography. Controls to detect endogenous β-glucuronidase should be included.

3.1.1. Radioactive Labeling and Saponin Extraction

All precautions regarding work with radioactive substances have to be considered. ^{35}S-Methionine is metabolized in cells to the gas H$_2$^{35}S. We recommend using sealed cell culture flasks or to putting cell culture dishes into a box filled with charcoal.

1. Wash cells twice with PBS.
2. Add cell culture medium containing 0.2 μCi ml ^{35}S-methionine. Methionine-free medium and dialyzed serum might be used to get a higher specific activity (*optional*).
3. Put cell culture dish in a box filled with charcoal.
4. Incubate cells for 1–3 h (37°C, 89% humidity, 5% CO_2).
5. Collect radioactive supernatant.
6. Wash three times with PBS and collect washing buffer.
7. Cover cells with 0.1% saponin for 10 min at room temperature (RT).
8. Collect saponin fraction containing soluble nonmembrane integrated enzyme.
9. Wash twice with PBS and collect radioactive supernatant.
10. Lyse cells in RIPA buffer (precooled on ice) for 5 min to extract membrane-integrated β-glucuronidase.

3.1.2. Immunoprecipitation and SDS–Gel Electrophoresis (Short Protocol)

11. Precool RIPA buffer on ice.
12. Mix 100 μL RIPA buffer to 200 μL of samples (saponin extract and cell lysates).
13. Add β-glucuronidase-specific antibody and incubate on ice for 1 h.
14. Add 40 μL protein A–sepharose prewashed with RIPA buffer and incubate on ice for at least 1 h. Mix carefully in between.
15. Wash pellet at least five times with RIPA buffer.
16. Add SDS sample buffer, boil for 2 min, and separate on a 7.5% acrylamide gel.
17. Dry gel and expose autoradiographic film.

In Fig. 2, an autoradiograph of a saponin extraction is shown. Cells transfected with constructs coding for a secreted form of β-glucuronidase (s-βGluc) or a transmembrane form (TM-βGluc) were labeled with ^{35}S-methionine and extracted with saponin, and the extracted proteins were separated on a polyacrylamide gel. Secreted and transmembrane forms of β-glucuronidase mainly appear in the saponin soluble and insoluble fraction, respectively. The saponin-insoluble β-glucuronidase in cells transfected with s-βGluc probably corresponds to β-glucuronidase attached to the endoplasmatic reticulum membrane.

3.2. 5-Bromo-4-Chloro-3-Indolyl β-D-Glucuronic Acid (X-gluc) for Chromogenic Staining of Cells in Culture and Histological Sections

β-Glucuronidase hydrolyzes β-linked D-glucuronides to D-glucuronic acid and aglycones. The substrates used for the detection of enzymatic activity in vitro and in vivo contain the sugar D-glucopyranosiduronic acid attached to a hydroxyl group of a chromogenic or fluorogenic molecule.

5-Bromo-4-chloro-3-indolyl β-D-glucuronic acid (X-gluc) provides a colorimetric method to localize β-glucuronidase activity in cell culture and in histological sections. β-Glucuronidase cleaves the colorless substrate to D-glucuronic acid and indoxyl derivatives. In the presence of oxidative reagents the released indoxyl molecules dimerize to the final indigo dye, which precipitates at the site of enzymatic cleavage (*see* **Fig. 3**).

3.2.1. Fixation

In order to preserve cell or tissue structure, samples are fixed before staining. Mild fixation conditions are used to keep a balance between optimal tissue preservation and retaining enzymatic activity (*see* **Notes 5** and **6**).

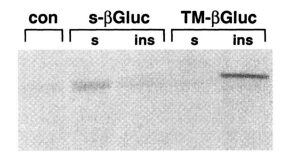

Fig. 2. Subcellular localization of s-βGluc and TM-βGluc. Saponin extractability of s-βGluc and TM-βGluc from ³⁵S-labeled COS-7 cells. Saponin-soluble (s) and saponin-insoluble (ins) βGluc protein was detected in cell extracts by immunoprecipitation.

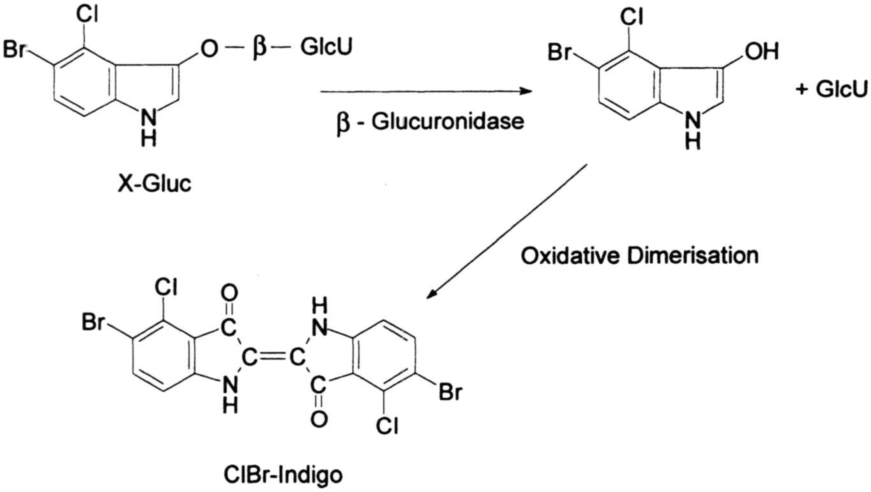

Fig. 3. Cleavage X-gluc by β-glucuronidase, followed by oxidative dimerization. GlcU, glucuronic acid; ClBr-Indigo, dichloro-dibromoindigo. [According to Stomp (89)].

3.2.1.1. FIXATION OF CELL CULTURE CELLS

1. Prepare working solution of 0.1% glutaraldehyde in PBS and keep on ice. Long-term storage of diluted glutaraldehyde solution is not recommended, because of oxidation of the aldehyde.
2. Rinse cells twice with PBS (*see* **Note 7**).
3. Cover cells with 0.1% glutaraldehyde and incubate for 10 min at room temperature.
4. Rinse cells three times with PBS.

3.2.1.2. Fixation of Histological Sections

1. Prepare frozen tissue sections.
2. Take a small box, where the cover slips can be arranged at a distance of roughly 2–3 cm to the bottom. Fill the box with formaldehyde (approx 1 cm).
3. Put the cover slips onto the box with the tissue section facing towards the formaldehyde.
4. Fix for 10–30 min in formaldehyde gas.

3.2.2. Staining and Post Fixation

The staining procedure is a modification of the protocol for *E. coli* β-galactosidase detection with X-gal *(90)*.

1. Prepare the staining solution:

	μL of stock solution	Final concentration
H₂O	440	
Acetate buffer	500	0.1 *M*
Ferricyanide	10	3 m*M*
Ferrocyanide	10	3 m*M*
X-gluc	40	0.08%

2. Cover fixed cells or frozen section with a minimal volume of staining solution and incubate at 37°C for 2–24 h.

In order to terminate the reaction:

3. remove the staining solution and
4. rinse twice with PBS.
5. Fix for 15 min with 3.7% formaldehyde/PBS for storage at 4°C.

An example of this staining technique is shown in **Fig. 4**.

3.3. Naphthol AS-BI β-ᴅ-Glucuronide
for Chromogenic Staining of Histological Sections

Naphthol AS-BI β-ᴅ-glucuronide is a substrate useful for histochemical detection of β-glucuronidase activity *(92–95)* (*see* **Fig. 5**). Upon hydrolysis the product naphthol AS-BI (6-bromo-2-hydroxy-3-naphthoyl-O-anisidine) reacts *in situ* with added New Fuchsin to a red precipitating azo dye.

3.3.1. Fixation

3.3.1.1. Acetone Fixation (Afterwards the Sections Can Be Stored at −80°C)

1. Prepare frozen sections (6 μm) on cover slips.
2. Air-dry for 30 min to 1 h.
3. Fix in acetone for 10 min.

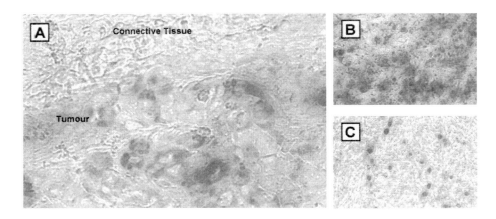

Fig. 4. Human A549 lung carcinoma cells were transduced with TM-βGluc and subcutane-ously injected into nude mice. Established tumors were removed and frozen in liquid nitrogen. Cryosections were fixed for 30 min in formaldehyde gas (**A** and **B**) or for 1 min in 3.7% form-aldehyde (**C**). Tumors established from untransduced cells were negative (data not shown).

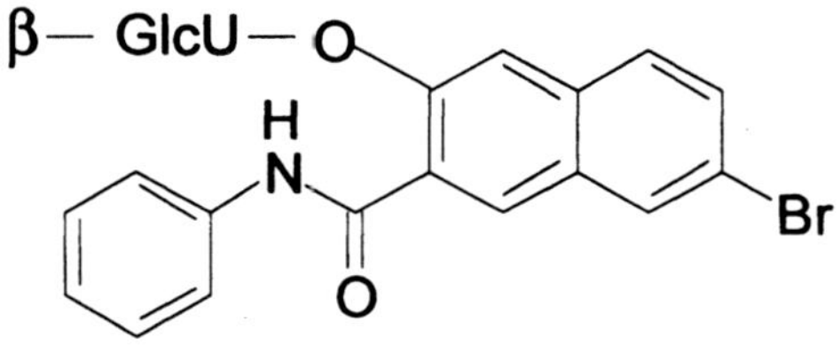

$$\beta-\text{GlcU}-O$$

Fig. 5. Chemical structure of naphthol AS-BI β-D-glucuronide.

4. Air-dry.
5. Store at –80°C.

3.3.1.2. FORMALDEHYDE FIXATION (AT THE DAY OF STAINING)

6. Air-dry frozen sections for at least 30 min.
7. Fix for 10 min in 4% formaldehyde in PBS (freshly diluted).
8. Water for 30 min with tap water and afterward for 5 min with aqua dest.

3.3.2. Staining

9. Freshly prepare the following stock solutions.
   a. 5% New Fuchsin solution (dissolve 30 mg New Fuchsin in 600 µL of 2 *N* HCl).
   b. 4% Sodium nitrite (dissolve 24 mg sodium nitrite in 600 µL H$_2$O).The solution can be stored at 4°C for 1 wk.
   c. 0.5 *M* Naphthol-AS-BI β-D-glucuronide pH 5 (dissolve 11 g Naphthol-AS-BI β-D-glucuronide in 20 mL of 0.2 *M* sodium acetate buffer pH 5 and add 20 ml H$_2$O).
10. Prepare the staining solution (should be used within 1 h):

	Stock solution	Final concentration
New Fuchsin	600 μL	2 mM
Sodium nitrite	600 μL	
	Mix and add to	
Naphthol–glucuronide	40 mL	0.5 mM
± Inhibitor:		
saccherolactone	2.1 mg/mL	10 mM

11. Cover tissue with staining solution and incubate at 45°–50°C (water bath) for 90 min.
12. Rinse with aqua dest.
13. Stain with hematoxylin for 90 s (or 5–7 min with hematoxylin diluted 1:10 in H$_2$O).
14. Water for 10 min with tap water and afterward for 10 min with aqua dest.
15. Air-dry.
16. Mount with Mowiol.

An example of this staining technique is shown in **Fig. 6**.

3.4. ELF-97 β-ᴅ-Glucuronide for Fluorimetric Staining of Histological Sections

Upon hydrolysis of ELF-97 β-ᴅ-glucuronide (*see* **Fig. 7**), this fluorogenic substrate produces a bright yellow-green fluorescent precipitate at the site of enzymatic activity. ELF-97 staining can be visualized using a fluorescence microscope equipped with a standard Hoechst/DAPI long-pass optical filter set. It is very photostable. Because the ELF-97 and Hoechst/DAPI fluorescence have distinct emission spectra, the two signals can be distinguished easily.

3.4.1. Fixation of Frozen Tissue Sections

1. Fix frozen tissue sections in 4% formaldehyde in PBS for 30 min.
2. Rinse in distilled water for at least 20 min.

3.4.2. Staining and Post Fixation

3. Freshly prepare the following solutions:
   a. Substrate solution: 0.25 mM ELF-97 β-ᴅ-glucuronide in sodium acetate buffer. Filtrate solution, for examples, with Millex columns from Millipore, SLGV 004 SL, PVDF membrane. For further details on ELF-97, we refer to Molecular Probes.
   b. Post fix solution: 2% formaldehyde, 2% BSA, in PBS.
   c. Hoechst 33258 solution for staining nuclei *(optional)*: Dilute Hoechst 33258 stock solution 1/1000 in PBS (final concentration: 2 μM).
4. Cover slides with sodium acetate buffer.
5. Tap off excess buffer.
6. Cover tissue with substrate solution.
7. Incubate at 37°C for 10 – 30 min.
8. Remove substrate solution.
9. Rinse briefly in distilled water (< 1 min).
10. Post fix for 30 min.

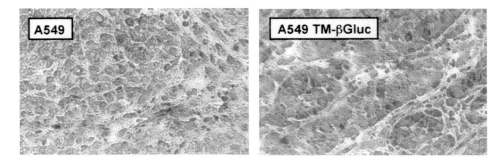

Fig. 6. Activity of β-glucuronidase in cryosections of tumors grown in nude mice after subcutaneous inoculation of control A549 lung carcinoma cells or TM-βGluc expressing A549 cells. β-Glucuronidase activity was visualized by the deposition of the water-insoluble red naphthol–New Fuchsin dye complex.

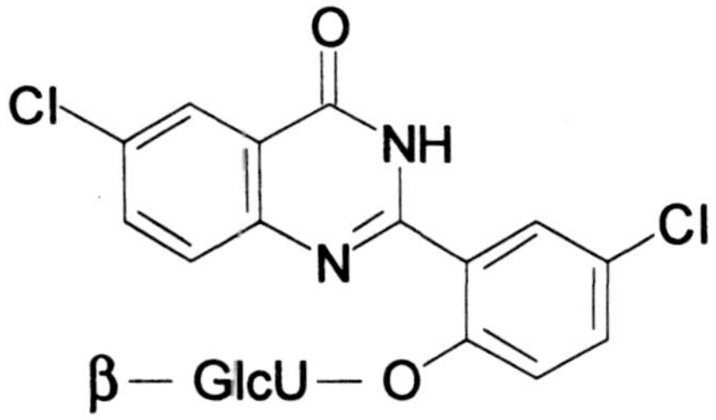

Fig. 7. Chemical structure of ELF-97 b-D-glucuronide.

11. Rinse twice with PBS.
12. Incubate for 5 – 10 min with Hoechst 33258 solution.
13. Rinse twice with PBS.
14. Rinse briefly in distilled water (< 1 min).
15. Cover with water based embedding solution (e.g. Mowiol).

An example of this staining technique is shown in **Fig. 8**.

3.5. 4-Methylumbelliferyl β-D-Glucuronic Acid for Fluorimetric Quantification

A sensitive fluorogenic assay to measure β-glucuronidase activity can be performed with the substrate 4-methylumbelliferyl β-D-glucuronic acid (4-MUG; *see* **Fig. 9**) *(96)*. It is used to detect enzymatic activity in cell culture supernatants, lysates, and organ homogenates. β-Glucuronidase hydrolyzes 4-MUG to the fluorochrome 4-methylumbelliferone and glucuronic acid. The fluorochrome can be excited at 350 nm and emission is measured at 455 nm. The fluorescence of 4-methylumbelliferone is pH sensitive as a result of the equilibrium between phenolic and phenoxide forms. The phenoxide form, which prevails at higher pH values, gives rise to maximal fluo-

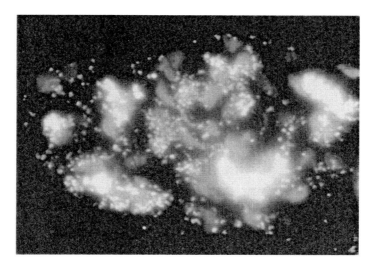

Fig. 8. Cryosections of JEG-3 choriocarcinoma tumors expressing β-glucuronidase transgene stained with ELF-97 β-D-glucuronide.

rescence. Therefore, the stop solution used to inhibit enzymatic activity by shifting the reaction conditions to higher pH values also leads to an increase in fluorescence intensity of the reaction product 4-methylumbelliferone. Standard solutions with the product 4-methylumbelliferone (4-MU) can be used to calibrate the data (*see* **Note 8**).

The amounts of enzymatically active β-glucuronidase extracted from cells in culture or from organs can be determined using the organ enzyme activity test (OEAT) *(5)*, a solid-phase enzyme-linked immunosorbent assay. The enzyme is indirectly attached to a surface via a coated human β-glucuronidase-specific antibody directed against the native enzyme. Afterward, the enzymatic activity is determined by 4-MUG conversion and measurement of fluorescence intensity.

3.5.1. Preparation of Cell or Organ Extracts

3.5.1.1. CELL EXTRACTS

1. Wash cells twice with PBS.
2. Lyse cells in 0.5% sodium deoxycholate (250 μL/3-cm dish) (go to **step 8**).

3.5.1.2. ORGAN EXTRACTS

1. Sacrifice animal.
2. Remove organ and weigh.
3. Add 2 mL BSA buffer.
4. Homogenize organs (5 mL potter).
5. Adjust to pH 4.2.
6. Centrifuge at 16,000*g* for 30 min.
7. Neutralize supernatant with 0.1 *N* NaOH.

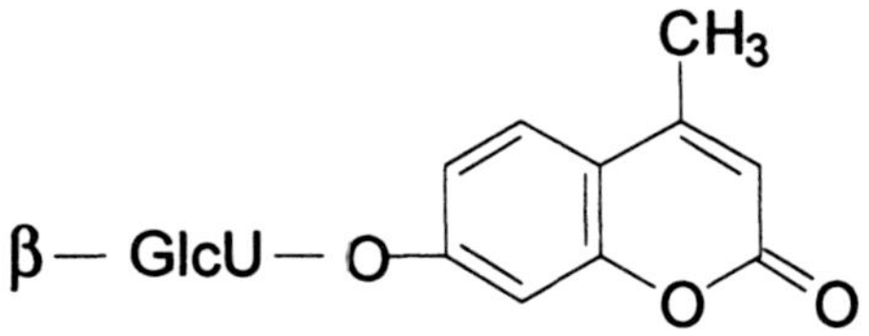

$$CH_3$$

$$\beta - GlcU - O \cdots$$

Fig. 9. Chemical structure of 4-methylumbelliferyl β-D-glucuronic acid.

3.5.2. Solid-Phase Enzyme-Linked Immunosorbent Assay

8. Freshly prepare the following solutions:
   a. Substrate solution: 2.5 mM 4-methylumbelliferyl β-D-glucuronic acid in sodium acetate buffer -/+ 10 mM saccherolactone.
   b. Standard: 2.5 mM 4-methylumbelliferone in sodium acetate buffer.
9. Coat antibody to flat-bottomed microtiter plates (depending on the source of the antibody, the amount of hybridoma supernatant or purified antibody has to be titrated; free-binding sites should not be limiting).
10. Wash three times with PBS.
11. Block nonspecific sites with 2% skim milk or 1% casein in PBS for at least 30 min at room temperature.
12. Wash three times with PBS.
13. Add 50 μL of β-glucuronidase-containing sample and incubate for 30 min at room temperature (*see* **Notes 9** and **10**). Use extraction buffer as blank value.
14. Wash extensively (at least five times) with PBS.
15. Add 50 μL of substrate solution and incubate for appropriate length of time at 37°C. The assay is linear over a broad time period (*see* **Note 9**).
16. Add 100 μl stop solution.
17. For quantification, prepare serial dilutions of the standard and add 100 μL stop solution.
18. Measure fluorescence: excitation at 350 nm and emission at 455 nm.

3.6. N-(4-β-Glucuronyl-3-Nitrobenzyloxycarbonyl)-Doxorubicin (HMR 1826) for Fluorimetric Staining of Transfected Cells

The prodrug *N*-(4-β-glucuronyl-3-nitrobenzyloxycarbonyl)-doxorubicin (HMR 1826; *see* **Fig. 10**) was developed by Florent et al. *(22)*. After cleavage of the glucuronic acid, the spacer is eliminated and the deliberated doxorubicin can pass cell membranes and intercalate into DNA. The nuclear autofluorescence of doxorubicin can be visualized under a fluorescence microscope. This staining method is not very sensitive and relatively high concentrations of prodrug have to be used to see nuclear fluorescence (5–15 μM). The advantage of this staining procedure is, however, the possibility to correlate prodrug conversion with β-glucuronidase expression detected by indirect immunofluorescence, to visualize the induction of apoptosis (nuclei with condensed chromatin), and to demonstrate a bystander effect.

1. Cover (transfected) cells with 5–15 μM of β-glucuronyl-doxorubicin prodrug in DMEM with reduced carbonate concentration (*see* **Notes 3** and **4**).

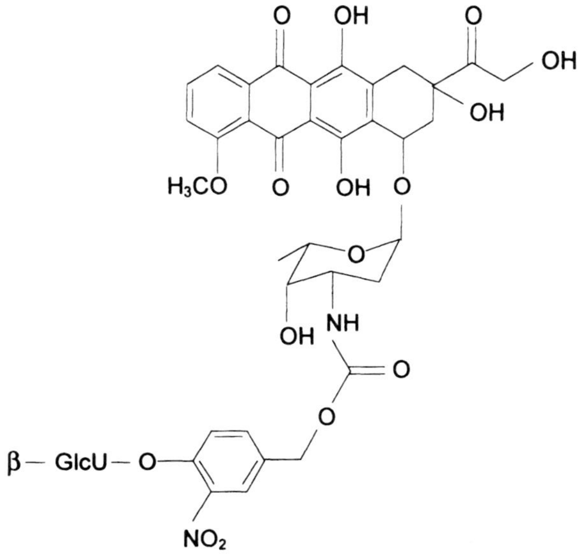

Fig. 10. Chemical structure of HMR 1826. (From refs. 5 and 22).

2. Incubate for 12–24 h at 37°C, 89% humidity, 7% CO_2 (with 1.2 g/L carbonate and 7% CO_2; the pH of the medium should be 7.0).
3. Wash three times with PBS.
4. Fix cells for 15 min with 4% formaldehyde in PBS.

Optional: Indirect immunofluorescence to detect β-glucuronidase expressing cells (**steps 5–10**).

5. Incubate with 0.2% Triton X-100 for 5 min.
6. Wash three times with PBS.
7. Incubate with first antibody diluted in PBS/0.5% Tween-20/0.5% BSA for at least 45 min.
8. Wash three times with PBS.
9. Incubate with second antibody diluted in PBS/ 0.5% Tween-20/ 0.5% BSA for at least 45 min.
10. Wash three times with PBS.

Optional: Staining of nuclei with Hoechst 33258 (**steps 11–13**).

11. Dilute Hoechst 33258 stock solution 1/1000 in PBS (final concentration: 2 μM).
12. Incubate with Hoechst 33258 for 5 min at RT.
13. Wash three times with PBS.
14. Rinse briefly in distilled water (< 1 min).
15. Cover with water based embedding solution (e.g. Mowiol).

An example of this staining technique is shown in **Fig. 11**. For additional literature about methods for β-glucuronidase detection is mentioned in **Note 11**.

4. Notes

1. We recommend adding protease inhibitors to RIPA buffer for lysis of the cells. Washing steps can be performed without the addition of protease inhibitors. In order to prevent

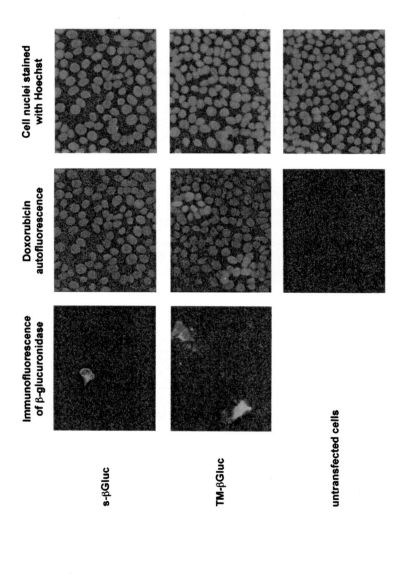

Fig. 11. Autofluorescence of doxorubicin intercalating into the DNA after extracellular prodrug cleavage. Two days after transfection with s-βGluc and TM-βGluc, cells were incubated for 16 h with 15 mM of the β-glucuronyl-doxorubicin prodrug HMR 1826 (obtained from Aventis-Pharma). Converted prodrug is seen as red doxorubicin autofluorescence. Transfected cells were detected by indirect immunofluorescence (green) and cell nuclei were visualized by staining with Hoechst 33258 (blue).

322

    protein degradation, it is more important to keep the sample on ice and to use precooled buffers rather than adding protease inhibitors.

2. We used the hybridoma supernatant 2118/157 from Aventis. This antibody is not commercially available.

3. In contrast to the substrate reactions mentioned earlier, which are performed in acetate buffer pH 5, the cleavage reaction of the prodrug HMR 1826 in this assay is carried out under more physiological conditions. Therefore, the pH of the cell culture medium needs special attention. The commonly used Dulbecco's modified Eagle's medium contains 3.7 g/L carbonate to buffer the acidic cell metabolites. In cell culture incubators with 5–10% CO_2 the pH of DMEM is between 7.6 at 5% and 7.3 at 10% CO_2. In order to achieve a physiological pH around 7, the carbonate concentration has to be reduced to 1.2 g/L and the CO_2 concentration must be adjusted to 7%. If it is necessary to use another cell culture medium, optimal carbonate and CO_2 concentrations have to be determined. An increase in CO_2 raises the H^+ concentration, an increase in HCO_3^- leads to a reduction of H^+.

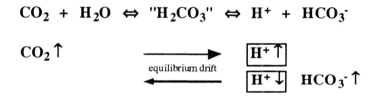

$$CO_2 + H_2O \Leftrightarrow \text{"}H_2CO_3\text{"} \Leftrightarrow H^+ + HCO_3^-$$

4. Concentrated minimal essential medium without carbonate (10 times concentrated MEM without $NaHCO_3$, e.g., Invitrogen 21430, Bio Whittaker 12-684) can be used to prepare a medium with reduced carbonate concentration. Dilute the stock medium in water (tissue culture grade) and add $NaCO_3$ as mentioned earlier.

5. The fixation method is very important for this relatively insensitive staining technique. An example of X-gluc staining of histological sections and the influence of the fixation method is shown in **Fig. 4**. Fixation of frozen sections (obtained from the same tumor) in formaldehyde gas (**Fig. 4A,B**) retains enzymatic activity much better than short incubation times in formaldehyde solution (**Fig. 4C**).

6. Matsumura et al. *(91)* have generated a glutaraldehyde resistant form of *E. coli* β-glucuronidase. No similar variant is known for the human form.

7. We recommend growing cells on cover slips and mounting the cells with, for example, Mowiol for long-term storage.

8. For quantification of enzymatic activity standard solutions with the product 4-MU can be used. One unit of enzyme activity is defined as the release of 1 nmol of 4-MU per hour. The pH of the standard has to be the same as the sample because of the pH-dependent fluorescence of 4-MU.

9. Different sample volumes can be used to ensure that the assay is linear with respect to β-glucuronidase concentration. Multiple time points (30 min to 24 h) can be used to show that the assay is linear with respect to time.

10. The assay can be used to determine β-glucuronidase activity in samples without prior binding to a solid phase bound antibody. In this case 5–25 mL of sample is mixed with 100 μL of substrate solution. When testing highly buffered solutions, like cell culture supernatant, the ratio of sample volume to substrate solution has to be reduced to ensure

optimal pH conditions for β-glucuronidase activity. The advantage of the OAET assay is that the substrate solution is added after removal of the sample extract and, therefore, the pH of the reaction buffer is constant and independent of sample preparation.

11. Additional Literature:
1. High-performance liquid chromatography (HPLC) of doxorubicin and doxorubicin prodrugs: (**refs. 5, 15, 21, 97**).
2. Fluorescence-activated cell-sorter-based assay for the quantitative analysis of β-glucuronidase activity in viable cells with the substrate fluorescein-di-β-D-glucuronide (FDGluc): (**refs. 98** and **99**).
3. For an overview about prodrug activating systems, I recommended *Enzyme–Prodrug Strategies for Cancer Therapy (100)*, and for addition technical advice, *GUS Protocols: Using the GUS Gene as a Reporter of Gene Expression (101)*.

Acknowledgments

I am grateful to Rolf Müller and Dagmar Heine for critically reading the manuscript and valuable suggestions, to Manfred Gerken and Hans-Harald Sedlacek (Aventis-Pharma) for prodrug HMR 1826, and to Klaus Bosslet for the monoclonal antibodies to β-glucuronidase, helpful discussions and advice. This work was supported by a grant from the Deutsche Forschungsgemeinschaft to SB (BR 1857/2).

References

1. Sharma, S. K., Bagshawe, K. D., Melton, R. G., and Sherwood, R. F. (1992) Human immune response to monoclonal antibody-enzyme conjugates in ADEPT pilot clinical trial. *Cell Biophys.* **21**, 109–120.
2. Achord, D. T., Brot, F. E., Bell, C. E., and Sly, W. S. (1978) Human beta–glucuronidase: in vivo clearance and in vitro uptake by a glycoprotein recognition system on reticuloendothelial cells. *Cell* **15**, 269–278.
3. Schlesinger, P. H., Rodman, J. S., Doebber, T. W., et al. (1980) The role of extra-hepatic tissues in the receptor-mediated plasma clearance of glycoproteins terminated by mannose or N-acetylglucosamine. *Biochemi. J.* **192**, 597–606.
4. Bosslet, K., Czech, J., Lorenz, P., Sedlacek, H. H., Schuermann, M., and Seemann, G. (1992) Molecular and functional characterisation of a fusion protein suited for tumor specific prodrug activation. *Br. J. Cancer.* **65**, 234–238.
5. Bosslet, K., Czech, J., and Hoffmann, D. (1994) Tumor-selective prodrug activation by fusion protein-mediated catalysis. *Cancer Res.* **54**, 2151–2159.
6. Houba, P. H., Boven, E., and Haisma, H. J. (1996) Improved characteristics of a human beta-glucuronidase-antibody conjugate after deglycosylation for use in antibody-directed enzyme–prodrug therapy. *Bioconjug. Chem.* **7**, 606–611.
7. Haisma, H. J., Sernee, M. F., Hooijberg, E., et al. (1998) Construction and characterization of a fusion protein of single-chain anti-CD20 antibody and human beta-glucuronidase for antibody-directed enzyme–prodrug therapy. *Blood* **92**, 184–190.
8. Houba, P. H., Boven, E., van der Meulen-Muileman, I. H., et al. (2001) Pronounced anti-tumor efficacy of doxorubicin when given as the prodrug DOX-GA3 in combination with a monoclonal antibody beta-glucuronidase conjugate. *Int. J. Cancer.* **91**, 550–554.
9. Weyel, D., Sedlacek, H. H., Müller, R., and Brüsselbach, S. (2000) Secreted human beta-glucuronidase: a novel tool for gene-directed enzyme–prodrug therapy. *Gene Ther.* **7**, 224–231.

10. Heine, D., Müller, R., and Brüsselbach, S. (2001) Cell surface display of a lysosomal enzyme for extracellular gene-directed enzyme–prodrug therapy. *Gene Ther.* **8,** 1005–1010.
11. Haisma, H. J., Boven, E., van Muijen, M., de Jong, J., van der Vijgh, W. J., and Pinedo, H. M. (1992) A monoclonal antibody-beta-glucuronidase conjugate as activator of the prodrug epirubicin-glucuronide for specific treatment of cancer. *Br. J. Cancer.* **66,** 474–478.
12. Haisma, H. J., van Muijen, M., Pinedo, H. M., and Boven, E. (1994) Comparison of two anthracycline-based prodrugs for activation by a monoclonal antibody-beta-glucuronidase conjugate in the specific treatment of cancer. *Cell Biophys.* **25,** 185–192.
13. Houba, P. H., Leenders, R. G., Boven, E., Scheeren, J. W., Pinedo, H. M., and Haisma, H. J. (1996) Characterization of novel anthracycline prodrugs activated by human beta-glucuronidase for use in antibody-directed enzyme–prodrug therapy. *Biochem Pharmacol.* **52,** 455–463.
14. Houba, P. H., Boven, E., Erkelens, C. A., et al. (1998) The efficacy of the anthracycline prodrug daunorubicin-GA3 in human ovarian cancer xenografts. *Br. J. Cancer.* **78,** 1600–1606.
15. Houba, P. H., Boven, E., van der Meulen-Muileman, I. H., Leenders, R. G., Scheeren, J. W., Pinedo, H. M., and Haisma, H. J. (1999) Distribution and pharmacokinetics of the prodrug daunorubicin-GA3 in nude mice bearing human ovarian cancer xenografts. *Biochem. Pharmacol.* **57,** 673–680.
16. Leenders, R. G., Damen, E. W., Bijsterveld, E. J., et al. (1999) Novel anthracycline-spacer-beta-glucuronide,-beta-glucoside, and -beta- galactoside prodrugs for application in selective chemotherapy. *Bioorg. Med. Chem.* **7,** 1597–1610.
17. Houba, P. H., Boven, E., van der Meulen-Muileman, I. H., et al. (2001) A novel doxorubicin-glucuronide prodrug DOX-GA3 for tumour-selective chemotherapy: distribution and efficacy in experimental human ovarian cancer. *Br. J. Cancer.* **84,** 550–557.
18. Bosslet, K., Czech, J., and Hoffmann, D. (1995) A novel one-step tumor-selective prodrug activation system. *Tumor Target.* **1,** 45–50.
19. Bosslet, K., Straub, R., Blumrich, M., et al. (1998) Elucidation of the mechanism enabling tumor selective prodrug monotherapy. *Cancer Res.* **58,** 1195–1201.
20. Bosslet, K., Czech, J., Seemann, G., Monneret, C., and Hoffmann, D. (1994) Fusion protein mediated prodrug activation (FMPA) in vivo. *Cell Biophys.* **25,** 51–63.
21. Murdter, T. E., Sperker, B., Kivisto, K. T., et al. (1997) Enhanced uptake of doxorubicin into bronchial carcinoma: beta- glucuronidase mediates release of doxorubicin from a glucuronide prodrug (HMR 1826) at the tumor site. *Cancer Res.* **57,** 2440–2445.
22. Florent, J. C., Dong, X., Gaudel, G., et al. (1998) Prodrugs of anthracyclines for use in antibody-directed enzyme–prodrug therapy. *J. Med. Chem.* **41,** 3572–3581.
23. Bakina, E., Wu, Z., Rosenblum, M., and Farquhar, D. (1997) Intensely cytotoxic anthracycline prodrugs: glucuronides. *J. Med. Chem.* **40,** 4013–4018.
24. Desbene, S., Van, H. D., Michel, S., et al. (1998) Doxorubicin prodrugs with reduced cytotoxicity suited for tumour- specific activation. Anticancer Drug Des. 13, 955–968.
25. Papot, S., Combaud, D., and Gesson, J. P. (1998) A new spacer group derived from arylmalonaldehydes for glucuronylated prodrugs. *Bioorg. Med. Chem. Lett.* **8,** 2545–2548.
26. Roffler, S. R., Wang, S. M., Chern, J. W., Yeh, M. Y., and Tung, E. (1991) Anti-neoplastic glucuronide prodrug treatment of human tumor cells targeted with a monoclonal antibody-enzyme conjugate. *Biochemi. Pharmacol.* **42,** 2062–2065.
27. Wang, S. M., Chern, J. W., Yeh, M. Y., Ng, J. C., Tung, E., and Roffler, S. R. (1992) Specific activation of glucuronide prodrugs by antibody-targeted enzyme conjugates for cancer therapy. *Cancer Res.* **52,** 4484–4491.

28. Lougerstay-Madec, R., Florent, J. C., Monneret, C., Nemati, F., and Poupon, M. F. (1998) Synthesis of self-immolative glucuronide-based prodrugs of a phenol mustard. *Anticancer Drug Des.* **13,** 995–1007.

29. Papot, S., Combaud, D., Bosslet, K., Gerken, M., Czech, J., and Gesson, J. P. (2000) Synthesis and cytotoxic activity of a glucuronylated prodrug of nornitrogen mustard. *Bioorg. Med. Chem. Lett.* **10,** 1835–1837.

30. Tietze, L. F., Seele, R., Leiting, B., and Krach, T. (1988) Stereoselective synthesis of (1-alkoxyalkyl) alpha- and beta-D-glucopyranosiduronates (acetal-glucopyranosiduronates): a new approach to specific cytostatics for the treatment of cancer. *Carbohydr. Res.* **180,** 253–262.

31. Albrecht, C. F., Theron, E. J., and Kruger, P. B. (1995) Morphological characterisation of the cell-growth inhibitory activity of rooperol and pharmacokinetic aspects of hypoxoside as an oral prodrug for cancer therapy. *S. Afr. Med. J.* **85,** 853–860.

32. de Bont, D. B., Leenders, R. G., Haisma, H. J., van der Meulen-Muileman, I., and Scheeren, H. W. (1997) Synthesis and biological activity of beta-glucuronyl carbamate-based prodrugs of paclitaxel as potential candidates for ADEPT. *Bioorg. Med. Chem.* **5,** 405–414.

33. Leu, Y. L., Roffler, S. R., and Chern, J. W. (1999) Design and synthesis of water-soluble glucuronide derivatives of camptothecin for cancer prodrug monotherapy and antibody-directed enzyme–prodrug therapy (ADEPT). *J. Med. Chem.* **42,** 3623–3628.

34. Guerquin-Kern, J. L., Volk, A., Chenu, E., et al. (2000) Direct in vivo observation of 5-fluorouracil release from a prodrug in human tumors heterotransplanted in nude mice: a magnetic resonance study. *NMR Biomed.* **13,** 306–310.

35. Desbene, S., Van, H. D., Michel, S., et al. (1999) Application of the ADEPT strategy to the MDR resistance in cancer chemotherapy. *Anticancer Drug Des.* **14,** 93–106.

36. Connors, T. A. and Whisson, M. E. (1966) Cure of mice bearing advanced plasma cell tumours with aniline mustard: the relationship between glucuronidase activity and tumour sensitivity. *Nature* **210,** 866–867.

37. Boyer, M. J. and Tannock, I. F. (1993) Lysosomes, lysosomal enzymes, and cancer. *Adv Cancer Res.* **60,** 269–291.

38. Paigen, K. (1989) Mammalian beta-glucuronidase: genetics, molecular biology, and cell biology. *Prog. Nucleic Acid. Res. Mol. Biol.* **37,** 155–205.

39. Brot, F. E., Bell, C. E., Jr., and Sly, W. S. (1978) Purification and properties of beta-glucuronidase from human placenta. Biochemistry 17, 385–391.

40. Jain, S., Drendel, W. B., Chen, Z. W., Mathews, F. S., Sly, W. S., and Grubb, J. H. (1996) Structure of human beta-glucuronidase reveals candidate lysosomal targeting and active-site motifs. *Nat. Struct. Biol.* **3,** 375–381.

41. Wong, A. W., He, S., Grubb, J. H., Sly, W. S., and Withers, S. G. (1998) Identification of Glu-540 as the catalytic nucleophile of human beta-glucuronidase using electrospray mass spectrometry. *J. Biol Chem.* **273,** 34,057–34,062.

42. Islam, M. R., Tomatsu, S., Shah, G. N., Grubb, J. H., Jain, S., and Sly, W. S. (1999) Active site residues of human beta-glucuronidase. Evidence for Glu(540) as the nucleophile and Glu(451) as the acid-base residue. *J. Biol. Chem.* **274,** 23,451–23,455.

43. Rosenfeld, M. G., Kreibich, G., Popov, D., Kato, K., and Sabatini, D. D. (1982) Biosynthesis of lysosomal hydrolases: their synthesis in bound polysomes and the role of co- and post-translational processing in determining their subcellular distribution. *J. Cell Biol.* **93,** 135–143.

44. Shipley, J. M., Grubb, J. H., and Sly, W. S. (1993) The role of glycosylation and phosphorylation in the expression of active human beta-glucuronidase. *J. Biol. Chem.* **268,** 12,193–12,198.
45. Islam, M. R., Grubb, J. H., and Sly, W. S. (1993) C-terminal processing of human beta-glucuronidase. The propeptide is required for full expression of catalytic activity, intracellular retention, and proper phosphorylation. *J. Biol. Chem.* **268,** 22,627–22,633.
46. Oshima, A., Kyle, J. W., Miller, R. D., et al. (1987) Cloning, sequencing, and expression of cDNA for human beta- glucuronidase. *Proc. Natl. Acad. Sci. USA.* **84,** 685–689.
47. Miller, R. D., Hoffmann, J. W., Powell, P. P., et al. (1990) Cloning and characterization of the human beta-glucuronidase gene. *Genomics.* **7,** 280–283.
48. Caygill, J. C. and Pitkeathly, D. A. (1966) A study of beta-acetylglucosaminase and acid phosphatase in pathological joint fluids. *Ann. Rheum. Dis.* **25,** 137–144.
49. Weissmann, G., Zurier, R. B., Spieler, P. J., and Goldstein, I. M. (1971) Mechanisms of lysosomal enzyme release from leukocytes exposed to immune complexes and other particles. *J. Exp. Med.* **134(Suppl.)** 149s.
50. Philpott, G. W., Bower, R. J., and Parker, C. W. (1973) Selective iodination and cytotoxicity of tumor cells with an antibody- enzyme conjugate. *Surgery.* **74,** 51–58.
51. Philpott, G. W., Shearer, W. T., Bower, R. J., and Parker, C. W. (1973) Selective cytotoxicity of hapten-substituted cells with an antibody- enzyme conjugate. *J. Immunol.* **111,** 921–929.
52. Bagshawe, K. D., Sharma, S. K., Springer, C. J., Antoniw, P., Boden, J. A., Rogers, G. T., Burke, P. J., Melton, R. G., and Sherwood, R. F. (1991) Antibody directed enzyme–prodrug therapy (ADEPT): clinical report. *Dis. Markers* **9,** 233–238.
53. Marais, R., Spooner, R. A., Stribbling, S. M., Light, Y., Martin, J., and Springer, C. J. (1997) A cell surface tethered enzyme improves efficiency in gene-directed enzyme–prodrug therapy. *Nature Biotechnol.* **15,** 1373–1377.
54. Sly, W. S., Quinton, B. A., McAlister, W. H., and Rimoin, D. L. (1973) Beta-glucuronidase deficiency: report of clinical, radiologic, and biochemical features of a new mucopolysaccharidosis. *J. Pediatr.* **82,** 249–257.
55. Brady, R. O. (1982) Lysosomal storage diseases. *Pharmacol. Ther.* **19,** 327–336.
56. Neufeld, E. F. and Muenzer, J. (1989) The mucopolysaccharidoses, in *The Metabolic Basis of Inherited Disease* (Scriver, C. R., Beaudet, A. L., Sly, W. S., and Valle, D., eds.), McGraw-Hill, New York, pp. 1565–1587.
57. Caillaud, C. and Poenaru, L. (2000) Gene therapy in lysosomal diseases. *Biomed. Pharmacother.* **54,** 505–512.
58. Sly, W. S. and Vogler, C. (1997) Gene therapy for lysosomal storage disease: a no-brainer? Transplants of fibroblasts secreting high levels of beta-glucuronidase decrease lesions in the brains of mice with Sly syndrome, a lysosomal storage disease. *Nature Med.* **3,** 719–720.
59. Birkenmeier, E. H., Davisson, M. T., Beamer, W. G., et al. (1989) Murine mucopolysaccharidosis type VII. Characterization of a mouse with beta-glucuronidase deficiency. *J. Clin. Invest.* **83,** 1258–1256.
60. Vogler, C., Birkenmeier, E. H., Sly, W. S. et al. (1990) A murine model of mucopolysaccharidosis VII. Gross and microscopic findings in beta-glucuronidase-deficient mice. *Am. J. Pathol.* **136,** 207–217.
61. Sands, M. S. and Birkenmeier, E. H. (1993) A single-base-pair deletion in the beta-glucuronidase gene accounts for the phenotype of murine mucopolysaccharidosis type VII. *Proc. Natl. Acad. Sci. USA.* **90,** 6567–6571.

62. Pastores, G. M., Sibille, A. R., and Grabowski, G. A. (1993) Enzyme therapy in Gaucher disease type 1: dosage efficacy and adverse effects in 33 patients treated for 6 to 24 months. *Blood* **82,** 408-416.
63. Sibille, A., Eng, C. M., Kim, S. J., Pastores, G., and Grabowski, G. A. (1993) Phenotype/ genotype correlations in Gaucher disease type I: clinical and therapeutic implications. *Am. J. Hum. Genet.* **52,** 1094–1101.
64. Vogler, C., Sands, M., Higgins, A., Levy, B., Grubb, J., Birkenmeier, E. H., and Sly, W. S. (1993) Enzyme replacement with recombinant beta-glucuronidase in the newborn mucopolysaccharidosis type VII mouse. *Pediatr. Res.* **34,** 837–840.
65. Sands, M. S., Vogler, C., Kyle, J. W., et al. (1994) Enzyme replacement therapy for murine mucopolysaccharidosis type VII. *J. Clin. Invest.* **93,** 2324–2331.
66. Vogler, C., Sands, M. S., Levy, B., Galvin, N., Birkenmeier, E. H., and Sly, W. S. (1996) Enzyme replacement with recombinant beta-glucuronidase in murine mucopolysaccharidosis type VII: impact of therapy during the first six weeks of life on subsequent lysosomal storage, growth, and survival. *Pediatr. Res.* **39,** 1050–1054.
67. Sands, M. S., Vogler, C., Torrey, A., et al. (1997) Murine mucopolysaccharidosis type VII: long term therapeutic effects of enzyme replacement and enzyme replacement followed by bone marrow transplantation. *J. Clin. Invest.* **99,** 1596–1605.
68. O'Connor, L. H., Erway, L. C., Vogler, C. A., et al. (1998) Enzyme replacement therapy for murine mucopolysaccharidosis type VII leads to improvements in behavior and auditory function. *J. Clin. Invest.* **101,** 1394–1400.
69. Vogler, C., Levy, B., Galvin, N. J., et al. (1999) Enzyme replacement in murine mucopolysaccharidosis type VII: neuronal and glial response to beta-glucuronidase requires early initiation of enzyme replacement therapy. *Pediatr. Res.* **45,** 838–844.
70. Birkenmeier, E. H., Barker, J. E., Vogler, C. A., et al. (1991) Increased life span and correction of metabolic defects in murine mucopolysaccharidosis type VII after syngeneic bone marrow transplantation. *Blood* **78,** 3081–3092.
71. Sands, M. S., Barker, J. E., Vogler, C., et al. (1993) Treatment of murine mucopolysaccharidosis type VII by syngeneic bone marrow transplantation in neonates. *Lab. Invest.* **68,** 676–686.
72. Bastedo, L., Sands, M. S., Lambert, D. T., Pisa, M. A., Birkenmeier, E., and Chang, P. L. (1994) Behavioral consequences of bone marrow transplantation in the treatment of murine mucopolysaccharidosis type VII. *J. Clin. Invest.* **94,** 1180–1186.
73. Sands, M. S., Erway, L. C., Vogler, C., Sly, W. S., and Birkenmeier, E. H. (1995) Syngeneic bone marrow transplantation reduces the hearing loss associated with murine mucopolysaccharidosis type VII. *Blood* **86,** 2033–2040.
74. Ohlemiller, K. K., Vogler, C. A., Roberts, M., Galvin, N., and Sands, M. S. (2000) Retinal function is improved in a murine model of a lysosomal storage disease following bone marrow transplantation. *Exp. Eye Res.* **71,** 469–481.
75. Birkenmeier, E. H. (1991) Correction of murine mucopolysaccharidosis type VII (MPS VII) by bone marrow transplantation and gene transfer therapy. *Hum. Gene Ther.* **2,** 113.
76. Wolfe, J. H., Sands, M. S., Barker, J. E., et al. (1992) Reversal of pathology in murine mucopolysaccharidosis type VII by somatic cell gene transfer. *Nature* **360,** 749–753.
77. Marechal, V., Naffakh, N., Danos, O., and Heard, J. M. (1993) Disappearance of lysosomal storage in spleen and liver of mucopolysaccharidosis VII mice after transplantation of genetically modified bone marrow cells. *Blood* **82,** 1358–1365.
78. Moullier, P., Bohl, D., Heard, J. M., and Danos, O. (1993) Correction of lysosomal storage in the liver and spleen of MPS VII mice by implantation of genetically modified skin fibroblasts. *Nat. Genet.* **4,** 154–159.

79. Snyder, E. Y., Taylor, R. M., and Wolfe, J. H. (1995) Neural progenitor cell engraftment corrects lysosomal storage throughout the MPS VII mouse brain. *Nature.* 374, 367–370.

80. Taylor, R. M. and Wolfe, J. H. (1997) Decreased lysosomal storage in the adult MPS VII mouse brain in the vicinity of grafts of retroviral vector-corrected fibroblasts secreting high levels of beta-glucuronidase. *Nature Med.* 3, 771–774.

81. Ohashi, T., Watabe, K., Uehara, K., Sly, W. S., Vogler, C., and Eto, Y. (1997) Adenovirus-mediated gene transfer and expression of human beta- glucuronidase gene in the liver, spleen, and central nervous system in mucopolysaccharidosis type VII mice. *Proc. Natl. Acad. Sci. USA.* 94, 1287–1292.

82. Stein, C. S., Ghodsi, A., Derksen, T., and Davidson, B. L. (1999) Systemic and central nervous system correction of lysosomal storage in mucopolysaccharidosis type VII mice. *J. Virol.* 73, 3424–3429.

83. Watson, G. L., Sayles, J. N., Chen, C., Elliger, S. S., Elliger, C. A., Raju, N. R., Kurtzman, G. J., and Podsakoff, G. M. (1998) Treatment of lysosomal storage disease in MPS VII mice using a recombinant adeno-associated virus. *Gene Ther.* 5, 1642–1649.

84. Ghodsi, A., Stein, C., Derksen, T., Yang, G., Anderson, R. D., and Davidson, B. L. (1998) Extensive beta-glucuronidase activity in murine central nervous system after adenovirus-mediated gene transfer to brain. *Hum. Gene Ther.* 9, 2331–2340.

85. Skorupa, A. F., Fisher, K. J., Wilson, J. M., Parente, M. K., and Wolfe, J. H. (1999) Sustained production of beta-glucuronidase from localized sites after AAV vector gene transfer results in widespread distribution of enzyme and reversal of lysosomal storage lesions in a large volume of brain in mucopolysaccharidosis VII mice. *Exp. Neurol.* 160, 17–27.

86. Elliger, S. S., Elliger, C. A., Aguilar, C. P., Raju, N. R., and Watson, G. L. (1999) Elimination of lysosomal storage in brains of MPS VII mice treated by intrathecal administration of an adeno-associated virus vector. *Gene Ther.* 6, 1175–1178.

87. Bosch, A., Perret, E., Desmaris, N., and Heard, J. M. (2000) Long-term and significant correction of brain lesions in adult mucopolysaccharidosis type VII mice using recombinant AAV vectors. *Mol. Ther.* 1, 63–70.

88. Bosch, A., Perret, E., Desmaris, N., Trono, D., and Heard, J. M. (2000) Reversal of pathology in the entire brain of mucopolysaccharidosis type VII mice after lentivirus-mediated gene transfer. *Hum. Gene Ther.* 11, 1139–1150.

89. Stomp, A.-M. (1992) Histochemical localization of beta-glucuronidase, in *GUS Protocols: Using the GUS Gene as a Reporter of Gene Expression* (Gallagher, S. R., ed.) Academic, Press, Inc., San Diego, CA, pp. 103–113.

90. Lojda, Z. (1970) Indigogenic methods for glycosidases. II. An improved method for beta-D-galactosidase and its application to localization studies of the enzymes in the intestine and in other tissues. *Histochemie* 23, 266–288.

91. Matsumura, I., Wallingford, J. B., Surana, N. K., Vize, P. D., and Ellington, A. D. (1999) Directed evolution of the surface chemistry of the reporter enzyme beta-glucuronidase. *Nature Biotechnol.* 17, 696–701.

92. Fishman, W. H. and Goldman, S. S. (1965) A postcoupling technique for beta-glucuronidase employing the substrate, naphthol AS-BI-beta-D-glucosiduronic acid. *J. Histochem. Cytochem.* 13, 441–447.

93. Hayashi, M., Shirahama, T., and Cohen, A. S. (1968) Combined cytochemical and electron microscopic demonstration of beta- glucuronidase activity in rat liver with the use of a simultaneous coupling azo dye technique. *J. Cell Biol.* 36, 289–297.

94. Hayashi, M. (1977) Comments on the cytochemical techniques using naphthol AS-BI substrates and hexazonium pararosanilin for the demonstration of acid phosphatase, beta-

glucuronidase and N-acetyl-beta-glucosaminidase activities. *J. Histochem. Cytochem.* **25,** 1021–1023.

95. Murray, G. I., Burke, M. D., and Ewen, S. W. (1989) Enzyme histochemistry on freeze-dried, resin-embedded tissue. *J. Histochem. Cytochem.* **37,** 643–652.

96. Glaser, J. H. and Sly, W. S. (1973) Beta-glucuronidase deficiency mucopolysaccharidosis: methods for enzymatic diagnosis. *J. Lab. Clin. Med.* **82,** 969–977.

97. Sperker, B., Murdter, T. E., Schick, M., Eckhardt, K., Bosslet, K., and Kroemer, H. K. (1997) Interindividual variability in expression and activity of human beta- glucuronidase in liver and kidney: consequences for drug metabolism. *J. Pharmacol. Exp. Ther.* **281,** 914–920.

98. Lorincz, M., Roederer, M., Diwu, Z., Herzenberg, L. A., and Nolan, G. P. (1996) Enzyme-generated intracellular fluorescence for single-cell reporter gene analysis utilizing Escherichia coli beta-glucuronidase. *Cytometry* **24,** 321–329.

99. Lorincz, M. C., Parente, M. K., Roederer, M., et al. (1999) Single cell analysis and selection of living retrovirus vector- corrected mucopolysaccharidosis VII cells using a fluorescence- activated cell sorting-based assay for mammalian beta-glucuronidase enzymatic activity. *J. Biol. Chem.* **274,** 657–665.

100. Melton, R. G. and Knox, R. J. (eds.). (1999) Enzyme–Prodrug Strategies for Cancer Therapy. Kluwer Academic/Plenum, New York.

101. Gallagher, S. R. (ed.) (1992) *GUS Protocols: Using the GUS Gene as a Reporter of Gene Expression.* Academic, San Diego, CA.

16

Enhancement of Suicide Gene Prodrug Activation by Random Mutagenesis

Jean-Emmanuel Kurtz and Margaret E. Black

1. Introduction

Suicide gene therapy provides a mechanism for sensitizing cells to normally non-toxic compounds or prodrugs. Genes are introduced into cancer cells thereby rendering them sensitive to prodrugs by virtue of the activity of the suicide gene product toward the prodrugs. The most widely investigated suicide genes and their respective prodrugs are the herpes simplex virus type I (HSV-1)–thymidine kinase (TK) with ganciclovir (GCV) and the *Escherichia coli* cytosine deaminase with 5-fluorocytosine (5-FC). Unfortunately, attempts to achieve high levels of antitumor activity with these systems have not been fully successful.

A major problem associated with these suicide gene–prodrug combinations is the low affinity displayed by the gene product toward the prodrugs. As such, high levels of prodrugs must be administered in order to achieve cell killing. HSV-1–TK has a K_m of 47 μM for GCV compared to a K_m of 0.4 μM it displays toward its normal substrate, thymidine *(1)*. Similarly, the K_m that the *E. coli* cytosine deaminase displays toward 5-FC is quite high at 17.9 mM *(2)*. Although prodrugs used in the genetic prodrug activation systems have a mild systemic toxicity, the plasmatic levels required to obtain a significant amount of active metabolites may lead to adverse effects. This is observed with 5-FC, whereas deamination by cytosine deaminase of bacterial intestine flora into 5-fluorouracil (5-FU) is responsible for side effects *(3)*.

There are several possible ways of improving the prodrug activation that would also reduce the amount of prodrug required for tumor ablation. For example, one may want to screen related enzymes from different species. With cytosine deaminase, the *Saccharomyces cerevisiae* gene *(FCY1)* displays a lower K_m (0.8 mM) toward 5-FC compared to the bacterial cytosine deaminase *(4)*. Alternatively, overexpression of the enzyme may prove beneficial. With HSV-1–TK such attempts have resulted in cytotoxicity in the absence of prodrug, although such approaches lack a bystander effect

From: *Methods in Molecular Medicine, Vol. 90, Suicide Gene Therapy: Methods and Reviews*
Edited by: C. J. Springer © Humana Press Inc., Totowa, NJ

and have not been shown to be hugely successful *(5)*. Because these suicide genes were not adapted to utilize these substrates by natural selection, techniques have been developed to create and identify suicide genes that have been optimized for prodrug activation. Furthermore, the use of new enzymes exhibiting a high affinity for prodrugs should minimize the side effects of the prodrug by reducing the amount necessary for tumor ablation. The application of engineered genes is likely to enhance the therapeutic efficacy of cancer suicide gene therapy.

In vitro DNA evolution accelerates the normal mutation rate of DNA and is used to create novel enzymes suited for prodrug activation. Techniques such as random sequence mutagenesis, error-prone polymerase chain reaction (PCR), and DNA shuffling are efficient tools of in vitro DNA evolution. In this chapter, we will focus on random sequence mutagenesis and the combination of error-prone PCR with DNA shuffling. Other techniques such as shuffling homologous genes from different species *(6)*, single-stranded DNA shuffling *(7)*, as well as the RACHITT *(8)* and StEP *(9)* procedures are variations of the error-prone PCR/DNA shuffling method and will not be discussed here.

Random sequence mutagenesis employs a plasmid backbone that encodes the gene of interest with restriction endonuclease sites flanking the sequence to be replaced by the target sequence. Homology alignments or structural information facilitates locating a putative active-site or target region. In the absence of such information, the degree of randomness and size of the region to be mutagenized may require that vast numbers of mutants be constructed and screened. To produce the random insert, two overlapping complementary oligonucleotides (one or both) containing random sequences are hybridized, extended with DNA polymerase to produce a duplex, amplified by the PCR, cut at restriction sites engineered into the ends of each oligonucleotide, and then ligated into a DNA vector (*see* **Fig. 1**). After ligation, the recombinant molecules are used to transform *E. coli*, and functional clones are identified on the basis of positive genetic complementation or screening. To identify mutants with improved prodrug activity, a secondary screening or negative selection system must be devised where cells expressing the wild-type gene grow but any mutant with increased activity toward the prodrug dies. This technique allows one to rapidly identify mutants in a very short period of time without protein purification or extensive biochemical or biophysical analyses.

In cases where there is little or no information regarding the position of the active site, techniques such as error-prone PCR and DNA shuffling have been developed and used with great success to introduce random mutations throughout the coding region of a gene *(6,10–12)*. Error prone PCR takes advantage of the infidelity of DNA polymerase under certain conditions such as the presence of manganese and an imbalance of dNTP pools. After amplification under error-prone conditions, the resulting fragment is subjected to a light DNase I treatment to produce small (25–100 bp) fragments (*see* **Fig. 2**). These fragments are gel purified and used to reassemble the gene using primerless PCR where the fragments themselves act as primers. Following reconstitution of the gene, the double-stranded DNA is restricted at sites flanking the gene and subcloned into compatible sites in an expression vector. Similar to random sequence

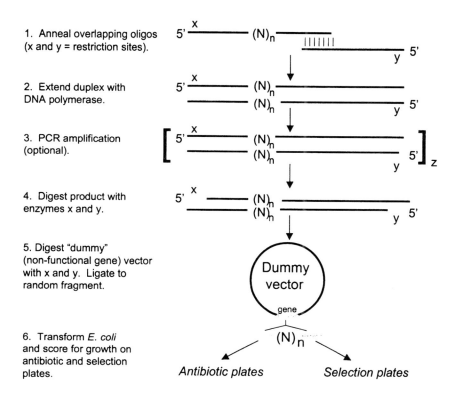

1. Anneal overlapping oligos (x and y = restriction sites).

2. Extend duplex with DNA polymerase.

3. PCR amplification (optional).

4. Digest product with enzymes x and y.

5. Digest "dummy" (non-functional gene) vector with x and y. Ligate to random fragment.

6. Transform *E. coli* and score for growth on antibiotic and selection plates.

Fig. 1. Outline of random sequence mutagenesis.

mutagenesis, the error-prone/shuffled library is used to transform *E. coli* and plated on selection plates to identify mutants of interest. Because the mutagenesis rate is fairly low (approx 0.6–2%), multiple rounds of error-prone PCR and DNA shuffling are often necessary, each round becoming more stringent by alterations in the selection or screening system *(13)*.

2. Materials

2.1. Preparation of Double-Stranded DNA From Oligonucleotides Containing Random Sequences

Store at –20°C unless otherwise stated.

1. 10X Annealing buffer: 70 mM tris-HCl, pH7.5/60 mM MgCl$_2$/200 mM NaCl.
2. 10 mM dNTPs: 10 mM of each dATP, dCTP, dGTP and dTTP.
3. 0.1 M dithiothreitol (DTT). Filter-sterilize.
4. *E. coli* DNA polymerase I, Klenow fragment (5 U/µL).
5. 10X PCR buffer: 200 mM Tris-HCl, pH 8.3, 250 mM KCl, 15 mM MgCl$_2$, 0.5% Tween-20.
6. BSA (bovine serum albumin): 10 mg/mL.
7. PCR primers (*see* **Note 1**).

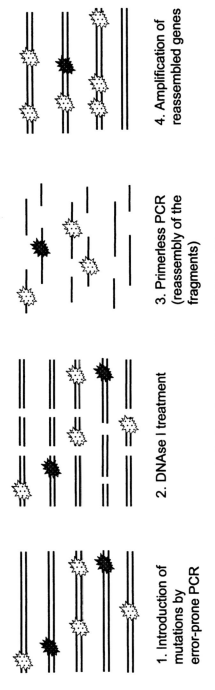

Fig. 2. Outline of error-prone PCR and DNA shuffling.

8. *Taq* polymerase: 5 U/μL (Perkin-Elmer Cetus).
9. Mineral oil for PCR overlay. Store at room temperature.
10. Restriction endonucleases. These depend on the cloning sites used (*see* **Note 2**).

2.2. Ligation, Preparation of Competent Cells, and Transformation

1. 10X Ligase buffer: 0.5 M Tris-HCl, pH 7.8, 0.1 M MgCl$_2$, 10 mM DTT, 10 mM ATP, 250 μg/mL BSA. This may also be provided with the purchase of DNA ligase. Store at –20°C.
2. *E. coli* strain (*see* **Note 3**).
3. 2 X YT medium: 16 g tryptone/10 g yeast extract/5 g NaCl per liter. For agar, add 15 g agar/L. Autoclave. Add appropriate antibiotic prior to pouring plates. Store at 4°C.
4. 10% glycerol. Filter-sterilize. Store at room temperature.
5. SOC: 2% tryptone, 0.5% yeast extract, 10 mM NaCl, 2.5 mM KCl, 10 mM MgCl$_2$, 10 mM MgSO$_4$, 20 mM glucose. Filter-sterilize. Store at 4°C.

2.3. Error-Prone PCR

Store at –20°C unless otherwise stated.

1. 10X PCR buffer: 100 mM Tris-HCl, pH 8.3, 500 mM KCl.
2. 50 mM MgCl$_2$.
3. 10 mM MnCl$_2$.
4. 10 mM dNTPs: 10 mM of each dATP, dCTP, dGTP, and dTTP.
5. PCR primers (*see* **Note 4**).
6. Template DNA (*see* **Note 5**).
7. *Taq* polymerase: 5 U/μL (Perkin-Elmer Cetus).
8. Mineral oil for PCR overlay, if needed (store at room temperature).

2.4. DNA Shuffling

Store at –20°C unless otherwise stated.

1. DNAse I: 0.02 U/μL (Gibco-BRL - 50–375 U/μL diluted to 0.2 U/μL).
2. 100 mM MgCl$_2$.
3. 200 mM EDTA.

2.5. Primerless PCR

1. 10 mM dNTPs: 10 mM of each dATP, dCTP, dGTP, and dTTP.
2. 10X PCR buffer: 100 mM Tris-HCl, pH 8.3, 500 mM KCl.
3. 50 mM MgCl$_2$.
4. *Taq* polymerase: 5 U/μL (Gibco-BRL).
5. Mineral oil for PCR overlay, if needed (store at room temperature).

3. Methods

3.1. Random Sequence Mutagenesis

3.1.1. Preparation of Double-Stranded DNA From Oligonucleotides

This annealing step involves hybridization of the two complementary, overlapping oligonucleotides (*see* **Fig. 1**). In order to form stable hybrids, the overlapping area of complementarity should be at least 12 to 15 nucleotides in length.

1. Combine equimolar concentrations of the oligonucleotides in a final volume of 40 μL (50 pmol of oligo #1, 50 pmol of oligo #2, 4 μL of 10X annealing buffer) (*see* **Note 6**).

2. Incubate the mixture at 95°C for 5 min.
3. Move the tube to a water bath or heating block at 65°C for 20 min.
4. Allow the reaction mixture to equilibrate to room temperature for a further 10 min.
5. Place the annealing reaction on ice.

3.1.2. Extension, Amplification, and Digestion

3.1.2.1. EXTENSION

By annealing the two oligonucleotides together, the two 3' hydroxy termini are immediately upstream from a region of the oligonucleotide that can serve as a template for chain elongation (*see* **Fig. 1**). In this step, the Klenow fragment of *E. coli* DNA Pol I is used to elongate the primer strands and thus synthesize a complete double-stranded oligonucleotide. The result of such a synthesis is a double-stranded fragment with complete complementarity, including the segments containing the random nucleotides. The entire library is random, but each individual molecule contains two complementary DNA strands. For large amounts of random inserts, the double-stranded fragment can be amplified by the PCR. Restriction with the appropriate endonucleases at sites proximal to the ends of each oligonucleotide (now the ends of the double-stranded DNA [dsDNA fragment]) is done to aid cloning efficiency and directionality.

1. For the extension reaction, add the following components to the 40 μL annealing reaction: 4 μL of 10X annealing buffer, 5.6 μL of 10 mM dNTPs, 1.6 μL of 0.1 M DTT, and 4.8 μL Klenow (5 U/μL) in a final volume of 80 μL.
2. Incubate the extension reaction at 37°C for 30 min.
3. Inactivate the DNA polymerase (Klenow fragment) by incubation for at least 10 min at 65°C.
4. Incubate the reaction for 10 min at room temperature to allow rehybridization of denatured duplexes.
5. *See* **Note 7**.

3.1.2.2. AMPLIFICATION

Amplification of the extended products can be achieved by using PCR (*see* **Fig. 1**). This is an optional step and can be omitted. We use a mixture of all the reagents except the extended products and aliquot the mixture into a number small microfuge tubes containing the extended products or a control that lacks template DNA. In this fashion, the same concentration level of all the reagents in relation to the template DNA is maintained (*see* **Note 8**).

1. Combine the following ingredients: 50 μL of 10X PCR buffer, 200 pmol of each PCR primer, 2 μL of 10 mg/mL BSA, 2.5 μL of 10 mM dNTPs, 2 μL *Taq* polymerase (5 U/μL), and H$_2$O in a final volume of 69.5 μL.
2. To each reaction tube add 13.9 μL of the mixture, 1–10 pmol of the extended product, and H$_2$O to a final volume of 100 μL.
3. Overlay the final reaction mixture with 1 drop of mineral oil if necessary for the PCR machine.
4. Run 30 cycles of amplification in a Perkin-Elmer Cetus DNA Thermal Cycler using cycles of 94°C for 1 min, 34°C for 2 min with a 7-min incubation at 72°C and left at 4°C (*see* **Note 9**).

5. Monitor the degree of amplification by running 1/10 the PCR reaction on a 2–3% agarose gel (1X TBE), a MetaPhor gel (*see* **Note 10**), or a 5–8% nondenaturing acrylamide (1X TBE) gel depending on the size of the expected product.

3.1.2.3. DIGESTION

Restriction endonucleases are used to digest at sites engineered into the 5' ends of the mutagenic oligonucleotides (*see* **Fig. 1**). This creates sticky ends for ligation and allows directional cloning into the prepared vector. At this stage, the fragments can be digested directly from the PCR reaction or precipitated with ethanol to concentrate prior to digestion with restriction enzymes.

1. Use approx 3–5 U of each endonuclease per microgram of DNA and incubate for 2–4 h at the appropriate temperature to ensure complete digestion.
2. To assess whether the digestion is complete, run a portion of the reaction mixture on a 8% acrylamide gel (nondenaturing) or 3–4% MetaPhor gel (1X TBE) alongside the uncut product and products digested individually with each of the endonucleases.

3.1.3. Vector Preparation

The next step is to prepare the vector containing the gene of interest by removing the DNA sequences between the restriction sites into which the pool of random fragments will be ligated. We use a "dummy" vector in place of a vector containing the full-length, functional gene in order to reduce the frequency of false positives resulting from incomplete digestion and religation.

1. Vector considerations (*see* **Note 11**).
2. Create a "dummy" vector (*see* **Note 12**).
3. Purify DNA by column chromatography such as the Qiagen tip-500 columns (Qiagen, Chatsworth, CA) (*see* **Note 13**).
4. We typically digest 10 µg of DNA in a 100 µL volume with 3–5 U of each enzyme per microgram of DNA at the appropriate temperature for 1–2 h.
5. Remove a small aliquot (2 µL) from the digestion mix and run it on a 1% agarose/1X TBE gel to confirm complete digestion.
6. When complete digestion is confirmed, pour a preparative agarose gel and electrophorese the remaining digested vector DNA.
7. Gel purify the fragment using GeneClean II (Bio 101, La Jolla, CA) or other similar DNA purification kits according to their protocols (*see* **Note 14**).
8. Determine the efficiency and quality of gel purification by optical density (OD_{260}) measurements and checking 0.2 µg of purified vector on a 1% agarose/1X TBE gel with the appropriate controls.

3.1.4. Ligation

Vector and insert DNAs are mixed and ligated together to create a pool of plasmids containing random sequences. This pool is then used to transform *E. coli* or other appropriated hosts that may be used for selection or screening (*see* **Fig. 1**).

1. Ligations are performed with roughly equimolar concentrations of insert and vector backbone in 1X ligase buffer and ligase (10 U/µL) in a 40-µL volume (*see* **Note 15**).
2. Incubate at 12–16°C overnight.

3. Check a small fraction (1/10) of the ligation on a 1% agarose/1X TBE gel. Also run approx 0.2 µg of cut vector and insert in neighboring lanes to serve as markers. Instead of distinct vector and insert bands, the DNA should look smeared, usually increasing in size from the vector DNA band.

3.1.5. Competent Cells and Transformation

In the case where *E. coli* is the system used for selection or screening, preparation of highly competent cells (at least 10^8 colony-forming untits [cfu]/µg DNA) is essential for creating very large libraries of random clones. Transformation is frequently the limiting step in the random mutagenesis procedure because of the inefficiency of many transformation protocols (10^7–10^8 cfu/µg DNA).

3.1.5.1. PREPARATION OF COMPETENT CELLS

1. Inoculate 1 L of 2X YT (16 g tryptone/10 g yeast extract/5 g NaCl for 1 L) with a 1/200 dilution of an overnight culture.
2. Grow the culture at 37°C (permissive temperature) until an OD_{600} of 0.5–0.8 is attained.
3. Transfer the culture to centrifuge bottles and chill on ice for 15–30 min.
4. Pellet the cells by centrifugation for 15 min at 4°C at 6000g.
5. Decant the supernatant and resuspend the cells in 1 L of ice-cold sterile H_2O. Be cautious at this point as the cell pellets can be loose and easily discarded with the supernatant.
6. Respin 15 min at 6000g and 4°C to pellet the cells.
7. Decant the supernatant and resuspend the cells in 500 mL of ice-cold sterile H_2O.
8. Centrifuge the cells again for 15 min at 6000g and 4°C. Resuspend them in 20 mL of 10% glycerol (chilled).
9. Transfer the resuspended cells to a 50-mL conical centrifuge tube and centrifuge again.
10. Resuspend the pellets a final time in 2.5 mL of 10% glycerol (chilled).
11. Aliquot 100–200 µL into 0.65-mL microfuge tubes on ice. Depending on the cuvet capacity, different aliquot volumes may be used.
12. Store the cells at –70°C. Cells prepared in this manner are competent for at least 6 mo.

3.1.5.2. TRANSFORMATION

1. Transform 50 µL of electroporation competent cells with 1–15 µL of ligation mix (depending on the cuvet capacity) using an electroporator according to the manufacturer's instructions (*see* **Note 16**).
2. After pulsing, immediately add 1 mL SOC (4°C) and transfer the transformation to a larger tube, such as a Falcon snap-cap tube. Shake for 1 h at 37°C (permissive temperature).
3. Plate a small portion of the transformation on nonselective medium to determine the total number of transformed cells. Plate the rest on selective medium.
4. Incubate the plates at the appropriate temperature.

3.1.6. Selection

The strength of random sequence selection is positive selection or genetic complementation. Active mutants can easily be identified using a stringent selection protocol. A poor selection system can lead to additional work. For example, the use of a temperature-sensitive strain able to grow efficiently at the permissive temperature but only marginally at the nonpermissive temperature may not be adequate for selection because it would be very difficult to distinguish a false positive (leaky wild type) from a true positive and requires retransformation to establish a plasmid-derived phenotype. The time spent in fine-tuning a selection system minimizes problems associated with the frequent recovery of false positives. Clearly, the selection step is one that must be devised with a particular question in mind as well as a knowledge about the bacterial strain and requirements for the identification of positive clones. Alternatively, a negative selection can be used but requires that every potential mutant must be plated individually on both selective (death) and nonselective (growth) plates in order to retrieve any functional clones—a formidable task. A secondary selection or screening system may be necessary to identify mutants with altered activities such as improved prodrug affinity. This is generally a negative selection in which prodrugs are added to selection plates at a concentration that permits growth of the wild-type (parental) gene, but mutants with improved activity toward the prodrugs are killed.

3.2. Error-Prone PCR and DNA Shuffling

Error-prone PCR is based on the infidelity of the *Taq* polymerase in the presence of an unbalanced mix of deoxynucleotides. Furthermore, the addition of manganese chloride stabilizes noncomplementary basepairs and promotes the introduction of random mutations throughout the amplified product *(13,14)*. In comparison to the spontaneous error rate of *Taq* polymerase of 0.001–0.02%, error-prone PCR yields a mutation rate between 0.6% and 2%, varying according to PCR conditions *(13,15)*. During the successive amplification cycles, mutations accumulate.

Given the fact that most mutations yield nonfunctional variants, the probability of obtaining two or more beneficial mutations in the same PCR product is very low. DNA shuffling involves the fragmentation of a library of mutants into 25- to 100-bp fragments using DNAse 1, followed by random reassembly that mimics natural DNA recombination (*see* **Fig. 2**). The final step of conventional PCR amplification allows the recovery of a variety of shuffled mutants *(10,11)*.

3.2.1. Error-Prone PCR

In this step, mutations are randomly introduced throughout the amplified region (*see* **Fig. 2**).

1. Combine the following ingredients: 5 μL of 10X PCR buffer, 3 μL of 50 mM MgCl$_2$, 5 μL of 10 mM dATP, 5 μL of 10 mM dGTP, 1 μL of 10 mM dCTP, 1 μL of 10 mM dTTP, 2.5 μL of 10 mM MnCl$_2$, 3 μL DNA template diluted to 1 ng/μL, 2 μL of each primer (25 pmol/μL), 0.4 μL *Taq* polymerase (5 U/μL), and water in a final volume of 50 μL.
2. Error-prone PCR should be run using the same time/temperature conditions as used for standard amplification of the wild-type sequence (*see* **Note 17**).

3.2.2. DNA Shuffling

DNA shuffling of the error-prone PCR requires three successive steps: (1) digestion by DNAse I, (2) primerless PCR to reassemble the fragments, and (3) final amplification using the 3' and 5' primers to recover the PCR product containing the shuffled DNA regions (*see* **Fig. 2**). In the first step, DNase I digestion of the error-prone PCR sample leads to the generation of small DNA fragments (from 25 to 100 bp).

1. Combine the following ingredients: 40 μL of the error-prone PCR product (approx 1 μg/ μL), 5 μL of 100 m*M* MgCl$_2$, and 5 μL DNAse I (0.02 U/μL) in a total volume of 50 μL.
2. Incubate at room temperature 2 min.
3. Stop the reaction by adding 5 μL of 200 m*M* EDTA followed by 5 min at 95°C.
4. Run 10–15 μL of the reaction on a 1.5% agarose gel to confirm digestion to the required degree. A DNA smear should be observed in the 25- to 100-bp range (*see* **Note 18**).
5. Gel isolate and purify the reaction products in the 25- to 100-bp size range (*see* **Note 19**).

3.2.3. Primerless PCR

In this PCR step, DNA fragments obtained by DNAse I digestion are reassembled by self-hybridization and gap filling by *Taq* polymerase (*see* **Fig. 2**).

1. The template DNA for this reaction is 10–30 ng/μL of DNA from the previous step (DNaseI treated and gel purified).
2. To the DNA add: 10 μL dNTP (10 m*M* each), 5 μL of 10X *Taq* buffer (100 m*M* Tris-HCl, pH 8.3/500 m*M* KCl), 3 μL of 50 m*M* MgCl$_2$, 0.5 μL *Taq* polymerase (5 U/μL), and H$_2$O in a final volume of 50 μL.
3. Reassemble the fragment using the time/temperature condition guidelines as follows: 95°C for 3 min. Perform 45 cycles of 95°C for 1 min, 60°C for 1 min, and 72°C for 1 min; repeat.
4. Run 10 μL of the primerless PCR products on a 1% or 1.5% agarose gel together with an aliquot from the error-prone PCR. A smear should be observed around the expected size of your starting fragment (*see* **Note 20**).

3.2.4. Reamplification

This next step involves amplification of the primerless PCR products (*see* **Fig. 2**).

1. Combine the PCR mix as follows: 5 μL dNTP (10 m*M* each), 5 μL of 10X *Taq* buffer (100 m*M* Tris-HCl, pH 8.3, and 500 m*M* KCl), 1.5 μL of 50 m*M* MgCl$_2$, 1 μL of 5' primer (25 pmol/μL), 1 μL of 3' primer (25 pmol/μL), 1–2 μL of template DNA (error-prone PCR product diluted 1 : 1000 in H$_2$O), 0.4 μL *Taq* polymerase (5 U/μL), and H$_2$O to a final volume of 50 μL (*see* **Note 21**).
2. Amplify the primerless PCR products using the following temperature/time selections as a guideline: 94°C for 3 min. Perform 25 cycles of 94°C for 30 s, 55°C for 30 s, 72°C for 40 s, and repeat. After the 25 cycles, leave the sample at 72°C for 3 min to ensure complete extension. Chill to 4°C.
3. Run 5 μL on a 1.5% agarose gel to confirm reassembly of the full-length product (*see* **Note 22**).

3.2.5. Vector Preparations

1. Vector considerations (*see* **Note 11**).
2. Preparation of vector DNA is described in **Subheading 3.1.3.**

3.2.6. Ligation, Transformation, and Selection

The basic methods for ligation of vector and insert, transformation of the ligation mixture and selection of mutants with the desired activities, are as described in **Subheading 3.1.**

4. Notes

1. Random sequence primer design is the most important aspect of creating a diverse library from which mutants with the desired characteristics will be derived. For each amino acid position, there are 20 possible amino acid substitutions. At the nucleotide level, the number of permutations for four amino acid residues (12 nucleotides) is 4^{12} or 1.7×10^7. Thus, a completely random library contains 20^4 or 1.6×10^5 different amino acid sequences. With six codons containing random nucleotide sequences, the number of clones with different nucleotide substitutions increases to 6.9×10^{10} and represents 6.4×10^7 different amino acid substitutions. Given a very efficient transformation protocol in concert with a strong selection system, it is feasible to examine this number of transformants and score for clones that contain inserts that code for active proteins. Stretches of larger numbers of random substitutions means that the total number of possible permutations cannot be analyzed simply for the reason that the capacity of the transformation system has been reached or exceeded. The major limitation to this procedure is the number of bacteria that can be successfully transformed. The number of codons randomized can be limited to a few residues in order to generate all possibilities at certain sites. Some investigators have mutagenized large regions of a polypeptide by creating many small libraries that span only two or three residues at a time *(16)*. Synthesis of the numbers of oligonucleotides required for such a study is very costly. One may want to consider constructing a 2–20% degenerative library initially and sequence a fair number of active clones. Although the absence of different amino acids substitutions does not necessarily mean that other residues are not permissible, it might also mean that not enough clones have been sequenced. In such a case, one may want to discern these two possibilities by generating a second library with 100% randomness. As a general approach, it is frequently advantageous to define the essentiality of different residues by utilizing a partially random sequence at specified positions.

   One way to reduce the complexity of possible permutations is to bias the mutagenesis toward the wild-type sequence (partially random). This slants the mutagenesis to favoring single mutations and also toward a higher frequency of clones that encode enzymatically active proteins because multiple mutations are more often nonfunctional than are single amino acid substitutions. For instance, if one desires single amino acid mutations at many residues, one might maintain a high percentage of wild-type sequences with a low percentage of non-wild-type sequences at each position. For example, a partially random sequence might be comprised of 80% wild-type and 20% of all other three nucleotides at each nucleotide position. This biased ratio ensures that a greater proportion of positively selected sequences are the result of single amino acid substitutions within the random array. Completely random sequence mutagenesis leads to a higher frequency of multiple amino acid replacements. It seems likely that multiple amino acid replacements would not have been adequately screening during evolution and may provide a fertile field for the discovery of new enzymatic activities.

   As with both random and partially random mutagenesis, the introduction of stop codons can be of concern depending on the number of nucleotides to be mutagenized. Some investigators use NNG/C (where N denotes all four nucleotides) instead of NNN to avoid the potential insertion of two stop codons among the random inserts while still allowing the coding of all possible amino acid residues *(17)*.

2. When designing the random oligonucleotides, be sure to take into account that restriction endonucleases require a specified number of nucleotides on either side of the restriction site for recognition. Moreover, the ends of oligonucleotides may fray and not be tightly hybridized. Thus, it is advantageous to incorporate a few extra G–C pairs at the ends of the oligonucleotides that contain the random sequences or to incorporate additional terminal nucleotides at the ends of primers that may be used for PCR amplification.

3. The *E. coli* strain used will depend on the selection scheme. Use a *rec*A-deficient cell line whenever possible to reduce nonhomologous recombination into the bacterial chromosome.

4. In order to subclone the error-prone PCR/DNA shuffled products, primers are designed to flank the gene with restriction sites that are compatible with restriction sites within the vector polylinker region.

5. Template DNA should be diluted to 1 ng/μL from a clean DNA preparation such as a Qiagen plasmid kit (Chatworth, CA). The amount of template DNA can be critical. Initially, try with about 2 ng of DNA. If no amplification is obtained, consider increasing the amount of template DNA to 5 ng.

6. The use of individual extinction coefficients in calculating oligonucleotide concentration provides a more accurate assessment than does a standard value for oligonucleotides. Generally, these are given on the specification sheet from the oligonucleotide synthesizer. If not, to determine the extinction coefficiency, the number of each nucleotide species is multiplied by the values for the individual nucleotides ($A=15.4 \times 10^3$, $C=7.5 \times 10^3$, $G=11.7 \times 10^3$, $T=7.4 \times 10^3$) and the sum totaled. For each random position use the average of all four values ($N=10.5 \times 10^3$). Division of the total OD_{260} reading by the oligonucleotide extinction coefficient gives moles per liter and then multiply by 10^6 to give picomoles per microliter.

7. The efficacy of annealing can be monitored by using radiolabeled oligonucleotides in a parallel annealing reaction followed by electrophoresis in a nondenaturing gel. When visualizing annealed and extended labeled oligonucleotides, do not heat denature prior to running the reactions on a nondenaturing polyacrylamide gel. If annealing is not complete, different (lower) temperatures and/or longer incubation times may be required.

8. At this point, if a scaled-up reaction has been done (i.e., no PCR amplification), the DNA is ethanol precipitated and restricted with the appropriate endonucleases. Completion of fragment digestion can be monitored by subjecting the cut and uncut DNA to electrophoresis on a nondenaturing 5–8% acrylamide gel.

9. This has worked for different primer–template combinations, but depending on the primers and template, the cycle times and/or temperatures may require modification.

10. As few as 4-bp differences can be resolved in a 3.5% MetaPhor (FMC BioProducts, Rockland, ME) agarose (1X TBE) gel with a range of 70–300 bp.

11. There are several important considerations in choosing a vector for cloning random sequences. The copy number of the plasmid is worth noting especially if the gene product is slightly toxic. By keeping the number of copies low, the toxic effects may be reduced. In the selection process, a low-copy-number plasmid might allow one to discern differential levels of mutant activities using selection plates containing a low concentration of substrates. A high-copy-number plasmid offers an additional advantage because sequencing is likely to involve double-stranded DNA and fair amounts of the DNA (2–3 μg) may be required. Furthermore, if a vector contains a single-stranded origin of replication, then sequencing is greatly simplified. Promoters are another consideration. For some situations, it is important to maintain tight control on expression levels. In some instances, promoters may be the target for random mutagenesis *(18)*.

12. By exchanging a stuffer fragment of DNA that is longer that the native fragment, a non-functional "dummy" vector can be constructed *(19)*. The stuffer fragment replaces the wild-type sequences and occupies the same position that the random sequences will. There are two important reasons for using a "dummy" vector: one can discern between singly- and doubly-cut, vector and, second, if the gel-isolated vector (double cut) is contaminated with some uncut vector, the selection would eliminate it as a nonfunctional clone, whereas the vector containing a wild-type gene would register as a positive clone. Alternatively, site-directed mutagenesis can be used to introduce a stop codon within the target region, thereby rendering the gene inactive. The inclusion of an internal restriction site within the oligonucleotides described here aids in discerning the wild-type-gene-containing vector from any recombinants. The use of a "dummy" vector removes the time-consuming step of performing restriction digests and running gels on all possible positives prior to sequencing. Generally, we only perform restriction analysis on the first 10–20 clones to confirm that the majority of the positive clones contain random sequence insertions.

13. Because the restricted vector DNA is gel purified, less clean DNA isolated from mini-preparations can be used if only a small library is required and will not cause difficulties at subsequent steps. The use of column-purified DNA is generally preferred for library constructions.

14. Other kits and techniques are available and can be used in a similar fashion to purify the vector DNA.

15. Several ratios of insert to vector ligations should be tried in pilot experiments in order to identify the best ligation conditions.

16. The volume of competent cells and ligation mix for maximal transformation efficiency needs to be determined for each strain and ligation. Furthermore, if arching occurs during electroporation, less of the ligation mix should be used or the DNA should be ethanol precipitated to remove excess salt.

17. The PCR conditions for standard amplifications may work for error-prone PCR. However, because of the unbalanced mix of dNTPs and the presence of manganese chloride, optimization of error-prone PCR conditions may be necessary. First consider the concentration of $MgCl_2$ and then that of $MnCl_2$.

18. If a DNA smear is not obtained, digestion has either not gone to completion or has not occurred at all. Titrate concentrations of $MgCl_2$ and DNase I to optimize DNAse I treatment conditions and/or extend the DNAseI treatment time.

19. If the whole DNA smear is in the range 25–100 bp, the gel purification step may be omitted. However, the DNase I mix contains EDTA that will chelate divalent cations necessary for *Taq* polymerase activity. To remove EDTA, perform a phenol extraction/ethanol precipitation or DNA elution through a spin column.

20. If the primerless PCR does not result in full-length fragments, try one or all of the following: (1) Alter the template DNA concentration. Concentrations up to 60 ng/mL work well in our hands. (2) Template DNA can be gel purified by either phenol extraction or a GeneClean II kit (Bio101). Alternatively, use a spin column kit such as the Qiaquick nucleotide removal kit from Qiagen (Chatworth, CA). (3) Decrease the annealing temperature to increase the fragment hybridization. Try to find the best annealing temperature, perhaps using a gradient PCR thermocycler.

21. The template DNA concentration may need to be increased to optimize reamplification of the gene.

22. In order to get good reamplification, you may need to titrate $MgCl_2$ concentration, for example, from 1.5 to 5 m*M*.

References

1. Kokoris, M. S., Sabo, P. S., Adman, E. T., and Black, M. E. (1999) Enhancement of tumor ablation by a selected HSV-1 thymidine kinase mutant. *Gene Ther.* **6,** 1415–1426.
2. Erbs, P., Exinger, F., and Jund, R. (1997) Characterization of the *Saccharomyces cerevisiae* FCY1 gene encoding cytosine deaminase and its homologue FCA1 of *Candida albicans*. *Curr. Genet.* **31,** 1–6.
3. Diasio, R., Lakings, D., and Benett, J. (1978) Evidence for conversion of 5-fluorocytosine to 5-fluorouracil in humans: possible factor in 5-fluorocytosine toxicity. *Antimicrob. Agents Chemother.* **41,** 903–908.
4. Kievit, E., Bershad, E., Ng, E., et al. (1999) Superiority of yeast over bacterial cytosine deaminase for enzyme/prodrug gene therapy in colon cancer xenografts. *Cancer Res.* **59,** 1417–1421.
5. Kim, Y. G., Bi, W., Feliciano, E. S., Drake, R. R., and Stambrook, P. J. (2000) Ganciclovir-mediated cell killing and bystander effect is enhanced in cells with two copies of the herpes simplex virus thymidine kinase gene. *Cancer Gene Ther.* **7,** 240–246.
6. Crameri A., Raillard S.-A., Bermudez E., and Stemmer P.C. (1998) DNA shuffling of a family of genes from diverse species accelerates directed evolution. *Nature* **391,** 288–291.
7. Kikuchi M., Ohnishi K., and Harayama S. (2000) An effective family shuffling method using single-stranded DNA. *Gene* **243,** 133–137.
8. Coco W. M., Levinson W. E., Crist M. J., et al. (2001) DNA shuffling method for generating highly recombined genes and evolved enzymes. *Nature Biotechnol.* **19,** 354–359.
9. Zhao H., Giver L., Shao Z., Affholter J. A., and Arnold F. H. (1998) Molecular evolution by staggered extension process (StEP) in vitro recombination. *Nature Biotechnol.* **16,** 258–261.
10. Stemmer, W. P. C. (1994) DNA shuffling by random fragmentation and reassembly: in vitro recombination for molecular evolution. *Proc. Natl. Acad. Sci. USA* **91,** 10,747–10,751.
11. Stemmer, W. P. C. (1994) Rapid evolution of a protein in vitro by DNA shuffling. *Nature* **370,** 389–391.
12. Zhang, J. H., Dawes, G., and Stemmer, W. P. C. (1997) Directed evolution of a fucosidase from a galactosidase by DNA shuffling and screening. *Proc. Natl. Acad. Sci. USA* **94,** 4504–4509.
13. Cadwell, R. C. and Joyce, G. F. (1992) Randomization of genes by PCR mutagenesis. *PCR Methods Applic.* **2,** 28–33.
14. Eckert, K. A. and Kunkel, T. A. (1990) High fidelity DNA synthesis by the *Thermus aquaticus* DNA polymerase. *Nucleic Acids Res.* **18,** 3739–3744.
15. Leung, D. W., Chen, E., and Goeddel, D. V. (1989) A method for random sequence mutagenesis of a defined DNA segment using a modified polymerase chain reaction. *Technique* **1,** 11–15.
16. Reidhaar-Olson, J. F. and Sauer, R. T. (1988) Combinatorial cassette mutagenesis as a probe of the informational content of protein sequences. *Science* **241,** 53–57.
17. Reidhaar-Olson, J. F., Bowie, J. U., Breyer, R. M., et al. (1991) Random mutagenesis of protein sequences using oligonucleotide cassettes. *Methods Enzymol.* **208,** 564–586.
18. Horwitz, M. S. and Loeb, L. A. (1986) Promoters selected from random DNA sequences. *Proc. Natl. Acad. Sci. USA* **83,** 7405–7409.
19. Black, M. E. and Loeb, L. A. (1993) Identification of important residues within the putative nucleoside binding site of HSV-1 thymidine kinase by random sequence selection: analysis of selected mutants *in vitro*. *Biochemistry* **32,** 11,618–11,626.

17

Combination Suicide Gene Therapy

Wolfgang Uckert, Brian Salmons, Christian Beltinger, Walter H. Günzburg, and Thomas Kammertöns

1. Introduction

Suicide genes (SG) can be viewed as negatively selectable marker genes. Their gene products convert otherwise nontoxic prodrugs (PD) into cytotoxic metabolites. The enzymatic conversion leads to high levels of the activated toxic drug within genetically modified cells and ultimately kills the cells. Several studies have shown that when SG-expressing tumor cells are mixed with parental, nongenetically modified cells, prodrug treatment induces toxic effects in the nonmodified cells. This phenomenon has been termed "bystander (killing) effect."

SG can be used as a safety modality to eliminate adoptively transferred cells in case of unwanted side effects. This safety approach has been used in a number of studies (1,2). More often, SG are used for the treatment of solid, inoperable tumors. Clinical trials have shown the limitations of SG therapy for the treatment of cancer and have indicated the need for more basic research efforts to improve SG efficacy, vector design, and target specificity.

One way of enhancing cell killing and thus SG efficiency is, similar to conventional chemotherapy, a combinatorial approach. Combining two SG/PD systems (1) can increase the efficiency of negative selection, (2) may allow the concentration of the PD to be reduced, and (3) may also diminish the likelihood of drug resistance. There are a number of studies that show that two SG/PD approaches can be combined to synergistically enhance their antitumor effects in vitro and in vivo (3–5).

To analyze the interactions of two SG, the choice of the model system is critical. It has been shown that the efficacy of negative selection varies with the cell model used. For example, the efficacy of *Escherichia coli* cytosine deaminase (CD) and the prodrug 5-fluorocytosine (5-FC) as well as herpes simplex virus thymidine kinase (HSV-TK) and ganciclovir (GCV) to kill cells varies considerably in the three murine cell lines NIH3T3, ESB, and TS/A (*see* **Fig. 1**). For the analysis of combinatorial effects of two SG, a cell line with intermediate sensitivity, allowing the detection of potential posi-

From: *Methods in Molecular Medicine, Vol. 90, Suicide Gene Therapy: Methods and Reviews*
Edited by: C. J. Springer © Humana Press Inc., Totowa, NJ

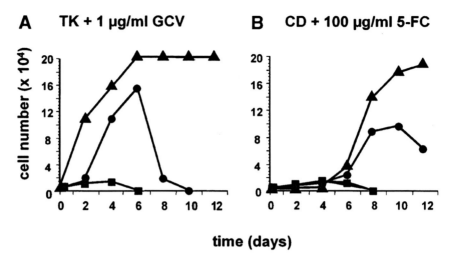

A TK + 1 µg/ml GCV   **B CD + 100 µg/ml 5-FC**

time (days)

Fig. 1. NIH 3T3 (squares), TS/A (circles), or ESB (triangles) cells were transduced with either pBabeTK (**A**) or pLCDSN (**B**). One thousand cells per well were seeded in 24-well plates and cultured in the presence of GCV (**A**) and 5-FC (**B**). At the time-points indicated, viable cells were counted by the trypan blue exclusion method.

tive as well as negative cooperative interactions, should be chosen. Therefore, of the cell lines depicted in **Fig. 1**, TS/A cells are best suited for the analysis of combinatorial effects between TK/GCV and CD/5-FC.

Cooperative interactions of two SG/PD systems can be measured directly by transducing a model cell line with both SG and evaluating single vs double PD treatment. Alternatively, cooperative effects, especially of the "bystander effect," can be measured by coculturing a cell line, which efficiently expresses the SG products of choice with target nonexpressing cells to establish cooperative toxic effects. There are a number of prerequisites for this indirect measurement. Both cell populations should be physically separated (e.g., either in a transwell system or by encapsulation of the SG-modified cells). Furthermore, this assay can only be used for those SG/PD approaches in which the toxic metabolites generated are freely diffusible.

In **Subheading 3.**, we provide one exemplary protocol for the evaluation of a direct cooperation between CD and TK in TS/A cells (*4*). Furthermore, we describe a protocol for the evaluation of "bystander effect" cooperation between the diffusible toxins hydroxyifosfamide produced after conversion of ifosfamide by cytochrome P450/2B1 and 5-fluorouracil produced from CD gene-modified and encapsulated CRFK cells (*5*).

2. Materials

2.1. Cell Lines

1. FLYA13 amphotropic retroviral packaging cells (*6*).
2. CRFK feline kidney cells (*7*).
3. TS/A murine mammary adenocarcinoma cells (*8*).

2.2. Vectors

1. The retroviral vectors pLCDSN and pBabeTK contain the bacterial CD gene together with the neomycin resistance gene and the herpes simplex virus-1–thymidine kinase gene in conjunction with the puromycin resistance gene, respectively. Both suicide genes are inserted into the vector so that they are placed under the control of the Moloney murine leukemia virus promoter while the expression of the selectable marker genes is driven by the simian virus 40 (SV40) early promoter *(4)*.
2. The plasmid vector pcDNA3 (Invitrogen, Groningen, The Netherlands) contains the rat cytochrome P450/2B1 gene under the control of the cytomegalovirus (CMV) immediate–early promoter *(9)*.

2.3. Cell Culture

1. Tissue culture media: Alpha-MEM, DMEM, RPMI 1640 (Life Technologies, Eggersheim, Germany). Tissue-culture media were always supplemented with 10% heat-inactivated (56°C, 1 h) fetal calf serum (FCS) (Biochrom, Berlin, Germany) unless otherwise indicated.
2. EDTA–trypsin.
3. Tissue culture flasks.
4. Multiwell tissue culture plates.
5. Roller tissue culture bottles (Costar, Bodenheim, Germany).
6. Disposable pipets (Costar).
7. 0.45-μm Disposable filter (Schleicher & Schuell, Dassel, Germany).

2.4. Solutions and Kits

1. Phosphate-buffered saline (PBS): 1% NaCl, 0.025% KCl, 0.14% Na_2HPO_4, 0.025% KH_2PO_4, pH 7.3; autoclaved.
2. G418 (Sigma, Deisenhofen, Germany); stock solution: 1 mg/mL in PBS.
3. Puromycin (Sigma); stock solution: 1 μg/mL in PBS.
4. 5-Fluorocytosine (5-FC) (Sigma); stock solution: 10 mg/mL in RPMI 1640 or DMEM.
5. Ganciclovir (GCV) (Syntex, Aachen, Germany); stock solution: 10 mg/mL in RPMI 1640 or DMEM.
6. Ifosfamide (IFO) (ASTA Medica, Frankfurt, Germany); prepare fresh each time.
7. Trypan blue (Sigma), 0.25% solution in PBS.
8. Polybrene (Sigma), stock solution: 1 mg/mL in PBS (*see* **Note 1**).
9. Mammalian DNA transfection kit (Pharmacia, Freiburg, Germany).
10. Plasmid DNA purification kit (Qiagen, Hilden, Germany).

2.5. Equipment

1. CO_2 incubator (Labotect, Göttingen, Germany).
2. Cell counter (Coulter, Krefeld, Germany).
3. Roller apparatus, Cellroll (Integra Biosciences, Fernwald, Germany).
4. Light microscope (Leitz, Wetzlar, Germany).
5. Hemocytometer

2.6. Encapsulated SG-Modified Cells

Encapsulation of SG-modified cells was performed as described *(5,9,10)*. 5×10^8 SG gene-modified or parental CRFK cells were mixed with 2–5% cellulose sulfate in 5 mL of Dulbecco's phosphate-buffered saline (D-PBS). Suspension droplets were allowed to form and these were collected in a polymerizing solution consisting of 3%

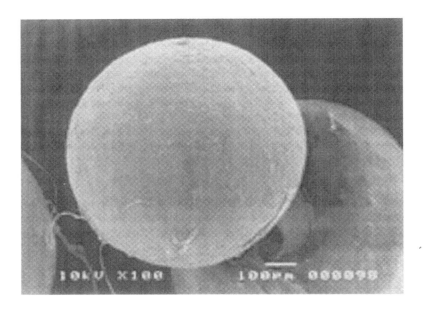

Fig. 2. Electron micrograph of cellulose sulfate capsule.

polydiallyldimethyl ammonium *(10)* in D-PBS using an Inotech apparatus (Dottikon, Switzerland). Polymerization of the outer cellulose layers of the capsules occurs immediately, generating capsules with an average diameter of 0.7±1 mm, harboring approx 1×10^4 cells (*see* **Fig. 2**). The capsules were washed twice with DMEM and kept either in culture (37°C, 5% CO_2) or at 4°C.

3. Methods

3.1. Transfection of Retroviral Plasmids into Packaging Cells

Plasmids carrying retroviral vectors were purified using a DNA purification kit according to the manufacturer's instruction (e.g., Qiagen).

1. **Day 1**: Plate 5×10^5 FLYA13 cells (or other amphotropic retroviral packaging cells) per 10-cm-diameter tissue culture dish with 10 mL DMEM. Grow cells at 37°C and 5% CO_2.
2. **Day 2**: Change medium and transfect cells with 10 µg of retroviral plasmid DNA, using calcium phosphate precipitation according to the supplier's instruction (e.g., Pharmacia, Stratagene).
3. **Day 3**: Wash cells twice with PBS, add fresh 10 mL of medium containing selection antibiotic (G418, 0.6 mg/mL; puromycin, 5 µg/mL).

Expand cell clones. Select for stable virus-producing cell lines and determine virus titer (*see* **Note 2**).

3.2. Generation of Retrovirus-Containing Supernatant

FLYA13 cells producing SG retroviruses were grown to confluency in roller tissue culture bottles (Costar) in 150 mL DMEM (without G418 or puromycin) at 37°C and

5% CO_2. Then, the medium was replaced by 40 mL fresh medium, the temperature was decreased to 32°C, and virus-containing supernatant was harvested in intervals of 24 h. Cells and debris were removed by filtration through a 0.45-μm disposable filter. Aliquots of virus supernatant were stored at –80°C (*see* **Note 3**).

3.3. Retroviral Transduction of Tumor Cells

1. **Day 1**: Plate 5×10^5 TS/A cells per 10-cm-diameter tissue culture dish with 10 mL RPMI 1640.
2. **Day 2**: Replace medium and add virus-containing supernatant (1×10^6 colony-forming untis [cfu]/mL) together with polybrene (4 μg/mL) (*see* **Note 4**).
3. **Day 3**: Change medium and propagate cells in the presence of G418 (0.6 μg/mL) and puromycin (1 μg/mL), respectively, until noninfected cells die (*see* **Note 5**).

Expand cells (bulk culture) or select individual clones.

3.4. Transfection of Tumor Cells

An alternative to the transduction of tumor cells with virus-containing supernatant is the transfection of the cells with plasmid DNA using the calcium phosphate method (*see* **Subheading 3.1.**).

3.5. In Vitro Cytotoxicity Assay

1. **Day 1**: Plate 1×10^3 single or double SG-transduced TS/A cells into each well of a six-well tissue culture plate in 2 mL of medium. Grow cells at 37°C and 5% CO_2.
2. **Day 2**: Replace medium and expose the cells to varying concentrations of 5-FC, GCV, and IFO alone or in combination for different periods of time (*see* **Note 6**).

Determine the number of viable cells using trypan blue solution and dye exclusion method or use a cell counter (*see* **Note 7**).

Determine the percentage of cell growth. To do so, non-genetically-modified cells that had not been treated with prodrugs were counted using a hemocytometer at the same time as SG-modified cells and the cell number obtained set at 100%. The relative percentage of cell growth was calculated for the other cells (for a typical result, *see* **Fig. 3**).

3.6. In Vitro Cytotoxicity Assay Using Encapsulated SG-Modified Cells (Bystander Effect)

This assay was performed to evaluate the potential interactions between activated toxins produced from encapsulated SG-modified CRFK cells and the toxic effects on a target cell line.

1. **Day 1**: Plate 1×10^4 nontransduced tumor cells per well into a 12-well tissue-culture plate in 2 mL of medium. Grow cells at 37°C and 5% CO_2.
2. **Day 2**: Add 30 capsules harboring CRFK SG-modified or parental CRFK cells. Add prodrugs, either alone or in combination (*see* **Note 6**).

Count viable tumor cells after 1 wk by the trypan blue dye exclusion method (for a typical result, *see* **Fig. 4**) (*see* **Note 7**).

4. Notes

1. All stock solutions were sterile filtered through a 0.45-μm disposable filter and frozen in aliquots at –20°C.

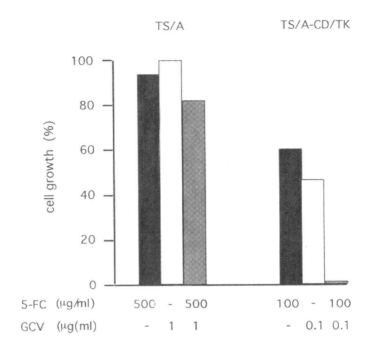

Fig. 3. TS/A cells were transduced with pBabeTK and pLCDSN subsequently. Cells coexpressing both SG (TS/A-CD/TK) and parental cells (TS/A) were seeded (1×10^3 cells/ well) into 6-well plates, and 24 h later, PD was added at the concentrations indicated. On d 5, cells were harvested and viable cells were determined by the trypan blue exclusion method. Cells not cultured in the presence of PD were counted and the value set as 100% cell growth. Black bars indicate treatment with 5-FC only, white bars indicate treatment with GCV, and gray bars indicate treatment with 5-FC and GCV.

2. After approx 14 d, cell clones appear and can be expanded to individual cell lines. The appropriate G418 and puromycin concentration used to select other packaging cell lines should be determined emperically. For human cells (FLYA13, BOSC23) and most NIH3T3 derivatives (PA317, ΨCRIP, GP+envAm12, ΨCRE, GP+E86), it is usually between 0.4 and 1 mg/mL for G418 and 2 and 5 µg/mL for puromycin, respectively. Virus titer should be determined using suitable indicator cells (e.g., NIH3T3, HeLa, HT1080, D17) by serial dilution of virus-containing supernatant *(11)*.

3. A detailed description of virus production in roller tissue culture bottles has been previously described *(11)*. If removal of cell debris by 0.45-µm filtration is difficult to perform, the virus-containing supernatant can be centrifuged for 10 min at 2000*g* at 4°C to remove most of the cells and debris before filtration.

4. Polybrene concentrations of 4 µg/mL can also be used without influencing the infection or transduction efficiency of FLYA13 or TS/A cells. Higher concentrations of polybrene than 8 µg/mL are not recommended because of potential harmful effects for the cells. Polybrene can be replaced by protamine sulfate, which is less toxic at the same concentration.

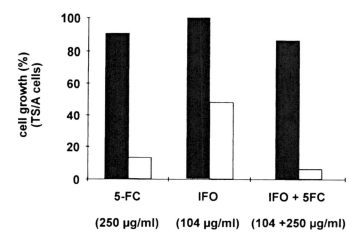

Fig. 4. TS/A cells were seeded at 1 × 10⁴ cells/well into 12-well plates. Thirty capsules harboring either parental CRFK cells (black bars), or SG-modified (2B1/CD) CRFK cells (white bars) were cocultured with 2 mL of medium. Twenty-four hours later, prodrugs were added at the concentrations indicated. On d 7, TS/A cells were harvested and viable cells were determined by the trypan blue exclusion method. Cells not cultured in the presence of PD were counted and set as 100% cell growth.

5. Transduction of target cells can either be done stepwise with the individual vector virus-containing supernatant or in parallel with both viruses. Stepwise transduction is more time-consuming because transduction with the second virus has to be started after establishing bulk cultures (or clones) from the transduction with the first virus. Parallel transduction with two viruses can be difficult to perform for some cell lines because of the double selection of cells with G418 and puromycin. In a single-selection protocol, nontransduced cells are dead after approx 14 d of selection.
6. The time of prodrug treatment as well as the concentration of prodrugs either used in combination or alone depends on the individual cell line and may differ considerably. Therefore, the optimal concentration to be used has to be determined in advance.
7. Whereas the application of a hemocytometer to count cells may be very time-consuming and eventually subjective, the utilization of a cell counter is more objective but requires a minimum amount of cells. Thus, the ratio of living/dead cells should be determined by the trypan blue exclusion method.

Acknowledgments

This work was supported by the Bundesministerium für Bildung, Wissenschaft, Forschung und Technologie (0311180 and 1220299). The authors thank Robert M. Saller and Peter Karle for help with this work.

References

1. Bonini, C., Ferrari, G., Verzeletti, S., et al. (1997) HSV-TK gene transfer into donor lymphocytes for control of allogeneic graft-versus-leukemia. *Science* **276**, 1719–1724.

2. Yee, C.,Thompson, J. A., Roche, P., et al. (2000) Melanocyte destruction after antigen-specific immunotherapy of melanoma: direct evidence of T cell-mediated vitiligo. *J. Exp. Med.* **192,** 1637–1644.

3. Rogulski, K. R., Kim, J. H., Kim, S. H., and Freytag, S. O. (1997) Glioma cells transduced with an *Escherichia coli* CD/HSV-1 TK fusion gene exhibit enhanced metabolic suicide and radiosensitivity. *Hum. Gene Ther.* **8,** 73–85 .

4. Uckert, W., Kammertöns, T., Haack, K., et al. (1998) Double suicide gene (cytosine deaminase and herpes simplex virus thymidine kinase) but not single gene transfer allows reliable elimination of tumor cells in vivo. *Hum. Gene Ther.* **9,** 855–865.

5. Kammertöns, T., Gelbmann, W., Karle, P., et al. (2000) Combined chemotherapy of murine mammary tumors by local activation of the prodrugs ifosfamide and 5-fluorocytosin. *Cancer Gene Ther.* **7,** 629–636.

6. Cosset, F.-L., Takeuchi, Y., Battini, J. L., Weiss, R. A., and Collins, M. K. (1995) High-titer packaging cells producing recombinant retrovirus resistant to human serum. *J. Virol.* **69,** 7400–7436.

7. Crandel, R. A., Fabricant, C. G., and Nelson, R. W. (1973) Development, characterization, and viral susceptibility of a feline (Felis catus) renal cell line (CRFK). *In Vitro* **9,** 176–185.

8. Nanni, P., de Giovanni, C., Lollini, P. L., Nicoletti, G., and Prodi, G. (1983) TS/A: a new metastasizing cell line from BALB/c spontaneous mammary adenocarcinoma. *Clin. Exp. Metastasis* **1,** 373–380.

9. Löhr, M., Müller, P., Karle, P., et al. (1998) Targeted chemotherapy by intratumoral injection of encapsulated cells engineered to produce CYP2B1, an ifosfamide activating cytochrome P450. *Gene Ther.* **5,** 1070–1078.

10. Dautzenberg, H., Schuldt, U., Grasnick, G., et al. (1999) Development of cellulose sulphate based polyelectrolyte complex microcapsules for medical applications. *Ann. NY Acad. Sci.* **875,** 46–63.

11. Uckert, W., Pedersen, L., and Günzburg, W. (2000) Green fluorescent protein retroviral vector: generation of high-titer producer cells and virus supernatant, in *Gene Therapy of Cancer: Methods and Protocols* (Walther, W. and Stein, U., eds.), Humana, Totowa, NJ, pp. 275–285.

18

Immune Response to Suicide Gene Therapy

Shigeki Kuriyama, Hirohisa Tsujinoue, and Hitoshi Yoshiji

1. Introduction

Many types of cancer become resistant to current chemotherapeutic and radiothera-peutic interventions. To overcome this situation, applications of gene therapy may be promising. Whereas many types of transgene, such as tumor suppressor genes and cytokine genes, have potential tumoricidal effects (*1*), genes encoding for prodrug-activating enzymes, the so-called suicide genes, are very promising and have been intensively investigated (*2,3*). The basic principle underlying suicide gene systems is intracellular conversion of a relatively nontoxic prodrug to a highly toxic drug by an enzyme that is not normally present in the cell. Viruses, bacteria, and fungi often use unique metabolic pathways not used by mammalian cells and contain genes for en-zymes that perform metabolic conversions that mammalian cells do not perform. Such distinctive enzymes have often been the targets of drugs developed for the treatment of infections. Such agents are lethal for the infecting microbes but do not harm the host cell because it lacks the enzyme system necessary to activate the drug (*4,5*). After genetically modifying tumor cells to express such enzymes, systemic prodrug treat-ment leads to the selective killing of tumor cells. The effectiveness of suicide gene–prodrug strategies against cancer has been shown in animal models carrying various types of cancer, and the transfer of a suicide gene into tumor cells followed by admin-istration of the appropriate prodrug is currently being used in various clinical gene therapy trials for the treatment of cancer (*6–10*).

2. Prototypic Suicide Gene Systems

There are a number of suicide gene–prodrug combinations (*3*). Among them, two of the best characterized systems are herpes simplex virus-thymidine kinase (*HSV-TK*)/ganciclovir (GCV) and *Escherichia coli* cytosine deaminase (*CD*)/5-fluorocytosine (5-FC). These suicide gene–prodrug systems are currently being evaluated in clinical trials. *HSV-TK* converts the antiviral drugs, such GCV and

From: *Methods in Molecular Medicine, Vol. 90, Suicide Gene Therapy: Methods and Reviews*
Edited by: C. J. Springer © Humana Press Inc., Totowa, NJ

acyclovir (ACV), to the monophosphorylated forms that are then metabolized to the toxic triphosphate forms by cellular phosphokinases. GCV–triphosphate and ACV–triphosphate interact with the cellular DNA polymerase, causing interference with DNA synthesis and thereby leading to the death of dividing cells *(11–13)*. Although both GCV and ACV are potent drugs for the destruction of cells infected with *HSV-TK*, GCV has been shown to be superior to ACV as a prodrug in the *HSV-TK*-mediated suicide gene system *(14,15)* and has been used in most of *HSV-TK* suicide gene therapy experiments of clinical trials as well as animal studies. *CD* is an enzyme found in many bacteria and fungi, but not in mammalian cells. Its normal function is to deaminate cytosine to uracil in times of nutritional stress *(16)*. In the treatment of fungal and bacterial infections, this metabolic step has been the target of the drug 5-FC, because *CD* converts 5-FC into the toxic anabolite 5-fluorouracil (5-FU), which is subsequently processed either to 5-fluorouracil triphosphate or to 5-fluoro-2'-deoxyuridine 5'-monophosphate. Whereas the former is incorporated into RNA and interferes with RNA processing, the latter irreversibly inhibits thymidylate synthase and thus interferes with DNA synthesis *(17)*.

3. Bystander Effect by the Suicide Gene–Prodrug Systems

Both the *HSV-TK*/GCV and *CD*/5-FC systems have been shown not only to kill transduced cells but also to exert toxic effects on neighboring untransduced cells. This phenomenon, termed the bystander effects, plays a crucial role in cancer gene therapy, because it appears impossible to transfer a suicide gene into all cells of a cancer by currently available techniques. Therefore, the success of gene therapy against cancer with the suicide/prodrug systems hinges on the strength of the bystander effect induced. The in vitro bystander effect caused by the *HSV-TK*/GCV system is mediated, at least in part, by metabolic cooperation in which metabolites of GCV phosphorylation are passed through gap junctions formed between physically contacted cells *(18–21)*. An alternative mechanism in which naive tumor cells phagocytose apoptotic vesicles produced by dying *HSV-TK*-transduced cells has been suggested *(22–24)*. These apoptotic vesicles may contain cytotoxic products, although the identity of the cytotoxic molecules in the vesicles is not clear. In contrast to phosphorylated forms of GCV, which cannot pass through the cellular membrane, 5-FU is freely diffusible across the cellular membrane and spreads from *CD*-transduced cells to adjacent tumor cells that do not express the *CD* gene. Therefore, the in vitro bystander effect induced by the *CD*/5-FC system has been shown not to be dependent on cell-to-cell contact *(25–27)*. The strength of the in vitro bystander effect induced by the *CD*/5-FC system has been shown to correlate very well with the levels of 5-FU generated from 5-FC by *CD*-transduced cells *(28,29)*.

4. Immune Responses Induced by the *HSV-TK*/GCV System

4.1. Involvement of Immunological Reactions

In addition to the events that are important in vitro, other factors may contribute to the bystander effect in vivo. Initial reports supported the notion that the immune system was not necessary for tumor rejection induced by the *HSV-TK*/GCV system

(30,31). However, recent evidence indicates that there is a contribution of the host's immune system to the in vivo bystander effect and that the complete elimination of tumor cells requires an intact immune system. We have shown that antitumor effects of the *HSV-TK*/GCV system demonstrated in vivo are somewhat unexpected compared with the results concerning the ability of in vitro neighboring cell killing using the same murine hepatocellular carcinoma (HCC) cells. We mixed *HSV-TK*-transduced murine HCC cells with parental cells at a ratio of 20% or 40% and subcutaneously implanted 1×10^6 cells into syngeneic BALB/c mice. With GCV treatment initiated 3 d after implantation, none of animals developed subcutaneous HCC tumors *(32–34)*. When the *HSV-TK*-transduced murine HCC cells were cultured together with parental HCC cells at ratios of 20% and 40% in the presence of GCV in a high cell population at which most cells were in contact with one another, approx 30% and 10%, respectively, of parental cells remained alive *(34–36)*. Parental HCC cells used in the experiments are highly tumorigenic, because even in the case of subcutaneous implantation of 5×10^4 cells, all animals developed tumors, indicating that if only 5% of implanted cells survive, tumor formation will occur in all animals. The discrepancy observed in the in vitro and in vivo experiments using the same HCC cell line indicates that some additional mechanism except the direct transfer of phosphorylated GCV from *HSV-TK*-transduced cells to untransduced cells via gap junctions may be at work in the in vivo bystander effect induced by the *HSV-TK*/GCV system.

We have also shown that when syngeneic immunocompetent mice were inoculated subcutaneously with murine HCC cells containing *HSV-TK*-transduced ones at a 50% ratio followed by GCV treatment, none of animals developed tumors. We then examined the inhibitory effect of the *HSV-TK*/GCV system on tumor formation using athymic nude mice that do not have an intact T-cell system. In marked contrast to the results obtained using syngeneic immunocompetent mice, when grafts inoculated into athymic nude mice contained *HSV-TK*-transduced cells at a 50% ratio, 8 of 10 mice developed subcutaneous tumors despite GCV treatment *(32,33)*. It has been shown that gap junctions play an essential role in the bystander effect caused by the *HSV-TK*/GCV system. However, the capacity for gap junctional intercellular communication has been lost in most cancer cells *(37)*. Although the gap-junctional status of HCC cells used in our study was not investigated, HCC tumors are supposed to have few gap junctions. Therefore, it is supposed that the transfer of phosphorylated GCV from *HSV-TK*-transduced cells to parental cells did not occur in subcutaneous HCC tumors because of the lack of gap junctions, resulting in no significant inhibition of the tumor development in athymic nude mice. Although subcutaneous HCC tumors of syngeneic immunocompetent mice did not have gap junctions either, parental HCC cells appeared to be eliminated by the host immunity elicited by the *HSV-TK*/GCV system.

Caruso et al. *(38)* have shown that immunological reactions are involved in tumor regression caused by the *HSV-TK*/GCV system. Syngeneic immunocompetent rats inoculated intrahepatically with rat colon carcinoma cells were given an intratumoral injection of retroviral packaging cells producing *HSV-TK*-expressing recombinant retroviral particles. With GCV treatment, a dramatic regression of the tumor volume was observed and the residual tumors were mostly made up of a massive fibrotic reaction. Furthermore, in some animals, the residual tumors were devoid of cancer cells. There was a moderate increase in the proportion of macrophages within the tumor mass of animals in the *HSV-TK*/GCV group compared with those in the control group. Furthermore, there was a dramatic infiltration of *CD4+* and *CD8+* lymphocytes in the tumor of animals in the *HSV-TK*/GCV group. These results indicate the involvement of host's immune responses in the antitumor effect induced by the *HSV-TK*/GCV system.

4.2. Induction of Tumor Immunity

It has been shown that the *HSV-TK*/GCV system can induce tumor immunity, and implantation of *HSV-TK*-transduced tumor cells followed by GCV treatment may work as a vaccination therapy against the parental tumor. Vile et al. *(39)* have shown that the antitumor effect induced by the *HSV-TK*/GCV system involved an immune component. They have shown that the number of established lung metastases of B16 melanoma in syngeneic C57BL mice treated with GCV was reduced compared with controls after multiple intravenous administrations of high-titer retroviral supernatant encoding the *HSV-TK* gene. The reduction in the number of experimental metastases in C57BL mice exceeded the anticipated extent of transduction of tumor cells, which is indicative of a marked in vivo bystander effect. This magnitude of reduction was not observed in immunodeficient athymic nude mice, indicating that the immune system plays some part in the in vivo bystander effect induced by the *HSV-TK*/GCV system. The authors have also shown that syngeneic immunocompetent animals treated with modified melanoma cells to express the *HSV-TK* gene followed by GCV treatment were resistant to later challenge with wild-type melanoma cells.

Barba et al. *(40)* have demonstrated that tumor immunity was induced after *HSV-TK* gene therapy. They implanted *HSV-TK*-carrying retroviral-producing cells into established 9L brain tumors in syngeneic immunocompetent rats. Significant tumor regression was seen following GCV treatment, with 7 of 32 animals being alive 90 d later. Histological examination of the brains of the successfully treated animals revealed residual tumor cells and inflammatory cells consisting predominantly of macrophages/microglia and T-cells in the hemisphere with the residual tumor cyst. Rats surviving 90 d rejected repeat tumor injections into the contralateral brain and flank, whereas identical tumor injections in naive animals resulted in both brain and flank tumors.

Gagandeep et al. *(41)* and Kianmanesh et al. *(42)* have shown that when grafts consisting of *HSV-TK*-transduced tumor cells were killed in vivo by GCV treatment, antitumor immunity was generated so that a subsequent challenge with untransduced parental tumor cells led to rejection. We have also shown that the *HSV-TK*/GCV system could induce tumor immunity to the wild-type parental tumor. Murine HCC cells transduced with the *HSV-TK* gene were mixed with parental cells at small ratios and implanted subcutaneously into syngeneic immunocompetent mice. Significant inhibition of tumor growth and even complete regression of established solid tumors were induced by GCV treatment. Tumor eradication rates were significant when established subcutaneous tumors contained *HSV-TK*-transduced ones at ratios of 10% or more. Furthermore, 18 of 22 animals that completely abrogated an established solid tumor containing *HSV-TK*-transduced cells at various ratios exhibited resistance to wild-type

HCC tumors. The 18 mice that rejected rechallenge of parental HCC cells were inoculated again with a tumorigenic dose of syngeneic murine colonic adenocarcinoma cells. There was no protection against the colonic adenocarcinoma cell challenge, and all mice developed subcutaneous solid tumors, with no significant delay of tumor formation compared with control animals. These results indicate that the tumor immunity induced by the *HSV-TK*/GCV system is tumor-cell-specific. The murine HCC cells used in our study appear not to be immunogenic, or at most to be weakly immunogenic, because vaccination with irradiated or mytomycin-treated parental HCC cells did not raise tumor immunity at all in syngeneic immunocompetent mice. These results indicate that the *HSV-TK*/GCV system can induce potent tumor immunity and may cause effective antitumor effects on metastatic lesions.

4.3. T-Cell-Mediated Immune Augmentation

The induction of antitumor-specific cytotoxic T-lymphocytes (CTLs) and an enhanced expression of the costimulatory molecules B7-1 and B7-2, intercellular adhesion molecule (ICAM), and major histocompatibility complex (MHC) suggest that cell killing following treatment with the *HSV-TK*/GCV system produces immunostimulatory signals, enabling the immune system of the host to recognize and eliminate the remaining tumor cells *(43–46)*. The results that the in vivo bystander effect of the *HSV-TK*/GCV system was not sufficient to restrain the tumor growth taking place in athymic nude mice *(33,34,41,47)* indicate that a T-cell-mediated immune mechanism appears to play an important role in tumor eradication caused by the *HSV-TK*/GCV strategy. We have demonstrated that marked infiltration of inflammatory cells was induced with GCV treatment in tumors containing *HSV-TK*-transduced cells at various ratios, but not in those containing no *HSV-TK*-transduced cells. Infiltrating cells were predominantly lymphocytes including *CD4*+ and *CD8*+ cells *(33)*.

Mullen et al. *(48)* have shown that syngeneic immunocompetent animals treated with *HSV-TK*-transduced tumors and GCV developed specific resistance to rechallenge with unmodified parental tumors. GCV treatment induced necrotic tumor death and a pronounced host inflammatory response consisting of both *CD4*+ and *CD8*+ lymphocytes and immunoregulatory cytokines, such as interleukin (IL)-12, in the tumor microenvironment. However, T-lymphocyte and cytokine responses induced by the *HSV-TK*/GCV-mediated necrosis was not observed in animals treated with the alkylating immunosuppressive agent cyclophosphamide, although both the traditional chemotherapy and the suicide gene treatment induced tumor necrosis. Inflammation-induced by the *HSV-TK*/GCV system could lead to more effective presentation of antigens from the necrotic tumor compared with an intact, progressively growing tumor. The polymorphonuclear cell release of degradative enzymes may produce higher local concentrations of potentially immunogenic proteins and peptides. Inflammation-induced vascular permeability may augment the entry of antigen-presenting cells and lymphocytes into the tumor microenvironment. Undefined paracrine factors in sites of inflammation may influence host cells to release immunoregulatory cytokines, which may shape the immune response to the released antigens. Although traditional chemotherapeutic agents also induce similar local necrosis, the severe systemic myelotoxicity and immunotoxicity of the chemotherapeutic agents may significantly impair the capability of the host to mount an effective immune response at the time the antigens are available, resulting in insufficient immune responses to the tumor.

Yamamoto et al. *(44)* subcutaneously implanted a tumorigenic dose of murine renal carcinoma cells transduced with the *HSV-TK* gene into syngeneic immunocompetent mice. After complete regression of inoculated tumors with GCV treatment, the animals were challenged with nontransduced tumor cells, resulting in rejection or significant growth inhibition of challenged tumor cells. In these animals, tumor-specific CTLs were efficiently induced and *CD*8+ cells were a main component in this CTL fraction. Expression of class I MHC antigens was increased in *HSV-TK*-transduced cells treated with GCV. These results indicate that systemic immunity observed after *HSV-TK*/GCV treatment may be established, in part, through increased expression of class I MHC antigen, which enhances the presentation of tumor antigens on the dying cells and induces the effective CTL response.

Vile et al. *(49)* have shown that *HSV-TK*/GCV-mediated cell killing in vivo stimulated a mononuclear cell infiltrate and a Th1-like profile of intratumoral cytokine expression. They implanted *HSV-TK*-transduced murine melanoma cells subcutaneously into syngeneic immunocompetent mice and observed an abundant intratumoral mononuclear cell infiltrate following GCV treatment. The infiltrate consisted of both *CD*4+ and *CD*8+ lymphocytes as well as a large number of macrophages at early time-points after GCV treatment. The authors have demonstrated that IL-2 and IL-12 mRNAs were present from an early stage and persisted through the period of tumor destruction. Other cytokines appeared more slowly at the tumor-site such as granulocyte–macrophage colony-stimulating factor (GM-CSF), interferon-γ (IFN-γ) and tumor necrosis factor-α (TNF-α). There were, however, no appreciable levels of IL-4 or IL-10 mRNA within the tumors at any stage, and IL-6 mRNA expression was initially present but was lost after 2–4 d of GCV treatment. This profile of cytokines within the tumor environment is characteristic of a Th1 immune response *(50)*, which is usually associated with the development of cell-mediated immunity and may also reflect the subsequent development of the antitumor immunity *(51)*.

Felzmann et al. *(52)* inoculated murine fibrosarcoma cells subcutaneously into syngeneic immunocompetent mice and transferred the *HSV-TK* gene *in situ* using recombinant adenoviruses. The tumors regressed in 80% of mice upon GCV treatment. Cured animals were protected from further challenge with wild-type tumor but not from challenge with an unrelated syngeneic tumor cell line. Although CTL responses induced by the *HSV-TK*/GCV system in their model were weak, enhanced secretion of GM-CSF, IL-2, IL-6, and IFN-γ from spleen cells of the treated animals was observed. The enhanced IFN-γ secretion with unchanged IL-4 secretion indicate that adenoviral-mediated transfer of the *HSV-TK* gene followed by GCV treatment may result in a predominantly Th1-mediated antitumor immune response. Taken collectively, these results suggest that *HSV-TK*/GCV-mediated cell killing in vivo elicits T-cell-mediated immune responses and creates a cytokine-rich immunostimulatory environment within the intratumoral regions, which are otherwise immunosilent in nonimmunogenic tumors, resulting in the potent antitumor effect and the induction of tumor immunity.

4.4. T-Cell-Independent Immune Augmentation

Tumor rejection in vivo involves tumor-specific CTL activity but may also involve other effectors, such as activated macrophages and natural killer (NK) cells. Ishii-Morita et al. *(21)* have shown that that antitumor effects induced by the *HSV-TK*/GCV system occur even in athymic nude mice. Roger et al. *(53)* have reported that when xenografts contained the cells expressing the *HSV-TK* gene at a 30% ratio, tumors regressed by GCV treatment even in severe combined immunodeficiency (SCID) mice. These results indicate that T-cell-independent immune responses can be elicited by the *HSV-TK*/GCV system and play an important role in the antitumor effect.

Hall et al. *(54)* have shown that NK cells were the major mediators of the in vivo antitumor effect induced by the *HSV-TK*/GCV system. They implanted a murine prostate tumor cell line orthotopically into syngeneic immunocompetent mice and adenovirally transferred the *HSV-TK* gene followed by GCV treatment. Freshly prepared tumor-infiltrating lymphocytes (TILs) generated significant in vitro lytic activity not only against the parental prostate cancer cell line but also against an unrelated prostate cancer cell line. In vitro antibody and complement depletion of *CD3+* T-cells and NK cells from TILs indicated that NK cell were the dominant mediator of the observed tumor cell lysis. Concurrently, no CTL activity was ascertained within spleen cells of treated animals. In vivo depletion of NK cells resulted in a 20% reduction in growth suppression within the primary tumor and complete abrogation of the inhibition of pre-established lung metastasis. In contrast, depletion of T-cells had no effect on either response.

4.5. Controversial Mechanism of Immune Responses

As described so far, elicitation of T-cell-dependent immune responses has been shown to play an essential role in the in vivo antitumor effect induced by the *HSV-TK*/GCV system in many animal experiments. Conversely, it has also been demonstrated in some animal experiments that T-cell-mediated immune responses is not necessary for tumor abrogation induced by the *HSV-TK*/GCV system or even that the T-cell-independent immune mechanism plays a substantial role in the antitumor effect. It is also controversial whether the death of tumor cells caused by the *HSV-TK*/GCV system occurs by apoptosis or by necrosis. Some reports demonstrated that apoptotic death of tumor cells was induced in vivo by the *HSV-TK*/GCV system *(33,47)*, whereas others demonstrated that *HSV-TK*-transduced tumor cells underwent necrosis but not apoptosis in vivo by GCV treatment *(48,49)*. Such discrepancies in determining the role of an immune response elicited by the *HSV-TK*/GCV system may be the result of the inherent immunogenicity of each cell line used in the experiments. Some tumor cell lines may be sufficiently immunogenic to induce immune responses even in immunodeficient animals but others may not be. Furthermore, it is possible that the transduction of an exogenous gene may alter the behavior of tumor cells with respect to immune responses. Uniquely, differential responses against the vector and transgene may also depend on the mouse strain and vector used in the experiments.

Thus, although the precise mechanism of immunological responses induced by the *HSV-TK*/GCV system remains to be determined, there are several plausible explanations for the immunological antitumor effects of the *HSV-TK*/GCV system. First, the death of genetically modified cells to express the *HSV-TK* gene leads to more effective antigen presentation. A correlation has been shown between regression of metastatic lesions and the infiltration of macrophages, *CD4+* and *CD8+* lymphocytes *(38)*. The inflammatory response to the dying cells could activate antigen-presenting cells, resulting in enhanced tumor immunity to wild-type cells. Second, the expression of the novel protein enhances the immune response against the tumor *(55)*. Although immunity directed against the protein expressed by a suicide gene will not lead to direct rejection of a wild-type tumor which does not express the suicide gene, the protein may function as a sort of superantigen leading to polyclonal activation of lymphocytes, some of which may be crossreactive with the tumor. Third, following transduction of the *HSV-TK* gene and a subsequent GCV treatment, immunity can develop against the untransduced parental tumor type *(40)*. We have shown an interesting result that mice pretreated with both *HSV-TK*-transduced and untransduced cells followed by GCV treatment developed tumors less frequently than those pretreated with only *HSV-TK*-transduced cells followed by GCV treatment *(32)*. This indicates that the existence of wild-type tumor cells, when suicide-gene-transduced cells are targeted by host immunity, may elicit a stronger protective immunity to wild-type tumors. Fourth, treatment by the *HSV-TK*/GCV system can elicit cytokine responses *(46,56)*, resulting in the enhancement of tumor immunity.

Bi et al. *(57)* have demonstrated noteworthy results concerning the antitumor effect of the *HSV-TK*/GCV system, using cells of human oral squamous cell carcinoma origin. Mixtures of *HSV-TK*-transduced and untransduced tumor cells were implanted subcutaneously in the left flank of athymic nude mice and untransduced parental cells were implanted subcutaneously in the right flank. With GCV treatment, the tumors composed of mixed cells in the left flank resolved. The naive tumors in the right flank either resolved or became cytostatic, showing little further growth compared with controls. An infiltration of lymphoid cells was observed in the regressing tumors. Concomitant treatment with an immunosuppressive agent dexamethasone impaired the antitumor effect on the contralateral side. When similar experiments were performed in SCID mice, there was a reduced antitumor effect on the ipsilateral flank and no antitumor response in the contralateral flank. Athymic nude mice are immuno-compromised primarily as a result of a deficiency in mature T-lymphocytes. However, they do have functional NK cells. Furthermore, compared with immunocompetent mice, nude mice have an enlarged monocyte/macrophage pool *(58)*. They can also produce antibody against nonprotein antigens *(59)*. Furthermore, older nude mice may develop some functional T-lymphocytes because of extrathymic T-cell maturation. Therefore, in principle, nude mice have the capacity to mount an immune response, albeit an incomplete one, against implanted tumor cells. Impairment of the immunity of nude mice by dexamethasone treatment resulted in the reduced bystander effect. No bystander effect was observed when similar experiments were carried out in SCID mice. These results indicate that the antitumor effect induced by the *HSV-TK*/GCV system requires immunocompetence.

Taken collectively, it appears apparent that the enhanced immunological responses but not the direct transfer of phosphorylated GCV into neighboring tumor cells play a substantial role in the antitumor effect induced by *HSV-TK* gene therapy. However, the mechanism of the antitumor effect is not fully understood or even controversial.

5. Immune Responses Induced by the CD/5-FC System

Localized in vivo generation of 5-FU as a new strategy for antitumor therapy was reported previously by Nishiyama et al. *(60)*. They implanted capsules containing *CD* into a rat glioma followed by systemic administration of 5-FC and demonstrated local 5-FU generation and antitumor activity. A similar strategy was achieved by a genetic approach *(61–63)*. Mullen et al. *(64)* and Huber et al. *(65)* genetically modified tumor cells to express *CD*. They implanted the modified cells into mice and demonstrated the local 5-FU generation and antitumor effects. We have shown that expression of the *CD* gene was not cytotoxic and *CD*-transduced murine HCC cells exhibited the same growth ratio compared with parental cells. In the presence of 5-FC, however, *CD*-transduced HCC cells were eliminated in vitro and showed more than 120-fold higher susceptibility to 5-FC compared with parental cells. On the other hand, *CD*-transduced cells showed the sensitivity to 5-FU similar to that of parental cells, indicating that there was no significant difference in the cells' inherent sensitivity to the toxic end product *(28,29)*. It has been shown that the marked bystander effect was induced by the *CD*/5-FC system not only in vitro but also in vivo *(28,65,66)*.

Consistent with the results obtained by the *HSV-TK*/GCV system *(33,34)*, we have shown that the bystander effect by the *CD*/5-FC system was induced more strongly in vivo than in vitro *(67)*. When as little as 5% of murine HCC cells expressing the *CD* gene were mixed with parental cells and inoculated subcutaneously into syngeneic immunocompetent mice, significant suppression of tumor formation was observed with 5-FC treatment. Furthermore, significant inhibition of tumor growth and even complete regression of established solid tumors containing *CD*-transduced cells at an only 5% ratio were induced by 5-FC treatment. These results indicate that significant antitumor activity could be induced when only a very small fraction of tumor was genetically modified to express the *CD* gene. These inhibitory rates are much higher than those observed in vitro *(28,29)*.

In contrast with the results obtained using syngeneic immunocompetent mice, when grafts inoculated into athymic nude mice contained *CD*-transduced cells at a ratio of 20% or 40%, all of the mice developed tumors despite 5-FC treatment. Furthermore, two of six nude mice inoculated with only *CD*-transduced cells developed tumors despite 5-FC treatment *(67)*. We have previously demonstrated that when cells transduced with the *HSV-TK* gene were inoculated into mice and developed established solid tumors, the *HSV-TK* gene was heavily methylated in some animals, resulting in no expression of the transduced *HSV-TK* gene *(32,68,69)*. It is, therefore, supposed that some populations of *CD*-transduced cells inoculated into mice did not express the *CD* gene because of methylation and that athymic nude mice could not eliminate the cells that lost *CD* gene expression and escaped from killing by 5-FU because of deficient immunity.

These results are inconsistent with the previous study reported by Huber et al. *(65)*. They mixed *CD*-transduced and parental human colorectal carcinoma cells at various ratios and implanted the cell mixtures subcutaneously into athymic nude mice. They demonstrated that significant tumor regressions were induced by 5-FC treatment in nude mice inoculated with xenografts containing *CD*-transduced cells at an only 2% ratio and that complete abrogation of established tumors was achieved in some of animals inoculated with xenografts containing *CD*-transduced cells at a ratio of 4% or more. Although they suggested that the transfer of 5-FU converted from 5-FC by *CD*-transduced cells resulted in significant antitumor effects in nude mice, our previous in vitro results demonstrated that even if *CD*-transduced cells were mixed with parental cells at a 20% ratio in the presence of 5-FC, 100% killing of parental cells was not achieved *(28)*. It is unlikely that the discrepancy is the result of the difference of sensitivity to 5-FU between the cell lines, because murine HCC cells used in our study are more susceptible to 5-FU than human colorectal carcinoma cells that Huber et al. used in their experiments (20 ng/mL vs 650 ng/mL as to the values of IC_{50}, defined as the dose required for 50% cytotoxicity). Although we do not know the exact reason for the discrepancy, it might be attributed to the difference of the immunogenicity of the cell lines used in the experiments. It is supposed that the T-cell-independent tumor immunity that athymic nude mice possess was sufficient to induce efficient antitumor effects against the human colorectal carcinoma cells that the investigators used but insufficient against the murine HCC cells used in our study.

It has been shown that the *CD*/5-FC system can induce protective immunity to wild-type tumor *(27,64,67)*. Uckert et al. *(70)* have shown that when murine mammary adenocarcinoma cells transduced with both the *CD* and *HSV-TK* genes were inoculated subcutaneously into syngeneic immunocompetent mice followed by a combination therapy of 5-FC and GCV, tumor development was completely inhibited. In athymic nude mice treated in the same way, however, most developed tumors, indicating that T-lymphocyte-mediated immune mechanisms appear to play an important role in suicide-gene-mediated tumor rejection. We have also demonstrated that marked infiltration of lymphocytes, including CD4+ and CD8+ lymphocytes, and macrophages was observed with 5-FC treatment in tumors consisting of both parental and *CD*-transduced cells but not in those containing no *CD*-transduced cells, and that mice that completely eradicated an established solid tumor consisting of parental and *CD*-transduced cells resisted subsequent rechallenge with untransduced wild-type tumor *(27,67)*.

Consalvo et al. *(71)* have shown that an immunological mechanism is involved in *CD*/5-FC-mediated cell killing in vivo. They transduced murine mammary adenocarcinoma cells with the *CD* gene and implanted the transduced cells into syngeneic immunocompetent mice. Intraperitoneal administration of 5-FC caused total regression of incipient and established tumors. Following regression, all mice were resistant to subsequent subcutaneous and intravenous lethal challenges with untransduced parental tumor cells. The authors then carried out the immunosuppression experiments using anti-CD4, anti-CD8, and antigranulocyte monoclonal antibodies. They demonstrated that removal of CD4+ cells did not impair the regression of *CD*-transduced tumors and all mice eventually rejected the tumors by 5-FC treatment, whereas the removal of

CD8+ cells or granulocytes substantially impaired the tumor regression. Although the tumor immunity elicited by the *CD*/5-FC system was dependent on *CD*4+ lymphocytes, its effector phase depended on both CD4+ and CD8+ lymphocytes.

It has been shown that NK cells play an important role in *CD*/5-FC-mediated tumor regression. Pierrefite-Clarle et al. *(72)* transduced the *CD* gene into a rat colon carcinoma cell line and injected the tumor-cells-expressing the *CD* gene intrahepatically into syngeneic immunocompetent rats. Treatment with 5-FC led to a 95% decrease in the mean tumor volume of *CD*-expressing tumors compared with control animals, with 7 of 11 treated animals being tumor-free. Intrahepatic injection of *CD*-expressing cells followed by 5-FC treatment rendered the treated animals resistant to challenge with wild-type tumor cells, with none of seven animals developing wild-type tumors in contrast to all control animals. Immunohistological analysis of experimental tumors revealed an infiltration of NK cells within the tumor, dependent on 5-FC treatment. In vivo depletion of NK cells substantially impaired the antitumor effect induced by the *CD*/5-FC system, indicating that NK cells were the major immune component involved in the antitumor effect.

Using a stable *CD* transfectant of a tumorigenic rat adenocarcinoma cell line, Haack et al. *(73)* have shown that regression of *CD*-transduced tumors occurred independently of 5-FC treatment in syngeneic immunocompetent animals and that 37% of these tumor-free animals rejected the subsequent challenge with tumorigenic doses of parental tumor cells. Immune rats contained lymphocytes able to specifically lyse the *CD*-transduced as well as the untransduced parental tumor cells in vitro, most likely contributing to the in vivo antitumor reaction. Thus, although the mechanism of immunological responses induced by the *CD*/5-FC system is also complicated and may differ from tumor to tumor, these results may offer the prospect that *CD*-transduced tumor cells and 5-FC can be used as components of a live antitumor vaccine.

6. Future Aspects of Suicide Gene Therapy

In conclusion, the results described in this chapter indicate that the host immune responses elicited by suicide gene/prodrug systems but not the direct transfer of the cytotoxic drug produced from the prodrug by suicide-gene-transduced tumor cells into untransduced ones appear to play a crucial role in the in vivo antitumor effect. These observations may have important implications for future clinical applications of suicide gene/prodrug systems, because the immune competence of patients with cancer appears to be a critical factor for achieving successful gene therapy against cancer using suicide gene/prodrug systems. The exact immunological mechanism of antitumor responses induced by suicide gene/prodrug systems is not clear and what makes it more complicated is that immunogenicity varies from tumor to tumor and immune competence also varies from host to host. Therefore, the effectiveness of cancer gene therapy with a suicide gene/prodrug system may differ from patient to patient. Furthermore, it should be noted that human tumors are less immunogenic and show a decreased immunity compared with the currently used experimental tumors *(74)*. Therefore, strategies aimed at augmenting the immune response of a suicide gene system by concomitantly transferring an immunostimulatory gene have been explored. It has been shown that a number of cytokine genes, such as IL-1, IL-2, IL-4, IL-6, IL-12, IFN-α, IFN-γ and GM-CSF, may be promising for the further enhancement of antitumor effects induced by suicide gene/prodrug systems *(75–86)*. Use of genes for costimulatory molecules, class I MHC antigens, and lymphoactins may also be attractive for the combination gene therapy *(87,88)*. As for experimental tumors, immunological characteristics of human tumors are not identical. It is difficult to identify the best immunostimulatory gene for each human tumor. Therefore, combinations of a suicide gene/prodrug system and plural immunostimulatory genes may be more effective and practical than those using a singular immunostimulatory gene for improving the therapeutic outcome of clinical cancer gene therapy. These combination gene therapies with a suicide gene and immunostimulatory genes may open up new avenues for the treatment of cancer.

References

1. Roth, J. A. and Cristiano, R. J. (1997) Gene therapy for cancer: what have we done and where are we going? *J. Natl. Cancer Inst.* **89**, 21–39.
2. Connors, T. A. (1995) The choice of prodrugs for gene directed enzyme prodrug therapy on cancer. *Gene Ther.* **2**, 702–709.
3. Aghi, M., Hochberg, F., and Breakefield, X. O. (2000) Prodrug activation enzymes in cancer gene therapy. *J. Gene Med.* **2**, 148–164.
4. Mullen, C. A. (1994) Metabolic suicide genes in gene therapy. *Pharmacol. Ther.* **63**, 199–207.
5. Moolten, F. L. (1994) Drug sensitivity ("suicide") genes for selective cancer chemotherapy. *Cancer Gene Ther.* **1**, 279–287.
6. Crystal, R. G. (1995) Transfer of genes to humans: early lessons and obstacles to success. *Science* **270**, 404–410.
7. Ross, G. (1996) Gene therapy in the United States: a five-year status report. *Hum. Gene Ther.* **7**, 1781–1790.
8. Marcel, T. and Grausz, J.D. (1996) The TMC worldwide gene therapy enrollment report (June 1996). *Hum. Gene Ther.* **7**, 2025–2046.
9. Smythe, W. R. (2000) Prodrug/drug sensitivity gene therapy: current status. *Curr. Oncol. Rep.* **2**, 17–22.
10. Human gene marker/therapy clinical protocols. (2000) *Hum. Gene Ther.* **11**, 2543–2617.
11. Elion, G. B., Furman, P. A., Fyfe, J. A., de Miranda, P., Beauchamp, L., and Schaeffer, H. J. (1977) Selectivity of action of an antiherpetic agent, 9-(2-hydroxyethoxymethyl) guanine. *Proc. Natl. Acad. Sci. USA* **74**, 5716–5720.
12. Field, A. K., Davies, M. E., DeWitt, C., et al. (1983) 9-{[2-Hydroxyl-1-(hydroxymethyl) ethoxy] methyl} guanine: a selective inhibitor of herpes group virus replication. *Proc. Natl. Acad. Sci. USA* **80**, 4139–4143.
13. Matthews, T. and Boehme, R. (1988) Antiviral activity and mechanism of action of ganciclovir. *Rev. Infect. Dis.* **10(Suppl. 3)**, 490–494.
14. Balzarini, J., Bohman, C., and De Clercq, E. (1993) Differential mechanism of cytostatic effect of (*E*)-5-(2-bromovinyl)-2'-deoxyuridine, 9-(1,3-dihydroxy-2-propoxymethyl) guanine, and other antiherpetic drugs on tumor cells transfected by the thymidine kinase gene of herpes simplex virus type 1 or type 2. *J. Biol. Chem.* **268**, 6332–6337.
15. Kuriyama, S., Nakatani, T., Masui, K., et al. (1996) Evaluation of prodrugs ability to induce effective ablation of cells transduced with viral thymidine kinase gene. *Anticancer Res.* **16**, 2623–2628.

16. Danielsen, S., Kilstrup, M., Barilla, K., Jochimsen, B., and Neuhard, J (1992) Characterization of the *Escherichia coli* codBA operon encoding cytosine permease and cytosine deaminase. *Mol. Microbiol.* **6**, 1335–1344.

17. Mullen, C. A., Kilstrup, M., and Blaese, R. M. (1992) Transfer of the bacterial gene for cytosine deaminase to mammalian cells confers lethal sensitivity to 5-fluorocytosine: a new negative selection system. *Proc. Natl. Acad. Sci. USA* **89**, 33–37.

18. Bi, W. L., Parysek, L. M., Warnick, R., and Stambrook, P. J. (1993) In vitro evidence that metabolic cooperation is responsible for the bystander effect observed with HSVtk retroviral gene therapy. *Hum. Gene Ther.* **4**, 725–731.

19. Mesnil, M., Piccoli, C., Tiraby, G., Willecke, K., and Yamasaki, H. (1996) Bystander killing of cancer cells by herpes simplex virus thymidine kinase gene is mediated by connexins. *Proc. Natl. Acad. Sci. USA* **93**, 1831–1835.

20. Elshami, A. A., Saavedra, A., Zhang, H., et al. (1996) Gap junctions play a role in the "bystander effect" of the herpes simplex virus thymidine kinase/ganciclovir system in vitro. *Gene Ther.* **3**, 85–92.

21. Ishii-Morita, H., Agbaria, R., Mullen, C. A., et al. (1997) Mechanism of "bystander effect" killing in the herpes simplex thymidine kinase gene therapy model of cancer treatment. *Gene Ther.* **4**, 244–251.

22. Freeman, S. M., Abboud, C. N., Whartenby, K. A., et al. (1993) The "bystander effect": tumor regression when a fraction of the tumor mass is genetically modified. *Cancer Res.* **53**, 5274–5283.

23. Samejima, Y. and Meruelo, D. (1995) "Bystander killing" induces apoptosis and is inhibited by forskolin. *Gene Ther.* **2**, 50–58.

24. Hamel, W., Magnelli, L., Chiarogi, V. P., and Israel, M. A. (1996) Herpes simplex virus thymidine kinase/ganciclovir-mediated apoptotic death of bystander cells. *Cancer Res.* **56**, 2696–2702.

25. Hirschowitz, E. A., Ohwada, A., Pascal, W. R., Russi, T. J., and Crystal, R. G. (1995) In vivo adenovirus-mediated gene transfer of the *Escherichia coli* cytosine deaminase gene to human colon carcinoma-derived tumors induces chemosensitivity to 5-fluorocytosine. *Hum. Gene Ther.* **6**, 1055–1063.

26. Dong, Y., Wen, P., Manome, Y., et al. (1996) In vivo replication-deficient adenovirus vector-mediated transduction of the cytosine deaminase gene sensitizes glioma cells to 5-fluorocytosine. *Hum. Gene Ther.* **7**, 713–720.

27. Kuriyama, S., Mitoro, A., Yamazaki, M., et al. (1999) Comparison of gene therapy with the herpes simplex virus thymidine kinase gene and the bacterial cytosine deaminase gene for the treatment of hepatocellular carcinoma. *Scand. J. Gastroenterol.* **34**, 1033–1041.

28. Kuriyama, S., Masui, K., Sakamoto, T., et al. (1995) Bacterial cytosine deaminase suicide gene transduction renders hepatocellular carcinoma sensitive to the prodrug 5-fluorocytosine. *Int. Hepatol. Commun.* **4**, 72–79.

29. Kuriyama, S., Masui, K., Sakamoto, T., et al. (1998) Bystander effect caused by cytosine deaminase gene and 5-fluorocytosine in vitro is substantially mediated by generated 5-fluorouracil. *Anticancer Res.* **18**, 3399–3406.

30. Ram, Z., Walbridge, S., Heiss, J. D., Culver, K. W., Blaese, R. M., and Oldfield, E. H. (1994) In vivo transfer of the human interleukin-2 gene: negative tumoricidal results in experimental brain tumors. *J. Neurosurg.* **80**, 535–540.

31. Dilber, M. S., Abedi, M. R., Christensson, B., et al. (1997) Gap junctions promote the bystander effect of herpes simplex virus thymidine kinase in vivo. *Cancer Res.* **57**, 1523–1528.

32. Kuriyama, S., Sakamoto, T., Masui, K., et al. (1997) Tissue-specific expression of *HSV-TK* gene can induce efficient antitumor effect and protective immunity to wild-type hepatocellular carcinoma. *Int. J. Cancer* **71**, 470–475.

33. Kuriyama, S., Kikukawa, M., Masui, K., et al. (1999) Cancer gene therapy with *HSV-TK/* GCV system depends on T-cell-mediated immune responses and causes apoptotic death of tumor cells in vivo. *Int. J. Cancer* **83**, 374–380.

34. Kuriyama, S., Tsujinoue, H., Nakatani, T., et al. (2000) Gene therapy for hepatocellular carcinoma, in *Molecular Target for Hematological Malignancies and Cancer* (Niho, Y., ed.), Kyushu University Press, Fukuoka, Japan, pp. 29–37.

35. Kuriyama, S., Yoshikawa, M., Tominaga, K., et al. (1993) Gene therapy for the treatment of hepatoma by retroviral-mediated gene transfer of the herpes simplex virus thymidine kinase. *Int. Hepatol. Commun.* **1**, 253–259.

36. Kuriyama, S., Nakatani, T., Masui, K., et al. (1995) Bystander effect caused by suicide gene expression indicates the feasibility of gene therapy for hepatocellular carcinoma. *Hepatology* **22**, 1838–1846.

37. Holder, J. W., Elmore, E., and Barrett, J. C. (1993) Gap junction function and cancer. *Cancer Res.* **53**, 3475–3485.

38. Caruso. M., Panis, Y., Gagandeep, S., Houssin, D., Salzmann, J. L., and Klatzmann, D. (1993) Regression of established macroscopic liver metastases after in situ transduction of a suicide gene. *Proc. Natl. Acad. Sci. USA* **90**, 7024–7028.

39. Vile, R. G., Nelson, J. A., Castleden, S., Chong, H., and Hart, I. R. (1994) Systemic gene therapy of murine melanoma using tissue specific expression of the HSVtk gene involves an immune component. *Cancer Res.* **54**, 6228–6234.

40. Barba, D., Hardin, J., Sadelain, M., and Gage, F. H. (1994) Development of anti-tumor immunity following thymidine kinase-mediated killing of experimental brain tumors. *Proc. Natl. Acad. Sci. USA* **91**, 4348–4352

41. Gagandeep, S., Brew, R., Green, B., et al. (1996) Prodrug-activated gene therapy: involvement of an immunological component in the "bystander effect." *Cancer Gene Ther.* **3**, 83–88.

42. Kianmanesh, A. R., Perrin, H., Panis, Y., et al. (1997) A "distant" bystander effect of suicide gene therapy: regression of nontransduced tumors together with a distant transduced tumor. *Hum. Gene Ther.* **8**, 1807–1814.

43. Freeman, S. M., Ramesh, R., and Marrogi, A. J. (1997) Immune system in suicide-gene therapy. *Lancet* **349**, 2–3.

44. Yamamoto, S., Suzuki, S., Hoshino, A., Akimoto, M., and Shimada, T. (1997) Herpes simplex virus thymidine kinase/ganciclovir-mediated killing of tumor cell induces tumor-specific cytotoxic T cells in mice. *Cancer Gene Ther.* **4**, 91–96.

45. Ramesh, R., Munshi, A., Abboud, C. N., Marrogi, A. J., and Freeman, S. M. (1996) Expression of costimulatory molecules: B7 and ICAM up-regulation after treatment with a suicide gene. *Cancer Gene Ther.* **3**, 373–384.

46. Ramesh, R., Marrogi, A. J., Munshi, A., Abbound, C. N., and Freeman, S. M. (1996) In vivo analysis of the "bystander effect": a cytokine cascade. *Exp. Hematol.* **24**, 829–838.

47. Colombo, B. M., Benedetti, S., Ottolenghi, S., et al. (1995) The "bystander effect": association of U-87 cell death with ganciclovir-mediated apoptosis of nearby cells and lack of effect in athymic mice. *Hum. Gene Ther.* **6**, 763–772.

48. Mullen, C. A., Anderson, L., Woods, K., Nishino, M., and Petropoulos, D. (1998) Ganciclovir chemoablation of herpes thymidine kinase suicide gene-modified tumors produces tumor necrosis and induces systemic immune responses. *Hum. Gene Ther.* **9**, 2019–2030.

49. Vile, R. G., Castleden, S., Marshall, J., Camplejohn, R., Upton, C., and Chong, H. (1997) Generation of an anti-tumour immune response in a non-immunogenic tumour: HSVtk

killing in vivo stimulates a mononuclear cell infiltrate and a Th1-like profile of intratumoral cytokine expression. *Int. J. Cancer* **71**, 267–274.

50. Seder, R. A. and Paul, W. E. (1994) Acquisition of lymphokine-producing phenotype by *CD4+* T cells. *Ann. Rev. Immunol.* **12**, 635–673.

51. Thompson, C. B. (1995) Distinct roles for the costimulatory ligands B7-1 and B7-2 in T helper cell differentiation. *Cell* **81**, 979–982.

52. Felzmann, T., Ramsey, W. J., and Blaese, R. M. (1997) Characterization of the antitumor immune response generated by treatment of murine tumors with recombinant adenoviruses expressing HSVtk, IL-2, IL-6 or B7-1. *Gene Ther.* **4**, 1322–1329.

53. Rogers, R. P., Ge, J.-Q., Holley-Guthrie, E., et al. (1996) Killing Epstein–Barr virus-positive B lymphocytes by gene therapy: comparing the efficacy of cytosine deaminase and herpes simplex virus thymidine kinase. *Hum. Gene Ther.* **7**, 2235–2245.

54. Hall, S. J., Sanford, M. A., Atkinson, G., and Chen, S.-H. (1998) Induction of potent antitumor natural killer cell activity by herpes simplex virus–thymidine kinase and ganciclovir therapy in an orthotopic mouse model of prostate cancer. *Cancer Res.* **58**, 3221–3225.

55. Tapscott, S. J., Miller, A. D., Olson, J. M., Berger, M. S., Groudine, M., and Spence, A. M. (1994) Gene therapy of rat 9L gliosarcoma tumors by transduction with selectable genes does not require drug selection. *Proc. Natl. Acad. Sci. USA* **91**, 8185–8189.

56. Freeman, S. M., Ramesh, R., Shastri, M., Munshi, A., Jensen, A. K., and Marrogi, A. J. (1995) The role of cytokines in mediating the bystander effect using HSVtk xenogeneic cells. *Cancer Lett.* **92**, 167–174.

57. Bi, W., Kim, Y. G., Feliciano, E. S., et al. (1997) An HSVtk-mediated local and distant antitumor bystander effect in tumors of head and neck origin in athymic mice. *Cancer Gene Ther.* **4**, 246–252.

58. Dziarski, R. (1984) Opposing effects of xid and nu mutations on proliferative and polyclonal antibody and autoantibody responses to peptidoglycan, LPS, protein A and PWM. *Immunology* **53**, 563–574.

59. Fidler, I. J., Murray, J. L., and Kleinerman, E. S. (1991) Systemic activation of macrophages by liposomes containing immunomodulators, in *Biologic Therapy of Cancer: Principles and Practice* (Hellman, S., DeVita, V. T. and Jr., Rosenberg, S. A., eds.), Lippincott, Philadelphia, pp. 730–742.

60. Nishiyama, T., Kawamura, Y., Kawamoto, K., et al. (1985) Antineoplastic effects in rats of 5-fluorocytosine in combination with cytosine deaminase capsules. *Cancer Res.* **45**, 1753–1761.

61. Cao, G., Kuriyama, S., Gao, J., et al. (1999) Effective and safe gene therapy for colorectal carcinoma using the cytosine deaminase gene directed by the carcinoembryonic antigen promoter. *Gene Ther.* **6**, 83–90.

62. Cao, G., Kuriyama, S., Cui, L., et al. (1999) Analysis of the human carcinoembryonic antigen promoter core region in colorectal carcinoma-selective cytosine deaminase gene therapy. *Cancer Gene Ther.* **6**, 572–580.

63. Cao, G., Kuriyama, S., Gao, J., et al. (1999) In vivo gene transfer of a suicide gene under the transcriptional control of the carcinoembryonic antigen promoter results in bone marrow transduction but can avoid bone marrow suppression. *Int. J. Oncol.* **15**, 107–112.

64. Mullen, C. A., Coale, M. M., Lowe, R., and Blaese, R. M. (1994) Tumors expressing the cytosine deaminase suicide gene can be eliminated in vivo with 5-fluorocytosine and induce protective immunity to wild type tumor. *Cancer Res.* **54**, 1503–1506.

65. Huber, B. E., Austin, E. A., Richards, C. A., Davis, S. T., and Good, S. S. (1994) Metabolism of 5-fluorocytosine to 5-fluorouracil in human colorectal tumor cells transduced with

the cytosine deaminase gene: significant antitumor effects when only a small percentage of tumor cells express cytosine deaminase. *Proc. Natl. Acad. Sci. USA* **91**, 8302–8306.

66. Rowley, S., Lindauer, M., Gebert, J. F., et al. (1996) Cytosine deaminase gene as a potential tool for the genetic therapy of colorectal cancer. *J. Surg. Oncol.* **61**, 42–48.

67. Kuriyama, S., Kikukawa, M., Masui, K., et al. (1999) Cytosine deaminase/5-fluorocytosine gene therapy can induce efficient anti-tumor effects and protective immunity in immunocompetent mice but not in athymic nude mice. *Int. J. Cancer* **81**, 592–597.

68. Kuriyama, S., Sakamoto, T., Kikukawa, M., et al. (1998) Expression of a retrovirally transduced gene under control of an internal housekeeping gene promoter does not persist due to methylation and is restored partially by 5-azacytidine treatment. *Gene Ther.* **5**, 1299–1305.

69. Kuriyama, S., Masui, K., Kikukawa, M., et al. (1999) Complete cure of established murine hepatocellular carcinoma is achievable by repeated injections of retroviruses carrying the herpes simplex virus thymidine kinase gene. *Gene Ther.* **6**, 525–533.

70. Uckert, W., Kammertöns, T., Haack, K., et al. (1998) Double suicide gene (cytosine deaminase and herpes simplex virus thymidine kinase) but not single gene transfer allows reliable elimination of tumor cells in vivo. *Hum. Gene Ther.* **9**, 855–865.

71. Consalvo, M., Mullen, C. A., Modesti, A., et al. (1995) 5-Fluorocytosine-induced eradication of murine adenocarcinomas engineered to express the cytosine deaminase suicide gene requires host immune competence and leaves an efficient memory. *J. Immunol.* **154**, 5302–5312.

72. Pierrefite-Carle, V., Baqué, P., Gavelli, A., et al. (1999) Cytosine deaminase/5-fluorocytosine-based vaccination against liver tumors: evidence of distant bystander effect. *J. Natl. Cancer Inst.* **91**, 2014–2019.

73. Haack, K., Linnebacher, M., Eisold, S., Zöller, M., von Knebel Doeberitz, M., and Gebert, J. (2000) Induction of protective immunity against syngeneic rat cancer cells by expression of the cytosine deaminase suicide gene. *Cancer Gene Ther.* **7**, 1357–1364.

74. Roszman, T., Elliott, L., and Brooks, W. (1991) Modulation of T-cell function by gliomas. *Immunol. Today* **12**, 370–374.

75. Chen, S.-H., Kosai, K., Xu, B. et al. (1996) Combination suicide and cytokine gene therapy for hepatic metastases of colon carcinoma: sustained antitumor immunity prolongs animal survival. *Cancer Res.* **56**, 3758–3762.

76. Mullen, C. A., Petropoulos, D., and Lowe, R. M. (1996) Treatment of microscopic pulmonary metastases with recombinant autologous tumor vaccine expressing interleukin 6 and *Escherichia coli* cytosine deaminase suicide genes. *Cancer Res.* **56**, 1361–1366.

77. O'Malley, B. W., Cope, K. A., Chen, S. H., Li, D., Schwarta, M. R., and Woo, S. L. (1996) Combination gene therapy for oral cancer in a murine model. *Cancer Res.* **56**, 1737–1741.

78. O'Malley, B. W., Jr., Sewell, D. A., Li, D., et al. (1997) The role of interleukin-2 in combination adenovirus gene therapy for head and neck cancer. *Mol. Endocrinol.* **11**, 667–673.

79. Coll, J.-L., Mesnil, M., Lefebvre, M.-F., Lancon, A., and Favrot, M. C. (1997) Long-term survival of immunocompetent rats with intraperitoneal colon carcinoma tumors using herpes simplex thymidine kinase/ganciclovir and IL-2 treatments. *Gene Ther.* **4**, 1160–1166.

80. Santodonato, L., Ferrantini, M., Gabriele, L., et al. (1996) Cure of mice established metastatic friend leukemia cell tumors by a combined therapy with tumor cells expressing both interferon-α1 and herpes simplex thymidine kinase followed by ganciclovir. *Hum. Gene Ther.* **7**, 1–10.

81. Santodonato, L., D'Agostino, G., Santini, S. M., et al. (1997) Local and systemic antitumor response after combined therapy of mouse metastatic tumors with tumor cells expressing IFN-α and HSVtk: perspectives for the generation of cancer vaccines. *Gene Ther.* **4**, 1246–1255.

82. Benedetti, S., Dimeco, F., Pollo, B., et al. (1997) Limited efficacy of the *HSV-TK*/GCV system for gene therapy of malignant gliomas and perspectives for the combined transduction of the interleukin-4 gene. *Hum. Gene Ther.* **8,** 1345–1353.
83. Nanni, P., De Giovanni, C., Nicoletti, G., et al. (1998) The immune response elicited by mammary adenocarcinoma cells transduced with interferon-γ and cytosine deaminase genes cures lung metastases by parental cells. *Hum. Gene Ther.* **9,** 217–224.
84. Cao, X., Ju, D. W., Tao, Q., et al. (1998) Adenovirus-mediated GM-CSF gene and cytosine deaminase gene transfer followed by 5-fluorocytosine administration elicit more potent antitumor response in tumor-bearing mice. *Gene Ther.* **5,** 1130–1136.
85. Okada, H., Giezeman-Smits, K. M., Tahara, H., et al. (1999) Effective cytokine gene therapy against an intracranial glioma using a retrovirally transduced IL-4 plus HSVtk tumor vaccine. *Gene Ther.* **6,** 219–226.
86. Toda, M., Martuza, R. L., and Rabkin, S. D. (2001) Combination suicide/cytokine gene therapy as adjuvants to a defective herpes simplex virus-based cancer vaccine. *Gene Ther.* **8,** 332–339.
87. Miller, P. W., Sharma, S., Stolina, M., et al. (1998) Dendritic cells augment granulocyte–macrophage colony-stimulating factor (GM-CSF)/herpes simplex virus thymidine kinase-mediated gene therapy of lung cancer. *Cancer Gene Ther.* **5,** 380–389.
88. Ju, D. W., Tao, Q., Cheng, D. S., et al. (2000) Adenovirus-mediated lymphotactin gene transfer improves therapeutic efficacy of cytosine deaminase suicide gene therapy in established murine colon carcinoma. *Gene Ther.* **7,** 329–338.

19

Targeting Cancer With Gene Therapy
Using Hypoxia as a Stimulus

Gabi U. Dachs, Olga Greco, and Gillian M. Tozer

1. Introduction
1.1. Tumor Hypoxia in the Clinic

Tumors are known to have an abnormal and chaotic vascular network, unable to effectively or reliably supply the whole tumor with oxygen and nutrients. Over the past years direct evidence has accumulated showing that reduced oxygen tension (hypoxia) is a common feature of both experimental and human solid tumors (1). For example, in a study of human breast cancer, the median tumor oxygen partial pressure (pO_2) for all stages of the disease was found to be around 28 mm Hg (3.9% O_2), compared with 65 mm Hg (8.7% O_2) for normal breast tissue. In the normal breast, pO_2 values less than 2.5 mm Hg (approx 0.3% O_2) could not be detected, whereas they were measured in about one-third of the breast cancer cases (2). Severe hypoxia has also been reported for head and neck cancer, cervical cancer, and melanomas (3–5).

Importantly, progress reports from clinical studies show that the most hypoxic tumors are consistently associated with poor treatment outcome. This was first shown in human cervix carcinomas (6) and soft-tissue sarcomas (7) and recently confirmed in a range of other tumor types. It is well known that the cellular response to radiation, chemotherapy, and cytokines is modified by oxygen tension. However, classical radioresistance of hypoxic cells is unlikely to be the only explanation, because tumor oxygen status is the most important prognostic factor for treatment outcome in cervical carcinoma, irrespective of the therapeutic modality (including surgery) (8). Unfortunately, methods aimed at overcoming treatment-resistant hypoxic cells have only achieved moderate success to date (9,10).

This clinical as well as experimental evidence is converging to suggest that tumor hypoxia acts to produce a phenotype that gives rise to more aggressive locoregional disease and enhanced invasive capacity. This is initially counterintuitive because, even though tumor cells can survive periods of hypoxia, severe hypoxia for extended periods eventually leads to cell death. Other factors, including hypoxic gene expression, are therefore likely to be important.

From: *Methods in Molecular Medicine, Vol. 90, Suicide Gene Therapy: Methods and Reviews*
Edited by: C. J. Springer © Humana Press Inc., Totowa, NJ

1.2. Gene Control Under Hypoxia

Hypoxia is an independent stimulus of gene expression, unrelated to ionizing radiation or heat shock. It can, to some extent, be mimicked by carbon monoxide, desferrioxamine, or cobalt, nickel, and manganese, via interference with the oxygen-sensing process (reviewed in **refs. 11** and **12**). Gene products upregulated by low oxygen generally aim to counteract the detrimental effects of hypoxia: Angiogenic factors attract new vasculature to increase oxygenation, vasodilators increase blood flow, glucose transporters and glycolytic enzymes allow the switch to energy-saving glycolysis, and oncoproteins give hypoxic tumor cells a growth advantage.

Gene expression can be regulated both at the transcriptional and posttranscriptional levels. To enhance or restrict transcription, transcription factors bind to particular DNA sequences, enhancers, or repressors that are located either within the promoter region or up to several kilobases upstream or downstream. Alternatively, the stability of mRNA and proteins can be modified to regulate the amount of final product.

The control of erythropoietin (EPO), the main regulator of red blood cell production, was studied as a model to gain an understanding of how cells sense and respond to changes in oxygen tension. Madan and Curtin (13) defined the minimal DNA region necessary for hypoxia response of the EPO gene as a 24-basepair (bp) sequence, able to regulate transcription regardless of orientation and distance of the coding region. Beck et al. (14) identified a 120-kDa protein that is upregulated by hypoxia and binds to the EPO hypoxia enhancer sequence. This nuclear transcription factor was defined as the hypoxia-inducible factor 1 (HIF-1) and found to be common to a variety of EPO-producing and EPO-nonproducing mammalian cells (15).

1.3. Hypoxia-Inducible Factor-1

Affinity purification and molecular cloning of HIF-1 showed it to function as a heterodimer, consisting of two basic helix–loop–helix proteins from the Per-aryl hydrocarbon receptor nuclear translocator-Sim (PAS) family of transcription factors: HIF-1α and HIF-1β {previously identified as aryl receptor nuclear translocator [ARNT], part of the xenobiotic response (16)}. HIF-1 is common to all mammalian cells tested to date and was also detected in all human tissue and organs assayed (17–19). Increased levels of HIF-1α protein in human prostate cancer cell lines correlated with increased metastatic potential (20). More importantly, 13/19 clinical tumor types were found to overexpress the HIF-1α protein subunit (21).

Hypoxia primarily upregulates the DNA-binding activity of HIF-1 (15). It is generally accepted that HIF-1β is not oxygen sensitive and that HIF-1α is hypoxia regulated at the posttranslational level. The amount of HIF-1α protein increases during hypoxia and is degraded within minutes during reoxygenation in intact cells (22). HIF-1α is polyubiquinated in air, targeting it to the ubiquitin–proteasome degradation pathway, whereas ubiquination is largely reduced under hypoxia (23,24). In addition, the hypoxic increase in HIF-1α protein depends on a redox-dependent increase in protein stabilization that, in turn, originates from a change in conformation upon dimerization with HIF-1β. Phosphorylation of HIF-1α via p42/p44 mitogen-activated protein kinase appears to also play a role in its activation pathway (25). Finally, the two subunits

Table 1
Hypoxia-Responsive Elements from Hypoxia-Inducible Genes of Different Origin

HRE core sequence	Gene
GGGCCCT**ACGTGC**TGCCTCGCATGGC	EPO mouse
GGGCCCT**ACGTGC**TGTCTCACACAGC	EPO human
ATTTGTC**ACGTCC**TGCACGACGCGAG	PGK-1 mouse
GCTGCAG**ACGTGC**GTGTG	PGK-1 human
CCAGCGG**ACGTGC**GGGAACCCACGTG	LDH-A mouse
TCCACAG**GCGTGC**CGTCTGACACGCA	GLUT-1 mouse
AGTGCAT**ACGTGG**GCTTCCACAGGTC	VEGF rat
AGTGCAT**ACGTGG**GCTCCAACAGGTC	VEGF human
TCGCTTC**ACGTGC**GGGGACCAGGGAC	ALD-A human
GGGCCGG**ACGTGG**GGCCCAGAGCGAC	ENO-1 human
CTGGCGT**ACGTGC**TGCAG	PFK-L mouse

Note: The HIF-1 binding site is underlined.

of HIF-1 bind in the cytosol and dimerization is required for stable association with the nuclear compartment *(26)*.

Recently the cellular oxygen sensor has been identified. Posttranslational hydroxylation of proline residues in HIF-1α has been shown to regulate HIF stabilization *(53,54)*. Under normoxic conditions, prolyl hydroxylation enables specific interaction with the von Hippel Lindau protein, which is part of the ubiquitin ligase complex. The enzyme responsible, HIF-1α–prolyl-hydroxylase, requires Fe^{2+} as a cofactor as well as molecular oxygen and 2-oxoglutarate to convert HIF-1α to the hydroxylated form. In the absense of oxygen the enzyme is inactive and posttranslational modification of HIF-1 does not occur.

1.4. Hypoxia-Responsive Elements

HIF-1 specifically binds to hypoxia-responsive elements (HREs), which contain the core sequence 5'-(A/G)CGT(G/C)(G/C)-3' and are localized at varying distances and orientations to the coding region of most hypoxia-regulated genes identified to date.

Table 1 shows a range of HRE sequences identified near genes encoding EPO, phosphoglycerate kinase (PGK) 1, lactate dehydrogenase (LDH) A, glucose transporter (GLUT) 1, vascular endothelial growth factor (VEGF), aldolase (ALD) A, enolase

(ENO) 1, and phosphofructokinase (PFK) L from different species *(27)*. The core sequence for HIF-1 binding is underlined.

1.5. Hypoxia-Targeted Gene Therapy

The high frequency of HIF-1 expression across many human tumors of diverse tissue origin represents a possible therapeutic target for HRE-directed gene therapy for the hypoxic environment. In a feasibility study, we demonstrated that marker gene expression regulated by the murine PGK-1 HRE in heterologous promoters could be induced by hypoxia in tumor cells *(28)*. Production of the marker protein CD2 in stably transfected human fibrosarcoma cells HT1080 increased with increasing length and severity of hypoxia. Compared to oxygen levels typical of normal tissues (2–5% O_2), radiobiologically relevant hypoxia (O_2 concentrations of less than 0.3%) induced an up to threefold increase in gene expression (*see* **Fig. 1**). Following anoxia and subsequent reoxygenation, a sevenfold to eightfold induction was observed. When the transfected tumor cells were grown as xenografts in nude mice, expression of the CD2 gene was limited to perinecrotic areas, which are indicative of hypoxia. To analyze this system on a single-cell basis, tumor-bearing mice were exposed to a bioreductive drug (which induces DNA crosslinks only in hypoxic cells) and X-rays (preferentially generating DNA strand breaks in oxic cells). By analyzing individual tumor cells ex vivo with the single-cell electrophoresis assay (the comet assay; *see* **Fig. 2**) combined with CD2 immunostaining, it could be demonstrated that increased CD2 expression was only seen in hypoxic tumor cells.

Other studies have subsequently shown similar findings. Murine C2C12 myoblasts manipulated to express the human EPO gene regulated by the murine PGK-1 promoter showed in vitro a 2.7-fold increase in gene expression in anoxia and a 3.2-fold induction at 1.3% O_2 *(29)*. In vivo, compared to controls kept at 21% O_2, a twofold increase in serum EPO levels was detected when mice with C2C12-EPO cells implanted in their dorsal flank were exposed to 7% O_2 *(29)*.

To increase the hypoxic/oxic induction ratio of hypoxia-responsive promoters, a series of DNA constructs containing fragments of the murine PGK-1, murine LDH-A, human EPO, and human ENO-1 genes were inserted into the basal simian virus 40 (SV40) promoter to control the reporter gene luciferase *(30)*. In transiently transfected human breast tumor T47D cells, the EPO-chimeric promoter exhibited the most stringent regulation in hypoxia (255-fold induction at 0.1% O_2), whereas the PGK-1 HREs showed the highest absolute levels of expression (more than the strong cytomegalovirus [CMV] promoter), at the expense of selective regulation (146-fold at 0.1% O_2; *see* **Fig. 3**). The hypoxic response was increased twofold by inserting at the C-terminus of the luciferase gene a 150-bp oligonucleotide spanning the 3' untranslated region (UTR) of VEGF, which is involved in hypoxia-induced mRNA stability. The PGK-1 HRE promoter was inserted in an adenoviral vector, and in a panel of transduced cell lines a low basal level of β-galactosidase (β-gal) transgene expression was observed, with levels of hypoxic induction comparable to the full-length CMV *(32)*.

In two studies on fibrosarcoma HT1080 cells transiently transfected with constructs containing fragments of the human EPO and VEGF genes, a significant differential

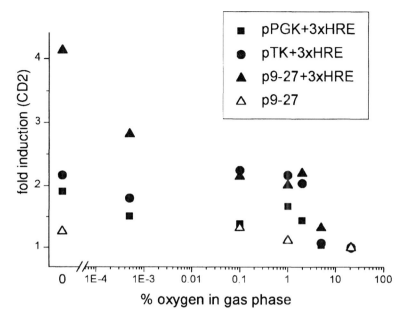

Fig. 1. Increased expression of CD2 under hypoxic conditions. Human fibrosarcoma cells HT1080 were stably transfected with DNA constructs containing three copies of the HRE from PGK-1 fused to the PGK-1 promoter, or the minimal thymidine kinase (TK) promoter or the 9–27 promoter. The hypoxic response was evaluated after 16 h of hypoxic treatment. Surface expression of CD2 protein was analyzed using immunostain followed by FACS analysis. The *y*-axis represents the ratio of hypoxic to normoxic CD2 production analyzed by FACS analysis.

response to hypoxia was obtained by combining five copies of the 35-bp VEGF HREs with the adenoviral E1b minimal promoter *(33,34)*. A 6-h hypoxic (0.02% O_2) incubation induced a 40- to 50-fold increase in luciferase activity *(33)* (*see* **Fig. 3**). An even higher hypoxic/aerobic ratio (approx 500) was obtained when the five VEGF HREs were linked to the minimal CMV, with luciferase activities similar to the full-length CMV *(34)* (*see* **Fig. 3**). In this study, the inclusion of the 3' VEGF UTR reduced hypoxic gene expression.

The cellular background appears to affect the hypoxic response system, because cell lines of diverse origin respond differently. For example, a study using the murine PGK-1 HRE controlling the β-gal encoding gene showed an 8.5-fold hypoxic increase in HS 906(d).Mu cells vs a 50-fold increase in SkMC cells *(32)*. Similarly, luciferase controlled by the human VEGF HRE increased expression in SCCVII cells 3.3-fold, vs 8.5-fold in HepG2 cells *(33)*.

It is not clear whether the large fold inductions by HRE-controlled genes in response to hypoxia in later reports *(31–34)* represent a clear improvement over the constructs used in earlier studies *(28)*, as transient rather than stable transfection methods were employed. Also, the end point in early studies was the immunological detection of a

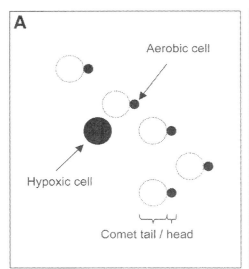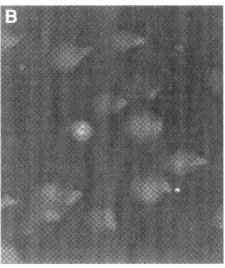

Fig. 2. Identification of single hypoxic cells in tumors. Cells derived from tumors treated with RSU1069 and 10 Gy of X-rays were subsequently analyzed with the alkaline comet assay. RSU 1069 induces the formation of DNA crosslinks in hypoxic cells only. In contrast, exposure to ionizing radiation results mainly in DNA strand breakage in aerobic cells. Anaerobic cells with damaged DNA appear as comets with a short tail and a big head. A schematic representation of a microscope slide (**A**) and a photograph of the propidium iodide-stained comets (**B**) are shown.

cell surface protein, whereas luciferase assays measure the conversion by the enzyme of many substrate molecules to light units. The luciferase assay therefore further amplifies any increase in transcription, making a direct comparison to other assays difficult. It is therefore important to analyze different reporter gene assays prior to selecting one for gene expression analysis.

1.6. Choice of Reporter Genes

The study of gene regulation and the development of optimized expression systems for gene therapy rely heavily on reporter genes. Reporter genes should display easily measurable phenotypes distinguishable above a background of endogenous proteins. Several genes are commonly used as reporters for gene transfer and expression studies: (1) the bacterial enzymes β-gal *(35)* and (2) chloramphenicol acetyltransferase (CAT) *(36)*, (3) the bioluminescent protein luciferase (also known as aequorin or mono-oxygenase) from firefly or sea pansy *(37)*, and (4) the green fluorescent protein (GFP) from jellyfish *(38)*. All of these systems have certain drawbacks.

Luciferase, β-gal and CAT are enzymes and thereby require substrates, such as luciferin, o-nitrophenyl-β-D-galactopyranoside (ONPG), and chloramphenicol, respectively, to produce detectable products *(39)*. This makes their use as real-time reporters for gene expression in vivo difficult and may overestimate the real increase in gene

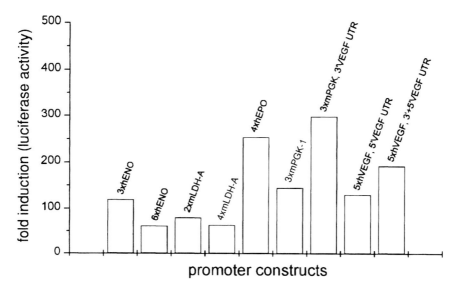

Fig. 3. Hypoxia-inducibility of HRE-containing promoters. The results of different in vitro studies of hypoxia-regulated transgene expression are indicated. The fold increase in luciferase activity after hypoxic treatment was normalized to the activity in normoxic cells. (Adapted from **ref. *31*.**)

induction. Luciferase is a monomeric protein that does not require posttranslational modification and its activity can therefore be assessed immediately following translation *(40)*. However, luciferase requires molecular oxygen and ATP at the time of activation of luciferin to produce luminescence, both of which are in limited supply in most solid, hypoxic tumors *(2)*. Additionally, the use of luciferase for gene regulation studies involving cyclic AMP- modulating agents has been questioned in the past *(41)*. It appeared, therefore, that GFP may be superior for studies under tumor conditions to other reporter genes currently available.

The GFP from the jellyfish *Aequorea victoria* and its mutagenized variants, with improved fluorescence intensity *(42)* and reduced half-life for transient gene expression studies *(43)*, are increasingly used as reporters. Although GFP does not require exogenous substrates or cofactors to produce the active fluorescent molecule *(44)*, it does require molecular oxygen to form the protein's fluorophore *(45)*. A posttranslational modification results from spontaneous cyclization and oxidation of the protein's aminoacids -Ser_{65} (or Thr_{65})-Tyr_{66}-Gly_{67}- *(45)*, which could represent a limitation when GFP is used as a reporter in hypoxic conditions.

1.7. Choice of Gene-Directed Enzyme–Prodrug Therapy Systems

The most well-known examples of enzyme–prodrug combinations in cancer gene-directed enzyme prodrug therapy (GDEPT) are herpes simplex virus-thymidine kinase (HSV-TK)/ganciclovir (GCV) and *Escherichia coli* cytosine deaminase (CD)/5-

fluorocytosine (5-FC) (reviewed in **ref. *46***). Because they interfere with DNA synthesis, both the HSV-TK/GCV and the CD/5-FC systems need cell proliferation for their action and are generally not suitable to target slowly dividing hypoxic cells. Although tumor cells transfected with a hypoxia-induced CD-encoding gene could be sensitised to 5-FC during subsequent drug exposure in air *(28)*, no cell kill could be detected when CD-expressing cells were treated in anoxia (own observation). Analogously, cells transfected with the HSV-TK gene could not be sensitized to GCV when exposed to the prodrug in anoxic conditions *(47)*. These observations suggest that cell-cycle-independent cytotoxins will be essential to successfully eradicate hypoxic tumor cells.

Therefore, we are developing a novel enzyme–prodrug system for GDEPT, consisting of the plant enzyme horseradish peroxidase (HRP) and the nontoxic plant hormone indole-3-acetic acid (IAA) *(47,48)*. The efficacy of the HRP/IAA system was evaluated in vitro by exposing a panel of human cell lines transfected with the HRP cDNA to IAA and derivatives. Significant cytotoxicity could be evoked after 2-h exposure only, and it was further increased after 24 h incubation. A substantial bystander effect resulting from the transfer of soluble toxic metabolites was also observed. Anoxic incubation did not reduce the efficacy of the system, indicating that the HRP/IAA combination has the potential to kill the hypoxic subpopulation in solid tumors.

2. Materials

2.1. Cell Culture

1. Dulbecco's modified Eagle's medium (DMEM; Life Technologies, Paisley, UK), supplemented with 10% fetal calf serum (FCS; Sigma, Gillingham, UK) and glutamine (2 m*M*; Life Technologies).
2. Trypsin/EDTA (Life Technologies).
3. Trypan blue (Sigma).

2.2. Hypoxic Conditions In Vitro

1. Permanox plastic dishes (Nalge Nunc International, Naperville, IL) (*see* **Note 1**).
2. Sealed gassing containers with sealed connections for gassing; gas-impermeable tubing.
3. Gas cylinders containing premixed certified gas mixtures (BOC Gases, London, UK).
4. Anaerobic glove cabinet with an atmosphere of 5% CO_2, 5% H_2, 90% N_2, with palladium catalyst (Don Whitley Scientific Ltd, Shipley, UK).

2.3. Hypoxia-Responsive Promoters

1. Plasmid DNA: pCI-neo (Promega, Southampton, UK), pEGFP-N1 (Clontech, Basingstoke, UK).
2. Enzymes and corresponding reaction buffers (Life Technologies; Promega): *Bgl*II, *Sgf*I, *Eco*RI, *Not*I, T4 DNA ligase.
3. Single-stranded oligonucleotides (MWG-Biotech, Milton Keynes, UK).
4. QIAquick PCR Purification kit; QIAfilter Plasmid Maxi kit (Quiagen, Crawley, UK).
5. TOP 10 *E. coli* competent cells (Invitrogen-Novex, Groningen, The Netherlands).

2.4. Transfection In Vitro

1. Plasmid DNA (at 1 mg/mL in water or Tris-EDTA buffer): pHDW9-27CD2, pDW9-27CD2 *(28)*; pHREGFPpuro, pCIGFPpuro, pRK34-HRP *(47)*.
2. Lipofectin (Life Technologies).

3. OptiMEM (Life Technologies), phosphate-buffered saline (PBS).
4. Integrin-targeted peptide (sequence K_{16}GACRRETAWACG, Institute of Child Health, London, UK) *(48)* at 0.1 mg/mL in OptiMEM.

2.5. Production of Transiently and Stably Transfected Cells

1. Neomycin analog G418 (Life Technologies).
2. Puromycin dihydrochloride (Sigma).
3. Dimethyl sulfoxide (DMSO) (Sigma).

2.6. Antibody Labeling of Cells for Analysis by Flow Cytometry

1. PBS, FCS.
2. Fluorescein isothiocyanate (FITC)-conjugated mouse IgG1 antihuman CD2 (Serotec, Oxford, UK).

2.7. Detection of Green Fluorescent Protein by Flow Cytometry

PBS, Hanks' balanced salt solution (HBSS, Life Technologies).

2.8. Alkaline Comet Assay

1. PBS, low-geling-temperature agarose (type VII, Sigma).
2. Bioreductive drug RSU 1069 *(50)*.
3. Lysis buffer 0.03 M NaOH, 1 M NaCl, 0.1% N-lauroylasarcosine.
4. Alkaline/tank buffer 0.03 M NaOH, 2 mM EDTA.
5. Propidium iodide (PI) (Sigma) stock at 2.5 mg/mL; use at 1/1000.

2.9. Combined Immunostain and Comet Assay

Materials as in **Subheadings 2.6.** and **2.8.**

2.10. Prodrug Activation (HRP/IAA Combination)

1. HBSS; PBS; isomethylated spirit (IMS).
2. Indole-3-acetic acid (IAA) (Aldrich, Gillingham, UK). IAA is light sensitive and could be stored at –20°C for up to 2 mo.
3. Crystal violet (Sigma).

3. Methods

3.1. Cell Culture

1. Obtain tumor cells from recognized cell banks such as the American Type Culture Collection (ATCC) or the European Collection of Cell Cultures (ECACC) (*see* **Note 2**).
2. Maintain cells of human or rodent origin in DMEM, or equivalent, in humidified air containing 5% CO_2 at 37°C.
3. Detach semiconfluent cells using trypsin/EDTA.
4. Count cells under a microscope using a hemocytometer.
5. Monitor cell growth and viability by cell counting and trypan blue exclusion assays. Suspend cells in media with a final concentration of trypan blue of 0.2%. Immediately count single cells under microscope. Only living cells exclude the dye.

3.2. Hypoxic Conditions In Vitro

1. Normoxia: Normoxia (21% O_2) is achieved by growing cells in a humidified 37°C incubator with 5% CO_2 in air.

2. Hypoxia: Ideally, all manipulations in hypoxic experiments should be carried out in an anaerobic glove cabinet to minimize the effect of oxygen and reoxygenation.
   a. Leave preconditioned (anoxic) media and all plastics to equilibrate in the anaerobic glove cabinet for at least 24 h prior to use.
   b. Bring Permanox dishes containing preplated cells into anaerobic glove cabinet.
   c. Replace normoxic media with a thin layer of preconditioned anoxic media (2 mL/6-cm dish) prior to the experiment.
   d. Place dishes into sealed gassing containers and move out of the glove cabinet.
   e. Flush sealed containers continuously with humidified gas containing different levels of oxygen ($0.1-5\%$ O_2) in 5% CO_2, with a balance of N_2 at $37°C$ for up to 24 h.
3. Anoxia: Two levels of anoxia are achievable under experimental conditions: either the less stringent anoxia, by gassing with a mixture of 5% CO_2 and 95% N_2 (a), or catalyst-induced anoxia (b) (*see* **Note 3**).
   a. Follow instructions as for hypoxic conditions and then flush sealed containers continuously with 5% CO_2 and 95% N_2, which is certified to contain $<0.0005\%$ O_2.
   b. Keep Permanox dishes in anaerobic glove cabinet to achieve catalyst-induced anoxia.

3.3. Hypoxia-Responsive Promoters

1. Anneal 10 µL of each single-stranded oligonucleotide (50 pmol/µL) at $55°C$ for 5 min. Incubate at room temperature (RT) overnight.
2. Digest 3 µg pCI-puro with 15 units *Bgl*II, 1X reaction buffer in a total volume of 20 µL.
3. Remove enzyme from digestion with the QIAquick PCR purification kit.
4. Digest the purified DNA with 15 units *Sgf*I, 1X reaction buffer.
5. To obtain pHREpuro, ligate 0.5 pmol double-stranded linkers and 200 ng *Bgl*II/*Sgf*I-digested vector using 10 units T4 DNA ligase and 1X reaction buffer in a total volume of 10 µL.
6. Amplify the DNA in TOP 10 *E. coli* as described by Sambrook et al. *(39)* and purify by using the QIAfilter Plasmid Maxi kit.
7. Excise the GFP gene from pEGFP-N1 by *Eco*RI/*Not*I digestion and insert the resulting fragment in pHREpuro or pCI-puro, linearized with the same restriction enzymes, to produce pHREGFPpuro or pCIGFPpuro, respectively.

3.4. Transfection In Vitro

1. Transfections are carried out as described by Hart et al. *(49)*. Transfection efficiencies vary depending on the cell line used. T24 bladder carcinoma cells, for example, are characterized by efficiencies of 60–70% on average.
2. Plate cells 24 h prior to transfection in air at $(1-5)\times10^5/6$-cm dish $[(4-18)\times10^3/cm^2])$, depending on the growth rate of the cell line.
3. Freshly prepare transfection mix containing a ratio of $0.75 : 1.8 : 1$ by weight of lipofectin, peptide, and plasmid DNA:

   > 1.5 µL lipofectin stock diluted in 200 µL OptiMEM;
   > 36 µL peptide stock;
   > 2 µL DNA stock diluted into 200 µL OptiMEM.

4. Mix together carefully in the above order. Leave to form complexes (*see* **Fig. 4**) for 2 h at RT. Prior to adding the mixture to the cells, add OptiMEM to a total volume of 1 mL.
5. Remove media and wash attached cells with excess PBS, followed by a wash in OptiMEM.
6. Add 1 mL of transfection mix per dish and incubate for 5–7 h at $37°C$ in humidified incubator.
7. Remove transfection mix and replace with DMEM.

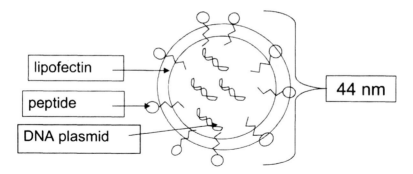

Fig. 4. Complexes of integrin-targeting peptides, lipofectin, and DNA. After 2 h incubation at RT, vesicles 44 nm in diameter containing plasmid DNA are formed. The peptide component contains a 16-lysine DNA-binding domain and an integrin-binding domain. The cationic charge properties of the complex, derived from the peptide, contribute to nonspecific cell-binding and transfection properties. The lipid component acts as an adjuvant to transfection by mediating endosomal escape of the plasmid component.

3.5. Production of Transiently and Stably Transfected Cells

1. Analyze transient transfectants within 48 h of transfection, prior to the integration of the transgene into the genome. No selection is necessary.
2. Select stable transfectants on G418 (0.5–1 mg active drug/mL) or puromycin dihydrochloride (1 μg/mL), depending on the plasmid vector used, for 7–30 d until clones have formed (*see* **Note 4**).
3. Pick separate clones using a fine pipet into 24-well culture dishes.
4. Expand cultures in the presence of selecting agent and test expression of transgene.
5. Test stable transfectants in the absence of selection, as gene expression can be lost.
6. Freeze clones in liquid nitrogen in 10% DMSO in FCS.

3.6. Antibody Labeling of Cells for Analysis by Flow Cytometry

Cell surface expression of transfected CD2 under the control of hypoxia-regulated promoters (pHDW9-27CD2, pDW9-27CD2) in stable transfectants can be analyzed using antibody staining followed by fluorescence-activated cell sorting (FACS) analysis.

1. Plate cells at $(1–5) \times 10^5$ cells/6-cm Permanox dish 24 h prior to hypoxia/anoxia treatment.
2. Incubate cells under hypoxia/anoxia for 0–24 h.
3. Harvest cells into ice-cold PBS by scraping with a rubber policeman. Avoid trypsin, as it destroys some surface antigens.
4. Wash cells twice in ice-cold PBS with 10% FCS.
5. Incubate single-cell suspension on ice with fluorescence-labeled antibodies (FITC-conjugated mouse IgG1 antihuman CD2) for 30 min.
6. Remove excess antibodies by washing with 1 mL ice-cold PBS with 10% FCS.
7. Resuspend in 0.5 mL cold PBS and transfer into FACS tubes.
8. Analyze relative fluorescence of the labeled cells using a fluorescent-activated cell sorter (FACScan, Becton Dickinson, UK), making sure cells are kept cold at all times.
9. Fluorescence, expressed in arbitrary units, is recorded as mean of the main peak. The fold increase in CD2 protein production is expressed as the ratio of the fluorescent signal of normoxic cells compared to that of hypoxic or anoxic cells.

3.7. Detection of Green Fluorescent Protein by Flow Cytometry

Green fluorescent protein (GFP) is widely used as a marker for transfection efficiencies and gene expression, although care should be taken when using it as a reporter of gene expression under hypoxia (see Note 5).

1. Detach transient or stable transfectants containing GFP using trypsin EDTA.
2. Wash once in PBS, then resuspend in HBSS at $(5-10) \times 10^5$ cells/mL.
3. Analyze relative fluorescence using a FACScan. Enhanced GFP has the following spectral characteristics: excitation maximum 488 nm, emission maximum 507 nm.
4. Fluorescence should be normalized to that of untransfected cells while thresholding against cell debris using forward vs side scatter (FCS vs SSC).

3.8. Alkaline Comet Assay

This protocol is derived from the method by Olive (51). The principle is based on the fact that aerobic cells are about three times more sensitive than hypoxic cells to ionizing radiation, which induces DNA damage in the form of strand breaks in individual cells. On the other hand, hypoxic cells are sensitive to the bioreductive agent RSU 1069 that, after enzymatic activation under hypoxia, causes intrastrand crosslinks in the DNA. The two populations of cells are distinguishable by visualizing single cells embedded in agarose after electrophoresis (see Fig. 2).

1. For in vivo studies, implant control and stably transfected cells into the hindleg of NuNu mice at 10^6 cells per animal. Allow the tumors to grow to about 8 mm diameter. Make certain that procedures are performed with approved protocols and strictly in accordance with the Scientific Procedures Act (1986).
2. Inject the mice with the hypoxia-selective drug RSU 1069 (80 mg/kg) 2 h prior to irradiation with 10-Gy X-rays.
3. Immediately excise the tumors and keep on ice. If tumor cells are allowed to warm up, DNA repair processes will interfere with the Comet assay.
4. Finely cut tumors and filter cells to obtain a single-cell suspension. Do not use enzymatic digestion at 37°C.
5. Count cells and adjust single-cell suspension to $(1-3) \times 10^4$ cells/mL in ice-cold PBS.
6. Prepare agarose and keep at 40°C. Label microscope slides.
7. Rapidly mix 1 mL cell suspension with 3 mL agarose.
8. Immediately pipet about 1.5 mL mixture onto labeled microscope slides. Keep slides horizontal at all times and allow agarose to set.
9. Place slides in sealable container with lysis buffer and allow cells to lyse in the dark at room temperature for 1 h.
10. Transfer slides to container with alkaline buffer, leave for total of 1 h with two changes of buffer. Take care not to lose the thin agarose gels in the process.
11. Place slides in horizontal electrophoresis tank in fresh alkaline/tank buffer. The buffer should be a few millimeters above agarose.
12. Electrophorese at 0.6 V/cm for 25–30 min; electric current should be about 40 mA.
13. Remove slides carefully and stain in sealed container for 15 min with PI.
14. Rinse slides with distilled water and keep in humidified sealed container in the dark until analysis by fluorescence microscopy.
15. Cells that were in hypoxic conditions at the time of drug and radiation treatment have most of their genome still within the nucleus because of extensive DNA crosslinking,

whereas cells originally under oxic conditions have most of their genome fragmented and contained in the comet tail because of DNA strand breaks (*see* **Fig. 2**).

3.9. Combined Immunostain and Comet Assay

1. Carry out alkaline Comet assay as described in **Subheading 3.8.**
2. Incubate slides simultaneously with PI and FITC-labeled anti-CD2 antibodies for 1–2 h at 37°C in 5 mL PBS with 10% FCS.
3. Wash thoroughly with PBS (>30 min). Add cover slip.
4. View slides with a fluorescent microscope. Cells that expressed the transfected CD2 surface antigen in hypoxic conditions stain positive following antibody staining and present a short comet tail and a big head.

3.10. Prodrug Activation (HRP/IAA Combination)

1. Preincubate all plastics and media for 24–48 h in the anaerobic glove cabinet.
2. Detach transient or stable HRP transfectants and control cells in air using trypsin/EDTA.
3. Count cells with a hemocytometer.
4. Transfer the cell suspension to the anaerobic cabinet and plate the cells at 10^2–10^5 cells per dish in anoxia.
5. Leave the cells to attach to the plates for 5–6 h in hypoxia/anoxia (*see* **Note 6**).
6. Prepare IAA solutions in HBSS in anoxia.
7. Remove media and replace with IAA-containing HBSS. Control plates are exposed to HBSS only.
8. After 2–24 h incubation, transfer plates to air, wash cells with PBS, and add complete DMEM.
9. To evaluate clonogenic survival, colonies are counted after 7–10 d by staining the cells with 2.5% crystal violet (w/v) in IMS. Surviving fractions are evaluated relative to HBSS-treated controls.

4. Notes

1. Permanox contains less dissolved oxygen than ordinary plastic, such as polystyrene, Perspex, polypropylene and polycarbonate. Plastic dishes retain oxygen for many hours, and attached cells can obtain oxygen from the support (*52*). Glass dishes, on the other hand, are not always a good alternative, because some cell lines do not attach as well as to plastic. In general, plastics and fluids should be preincubated in anoxic conditions for 24–48 h prior to hypoxic/anoxic experiments to remove residual oxygen.
2. Only use cells tested negative for mycoplasma infection. Mycoplasma infection interferes with transfection efficiency, gene regulation, and other assays, especially under hypoxia. The presence of mycoplasma can be identified using the MycoTect kit (Life Technologies). If needed, the most important clones can be cleaned by using Mycoplasma Removal Agent (ICN Biomedicals Ltd., Thame, UK). Also, culture cells routinely in the absence of antibiotics that otherwise could hide the presence of low-level infections.
3. The anoxia achieved in anaerobic glove cabinets was found to be more severe than that induced by gassing with CO_2 and N_2, and differences could be detected for gene regulation, drug sensitivity, and other assays (*28*). Glove cabinets were designed for culturing obligate anaerobic bacteria and can maintain stringent anoxic conditions. They allow manipulations under anoxia such as changing media, trypsinizing, and plating cells. The palladium catalyst combines any incoming oxygen with H_2 to form water vapor, which is removed using silica gel. However, it is good practice to continuously monitor the pres-

ence of oxygen in the anaerobic cabinet with O_2 indicators that can be inserted in the chamber, such as the anaerobic indicator BR55 (Oxoid Ltd., Basingstoke, UK).

4. Before starting the selection of stable clones, evaluate the sensitivity of the cells to the selecting agent, as some lines can develop spontaneous resistance to G418 or puromycin. Drug-sensitivity analysis should be performed for each new batch of agent, because it may vary. Only culture stable clones continuously for short periods of time, as the phenotype is easily lost, even in the presence of selection. Therefore, freeze-down several vials of the original clones and, when defrosting, keep testing the expression of the transgene. When using transient transfectants, it is important to note that the inducibility of hypoxia-responsive promoters can be affected by the transfection efficiency. The transfection efficiency and the hypoxic induction depend on the cell line; therefore, preliminary experiments should be performed to assess the transfection method of choice.

5. We have shown that the requirement of molecular oxygen to form the fluorophore is a problem when GFP is used as reporter in hypoxic biological systems (unpublished). For gene regulation studies, conclusions about the rate of transcription are drawn by analyzing the strength of the fluorescence signal. Final fluorescence is used as a surrogate marker for a long and complex pathway starting with the rate of transcription, translation, and posttranslational modifications, and resulting in the emission of green fluorescence. We demonstrated that fluorescence under anoxia was absent, and under radiobiological hypoxic conditions (<0.3% O_2), it was significantly lower (by more than 50%) when compared to physiologic conditions (2% and 5% O_2). After 5–10 h of reoxygenation, a full recovery of the fluorescence signal was observed. These findings suggest that it may be problematic to analyze hypoxia-regulated gene expression using GFP and that, after hypoxic/anoxic exposure, it is necessary to incubate the cells in normoxia for about 10 h prior to fluorescence analysis.

6. Some cell lines plated in anoxic conditions are characterized by a reduced plating efficiency compared to normoxia. Also, they require a longer time interval to attach to plastics. Therefore, it is advisable to perform a brief preliminary experiment to evaluate the anoxic plating efficiency and the optimal number of cells to be plated for the survival assay chosen. Generally, cells should not be kept under hypoxic or anoxic conditions for more than 24 h, as prolonged incubations may result in loss of viability. T24 human bladder carcinoma cells and FaDu squamous carcinoma cells of the head and neck, for example, showed 7–13% loss of viability after 31 h anoxic incubation. Also, the media pH should be monitored. We found it to be the same in air and anoxic conditions (pH 7.5).

Acknowledgments

The authors are grateful to Dr. Simon Scott for technical help in the synthesis of hypoxia-responsive promoters and to Mrs. Claudia Coralli for information on GFP activity in hypoxic conditions. This work is supported by the Cancer Research Campaign (CRC) and the Gray Laboratory Cancer Research Trust.

References

1. Vaupel, P. and Kelleher, D. K. (eds.) (1999) *Tumour Hypoxia: Pathophysiology, Clinical Significance and Therapeutic Perspectives.* Wissenschaftliche Verlagsgesellschaft, Stuttgart.
2. Vaupel, P. W. (ed.) (1994) *Blood Flow, Oxygenation, Tissue pH Distribution and Bioenergetic Status of Tumors.* Ernst Schering Research Foundation, Berlin.

3. Nordsmark, M., Bentzen, S. M., and Overgaard, J. (1994) Measurement of human tumor oxygenation status by a polarographic needle electrode. An analysis of inter- and intratumor heterogeneity. *Acta Oncol.* **33**, 383–389.
4. Hoeckel, M., Schlenger, K., Knoop, C., and Vaupel, P. (1991) Oxygenation of carcinoma of the uterine cervix: evaluation by computerized O_2 tension measurements. *Cancer Res.* **51**, 6098–6102.
5. Lartigau, E., Randrianarivelo, H., Avril, M. F., et al. (1997) Intratumoral oxygen tension in metastatic melanoma. *Melanoma Res.* **7**, 400–406.
6. Hoeckel, M., Schlenger, K., Aral, B., Mitze, M., Schaeffer, U., and Vaupel, P. (1996) Association between tumour hypoxia and malignant progression in advanced cancer of the uterine cervix. *Cancer Res.* **56**, 4509–4515.
7. Brizel, D. M., Scully, S. P., Harrelson, J. M., et al. (1996) Tumor oxygenation predicts for the likelihood of distant metastases in human soft tissue sarcoma. *Cancer Res.* **56**, 941–943.
8. Hoeckel, M., Schlenger, K., Hoeckel, S., and Vaupel, P. (1999) Hypoxic cervical cancers with low apoptotic index are highly aggressive. *Cancer Res.* **59**, 4525–4528.
9. Overgaard, J. (1994) Clinical evaluation of nitroimidazoles as modifiers of hypoxia in solid tumors. *Oncol. Res.* **6**, 509–518.
10. Lee, D. J., Moini, M., Giuliano, J., and Westra, W. H. (1996) Hypoxic sensitizer and cytotoxin for head and neck cancer. *Ann. Acad. Med. Singapore* **25**, 397–404.
11. Bunn, H. F. and Poyton, R. O. (1996) Oxygen sensing and molecular adaptation to hypoxia. *Physiol. Rev.* **76**, 839–885.
12. Dachs, G. U. and Chaplin, D. J. (1998) Microenvironmental control of gene expression: implications for tumour angiogenesis, progression, and metastasis. *Semin. Radiat. Oncol.* **8**, 208–216.
13. Madan, A. and Curtin, P. T. (1993) A 24-base-pair sequence 3' to the human erythropoietin gene contains a hypoxia-responsive transcriptional enhancer. *Proc. Natl. Acad. Sci. USA* **90**, 3928–3932.
14. Beck, I., Weinmann, R., and Caro, J. (1993) Characterisation of hypoxia-responsive enhancer in the human erythropoietin gene shows presence of hypoxia-inducible 120-kD nuclear DNA-binding protein in erythropoietin-producing and nonproducing cells. *Blood* **82**, 704–711.
15. Wang, G. L. and Semenza, G. L. (1993). General involvement of hypoxia-inducible factor-1 in transcriptional response to hypoxia. *Proc. Natl. Acad. Sci. USA* **90**, 4304–4308.
16. Wang, G. L., Jiang, B. H., Rue, E. A., and Semenza, G. L. (1995) Hypoxia-inducible factor 1 is a basic-helix–loop–helix–PAS heterodimer regulated by cellular O_2 tension. *Proc. Natl. Acad. Sci. USA* **92**, 5510–5514.
17. Wang, G. L. and Semenza, G. L. (1993) Characterization of hypoxia-inducible factor-1 and regulation of DNA-binding activity by hypoxia. *J. Biol. Chem.* **268**, 21,513–21,518.
18. Maxwell, P. H., Pugh, C. W., and Ratcliffe, P. J. (1993) Inducible operation of the erythopoietin 3' enhancer in multiple cell lines: evidence for a widespread oxygen sensing mechanism. *Proc. Natl. Acad. Sci. USA* **90**, 2423–2427.
19. Wiener, C. M., Booth, G., and Semenza, G. L. (1996) In vivo expression of messenger RNAs encoding hypoxia inducible factor-1. *Biochem. Biophys. Res. Commun.* **225**, 485–488.
20. Zhong, H., Agani, F., Baccala, A. A., et al. (1998) Increased expression of hypoxia inducible factor 1_ in rat and human prostate cancer. *Cancer Res.* **58**, 5280–5284.
21. Zhong, H., De Marzo, A. M., Laughner, E., et al. (1999) Overexpression of hypoxia-inducible factor 1κ in common human cancers and their metastasis. *Cancer Res.* **59**, 5830–5835.

22. Huang, L. E., Arany, Z., Livingston, D. M., and Bunn, H. F. (1996) Activation of hypoxia inducible transcription factor depends primarily upon redox-sensitive stabilization of its alpha subunit. *J. Biol. Chem.* **271,** 32,253–32,259.

23. Huang, L. E., Gu, J., Schau, M., and Bunn, H. F. (1998) Regulation of hypoxia-inducible factor 1α is mediated by an O_2-dependent degradation domain via the ubiquitin-proteasome pathway. *Proc. Natl. Acad. Sci. USA* **95,** 7987–7992.

24. Kallio, P. J., Wilson, W. J., Obrien, S., Makino, Y., and Poellinger. L. (1999) Regulation of the hypoxia-inducible factor-1α by the ubiquitin–proteasome pathway. *J. Biol. Chem.* **274,** 6519–6525.

25. Richard, D. E., Berra, E., Gothie, E., Roux, D., and Pouyssegur, J. (1999) p42/p44 Mitogen activated protein kinases phosphorylate hypoxia-inducible factor 1α (HIF-1α) and enhance the transcriptional activity of HIF-1. *J. Biol. Chem.* **274,** 32,631–32,637.

26. Chilov, D., Camenish, G., Kvietikova, I., Ziegler, U., Gassmann, M., and Wenger, R. H. (1999) Induction and nuclear translocation of hypoxia-inducible factor-1 (HIF-1): heterodimerisation with ARNT is not necessary for nuclear accumulation of HIF-1α. *J. Cell. Sci.* **112,** 1203–1212.

27. Wang, G. L. and Semenza, G. L. (1996). Oxygen sensing and response to hypoxia by mammalian cells. *Redox Rep.* **2,** 89–96.

28. Dachs, G. U., Patterson, A. V., Firth, J. D, et al. (1997) Targeting gene expression to hypoxic tumour cells. *Nature Med.* **3,** 515–520.

29. Rinsch, C., Régulier, E., Déglon, N., Dalle, B., Beuzard, Y., and Aebischer, P. (1997) A gene therapy approach to regulated delivery of erythropoietin as a function of oxygen tension. *Hum. Gene Ther.* **8,** 1881–1889.

30. Boast, K., Binley, K., Iqball, S., et al. (1999) Characterization of physiologically regulated vectors for the treatment of ischemic disease. *Hum. Gene Ther.* **10,** 2197–2208.

31. Greco, O., Patterson, A. V., and Dachs, G. U. (2000) Can gene therapy overcome the problem of hypoxia in radiotherapy? *J. Radiat. Res.* **41,** 201–212.

32. Binley, K., Iqball, S., Kingsman, S., and Naylor, S. (1999) An adenoviral vector regulated by hypoxia for the treatment of ischemic disease and cancer. *Gene Ther.* **6,** 1721–1727.

33. Shibata, T., Akiyama, N., Noda, M., Sasai, K., and Hiraoka, M. (1998) Enhancement of gene expression under hypoxic conditions using fragments of the human vascular endothelial growth factor and the erythropoietin genes. *Int. J. Radiat. Oncol. Biol. Phys.* **42,** 913–916.

34. Shibata, T., Giaccia, A. J., and Brown, J. M. (2000) Development of a hypoxia-responsive vector for tumor-specific gene therapy. *Gene Ther.* **7,** 493–498.

35. Hall, C. V., Jacob, P. E., Ringold, G. M., and Lee, F. (1983) Expression and regulation of *Escherichia coli* lacZ gene fusions in mammalian cells. *J. Mol. Appl. Genet.* **2,** 101–109.

36. Gorman, C. M., Moffat, L. F., and Howard, B. H. (1982) Recombinant genomes which express chloramphenicol acetyltransferase in mammalian cells. *Mol. Cell. Biol.* **2,** 1044–1051.

37. Brasier, A. R., Tate, J. E., and Habener, J. F. (1989) Optimized use of the firefly luciferase assay as a reporter gene in mammalian cell lines. *BioTechniques* **7,** 1116–1122.

38. Cubitt, A. B., Heim, R., Adams, S. R., Boyd, A. E., Gross, L. A., and Tsien, R. Y. (1995) Understanding, improving and using green fluorescent proteins. *Trends Biochem. Sci.* **20,** 448–455.

39. Sambrook, J., Fritsch, E. F., and Maniatis, T. (eds.) (1989) *Molecular Cloning. A Laboratory Manual.* Cold Spring Harbor Laboratory, Cold Spring Harbor, New York.

40. de Wet, J. R., Wood, K. V., Helinski, D. R., and DeLuca, M. (1985) Cloning of firefly luciferase cDNA and the expression of active luciferase in *Escherichia coli. Proc. Natl. Acad. Sci. USA* **82,** 7870–7873.
41. Benzakour, O., Kanthou, C., Dennehy, U., et al. (1995) Evaluation of the use of the luciferase-reporter-gene system for gene-regulation studies involving cyclic AMP-elevating agents. *Biochem. J.* **309,** 385–387.
42. Heim, R. and Tsien, R. Y. (1996) Engineering green fluorescent protein for improved brightness, longer wavelenghts and fluorescence resonance energy transfer. *Curr. Biol.* **6,** 178–182.
43. Li, X., Zhao, X., Fang, Y., et al. (1998) Generation of destabilized green fluorescent protein as a transcription reporter. *J. Biol. Chem.* **273,** 34,970–34,975.
44. Chalfie, M., Tu, Y., Euskirchen, G., Ward, W. W., and Prasher, D. C. (1994) Green fluorescent protein as a marker for gene expression. *Science* **263,** 802–805.
45. Heim, R., Prasher, D. C., and Tsien, R. Y. (1994) Wavelength mutations and posttranslational autoxidation of green fluorescent protein. *Proc. Natl. Acad. Sci. USA* **91,** 12,501–12,504.
46. Springer, C. J. and Niculescu-Duvaz, I. (1996) Gene-directed enzyme prodrug therapy (GDEPT): choice of prodrugs. *Adv. Drug Delivery Rev.* **22,** 351–364.
47. Greco, O., Folkes, L. K., Wardman, P., Tozer, G. M., and Dachs, G. U. (2000) Development of a novel enzyme–prodrug combination for gene therapy of cancer: horseradish peroxidase/indole-3-acetic acid. *Cancer Gene Ther.* **7,** 1414–1420.
48. Greco, O., Tozer, G. M., Folkes, L. K., Rossiter, S., Wardman, P., and Dachs, G. U. (2000) Horseradish peroxidase (HRP)/indole-3-acetic acid (IAA): use of IAA and analogues in oxic and anoxic tumor conditions. *Cancer Gene Ther.* **7,** S19.
49. Hart, S. L., Arancibia-Cárcamo, C. V., Wolfert, M. A., et al. (1998) Lipid-mediated enhancement of transfection by a nonviral integrin-targeting vector. *Hum. Gene Ther.* **9,** 575–585.
50. Adams, G. E., Ahmed, I., Sheldon, P. W., and Stratford, I. J. (1984). Radiation sensitisation and chemopotentiation: RSU-1069, a compound more efficient than misonidazole in vitro and in vivo. *Br. J. Cancer* **49,** 571–577.
51. Olive, P. L. (1995) Detection of hypoxia by measurement of DNA damage in individual cells from spheroid and murine tumours exposed to bioreductive drugs. II. RSU1069. *Br. J. Cancer* **71,** 537–542.
52. Chapman, J. D., Sturrock, J, Boag, J. W., and Crookall, J. O. (1970) Factors affecting the oxygen tension around cells growing in plastic Petri dishes. *Int. J. Radiat. Biol.* **17,** 305–328.
53. Ivan, M., Kondo, K., Yang, H., et al. (2001) HIFα targeted for VHL-mediated destruction by proline hydroxylation: implications for O_2 sensing. *Science* **292,** 464–468.
54. Jaakkola, P., Mole, D. R., Tian, Y. M., et al. (2001) Targeting of HIF-α to the von Hippel-Lindau ubiquitylation complex by O_2-regulated prolyl hydroxylation. *Science* **292,** 468–472.
55. Coralli, C., Cemazar, M., Tozer, G. M., Dachs, G. U. (2001) Limitations of the reporter green fluorescent protein under simulated tumour conditions. *Cancer Res.* **61,** 4784–4790.

20

Radiation-Activated Antitumor Vectors

Simon D. Scott and Brian Marples

1. Introduction
1.1. Radiotherapy

Radiotherapy (RT) is a primary treatment modality for the majority of solid tumors. The objective is to destroy the tumor mass by exposure to ionizing radiation (IR) from an external beam or isotopic source. IR causes DNA damage directly and indirectly via the production of reactive oxygen intermediates (ROIs). Accumulation of sufficient damage leads to tumor cell death. The efficacy of RT is usually governed by the radiation dose given, the main limitation being the need to avoid injury to the surrounding normal tissues. To address the latter problem, physical techniques such as conformal and intensity-modulated radiotherapy have been developed to improve the precision of dose delivery to the tumor volume. However, some tumors prove refractory to conventional radiotherapy treatments, as insufficient dose can be delivered to the tumor. In such cases, other therapeutic strategies, such as chemotherapy, can be used in combination, particularly if such drugs lead to increased tumor radiosensitization. Nevertheless, many tumor types, (e.g., glioblastoma) are often resistant to even these combined approaches. Consequently, there is a need for new strategies that can improve the effectiveness of current radiotherapy regimens. Gene therapy offers the exciting possibility of significantly improving the efficacy of radiotherapy without the need for IR-dose escalation or undue increases in normal tissue morbidity. Furthermore, the potential to spatially and temporally target the activation of gene therapy vectors using clinically relevant IR doses provides a particularly attractive prospect.

1.2. Gene Expression Induced by Ionizing Radiation

The expression of a number of genes is known to be upregulated in response to cellular exposure to IR (1–4). Many of these "immediate–early response" genes are involved in DNA damage-sensing, repair, and cell cycle progression pathways. The promoter regions of some of these genes have been used to drive expression of heter-

From: *Methods in Molecular Medicine, Vol. 90, Suicide Gene Therapy: Methods and Reviews*
Edited by: C. J. Springer © Humana Press Inc., Totowa, NJ

ologous coding sequences (including suicide genes). These include the p21 (WAF1/ CIP1) and early growth response 1 (*Egr1*) promoters *(5–7)*. However, some of these early response genes have been shown to operate within p53-dependent pathways [e.g., WAF1 *(5)*, GADD45 *(8)*] and thus may not function efficiently in the many tumor cell types exhibiting mutant p53 phenotypes. Consequently, much attention has focused on the promoter region of the p53-independent *Egr1* gene.

1.3. Radiation-Responsive Gene Therapy Vectors

Weichselbaum et al. *(7)* showed that a 425 nucleotide region (E425) *(9)* located upstream of the coding sequence in the murine *Egr1* gene, when placed in a plasmid vector, could control expression of the downstream tumor necrosis factor-α coding sequence (TNF-α CDS) following 20-Gy X-rays. This cytokine construct was also used in vivo to control the growth of tumor xenografts when combined with single or fractionated dosing *(7,10)*. Similarly, this *Egr1* promoter has been used for gene-directed enzyme–prodrug therapy (GDEPT). Joki et al. *(11)* employed the *Egr1* promoter for IR-controlled expression of the herpes simplex virus type 1–thymidine kinase (HSV-TK) suicide gene. The HSV-TK enzyme is able to convert the relatively nontoxic nucleoside prodrug ganciclovir (GCV) to its monophosphate form. Further phosphorylation of GCV by cellular kinases produces the cytotoxic triphosphate form (GCVtriP). A major advantage of this suicide gene system for combined radiation + gene therapy ("radiogenetic therapy") is that GCVtriP is a potent radiosensitizer, as it is incorporated into the DNA strand breaks caused by ionizing radiation. In addition, the HSV-TK/GCV system exhibits the "bystander effect," whereby the toxic GCVtriP metabolite is able to pass from vector-transfected cells into neighboring cells, via gap junctions, often leading to the death of these nontransfected bystander cells *(12)*.

1.4. Radiation-Responsive Gene Promoter Sequences

To further delineate the sequences involved in the IR activation of the *Egr1* promoter, Datta et al. *(13)* examined a series of deletion mutants, using those to drive expression of the chloramphenicol acetyl-transferase (CAT) reporter gene. This identified the essential sequences for IR induction as being 10 nucleotide motifs of the consensus sequence $CC(A/T)_6GG$, also known as CArG elements or boxes. That ROIs were important in the induction was demonstrated by the fact that hydrogen peroxide was also able to activate the *Egr1* promoter *(14)*. These motifs had previously been shown to be important in the downregulation of *Egr1* expression by the product of the c-*fos* gene, following mitogenic stimulation with fetal calf serum *(9)*. Hence, CArG sequences are frequently also called serum-response elements (SREs). Indeed, mitogenic induction of *Egr1* gene expression has also been independently reported *(15)*. Furthermore, the human and murine *Egr1* promoters also contain putative binding sites for the Sp1 transcription factor, AP-1 (the Fos–Jun heterodimer) as well as for cyclic AMP and Egr1 itself *(16–18)*, all of which may influence promoter induction.

1.5. Synthetic Gene Promoters

In order to produce an IR-responsive promoter without the presence of these potentially antagonistic binding sites, as well as the capacity for adaptation and improvement, we have been developing synthetic alternatives based on isolated CArG elements *(19)*. These promoters consist of an enhancer region, containing the CArG elements themselves, adjacent to a basal promoter (i.e., from the cytomegalovirus immediate early, CMV IE, gene) containing the essential transcriptional initiation apparatus such as the CCAAT/TATA boxes (*see* **Fig. 1**). The enhancer is produced by cloning complementary, single-stranded, oligo-deoxyribonucleotides (ODNs), containing the CArG element sequences. The chimeric synthetic promoter is positioned directly upstream of the coding sequence of the enhanced green fluorescent protein (EGFP) reporter gene in a plasmid vector. Target cells are transfected with the plasmid construct and irradiated, and subsequent EGFP production is measured by flow cytometry.

By this methodology, we demonstrated that a synthetic promoter, containing an enhancer containing four directly repeated CArG elements of the same sequence, was significantly more IR responsive than the wild-type enhancer *(19)*. This was confimed using the HSV-TK/GCV suicide gene system and a tumor cell growth-inhibition assay. In addition, we have demonstrated the capacity for improving the induction response by the addition of more CArG elements and by alterations to the core sequence. Importantly, we have also been able to amplify and maintain target gene expression using vectors incorporating a novel "molecular switch" system *(20)*.

The following protocol details the procedure needed to produce and assay vectors containing natural or synthetic enhancer/promoters for their initiation of induced transcription by ionizing radiation (1–5 Gy). We recommend initial screening of novel promoters by EGFP reporter gene assay, the best promoters being taken forward for assessment using a suicide gene assay system such as described in this chapter.

The major procedures involved in the procedure are as follows:

1. Growth and maintenance of human tumor cell lines.
2. Subcloning of EGFP reporter gene into gene therapy plasmid vector.
3. Cloning of IR-responsive promoter sequences from polymerase chain reaction (PCR) products or oligonucleotides.
4. Assaying IR induction of EGFP expression by flow cytometry following transient transfection of tumor cells.
5. Cloning of HSV-TK suicide gene into IR-responsive vector.
6. Assaying growth inhibition of tumor cell cultures transfected with suicide vector.

2. Materials

2.1. Cell Culture

1. RPMI 1640 culture medium (Life Technologies, Paisley, Scotland, UK) supplemented with 10% fetal calf serum (FCS) (Sigma, Poole, UK), L-glutamine (2 m*M*) (Sigma), and sodium pyruvate (1 m*M*) (Sigma). This "complete medium" is made up fresh each day.
2. Cell lines (European Collection of Cell Cultures, Salisbury, UK); human MCF-7 breast adenocarcinoma (ECACC 86012803), U87- and U373-MG glioblastoma–astrocytoma (ECACC 89081402 and 89081403, respectively). Store stocks in 2 mL cryotubes (Greiner, Stonehouse, UK) in complete cell culture medium (20% FCS) with 10% dimethyl sulfoxide solution (DMSO) (Sigma) in the gaseous phase of liquid nitrogen.

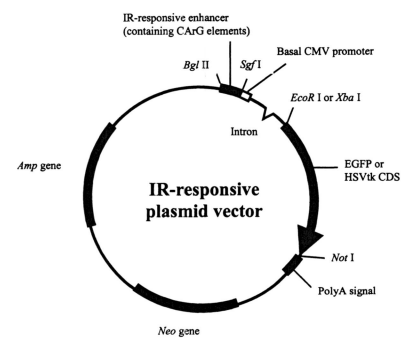

Fig. 1. Schematic of IR-responsive plasmid vector (based on PCI-neo; Promega) showing chimeric enhancer/promoter and reporter or suicide genes. Restriction sites used for cloning components are italicized. The intron is present to increase expression of the CDS immediately downstream. The SV40 polyadenylation signal allows efficient processing of RNA transcripts. *Amp* and *Neo* genes are used as selectable markers for establishing clones in bacterial and mammalian cell cultures, respectively.

3. T25 cell culture flasks (Helena Biosciences, Sunderland, UK).
4. Trypsin /EDTA (Sigma).

2.2. Molecular Biology

1. Plasmid (p) DNA; pCIneo (Promega, Southhampton, UK), pEGFP1 (Clontech, Basingstoke, UK), and phSV-TK (cloned *Bam*HI fragment of HSV genomic DNA; kind gift of the Virology Unit, Glasgow University). All stored at –20°C in ultrapure water (water purifier USF ELGA Option 4, High Wycombe, UK). Also, 1.5-mL reaction tubes (Anachem, Luton, UK). Sterilize water and tubes by autoclaving.
2. Seakem LE (FMC, Rockland, ME) and GTG electrophoresis agarose (Helena Biosciences, Sunderland, UK). TAE buffer, pH 7.7; 0.04 *M* Tris-acetate (Trizma base; Sigma), 0.02 *M* glacial acetic acid (Fischer, Loughborough, UK), 0.001 *M* EDTA (Sigma). DNA size ladders (1 kb and 100 bp; Life Technologies). 6X Loading dye (Life Technologies).
3. Custom-made, single-stranded ODNs with additional 5' phosphate modification for cloning, IRD800 end label for DNA sequencing or with no additional modification for use in PCR (MWG-Biotech, Milton Keynes, UK).

EGFP PCR primer 1: 5'-GGTCGAGCTGGACGGCGACG
EGFP PCR primer 2: 5'-TCACGAACTCCAGCAGGACC;
T3d PCR/sequencing primer: 5'-CCCACATCTCCCCCTGAACC
T7c PCR/sequencing primer: 5'-GGCACCTATTGGTCTTACTGAC;
Egr1 enhancer PCR primer 1: 5'-TCCAGATCTCAGCCGCTCCTCCCCCGCAC-3'
Egr1 enhancer PCR primer 2: 5'ACTGCGATCGCGGGCCCGGCCCGGCCCGCATCC-3';
4 CArG element ODN1: 5'-GATCT(CCTTATTTGG)$_4$CGAT-3'
4 CArG element ODN2: 5'-A(GGAATAAACC)$_4$CGC-3';
PCIN2 PCR/sequencing primer: 5'-CCACCTCTGACTTGAGCGTCG
CMVRev PCR/sequencing primer: 5'-GGTTCACTAAACGAGCTCTGC;
HSV-TK PCR primer 1: 5'-GCTCTAGAGTCGACATGGCTTCGTACCCCGGC-3'
HSV-TK PCR primer 2: 5'-CCATCGATCTCCTTCCGTGTTTCAGTTAGC-3'.

4. Reddy-load PCR master mix (Advanced Biotechnologies, Epsom, UK). Platinum *Pfx* DNA polymerase kit (Life Technologies).
5. Restriction and modifying enzymes and reaction buffers; *Bgl*II, *Eco*RI, *Not*I, *Xba*I, calf intestinal alkaline phosphatase (CIAP), T4 DNA ligase (MBI Fermentas; UK distributors: Helena Biosciences), *Sgf*I (Promega, Southampton, UK).
6. QIAquick PCR Purification Kit, QIAquick Gel Extraction Kit, HiSpeed Plasmid Mini Kit, and QIAfilter Plasmid Maxi Kits (Qiagen, Crawley, UK). Genomic G1 DNA Extraction kit (Helena Biosciences).
7. TOP 10 *Escherichia coli* competent cells and SOC bacterial culture medium (Invitrogen–Novex, Groningen, Netherlands). Luria broth (LB) base (Sigma), agar-select (1.5% [w/v] for bacterial plates) (Sigma), Ampicillin (100 µg/mL final concentration in plates) (Sigma).
8. "BioPhotometer" spectrophotometer (Eppendorf, Cambridge, UK).
9. PTC 100 thermocycler (Biometra, Maidstone, UK). Thin-walled 0.2-µL PCR tubes (Anachem).
10. Licor DNA analyzer (Licor, Lincoln, NE), SeqiTherm Excel II DNA sequencing kit LC (Cambio, Cambridge, UK).

2.3. Cell Transfection

1. Lipofectamine (Life Technologies).
2. Phosphate-buffered saline, pH 7.5 (PBS) (Oxoid, Basingstoke, UK).
3. 1.5-mL Reaction tubes (Anachem), six-well plates (Helena Biosciences).
4. Geneticin (Life Technologies).

2.4. Irradiation

1. 240 kVp X-ray set (Pantak, Reading, UK).
2. Samples were irradiated at 37°C in an in-house constructed thermostatically controlled Perspex® incubator.

2.5. GFP Assay

1. FACscan II flow cytometer and CellQuest data analysis program (Becton Dickinson, Oxford, UK).
2. PBS, complete medium.
3. 5-mL Falcon tubes (Becton Dickinson).

2.6. Cell Growth Inhibition Assay

1. 96-Well plates (Helena Biosciences).
2. Complete medium + Cymevene (GCV; 50 μ*M*) (Roche, Welwyn Garden City, UK).
3. 3-(4,5-Dimethylthiazol-2-yl)-5-(3-carboxymethoxyphenyl)-2-(4-sulfophenyl)-2*H*-tetra-zolium (MTS), filter-sterilized (Promega).
4. PMS: Phenazine methosulfate (Promega).
5. Multiskan biochromatic multiplate reader, Genesis II platereader software (Labsystems, Basingstoke, UK).

3. Methods

3.1. Cell Culture

1. Maintain cells as subconfluent monolayers in complete medium in vented tissue culture flasks or dishes at 37°C in a water-saturated atmosphere of 90% N_2 : 5% O_2: 5% CO_2. Replace culture medium twice weekly and reseed weekly.
2. Remove cells from near-confluent culture by incubation of PBS-washed (2 mL, 37°C) cell monolayer with 0.5 mL 37°C trypsin/EDTA per T25 culture flask by incubating for approx 2 min at 37°C (*see* **Note 1**). Stop reaction by adding 5 mL of fresh, prewarmed (37°C) complete medium.
3. Centrifuge and resuspend cell pellet in prewarmed complete medium. Reseed new culture from this stock, routinely making a 1 in 6–10 dilution.

3.2. Molecular Biology

3.2.1. EGFP Reporter Gene Cloning

3.2.1.1. DNA Manipulation

1. To subclone the reporter gene coding sequence (CDS) from pEGFP into pCI-neo, first incubate 5 μg of pEGFP and 3 μg of pCI-neo (measured using 1 in 20 dilutions by spectrophotometry) at 37°C for 4 h with 25 and 15 units of *Eco*RI and diluted reaction buffer, respectively, in total volumes of 10–50 μL. Purify the digested DNA using the PCR purification kit. Repeat the procedure with *Not*I (*see* **Note 2**), then repurify the vector DNA.
2. Load the pEGFP double-digest (+ loading dye) onto a 1% GTG agarose gel and electrophorese at 0.5–0.7 V/cm for 1 h (alongside the 1-kb ladder) to separate the vector and insert bands. Excise the approx 800-bp EGFP band under ultraviolet (UV) transillumination using a clean scalpel and purify using the gel extraction kit.
3. Measure concentration of DNA eluted from the respective purifications by spectrophotometry. Next, 20 ng *Eco*RI/*Not*I-digested pCIneo is added to approx 15 ng of the EGFP fragment and incubated overnight at 22°C with 1 μL (10 units) of T4 DNA ligase and 10X reaction buffer in a volume of 10–20 μL (*see also* **Note 3**). The amount of insert (EGFP) DNA used in the ligation is calculated using the formula (Mass of vector × Size of insert)/Size of vector × 3. This gives a 1 : 3 molar ratio of vector : insert. A negative control reaction is also set up where the insert is omitted and replaced with the equivalent volume of ultrapure water.

3.2.1.2. Transformation

1. Carefully pipet 25 μL of competent cells into precooled 1.5-mL reaction tubes placed on wet ice. Add 2.5 μL of each ligation reaction into separate tubes and mix slowly with the pipet tip and leave for 30 min.

2. Heat shock the cell/DNA mixture for 20 s in a 42°C waterbath, then place immediately back on ice for >1min.
3. Add 250 μL of super optimal catabolite growth medium (SOC) to each sample and place in an orbital shaker at 37°C and 225 rpm for 1 h. Spread 50 μL of each culture onto 90-mm-diameter LB–ampicillin agar plates and incubate overnight at 37°C.

3.2.1.3. SCREENING CLONES

If the colony number on the vector+insert ligation plate is at least double that on the control, the former clones can be screened for the presence of the insert DNA. The best method is by PCR assay, using either primers specific to the insert sequences (i.e., EGFP) or in the vectors "arms" (i.e., based on T3 and T7 polymerase promoter sequences). Positive, negative, and water controls should be included in all PCR screenings (*see* **Note 4**).

1. Pick test colonies onto fresh LB–ampicillin plates in a numbered grid pattern and incubate from 6 to 18 h at 37°C (*see also* **Note 4**).
2. Transfer visible amount of bacterial cells, using a sterile loop, into 0.5-mL Eppendorf tubes each containing 100 μL ultrapure water. Lyse cells at 95°C for 3 min to release DNA into solution. Prepare PCR reaction mixture containing 38 μL of PCR master mix + 1 μL (100 ng) of each PCR primer per sample, and add 40 μL aliquots to 10 μL of each lysis mix per PCR tube. Place samples in thermocycler and run the following program: 1× 2 min, 94°C; 30× 1 min 94°C + 1 min, 55°C + 1 min, 72°C; 1× 5 min, 72°C (*see* **Note 5**).
3. Run 10-μL volumes of each reaction on 1% Seakem LE gel to reveal from which gridded clones the appropriate-sized PCR products derive. Purify DNA from clones (i.e., pCI-EGFP) using Mini (for sequencing) or Maxi kits (for transfection). Determine DNA sequence of new regions for all clones to verify integrity using T3d and T7c primers (*see* **Note 6**).

3.2.2. IR-Responsive Gene Enhancer Cloning

3.2.2.1. VECTOR PREPARATION

1. Digest pCI-EGFP as described in **Subheading 3.2.1.1.** using *Bgl*II and *Sgf*I restriction enzymes.
2. Gel purify double-digested vector DNA, leaving the approx 650-bp CMV IE enhancer fragment in the gel (*see* **Subheading 3.2.1.1.**).
3. If additional enhancer fragments (e.g., more CArG elements) are to be placed in tandem with the primary enhancer sequence cloned, this construct should be linearized using *Bgl*II or *Sgf*I. The digested DNA should then be treated with CIAP as follows (this removes 5'-terminal phosphates, preventing vector self-ligation): 43 μL (1–2 μg) purified vector DNA + 5 μL 10X reaction buffer + 2 μL (2 units) CIAP, 30 min, 37°C. Repurify DNA with PCR purification kit.

3.2.2.2. WILD-TYPE GENE ENHANCERS

To clone enhancer sequences (e.g., *Egr1*) from genomic DNA, PCR primer pairs (containing *Bgl*II and *Sgf*I restriction enzyme sites, respectively) encompassing the enhancer region are designed (*see* **Note 5**).

1. Extract DNA from pellet of approx 1 × 10^5 PBS-washed cells using the Genomic DNA purification kit and assess concentration by spectrophotometry.

2. Amplify enhancer sequences by setting up the following PCR reaction: 1 µL (100 ng) genomic DNA + 1 µL of 50 m*M* magnesium sulfate + 1.5 µL of 10 m*M* dNTP mix + 5 µL of *Pfx* reaction buffer + 1 µL (100 ng) PCR primer 1 + 1 µL (100 ng) PCR primer 2 + 38.5 µL ultrapure water + 1 µL (2.5 U) *Pfx* (a proof-reading DNA polymerase). Place in thermocycler and run the following program: 1X 2 min, 94°C; 30X 15 s, 94°C; + 30 s, 55°C; 1 min, 68°C; 1X 5 min, 68°C (*see* **Note 5**).
3. Electrophorese on 1% GTG gel and purify PCR product (*see* **Subheading 3.2.1.1.**).
4. *Bgl*II/*Sgf*I-digest and purify PCR fragment before final ligation into the purified pCI-EGFP *Bgl*II/*Sgf*I-digested vector (*see* **Subheadings 3.2.1.1. and 3.2.2.1.**).
5. Transform and PCR screen using the same enhancer PCR primer pair (e.g., the PCR product for the *Egr1* enhancer is 425 bp; *see* **Subheading 1.3.**).
6. Determine DNA sequence of cloned enhancer (*see* **Note 6**).

3.2.2.3. SYNTHETIC GENE ENHANCERS

1. To produce double-stranded linker molecules containing enhancer sequences for cloning, anneal 10-pmol mixtures of each oligonucleotide pair in a volume of 5 µL, first by heating to 55°C and then allowing to cool and leaving overnight at room temperature (*see* **Subheading 1.5. and Note 6**).
2. To this annealed oligonucleotide mix is added 50 ng of compatibly digested vector DNA (e.g., pCI-EGFP *Bgl*II/*Sgf*I) + 1 µL 10X reaction buffer + 1 µL (10 units) T4 DNA ligase + ultrapure water to a final volume of 10 µL. Incubate at 22°C overnight and then transform (*see* **Subheading 3.2.1.2.**). PCR screen colonies using vector arm primers (e.g., PCIN2 and CMVRev) and analyze products on 1.8% LE gel (*see* **Subheading 3.2.1.3.**).
3. Sequence putative cloned promoters using PCIN2 and CMVREV primers (*see* **Note 6**).

3.2.3. Suicide Gene Cloning

1. Digest pCI-neo with *Xba*I and *Not*I as described in **Subheading 3.2.1.1.** (*see also* **Note 2**).
2. Amplify HSV-TK coding sequence by PCR from pHSV-TK plasmid by the method described in **Subheading 3.2.2.2.** (*see also* **Note 5**).
3. Electrophorese on 1% GTG gel and purify PCR product (*see* **Subheading 3.2.1.1.**).
4. *Xba*I/*Not*I digest and purify HSV-TK PCR product before ligation into pCI-neo (*see* **Subheadings 3.2.1.1. and 3.2.2.**).
5. Transform and PCR screen using the same HSV-TK PCR primer pair (*Note*: The PCR product for the HSV-TK is approx 1.2 kbp; *see* **Subheading 1.3.**).

3.3. Cell Transfection

1. Seed cells in complete medium into six-well plates to ensure 40–50% confluence within 24 h.
2. Measure plasmid DNA concentrations using 1 : 20 dilutions via spectrophotometry at 260 nm.
3. Add 5 µg of each test or control (*see* **Note 7**) plasmid DNA (in 10 µL sterile ultrapure water) to 90 µL (37°C) serum-free medium (SFM). Mix 15 µL lipofectamine (2 mg/mL) with 85 µL SFM. Combine DNA and lipofectamine mixtures in 1.5-mL reaction tubes and incubate at room temperature for 30–45 min, mixing occasionally using a pipet tip.
4. Remove complete medium from cell monolayers in six-well plates and carefully wash twice with 2 mL of 37°C SFM. Add 200 µL DNA mixture to each sample well and gently swirl to ensure even coverage. Add 800 µL of 37°C 5% FCS medium to each well. Place

in 37°C incubator for 4 h. Then, replace DNA/5% FCS medium mixture with 37°C complete medium, return to incubator, and culture as normal.

5. Plasmid-containing cell lines (e.g., for further experimention, tumor xenografts) can be established by selection using the selectable marker *Neo* (*see* **Fig. 1**), by growth and maintenance in geneticin (0.1–1 μ*M*, depending on cell line). Control nontransfected cultures should be treated in parallel and will die within 3–4 wk. Individual resistant clones can then be isolated in fresh cultures by removal with a pipet tip.

3.4. Irradiation

1. Eight to 24 h following transfection, irradiate the attached cell monolayers at 37°C (typical dose rate of 0.5–2 Gy/min; *see* **Subheading 2.4.**). Include mock-irradiated and transfection controls in all experiments (*see* **Note 7**).
2. Return to 37°C incubator for 24–48 h; then, trypsinize cells to single-cell suspensions and assay for GFP expression.

3.5. GFP Assay

1. Remove medium from cell monolayers, wash twice with 2 mL PBS, and trypsinize to give single-cell suspension.
2. Wash cells three times with 2 mL of 4°C PBS by centrifugation (200*g*, 4 min) and resuspension. Finally, resuspend in 0.5 mL of 4°C PBS for flow cytometry analysis.
3. Analyze 40,000 cells for each sample, with an excitation wavelength of 488 nm and FITC collection wavelength using a bandpass filter at 530 ± 15 nm. Gate out dead cells by forward and side scatter (*see* **Fig. 2**). Use the control plasmid-transfected cells to configure data acquisition ensuring that the GFP negative cells do not exceed the 10^{-2} FL1 (fluorescence intensity) boundary using the data analysis program; plot FL1 on a 4-log scale (*see* **Fig 2**). Therefore, any cells exhibiting fluorescence exceeding that of unirradiated controls are considered positive for radiation induction. Fold-induction is calculated as a ratio of "fluorescence of irradiated cells/fluorescence of unirradiated cells" above the fluorescence threshold.

3.6. Cell Growth Inhibition Assay

When positive IR induction has been demonstrated for a test promoter construct using the GFP assay, the ability to drive radiation-controlled suicide gene killing of tumor cells is assessed. We have used the HSV-TK/GCV system, primarily because of the radiosensitizing and bystander effects (*see* **Subheading 1.3.**). The efficacy of tumor cell killing is measured by the ability to inhibit tumor cell growth of an irradiated, plasmid-transfected population in the presence of the GCV prodrug. Cell growth is determined by the intensity change of a colormetric reagent (MTS) placed on the cells.

1. Transfect cells with the test and control constructs in duplicate (i.e., IR-inducible promoter regulating HSV-TK expression) (*see* **Subheading 3.3.**).
2. After 24 h, remove cells with trypsin and reseed 200–400 cells into each well of a 96-well plates in 200 μL of complete medium, with or without 50 μ*M* GCV.
3. After a further 3 h, irradiate (or mock-irradiate) cells, then incubate at 37°C.
4. After 24 h incubation, add 40 μL of MTS solution mix (*see* **Note 8**) to each well and reincubate for 4 h at 37°C to allow formazan reaction.
5. Read fluorescence at 490 nm to quantify formazan product.

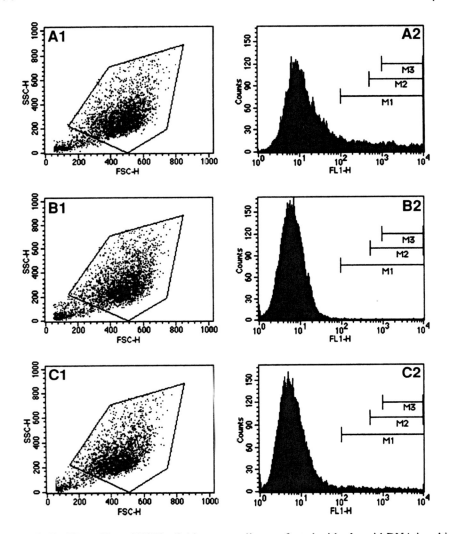

Fig. 2. FACS profiles of U373 glioblastoma cells transfected with plasmid DNA in which EGFP expression is regulated by the strong CMV IE promoter **(A1,A2)** and IR-responsive CArG promoter, 48 h after mock-irradiation **(B1,B2)** and a single 5-Gy X-ray dose **(C1,C2)**. The dotplots shown in panels A1–C1 are used to exclude dead cells and from the analysis using forward (FSC-H) and side-scatter (SSC-H) parameters. The histograms shown in panels A2–C2 depict only those events within the boundary shown in panels A1–C1. Panel A2 illustrates a cell population with a high proportion of GFP-positive cells indicated by marked fluorescence above an intensity 10^{-2} (FL1-H scale). Panel B2 shows very few fluorescent cells in the nonirradiated cell population transfected with an IR-responsive construct. This represents the "leakiness" of the test promoter. In contrast, a large fluorescent population of cells is evident following radiation treatment **(C2)**. Fold-induction is calculated as the ratio of C2/B2. FACS profiles are also required (not shown) from a nontransfected cell population to define the default SSC-H, FSC-H, and FL1-H parameters.

4. Notes

1. The duration of trypsin exposure is cell line dependent. Do not overexpose cells to trypsin, as this causes undue stress to the cell membranes and will reduce reseeding and transfection efficiency. As soon as the cells begin to round-up and detach from the plastic surface of the culture plates, quench reaction with medium (containing 10% FCS). Mechanical detachment of cells can also be used by tapping plates on the side during trypsinization.

2. All double-digests should be performed in their optimal buffers, rather than universal buffers, as even small quantities of uncut or singly digested vector DNA resulting from incomplete digestions can result in large numbers of background colonies on transformation. This makes screening much more time-consuming.

3. Heat-killing the ligase reaction for 10 min at 75°C often improves later transformation efficiencies.

4. The number of colonies to be screened depends on colony numbers on ligation plates. Usually, the greater the true ligation : control ratio, less screening is necessary. Typically, screen 20–60 colonies, in batches of 20. Positive and negative control colonies should be included on all grid plates and PCR screenings. Positive controls should be the original clone from where the insert derived (if using gene-specific PCR primers) or another pCIneo clone containing a similar-sized insert (if using primers based on vector arm sequences). A negative control colony can be taken from the ligation control plate. The water control contains all components except template DNA.

5. The PCR primers are designed to encompass the complete region of interest (i.e., 5' and 3' ends of promoter or coding sequences). Primers should be complementary to 20- to 30-bp regions of target sequence and have approximately equal A/T : G/C ratios. However, a concentration of G/Cs at the 3' termini (a "G/C clamp") can help stable binding of the primer to the target sequence. Palindromic sequences of more than three bases should be avoided throughout. Restriction enzyme sites (for later cloning purposes) should be included at the 5' termini. Furthermore, a few extra bases can be added to aid efficient restriction digest of the PCR product (e.g., see table in Restriction Enzyme Properties appendix of the New England Biolabs catalog or www.neb.com/neb/frame_tech. for suitable choices). Annealing temperatures will be different for various primers, primarily depending on G/C content. This temperature, along with the magnesium ion concentration, can be altered to improve the specificity and efficacy of results. The elongation time may also have to be increased for longer PCR products.

6. Double-stranded linker molecules containing IR-responsive (CArG) elements are composed of complementary ODNs. These should be designed so that when annealed, the termini formed are immediately ready for ligation to compatibly digested vector DNA (*see* **Fig. 3**). We have noted reduced cloning efficiency with longer ODNs (>70 bp). Furthermore, even when these linkers successfully ligate into vectors, we frequently see sequence rearrangements. This may be the result of homologous recombination between the identical sequences of the responsive elements. To overcome this, it is often better to clone a succession of smaller linkers (e.g., <60 bp). If restriction sites are limited (as is the case in the promoter regions of most vectors), a series of "locks" can be incorporated into the ODN design, so that after ligation, only one end of the linker retains an intact restriction site available for subsequent cloning (*see* **Fig. 3**). Finally, it is essential to sequence newly cloned inserts, preferably on both DNA strands for accuracy. This is particularly important for PCR products that may have incorporated nucleotide mutations in the amplification process (resulting from inefficiencies in the proof-reading ability of the DNA polymerase) and for linkers to determine orientation and check for rearrange-

A   Ligation of linker into vector

Vector arm   Linker   Existing linker/vector arm

     Bgl II   *Bgl* II
GGCTCGACA   GATCT(CCTTATTTGG)$_n$ *GATCTTCAATA*
CCGAGCTG*TCTAG*   A(GGAATAAACC)$_n$ AAGTTAT

B   Ligated DNA

     Bgl II   <u>*Bgl* II</u>
GGCTCGAC*AGATCT*(CCTTATTTG<u>**G**)</u>$_n$<u>GATCT</u>TCAATA
CCGAGCTG*TCTAGA*(GGAATAAAC<u>**C**)</u>$_n$<u>CTAGA</u>AGTTAT

C   Recleavage of vector for additional linker ligation

  Bgl II   *Bgl* II   <u>*Bgl* II</u>
GGCTCGACA   *GATCT*(CCTTATTTG<u>**G**)</u>$_n$<u>GATCT</u>TCAATA .
CCGAGCTG*TCTAG*   A(GGAATAAAC<u>**C**)</u>$_n$<u>CTAGA</u>AGTTAT

Fig. 3. Design and ligation of multiple linkers, containing n numbers of IR-responsive CArG elements, into vector DNA. After annealing ODNs to form the double-stranded linker molecules, these are ligated into vector DNA digested with compatible restriction enzymes (**A**). Linkers are designed such that the ligation process produces DNA possessing one intact and one "locked" restriction site (**B**). Treatment of this DNA with the same enzyme will result in restriction only at the intact site (**C**), thus allowing the addition of further linkers without displacement of those previously inserted. Intact and digested restriction sites (*Bgl*II) are shown in italic. The "locked" restriction site is shown underlined, with the nucleotides producing this nonrecleavable lock shown in bold.

    ments for the reasons outlined. Even small sequence alterations can substantially alter promoter or gene efficacy. Use PCIN2 and CMVREV for sequencing enhancer regions. T3d and T7c primers are longer versions of the commercially available T3 and T7 primers, which give better sequencing results at the 48°C annealing temperature used for our standard sequencing reactions.

7. All experiments should include a series of "control" vector transfections. First, an untransfected cell population is required in order to set up the default intensity profiles for the FACS machine. Second, a population of cells transfected with an "empty" vector containing no reporter gene (or controlling promoter) is also needed, as this allows the effect of the transfection process to be ascertained. Transfection with a plasmid in which the reporter gene is under the control of a strong constitutive promoter (e.g., CMV) allows the transfection efficiency to be determined, which is necessary for interexperimental comparison. In addition, irradiated and mock-irradiated samples are required for all test samples and controls, preferably in duplicate within each experiment. This allows radio-inducibility to be calculated.

8. The MTS colorimetric assay is a method for determining the number of proliferating cells in a population. The assay utilizes solutions of tetrazolium compound (MTS) and the electron-coupling reagent phenazine methosulfate (PMS). MTS is bioreduced by cells into a

formazan compound that is soluble in tissue culture medium and can be directly measured at 490 nm. Dehydrogenase enzymes found in metabolically active cells carry out this conversion. The concentration of MTS/PMS is cell line dependent. For wells containing 100 µL of medium [with (5–20) × 10⁴ cells], we recommend using 20 µL MTS/PMS solution; this results in final concentrations of 333 µg/mL MTS and 25 µM PMS (*see* the Promega catalog or www.promega.com/tbs/tb169/tb169. for further details).

Acknowledgments

The authors would like to thank Professor Mike Joiner, Mrs. Sara Bourne, Ms. Amanda Walker, and Ms. Sheena Balroop for their contributions to the preparation of the work detailed within this chapter. The work described was supported by the Cancer Research Campaign and the Gray Laboratory Cancer Research Trust.

References

1. Boothman, D. A., Bouvard, I., and Hughes, E. N. (1989) Identification and characterization of X-ray-induced proteins in human cells. *Cancer Res.* **49**, 2871–2878.
2. Fornace, A. J. (1992) Mammalian genes induced by radiation; activation of genes associated with growth control. *Annu. Rev. Genet.* **26**, 507–526.
3. Weichselbaum, R. R., Hallahan, D., Fuks, Z., and Kufe, D. (1994) Radiation induction of immediate early genes: effectors of the radiation-stress response. *Int. J. Radiat. Oncol. Biol. Phys.* **30(1)**, 229–234.
4. Amundson, S. A., Do, K. T., and Fornace, A. J., Jr. (1999) Induction of stress genes by low doses of gamma rays. *Radiat. Res.* **152(3)**, 225–231.
5. El-diery, W. S. Tokino, T., Velculescu, V. E., et al. (1993) WAF1, a potential mediator of p53 tumor suppression. *Cell* **75(4)**, 817–825.
6. Worthington, J. Robson, T., Murray, M., O'Rourke, M., Keilty, G., and Hirst, D. G. (2000) Modification of vascular tone using iNOS under the control of a radiation-inducible promoter. *Gene Ther.* **7**, 1126–1131.
7. Weichselbaum, R. R., Hallahan, D. E., Beckett, M. A., et al. (1994) Gene therapy targeted by radiation preferentially radiosensitizes tumor cells. *Cancer Res.* **54**, 4266–4269.
8. Kastan, M. B., Zhan Q., el-Deiry, W. S., et al. (1992) A mammalian cell cycle checkpoint pathway utilizing p53 and GADD45 is defective in ataxia telangiectasia. *Cell* **71(4)**, 587–597.
9. Gius, D., Cao, X., Rauscher, F. J., III, Cohen, D. R., Curran, T., and Sukhatme, V. P. (1990) Transcriptional activation and repression by Fos are independent functions: the C terminus represses immediate–early gene expression via CArG elements. *Mol. Cell. Biol.* **10(8)**, 4243–4255.
10. Hallahan, D. E., Mauceri, H. J., Seung, L. P., et al. (1995) Spatial and temporal control of gene therapy using ionising radiation. *Nature Med.* **1(8)**, 786–791.
11. Joki, T., Nakamura, M., and Ohno, T. (1995) Activation of the radiosensitive EGR-1 promoter induces expression of the herpes simplex virus thymidine kinase gene and sensitivity of human glioma cells to ganciclovir. *Hum. Gene Ther.* **6**, 1507–1513.
12. Mesnil, M. and Yamasaki, H. (2000) Bystander effect in herpes simplex virus-thymidine kinase/ganciclovir cancer gene therapy: role of gap-junctional intercellular communication. *Cancer Res.* **60**, 3989–3999.
13. Datta, R, Rubin, E., Sukhatme, V., et al. (1992) Ionizing radiation activates transcription of the EGR1 gene via CArG elements. *Proc. Natl. Acad. Sci. USA* **89**, 10,149–10,153.

14. Datta, R., Taneja, N., Sukhatme, V. P., Qureshi, S. A., Weichselbaum, R., and Kufe, D. W. (1993) Reactive oxygen intermediates target CC(A/T)$_6$GG sequences to mediate activation of the early growth response 1 transcription factor gene by ionizing radiation. *Proc. Natl. Acad. Sci. USA* **90**, 2419–2422.

15. Sukhatme, V. P., Kartha, S., Toback, F. G., Taub, R., Hoover, R. G., and Tsai-Morris, C.-H. (1988) A novel early growth response gene rapidly induced by fibroblast, epithelial cell and lymphocyte mitogens. *Oncogene Res.* **1**, 343–355.

16. Tsai-Morris, C. -H., Cao, X., and Sukhatme, V. P. (1988) 5' Flanking sequence and genomic structure of Egr-1, a murine mitogen inducible zinc finger encoding gene. *Nucleic Acids Res.* **16(18)**, 8835–8846.

17. Christy, B. and Nathans, D (1989) DNA binding site of the growth-factor-inducible protein Zif268. *Proc. Natl. Acad. Sci. USA* **86**, 8737–8741.

18. Sakamoto, K. M., Bardeleben, C., Yates, K. E., Raines, M. A., Golde, D. W., and Gasson, J. C. (1991) 5' Upstream sequence and genomic structure of the human primary response gene, EGR-1/TIS8. *Oncogene* **6**, 867–871.

19. Marples, B., Scott, S. D., Hendry, J. H., Embleton, M. J., Lashford, L. S., and Margison G. P. (2000) Development of synthetic promoters for radiation-mediated gene therapy. *Gene Ther.* **7**, 511–517.

20. Scott, S. D., Marples, B., Hendry, J. H., et al. (2000) A radiation-controlled molecular switch for use in gene therapy of cancer. *Gene Ther.* **7**, 1121–1125.

21

In Vitro and In Vivo Models for Evaluation of GDEPT

Quantifying Bystander Killing in Cell Cultures and Tumors

William R. Wilson, Susan M. Pullen, Alison Hogg, Stephen M. Hobbs, Frederik B. Pruijn, and Kevin O. Hicks

1. Introduction

The vectors currently available for gene therapy of cancer rarely achieve expression of therapeutic genes in more than a small fraction of the cells in solid tumors. This makes therapeutic success critically dependent on secondary events, known as bystander effects, by which transgene expression leads to the death of nontransduced tumor cells. An efficient bystander effect has the potential to compensate for spatially nonuniform expression of therapeutic genes, and its optimization is therefore an important goal in gene therapy of cancer. Here, we describe protocols for quantifying bystander effects using in vitro and in vivo experimental models.

The generation of efficient bystander killing is the key rationale for gene-dependent enzyme–prodrug therapy (GDEPT), in which a suicide gene codes for a prodrug-activating enzyme (PAE) that generates a diffusible cytotoxin. In a well-studied example, the prodrug ganciclovir (GCV) is activated by herpes simplex virus-thymidine kinase (HSV-TK) to form a phosphorylated metabolite that diffuses between cells via gap junctions *(1,2)*. In other cases, the bystander metabolite can diffuse across cell membranes, as for 5-fluorouracil (5-FU) generated from 5-fluorocytosine (5-FC) by bacterial or yeast cytosine deaminase (CD) *(3,4)*. Several newer GDEPT systems generate freely diffusible (membrane-permeable) alkylating metabolites with the added attractive feature of killing noncycling as well as cycling tumor cells; these include oxidation of cyclophosphamide and other oxazaphosphorines by cytochrome P450 2B1/cytochrome P450 reductase *(5)*, hydrolysis of glutamate derivatives of aromatic nitrogen mustards (prodrugs CMDA and ZD2767P) by *Pseudomonas* carboxypeptidase G2 *(6,7)*, and reduction of the dinitrobenzamide CB 1954 *(see* **Fig. 1**) to its 4-hydroxylamine by the *Escherichia coli* aerobic nitroreductase NTR *(8–10)*. The CB 1954/NTR

From: *Methods in Molecular Medicine, Vol. 90, Suicide Gene Therapy: Methods and Reviews*
Edited by: C. J. Springer © Humana Press Inc., Totowa, NJ

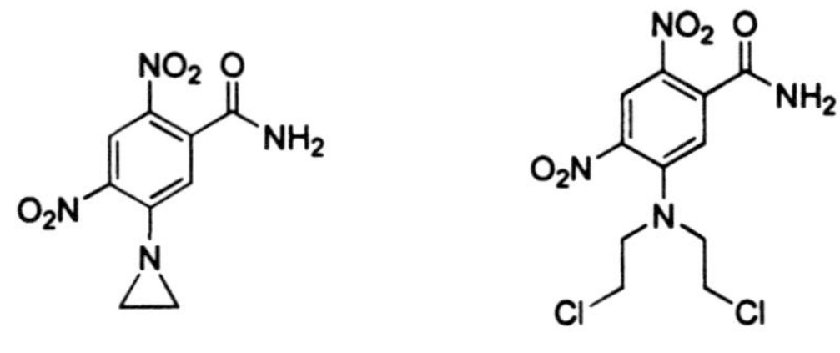

Fig. 1. Dinitrobenzamide prodrugs activated by the *E. coli* nitroreductase NTR, used as examples in these protocols.

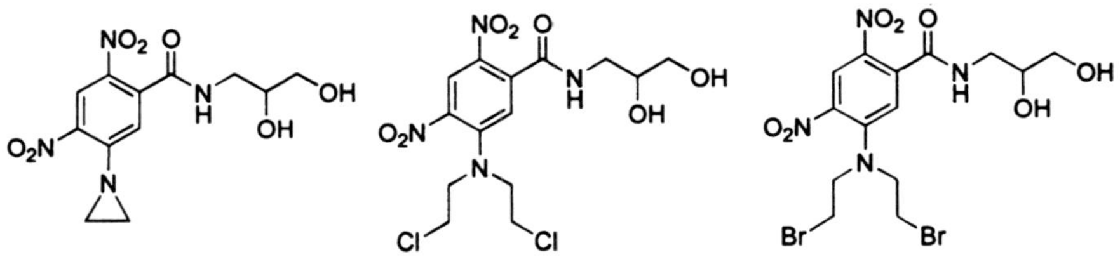

system provides very large differential toxicities between PAE-expressing and PAE-non-expressing cells in vitro and in vivo *(11–16)* and is in clinical trial in conjunction with adenoviral vectors *(17)*. We are currently optimizing dinitrobenzamide mustards related to CB 1954 (e.g., *see* **Fig. 1**) as NTR prodrugs and will use this system as an example in the following protocols.

There are three broad bystander mechanisms by which killing can be transmitted from genetically transduced to nontransduced cells in tumors:

1. Cell-to-cell transfer of cytotoxicity, usually through diffusion of a cytotoxic drug metabolite as discussed earlier. In GDEPT, cytotoxicity can also be transferred through recycling of the PAE and metabolites via local uptake of apoptotic bodies *(18)*. In addition, the potential exists for transmission of cytotoxicity via cell-to-cell signaling, as illustrated by bystander killing of adjacent cells after passage of an ionizing radiation track *(19)*, although the significance of this phenomenon in GDEPT is not yet known.

2. Immunological effects, as illustrated by regression of distant tumors following expression of the T-cell costimulator molecule B7.1 *(20)* and the antitumor activity of vectors expressing cytokines such as interleukin (IL)-2 *(21)*. Immunological mechanisms are also important in the GCV-HSV-TK GDEPT paradigm, as demonstrated by the lack of bystander effects in immunodeficient hosts *(18,22)*.

3. Antivascular effects, in which damage to microvascular endothelium in tumors results in loss of blood flow and death of the tumor cells dependent on the affected vessel. There is current interest in targeting endothelium in gene therapy to exploit this effect *(23,24)*. In addition, the bystander effect resulting from GCV-HSV-TK, even when not specifically targeted to endothelium, is in part the result of vascular damage as demonstrated by GCV-dependent prompt hemorrhagic necrosis after intratumoral injection of HSV-TK retroviral

producer cells *(25)*. Such effects may be elicited by the release of pro-inflammatory cytokines such as tumor necrosis factor (TNF) and IL-1 *(22)* as well as by direct endothelial cell toxicity.

Given this multiplicity of mechanisms, it is useful to have access to a range of experimental models to dissect and quantify bystander effects. In this respect, in vitro and in vivo models perform complementary functions. In vitro methods are valuable for examining cell-to-cell cytotoxicity transfer in isolation from the immunological or antivascular effects that may make a contribution in vivo and have a potentially important role to play in optimization of bystander effects through prodrug design. In vitro models also allow flexible manipulation of experimental conditions in order to address specific mechanistic questions.

Investigation of GDEPT paradigms has been greatly facilitated by use of cell lines that have been transfected in vitro and selected for stable expression of the PAE. These can be used to grow mixed cultures, or mixed tumors, containing PAE-expressing cells ("activators") and nonexpressing "targets" for investigation of bystander effects. In most published studies, bystander killing is inferred from the ability of activator cells to inhibit overall growth of the culture (or tumor) to a greater extent than can be accounted for by inhibition of the activator cells only *(1,12,15,26–28)*.

The protocols described here represent a variation on the above theme, in which antibiotic resistant marker(s) introduced at the time of selecting stable PAE transfectants, along with additional markers on the target cells, are used to discriminate the two populations unambiguously. The methods are based on the measurement of cell killing by clonogenic assay (i.e., cell sterilization) that integrates the contribution of all cell death pathways (prompt and delayed apoptosis, necrosis). Although stable transfectants provide useful models, it should be noted that the distances over which activated metabolites need to diffuse will depend on the spatial distribution of PAE expression in tumors and that this may not be adequately represented by the intimate cell mixtures investigated in these protocols. This limitation can be partially addressed by manipulating the experimental models, but studies with stable transfectants ultimately need to be complemented by investigations with gene therapy vectors administered using the same regime as in the clinical setting.

An important limitation with most experimental studies of bystander effects in cell culture has been the reliance on oversimplified models that poorly represent the physiology of tumors. In particular, most studies use low-cell-density monolayer cocultures of activators and targets *(13,27–32)* or bioassay medium from cultures of activators after exposure to prodrugs *(29,32)*. Although these models are qualitatively useful in demonstrating transfer of active metabolites between cells (either cell to cell or via the medium), their ability to rank in vivo bystander effects meaningfully within a series of prodrugs remains unproven. It would be reasonable to expect three-dimensional (3D) cell cultures, such as multicellular spheroids, to provide superior models for GDEPT bystander effects; they more faithfully represent the microenvironment of the extravascular compartment of solid tumors *(33,34)*, and there is much evidence that cells in 3D contact with extracellular matrix and with other cells are phenotypically different from cells in monolayers *(35–37)*. Regrettably, as yet, 3D cultures have received little attention as GDEPT models.

We *(38–42)* and others *(43–46)* have developed methods for culturing tumor cell lines in an alternate 3D format by growing them as multicellular layers (MCLs) (illustrated in **Fig. 2E**). The MCL model was initially developed to quantify extravascular transport of therapeutic agents *(38)* for which purpose it has technical advantages over spheroids. However, MCLs also have advantages for quantifying bystander effects (of the cytotoxicity transfer type) because a wider range of cell lines can be grown as MCLs than as spheroids and preparation of cocultures is much more straightforward. We have recently shown that the NTR/CB 1954 bystander effect is more efficient in MCLs than in monolayers, that NTR prodrug structure–activity relationships for bystander killing are different in the two models, and that bystander effects in MCLs grown from mixtures of NTR+ve and –ve WiDr cells predict for those in tumors of the same cell types *(16)*.

Multicellular layers are grown on commercially-available microporous membranes in cell culture inserts of the kind used for the culture of transporting epithelia. We use Millicell CM inserts (Millipore Corporation) (*see* **Fig. 2A**), which contain a Teflon microporous membrane (Biopore™, 0.4 -μm pore size, 30-μm thickness). Coating with collagen is required for cell attachment. The membranes are transparent when wet, facilitating visualization of cells by phase-contrast microscopy. The key technical modification to the standard methods for epithelial cultures in such inserts is to provide an efficient nutrient supply to both faces of the cellular layer, allowing proliferation to form a diffusion-limited MCL which eventually becomes hypoxic and necrotic in the centrer *(38,43)*. In our laboratory, this is achieved simply by submerging the inserts in a large reservoir of stirred culture medium (*see* **Fig. 2C,D**).

The following protocols provide methods for growing mixtures of NTR+ve activators and NTR–ve targets as MCLs and tumors and for quantifying bystander effects by differential plating assays in which clonogenic cell survival of activators and targets can be quantified separately. The protocols discuss three activator–target pairs recently investigated in this laboratory (*see* **Table 1**), but can readily be adapted to other cell lines that grow well as MCLs and/or tumors. Some of the human carcinoma lines currently in use in our laboratory for MCL studies are listed in **Table 2**.

2. Materials

2.1. Multicellular Layer Cultures

1. Conventional monolayer (T-flask) cell cultures (require 10^6 cells for each MCL initiated).
2. Polymerase chain reaction–enzyme-linked immunosorbent assay (PCR-ELISA) kit (Roche; cat. no. 1 663 925) for mycoplasma testing.
3. 0.07% Trypsin (Difco Laboratories; cat. no. 0152-13) dissolved in citrate–saline buffer (2.2 g/L trisodium citrate monohydrate, 10 g/L KCl, adjusted to pH 7.6 and autoclaved for storage). Filter-sterilize and store at –20°C.
4. Millicell-CM cell culture inserts, 0.4-μm pore size, 12-mm outer diameter, with uncoated Teflon membranes (Millipore Corporation; cat. no. PICM 01250).
5. Sigma calf skin collagen type III, acid soluble (Sigma; cat. no. C3511), stored in desiccator.
6. 0.01 *N* HCl.
7. 60% and 70% Ethanol/water mixtures.
8. Disposable bacteriological Petri dishes (100-mm diameter).

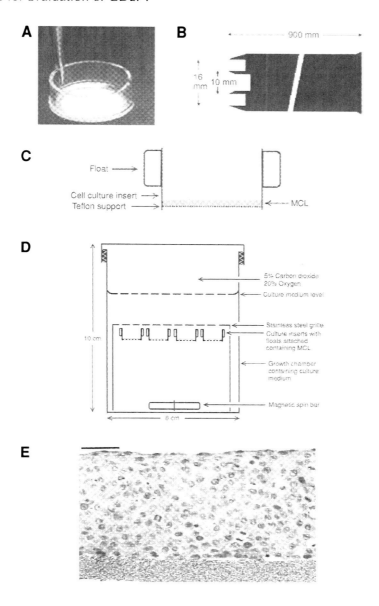

Fig. 2. Growth of MCL cultures. (**A**) Millicell-CM cell culture insert; (**B**) tool (stainless-steel punch) for cutting "floats" from expanded polyethylene sheet, in longitudinal section; (**C**) culture insert with added float; (**D**) culture of MCLs, following a period of cell attachment (see text), by submerging in stirred culture medium in a 500-mL jar, allowing efficient supply of nutrients to both sides of the cellular layer; (**E**) histology (4-µm paraffin section, stained with H&E) of a typical WiDr MCL after seeding 10^6 cells, allowing attachment for 4 h, then growing submerged for a further 3 d. The Teflon support membrane (Biopore™) is seen at the bottom of the image. The bar represents 50 µm.

Table 1

Characteristics of NTR Transfectants (Activators) and Their Non-NTR-Expressing Counterparts (Targets) Used in These Protocols

Cell type	Chinese hamster fibroblast	Human colon carcinoma	Mouse mammary carcinoma
NTR–ve targets	V79[oua][a]	WiDr[b]	EMT6[c]
NTR+ve activators			
Cell line name	V79-NTR[puro]	WiDr-NTR[neo]	EMT6-NTR[puro]
Synonym	T79-A3	WC14	EN2A
Origin	**ref. 51**	**ref. 13**	This lab[d]
Expression	CMV promoter,	CMV promoter,	EF-1α promoter,
cassette	monocistronic	monocistronic	bicistronic (vector
	(vector F8i3 from	(vector pCDNA3-	F399)[e]
	pRc/CMV)	NTR)	
Selection	15 μM puromycin	300 μg/mL G418	5 μM puromycin[f]
Doubling time in monolayer cultures (h)			
Activators	8	28	12
Targets	8	25	10
IC_{50} ratio (IC_{50} targets/IC_{50} activators)[g]			
CB 1954[h]	2,020 ± 210 (87)[i]	51 ± 2 (84)	930 ± 140 (28)
SN 23862	42 ± 6 (14)	93 ± 13 (16)	261 ± 26 (12)
SN 26634	381 ± 79 (5)	49 ± 6 (4)	86 ± 13 (3)
SN 25261	135 ± 22 (7)	79 ± 19 (4)	800 ± 130 (2)
SN 27217	828 ± 150 (2)	313 ± 107 (2)	1670 ± 230 (3)

[a]A spontaneous ouabain-resistant clone was selected from V79-379A cells (the same parental line as for T79-A3) by plating in 1 mM ouabain.

[b]Obtained from ATCC, Manassas, VA.

[c]Generously provided by Professor P.L. Olive, British Columbia Cancer Centre, Vancouver.

[d]EMT6 cells were transfected with F399 using Lipofectamine Plus™ according to the manufacturer's instructions (Invitrogen). 5×10^5 cells were transfected in 2 mL serum-free medium in a T25 flask for 3 h, with a final plasmid concentration of 4 μg/mL. Cells were grown (with 5% FBS) for 24 h, plated in the same medium at low density, and grown for a further 24 h without selection. Puromycin was then added to 5 μM, and a clone (EN2) was selected 6 d later and recloned to give EN2A. This clone retained CB 1954 sensitivity and puromycin resistance when grown in the absence of puromycin for 4 wk.

[e]Constructed from pEFIRES-P *(55)*.

[f]A lower puromycin concentration (3 μM) is optimal for the discrimination of activators and targets in clonogenic assays.

[g]Prodrug concentration for 50% inhibition of cell growth following 18 h exposure of log-phase cells. Cells were seeded into 96-well plates 24 h before the addition of prodrugs, at 50, 800, or 75 cells/well (V79, WiDr, and EMT6 lines, respectively). After washing out the prodrugs, cultures were grown for a further 3 d (V79, EMT6 lines) or 4 d (WiDr lines) before staining with sulforhodamine B *(56)*.

[h]For structures, *see* **Fig 1**.

[i]Mean ± SEM, with number of experiments in parentheses.

9. Expanded polyethylene sheet (5-mm thickness).
10. Custom-made stainless steel tool (punch), to cut out floatation rings (inner diameter, 10 mm; outer diameter, 16 mm) from polyethylene sheet. *See* **Fig. 2B**.

Table 2
Growth of (Nontransfected) Human Tumor Cell Lines as MCLs, and Diffusion Coefficients of Flux Markers (Urea and Mannitol) Through MCLs

Cell line	MCL formation[a]	Cell number /MCL[b] (× 10⁻⁶)	MCL thickness[c] (μm)	Dm[d] for ^{14}C-urea (cm²/s) × 10⁷	Dm[d] for ^{3}H-mannitol (cm²/s) × 10⁷
HCT-8	+	3.65 ± 0.05	257 ± 36 (8)	1.56 ± 0.08 (8)	0.40 ± 0.03 (8)
HT-29	++	7.4 ± 0.2	291 ± 24 (3)	6.36 ± 0.49 (4)	2.91 ± 0.24 (4)
SW620	+	9.6	n.d.[e]	n.d.[e]	n.d.[e]
HCT 116	++	9.7 ± 0.7	219	3.64	1.38
LoVo	+	6.5 ± 0.0	298 ± 21 (6)	5.0 ± 0.6 (4)	2.29 ± 0.25 (4)
SiHa	++	5.1 ± 0.6	171 ± 18 (5)	3.72 ± 0.26 (4)	1.71 ± 0.02 (5)
C-33 A	+	5.1 ± 0.1	n.d.[e]	n.d.[e]	n.d.[e]
SKOV-3	++	2.1 ± 0.6	81 ± 21 (5)	7.1 ± 1.1 (4)	2.7 ± 0.8 (4)
A549	++	5 ± 1	194 ± 19 (4)	4.78 ± 0.44 (4)	2.14 ± 0.20 (4)
NCI-H460	+	11.5 ± 1.5	405 ± 30 (3)	4.40 ± 0.31 (3)	1.76 ± 0.12 (3)
NCI-H1299	±	3.4 ± 0.2	305 ± 28 (6)	7.25 ± 0.75 (4)	4.08 ± 0.62 (4)
MGH-U1	++	3.6 ± 0.8	142 ± 43 (4)	18.7 ± 2.4 (4)	9.3 ± 1.9 (2)

Note: For this comparison, all MCLs were initiated using 1 × 10⁶ cells per culture insert and grown submerged for 4 d in culture medium containing 10% FBS.

[a]Observed under a phase-contrast microscope. ±: incomplete coverage of Teflon support membrane; +: complete but nonuniform coverage; ++: uniform MCL.

[b]Determined by trypsinization as described in **Subheading 3.3.1.** Values are mean and range for two MCLs.

[c]Measured on H&E-stained frozen sections after the flux experiment. Values are the mean ± SD, with the number of MCLs in parentheses.

[d]Diffusion coefficient in the MCL. Determined by fitting the flux kinetics to Fick's second law, for MCLs of known thickness, as described (*41*). Values are mean ± SEM, with the number of MCLs in parentheses.

[e]Not determined because MCLs were too unstable for flux studies.

11. Standard tissue culture facilities including inverted phase-contrast microscope, laminar-flow hood, and 5% CO_2 incubator.
12. Phosphate-buffered saline (PBS): 40 g NaCl, 1 g KCl, 1 g KH_2PO_4 (anhydrous), 5.75 g Na_2HPO_4 (anhydrous), 5 L analytical-grade (e.g., MilliQ) water.
13. Deoxyribonuclease I (Sigma; cat. no. DN-25). Prepare 10X stock at 1 mg/mL in PBS containing Ca^{2+} and Mg^{2+} (add $CaCl_2$ and $MgCl_2 \cdot 6H_2O$ to 0.1 g/L each, final concentration in PBS), filter-sterilize, and store at $-20°C$.
14. 250- or 500-mL sterile, disposable polystyrene screw-top specimen jars (Labserv Ltd, Auckland) with 40-mm spin bar (*see* **Fig. 2D**).
15. Stainless-steel (marine grade) grill cut and bent to fit into above jars (*see* **Fig. 2D**).
16. Magnetic stirrer for jars, under water bath or in dry-air incubator (37°C).

2.2. Characterization of Multicellular Layers

1. ^{14}C-urea (Amersham Pharmacia Biotech; cat. no CFA41). Requires stock solution at approx 0.75 MBq/mL and approx 40 MBq/mmol in sterile saline or PBS. Dilute 100-fold into donor compartment to investigate flux through MCLs.
2. ^3H-mannitol (ICN Pharmaceuticals; cat. no. 27040). Requires stock solution at approx 2 MBq/mL and approx 40 GBq/mmol in sterile saline or PBS. Dilute 100-fold into donor compartment to investigate flux through MCLs.
3. Water-accepting scintillation cocktail; for example, Emulsifier-Safe™ (Packard BioScience; cat. no. 6013389).
4. 10% Neutral buffered formalin (NBF): 4 g $NaH_2PO_4 \cdot H_2O$, 6 g Na_2HPO_4 (anhydrous), 100 mL formaldehyde solution (40%), 900 mL analytical-grade (e.g., Milli-Q) water.
5. Aluminum foil.
6. Tissue-Tek O.C.T. Compound 4583 (Sakura).
7. Scalpel blade #11.
8. Open liquid-nitrogen Dewar (bowl type).
9. Isopentane (approx 150 mL in 250-mL glass beaker, inside Dewar).
10. Liquid nitrogen, in Dewar, to below the level of the isopentane.
11. Paper towels.
12. Eppendorf tube rack.
13. Clamp scissors.
14. Pair of fine tweezers.
15. Pair of large tweezers.
16. Plastic cups for O.C.T. embedding.
17. Cryomicrotome.
18. Superfrost Plus microscope slides (BDH Labs).
19. Automated tissue processor (e.g., Tissue Tek VIP, Miles Scientific Ltd)
20. Scott's Tap Water Substitute (2 g sodium bicarbonate and 20 g magnesium sulfate dissolved in 1 L of analytical-grade water, plus one to three crystals of thymol to retard mold growth).
21. Xylol.
22. Paraplast paraffin wax (Oxford Labware).
23. Silane-coated microscope slides (Acros Organics, NJ).
24. DPX mounting solution (BDH labs).
25. Gill's Hematoxylin II: 250 mL ethylene glycol, 4 g hematoxylin, 0.4 g sodium iodate, 70.4 g aluminum sulfate, 20 mL glacial acetic acid, or 1 g citric acid.
26. Eosin (BDH Labs).

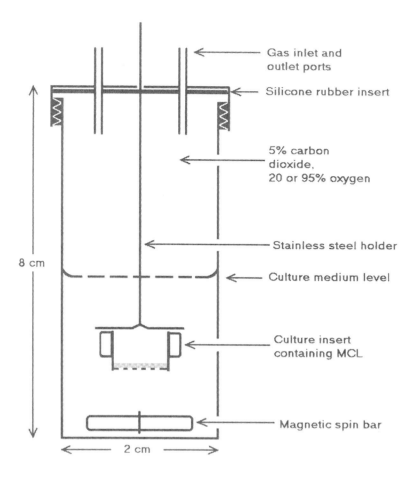

Fig. 3. Vessel for drug exposure of MCL. The MCL is held below the surface of the stirred medium using a stainless-steel holder (shaft with cross-piece on end). The shaft protrudes through a hole in the lid and silicone rubber liner allowing adjustment of height according to liquid level. Gas inlet and exit ports are used to flush continuously with the appropriate gas phase (usually 5% CO_2 in air or O_2) during drug exposure.

2.3. Bystander Measurements in Multicellular Layers

1. Custom vessels for exposure of MCLs to prodrugs, as illustrated in **Fig 3**. These are prepared by modifying the lids of standard glass Universal bottles (or similar bottles with a volume of approx 25 mL) and by fabricating a stainless-steel rod with a cross-piece that is inserted through the lid as shown.
2. 5% CO_2 in air or 5% CO_2 in O_2 (carbogen).
3. Drechsel bottle for humidification of gas.
4. Prodrugs, as appropriate, in sterile stock solution at approx 100X final concentration.

5. Positive displacement pipettor (e.g., Socorex micropipet 841).
6. Sterile, disposable 14-mL tubes with caps (Becton Dickinson Labware, Falcon 2057).
7. 60-mm-Diameter tissue culture dishes (P-60; e.g. Becton Dickinson Labware, Falcon 3002).
8. Puromycin (Sigma; cat. no. P-7255).
9. Geneticin (G418; Invitrogen, cat. no. 1181-031).
10. Ouabain (Serva; cat. no. 77647).
11. Methylene blue (BDH; cat. no. 621887), 2 g/L in 50% aqueous ethanol.

2.4. Tumor Xenografts

1. T175 flasks (e.g., Becton Dickinson Labware, Falcon 3112).
2. Culture medium, trypsin, DNAase I as in **Subheading 2.1.**
3. Trypan blue stain, 0.4% in 0.85% saline (Gibco BRL; cat. no. 15250-061).
4. Hemocytometer (e.g., Kova Glasstic disposable hemocytometers from Hycor Biomedical Inc, CA).
5. CD-1 nude mice of either sex, 20–25 g in weight.
6. 27-Gauge needles plus 1-mL tuberculin syringes (Terumo) for sc tumor inoculation.
7. Avertin anaesthetic. Stock solution: 2 g of 2,2,2-tribromoethanol in 1.24 mL tertiary amyl alcohol. Store in dark (with foil or amber bottle) at 4°C. Make fresh every 3 mo. Working solution: Dilute 100 µL of stock solution to 5 mL with isotonic saline. Warm to 40°C, shake vigorously, and then store in dark at 4°C. Use within 2 wk.
8. Ear tags for mice (National Band and Tag Co., Newport, KY).
9. Electronic calipers for tumor measurement (Mitutoyo America Corp. IL; model 500-474 Solar Absolute MyCal Digimatic Caliper).
10. 26-Gage needles plus tuberculin syringes for ip prodrug injection.
11. Hamilton syringes for ip prodrug injection (Hamilton Co., Reno, NV).
12. Animal balance (e.g., Sartorius model SARCP622).
13. Dissection equipment (tweezers, scissors, No. 21 scalpels).
14. Tissue culture dishes, 60 mm in diameter (BD Labware, Falcon 3002).
15. 14-mL Sterile disposable polystyrene tubes (BD Labware, Falcon 2057).
16. Magnetic spin bars, 10 mm.
17. Pronase (Sigma; cat. no. P-5147).
18. Collagenase (Sigma; cat. no. C-5138).
19. 37°C Waterbath over a magnetic stirrer.
20. Puromycin (Sigma; cat. no. P-7255).
21. Methylene blue (BDH; cat. no. 621887), 2 g/L in 50% aqueous ethanol.
22. Software for statistical analysis (e.g., Sigmastat version 2, Jandel Scientific, CA).

3. Methods

3.1. Validation of Differential Plating Assays (Selection Conditions)

The ability to discriminate activators and targets in mixed-cell suspensions from MCLs or tumors is central to the measurement of bystander effects in these protocols. The appropriate selection conditions should be established by performing experiments that reconstruct the selection using known ratios of activators and targets. Such a validation experiment is illustrated in **Fig. 4**, which demonstrates reliable quantitation of V79-NTR^{puro} (NTR+ve activators) and V79^{oua} (NTR–ve targets) within mixtures containing up to a 1000-fold excess of the other cell type.

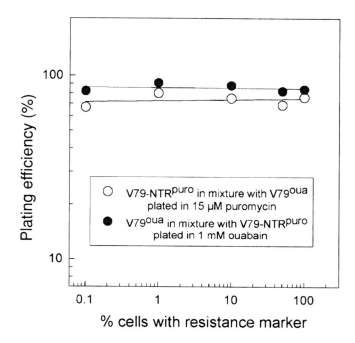

Fig. 4. Validation of differential plating assay for quantifying survival of activator cells and target cells in mixtures of both cell types. The indicated cell mixtures were plated in 15 μM puromycin (to measure V79-NTR^{puro}) and 1 mM ouabain (to measure V79^{oua}). The number of colonies recovered, expressed as the plating efficiency, was unaffected by a large excess of the other cell type.

3.2. Growth of Multicellular Layers

3.2.1. Preparation of Collagen-Coated Inserts With Polyethylene Floats

1. Dissolve collagen in 0.01 N HCl at 3 mg/mL by stirring magnetically at 37°C. May be stored for a few days at 4°C before use.
2. Place Millicell CM inserts in Petri dishes in a laminar-flow hood (approx 10 inserts per 100-mm dish).
3. Gently mix 1 part collagen solution with 4 parts 60% ethanol, taking care not to introduce air bubbles into the mixture.
4. Aliquot 100 μL of mixture into each insert, ensuring that the entire support membrane becomes coated. The membranes should become transparent; discard any that do not.
5. Leave to dry in the laminar-flow hood overnight (no lids on the Petri dishes), until the membranes change to chalky white. Store coated inserts in a sterile jar at room temperature until required (storage for at least 1 yr is acceptable) (*see* **Note 1**).
6. Use the float-cutting tool (*see* **Subheading 2.**) to cut rings ("floats") from a sheet of polyethylene closed cell foam (5 mm thickness). The floats should have in inner diameter of 10 mm and outer diameter of 16 mm.
7. Sterilize the floats by immersion in 70% ethanol for at least 24 h (can be left in ethanol indefinitely until use).

8. Working in a sterile hood, place sterilized floats in a 100-mm Petri dish, and while still wet with ethanol, use forceps to place the floats on the collagen-coated inserts, as shown in **Fig. 2C**.

9. Leave to dry in the laminar-flow hood overnight, and store in a sterile jar until use.

3.2.2. Seeding and Growth of MCL

1. Passage cell lines as conventional monolayer cultures in T-flasks, without antibiotics, and reinitiate from frozen stocks (liquid N_2) at intervals of not more than 3 mo. All cell lines should be confirmed free of mycoplasma (e.g., by cytochemical staining) *(47)* and PCR-ELISA (according to the kit manufacturer's protocol; *see* **Subheading 2.**).

2. Prepare culture medium for MCL cultures (usually the same as for monolayers). For V79, WiDr, and their NTR transfectants, MCLs are grown in αMEM containing 5% heat-inactivated fetal bovine serum (FBS), and antibiotics (penicillin 100 units/mL, streptomycin 100 μg/mL, with optional fungizone [amphotericin B] 1 μg/mL; *see* **Note 2**).

3. Prepare single-cell suspensions by standard methods; for example, rinse the monolayer with Ca/Mg-free PBS and then incubate with 0.07% trypsin in citrate–saline buffer (1 mL/25cm^2) for approx 5–10 min at 37°C. When the cells have rounded and detached from the substrate, quench trypsin by adding at least an equal volume of medium containing serum, then pipet vigorously to break up cell clumps. The addition of DNAse I to 0.1 mg/mL is advised if a significant amount of DNA is released; this can compromise the uniformity of seeding of the inserts. Incubate for 5–10 min at 37°C until DNA fibers have disappeared, then centrifuge and resuspend in fresh growth medium, mixing cell lines (if required) to give a total cell density of 2×10^6/mL.

4. Wet the collagen-coated inserts (**Subheading 3.2.1.**) by placing them in a 100-mm Petri dish containing 15 mL culture medium. Discard any inserts with membranes that do not become completely transparent upon wetting.

5. Seed 0.5-mL aliquots of the cell suspension (10^6 cells) into the inserts.

6. Allow cells to attach to the collagen-coated support membrane by incubating in a CO_2 incubator at 37°C, in Petri dishes, for at least 4 h (longer may be required for some cell lines). Confirm that cells are attached and uniformly distributed on the support membrane under an inverted phase-contrast microscope (*see* **Note 3**).

7. Float the inserts on a large reservoir (approx 350 mL) of culture medium, pre-equilibrated at 37°C in a 5% CO_2 incubator in a sterile polystyrene screw-top specimen jar (500 mL). Allow 60 mL medium/insert, with up to six inserts per jar. Then, gently fill the inserts with culture medium by turning them on their side using sterile tweezers, and submerge by lowering a stainless-steel (marine grade) grill into the jar as shown in **Fig. 2D**. This allows supply of nutrients from both sides of the cell layer. Flush the jars with 5% CO_2/air and seal.

8. Incubate at 37°C with magnetic stirring, typically for 3–5 d depending on the growth rate of cell line and intended purpose. For bystander studies with V79 or WiDr MCLs, growth for 3 or 4–5 d, respectively, provides MCLs with little or no central necrosis, with cell numbers in the range $(6–8) \times 10^6$ cells/MCL.

9. Prior to use, examine MCLs by phase-contrast microscopy to check for uniformity. A more detailed characterization may be undertaken prior to investigating bystander effects, or at the end of the prodrug exposure period, using destructive methods (enzymatic dissociation, histology) or nondestructive methods (flux markers, impedance spectroscopy) as discussed in **Subheading 3.3.**

3.3. Characterization of Multicellular Layers

3.3.1. Cell Number

Dissociation of most MCLs, including V79 and WiDr, to give a single-cell suspension for counting can be achieved using the following method:

1. Carefully aspirate the medium from the insert. Do not rinse.
2. Place the whole culture insert into 6 mL of citrate–saline buffer containing 0.07% trypsin and stir magnetically at 37°C for 10 min.
3. Terminate trypsinization by adding an equal volume of culture medium with 10% FBS and pipet vigorously to break up cell clumps. Add DNAase I if necessary, to 0.1 mg/mL, and incubate for a further 10 min.
4. Viable or total cells are enumerated by standard techniques (hemocytometer with trypan blue or eosin Y dye exclusion, electronic particle counter, clonogenic assay, etc.).

3.3.2. Flux Markers

The integrity and thickness of MCLs can be assessed nondestructively by examining the transport of markers with known diffusion coefficient in the MCLs. The flux of markers is determined using a diffusion chamber in which the insert (and MCL) separates two well-stirred compartments (approx 7 mL each). Details of this method are given in **ref. 41**. Briefly, the flux markers ^{3}H-mannitol (which marks the paracellular transport route) and ^{14}C-urea (which is transported via both the paracellular and transcellular route in most MCLs) are added together to the "donor" compartment, and the concentrations in the donor and "receiver" compartments are determined by sampling 50 µL and counting radioactivity in a water-accepting scintillation cocktail (5 mL). The concentration–time profiles in the donor and receiver are fitted to Fick's second law to estimate MCL thickness, providing a weighted mean over the whole MCL. Determination of flux over a 2-h period is sufficient for this purpose.

Measurement of absolute thicknesses by this method requires knowledge of diffusion coefficients of the markers in MCLs (D_{MCL}) of the cell line of interest. These values are determined calibrating flux against thicknesses measured by histology (*see* **Note 4**). Values of D_{MCL} for urea and mannitol for several cell lines, determined in this manner, are shown in Table 2 (*see* **Note 5**).

3.3.3. Electrical Impedance Spectroscopy

Kyle et al. (**48**) have shown that electrical impedance spectroscopy provides an alternative non-destructive method for monitoring MCL thickness and integrity. As with flux marker diffusion, this requires calibration against histological sections, but is a rapid method which is well suited to characterization of MCLs before (or even during) use. It requires specialized equipment, although useful characterization could be achieved using simplified approaches such as measurement of impedance at a single frequency or of ac resistance with a Millicell Electrical Resistance System (Millipore; cat. no. MERS 000 01). The latter is widely employed to determine transepithelial electrical resistance of caco-2 monolayers in culture inserts (e.g., **ref. 49**).

3.3.4. Histology: Frozen Sections

Paraffin sections provide superior histology to frozen sections, but the latter are more easily processed without dislodging the MCL from its support. Frozen sections are therefore preferable for measurement of thickness and, depending on the epitope, are sometimes preferable for immunostaining for hypoxia *(40)* or PAE expression *(16)*. The same initial fixation method (**steps 1–4** following) can be used for both paraffin and frozen sections.

1. Drain medium from culture inserts. Fix MCLs by submerging very gently in 10% neutral-buffered formalin (NBF) and holding at room temperature for 24 h. Transfer to PBS for longer-term storage (satisfactory for up to at least 3 mo) at 4°C.
2. Drain PBS from the culture inserts and remove excess liquid by inverting onto a paper towel.
3. Immediately cut out the coated support membrane and attached MCL using a scalpel blade and fine tweezers. This requires clamping the insert firmly, which can be achieved by placing a paper towel over a microcentrifuge tube rack and tightly fitting the insert, upside down, into the rack.
4. Carefully insert the scalpel tip through the support membrane and MCL at one edge. Make a small cut, grip the membrane near the cut edge with fine tweezers, and cut around the inside of the insert wall.
5. Using the tweezers, gently place the MCL face down (cell side down) on top of the O.C.T. freezing mixture in a plastic cup, taking care not to introduce bubbles or let the membrane to fold back on itself.
6. Slowly add 2 drops of O.C.T. freezing mixture to submerge the insert until it is located in the center of the plastic cup.
7. Holding the cup with scissor tongs, lower into the cold isopentane bath in liquid nitrogen (in an open Dewar flask). Hold the cup in the liquid (not submerged) until the O.C.T. is frozen; then, submerge the cup to ensure freezing through the block. Keep the cup as horizontal as possible during freezing so that the insert freezes straight in the O.C.T block.
8. Transfer the cup onto a piece of aluminum foil labeled with the sample code. As the cup warms slightly, squeeze the frozen block out of the cup. Wrap quickly in the foil and hold at –20°C for temporary storage or –80°C for longer-term storage.
9. Cut 14-μm transverse sections with a cryomicrotome. Typically, sections are cut at several different positions through the MCL.
10. Collect the sections on Superfrost Plus microscope slides, which are electrostatically charged for improved binding, and store at –20°C in sealed containers.

3.3.5. Histology: Paraffin Sections

Multicellular layers are fixed in neutral-buffered formalin as for frozen sections, laid between two biopsy sponges in a standard cassette, and embedded in paraffin in an automated histology processor using the following program:

1. Neutral-buffered formalin.
2. 70% Ethanol, 30 min.
3. 95% Ethanol, 30 min.
4. 95% Ethanol, 30 min.
5. 100% Ethanol, 60 min.
6. 100% Ethanol, 60 min.

7. Xylol, 20 min.
8. Xylol, 40 min.
9. Paraffin wax, 30 min.
10. Paraffin wax, 30 min.
11. Paraffin wax, 40 min.

The blocks are then cut at 4 μm with a hand-operated microtome and floated onto silane-coated slides.

3.3.6. Histology: H&E Staining

Frozen sections are brought to room temperature (at least 4 min) and hydrated with a quick dip in tap water. Rehydration of paraffin sections is performed using the following protocol:

1. Dewax in xylol, mins.
2. Dewax in xylol, 5 mins.
3. Absolute alcohol, 6 dips.
4. 95% alcohol, 6 dips.
5. 95% alcohol, 6 dips.
6. 70% alcohol, 6 dips.
7. Tap water, wash.

Sections are then stained with H&E using the following protocol:

1. Gill's Haematoxylin II, 1 min.
2. Tap water, wash.
3. Scott's tap water substitute, 8 dips.
4. Tap water, wash.
5. Eosin, 1 min.
6. Tap water, wash.
7. 95% Alcohol, 6 dips.
8. 95% Alcohol, 6 dips.
9. Absolute alcohol, 6 dips.
10. 50/50 Absolute alcohol + xylol, 12 dips.
11. Xylol, 12 dips.
12. Xylol, 2 mins.

Mount paraffin sections with DPX or Histomount and cover slip.

3.4. Measurement of GDEPT Bystander Effects in Multicellular Layers

1. Initiate and grow MCLs as in **Subheading 3.2.2.**, using known mixtures of "activator" (i.e., PAE-expressing) and "target" (i.e., nonexpressing) cells. For the example shown in **Fig. 5**, mixed MCLs were established by seeding 3×10^4 V79-NTR^{puro} cells (NTR-expressing activators) and 9.7×10^5 V79^{oua} cells (nonNTR-expressing targets) on collagen-coated Teflon membranes. Separate MCLs with target cells only were prepared by seeding 10^6 V79^{oua} cells.

2. When MCLs have grown to the appropriate thicknesss, examine by phase-contrast microscopy (without removing the culture medium within the insert) and select inserts with uniform MCLs (*see* **Notes 5** and **6**).

3. Place MCLs in exposure vessels (*see* **Fig. 3**) containing 9.5 mL fresh culture medium (final volume 10 mL, including 0.5 mL in the insert). Connect to a humidified gas line, typically 5% CO_2 in air or oxygen (*see* **Note 7**) scrubbed through a Drechsel bottle containing sterile water to minimize evaporation.

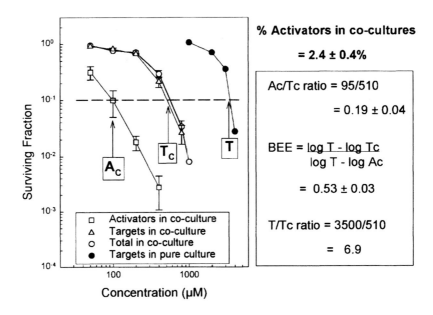

% Activators in co-cultures

= 2.4 ± 0.4%

Ac/Tc ratio = 95/510

= 0.19 ± 0.04

$$BEE = \frac{\log T - \log Tc}{\log T - \log Ac}$$

= 0.53 ± 0.03

T/Tc ratio = 3500/510

= 6.9

Fig. 5. Example of measurement of bystander killing in MCLs. Cell mixtures comprising 3% V79-NTR[puro] (NTR-expressing "activator" cells) and 97% V79[oua] targets (NTR –ve) were grown as MCL cocultures (open symbols) for 3 d and compared to MCLs grown from V79[oua] targets only (filled symbols) under the same conditions. MCLs were exposed to the NTR prodrug SN 25261 for 5 h under 5% CO_2/95% O_2 (to suppress any activation by endogenous oxygen-sensitive reductases), dissociated with trypsin, and assayed for clonogenicity. Cells were plated in nonselective medium (circles) to measure total cell survival, in medium containing 1 mM ouabain (triangles) to measure target cell survival, and in medium containing 15 µM puromycin (squares) to measure activator cell survival. Surviving fractions are ratios of plating efficiency of treated/control (no prodrug). Values are mean ± range for two independent experiments, each with a single MCL at each prodrug concentration. Drug concentrations for 10% cell survival for activators in cocultures (Ac), targets in cocultures (Tc), and targets in pure cultures (T) were determined by interpolation. Three parameters useful for quantifying different aspects of the bystander effect (Ac/Tc ratio, bystander effect efficiency (BEE), T/Tc ratio) are illustrated (*see* text for discussion).

4. Equilibrate with magnetic stirring at 37°C for 30 min.
5. Add prodrugs to initiate exposure by inserting a positive displacement pipettor through the gas exit port and adding 10–100 µL of prodrug stock solution in a suitable solvent (with inclusion of appropriate controls for potential solvent effects).
6. Incubate for the required prodrug exposure period (in **Fig. 5**, for 5 h) while maintaining gassing continuously at a low flow rate (30–50 mL/min).
7. Enzymatically dissociate to single-cell suspensions as in **Subheading 3.3.1.** for clonogenic assay of cell survival.
8. Determine cell density of suspensions and make 10-fold serial dilutions (10^2–10^5 cells/mL) in 14-mL tubes.

9. Plate 1-mL aliquots of appropriate dilutions (depending on expected cell survival) in 60-mm Petri dishes containing 4.5 mL culture medium, in triplicate, in three different series:
   a. Nonselective medium (to determine total clonogenic cells).
   b. Selective medium containing the antibiotic to which activator cells are resistant. For V79-NTR^{puro} activators, use 15 μM puromycin. For WiDr-NTR^{neo} activators, use 0.3 mg/mL G418.
   c. (*Optional*) Selective medium for target cells. For V79^{oua} targets use 1 mM ouabain (*see* **Note 8**).

10. Incubate the Petri dishes until macroscopic colonies are evident (7 d for V79, 14 d for WiDr); then, stain with methylene blue after decanting the medium.

11. Count colonies containing >50 cells (*see* **Note 9**) and calculate plating efficiency (colonies/cells plated) for both cell types in the mixture. For activators, this is determined using the appropriate selective plates (**step 9b**). For targets, this can also be determined using selection (**step 9c**) or by the difference between total clonogens (**step 9a**) and activators (**step 9b**) (*see* **Note 10**).

12. The control (nonprodrug-treated MCL) plating efficiencies from such experiments provide an estimate of the proportion of activator cells in the MCL cocultures. This is calculated as PE_{Ac} /(PE_{Ac} + PE_{Tc}), where PE_{Ac} and PE_{Tc} are the plating efficiencies of the activators and targets, respectively, from the MCL cocultures. This calculation requires modification if the plating efficiencies of the initial activator and target cell lines are different (*see* **Note 11**). For V79 and WiDr MCLs seeded with mixtures of activators (V79-NTR^{puro} and WiDr-NTR^{neo}) and targets (V79^{oua} and WiDr), the ratio of activators to targets in established MCLs, by this method, was indistinguishable from that in the seeding mixture over an extended series of experiments (*16*).

13. Determine the clonogenic surviving fraction (ratio of plating efficiency of treated/control) for both cell types in the mixture and plot as a function of prodrug concentration (e.g., **Fig. 5**). **Figure 5** shows representative data for the NTR prodrug SN 25261 (*see* **Fig. 1**), which is a hydrophilic analog of the nitrogen mustard SN 23862. Note that the survival curves for target cells in the cocultures are indistinguishable whether determined by plating in ouabain (to eliminate activators) or in nonselective medium because the proportion of activators in the treated MCLs is extremely low in this case. The presence of a bystander effect is demonstrated by the shift in the target cell survival curve when activator cells are present, with the prodrug concentration for 10% survival (C_{10}) decreasing from 3500 μM in MCLs of pure targets (T) to 510 μM for targets in the cocultures (Tc). Unmasking the surviving activator cells by plating in puromycin demonstrates a C_{10} of 95 μM in the cocultures (A_C); thus, the bystander effect is not fully efficient because the sensitivity of targets in the cocultures is less than for the activators.

14. Parameters for quantifying bystander effects can be derived from the survival curves using the C_{10} values defined in **step 14**, as illustrated in **Fig. 5**. Each parameter is appropriate for addressing a separate question:

   a. The Ac/Tc ratio assesses bystander efficiency in terms of how closely the target cell survival curve approaches that of the activators in cocultures. For a perfect bystander effect, Ac/Tc reaches unity (*see* **Note 12**). However, this parameter does not take into account the differential in sensitivity between activators and targets in the absence of a bystander effect. For example, a poor NTR substrate might give an Ac/Tc ratio close to unity simply because activation by the *E. coli* NTR is insignificant relative to activation by endogenous nitroreductases in both activators and targets (rather than because of an efficient bystander effect).

b. The bystander effect efficiency (BEE), defined by the formula in **Fig. 5**, avoids the latter problem. This parameter quantifies the shift in apparent sensitivity of targets, because of the presence of activators, normalizing this against the difference in sensitivity of targets in pure cultures (T) and activators in cocultures (Ac). For SN 25261, the BEE is 0.53, indicating that the target curve is shifted just over half of the "distance" (log concentration) required for a full bystander effect (BEE = 1), in which case the target curve would be superimposed on the activator curve. This is an appropriate parameter for comparing the efficiency of the transmission of cytotoxic metabolites of different prodrugs, or PAE/prodrug systems, and it isolates this aspect of the phenomenon. It is useful in structure–activity studies that seek to relate properties of bystander metabolites to the efficiency of transmission in tissue; for prodrug series with similarly large Ac vs T differentials, BEE and Ac/Tc will correlate, and we have shown a close relationship between the latter parameter and lipophilicity for NTR prodrugs in MCLs (*16*). However, for therapeutic ranking of enzyme/prodrug systems, it is not just transmissibility of effects (as measured by Ac/Tc and BEE) that is important.

c. The T/Tc ratio is perhaps the most therapeutically relevant, as it measures the overall shift in sensitivity of targets due to the bystander effect. This will reflect bystander efficiency, as defined in **step 14b** (i.e.. transmissibility), but it will also be influenced by the rate of generation of the diffusing metabolite and its cytotoxic potency. Rapid formation of potent metabolites will shift Ac to lower values; even if Ac/Tc or BEE is not improved, this will have a beneficial effect by displacing Tc to lower values (which is the key therapeutic goal in GDEPT). This net bystander effect (resulting from the efficient formation of potent metabolites and their efficient transmission to nearby cells) is conveniently measured as the T/Tc ratio, which should be as high as possible (*see* **Note 13**).

3.5. Bystander Effect in Tumors

Investigations of GDEPT bystander effects in tumors have primarily focused on human tumor xenografts grown from mixtures of wild-type tumor lines and PAE-expressing stable transfectants in immunodeficient mice (*see* **Note 14**). Almost without exception, these studies employ tumor growth inhibition/cure end points, which have obvious relevance to the clinical setting and make it possible to evaluate contributions from multiple bystander mechanisms. The drawback with such studies for prodrug screening is that investigations are protracted (typically 4–6 mo from tumor inoculation to end point), expensive, and provide little information about underlying mechanisms. In these respects, evaluation of cell killing at early times after treatment by clonogenic assays provides a useful complement and offers the possibility of assessing response of both activator and target cells using the same general approaches as for MCLs (*see* **Subheading 3.4.**).

The following protocol describes a relatively rapid assay for bystander effects (and overall therapeutic utility) of NTR prodrugs based on differential clonogenic assay of activators and targets in a murine breast carcinoma (EMT6), using the NTR transfectant EMT6-NTR[puro] as activators. The latter cell line was derived from EMT6 using a bicistronic pEFIRES-P plasmid in which both *NTR* and the puromycin *N*-acetyltransferase (*pac*) resistance marker gene are transcribed from a single EF-1α promoter (*see* **Table 1**). Translation of the NTR gene is cap dependent, whereas translation of *pac* occurs via an internal ribosome entry site (IRES) derived from encephalomyocarditis virus. The number of surviving activator cells in the treated tumors is determined by plating in medium containing puromycin at a concentration high enough to eliminate EMT6 cells (3 μM). The number of surviving target cells is determined by plating in nonselective media and subtracting the (usually small) number of surviving activators.

The method is described for tumors in CD-1 nude mice, but can also be used with immunocompetent Balb/c hosts in order to include immunological mechanisms (although this would require excision of tumors at later times to allow for the slower kinetics of killing by such pathways). Quantities are indicated for a typical screening experiment comparing three compounds against two different tumor types (inoculated using targets only, and 2 : 1 activator : target mixtures), with five tumors/group. Approximately 30 mice should be inoculated with each of these tumor cell preparations to obtain 20 tumors of each type sufficiently similar in size (9 ± 1 mm mean diameter) to be treated on the same day. The latter requirement is important with the EMT6/EMT6-NTR^{puro} model because of time-dependent changes in the ratio of activators : targets during tumor growth (*see* **Subheading 14.** and **Fig. 6**).

1. Harvest subconfluent monolayers of EMT6 cells (passaged in αMEM + 5% FBS + penicillin [100 IU/mL] + streptomycin [100 μg/mL]) and EMT6-NTR^{puro} cells (passaged in same medium + 5 μM puromycin). For each line, seed three T175 flasks with 10^4 cells each (50 mL/flask) using the appropriate medium.

2. Seven days later, the cultures should be approx 50–75% confluent. Harvest with 0.07% trypsin in citrate–saline for 5 min at 37°C. Quench trypsin with medium containing serum, add DNAase I to 0.1 mg/mL, and incubate for 5–10 min until DNA has disappeared. Collect cells by refrigerated low-speed centrifugation, resuspending the pellet as soon as the centrifuge stops using 1 mL medium/flask. Dilute a sample 100-fold in medium or PBS and transfer 100 μL to 40 μL of 0.4% trypan blue. Use a hemocytometer to determine viability and cell density. Dilute EMT6 to 3 × 10^7 cells/mL in αMEM with 5% FBS (for 100% EMT6 tumors) and to 2 × 10^7 cells/mL for mixed tumors. Dilute EMT6-NTR^{puro} to 4 × 10^7 cells/mL and mix with an equal volume of the EMT6 suspension at 2 × 10^7/mL to give a 1 : 2 mixture of EMT6/EMT6-NTR^{puro} at an overall density of 3 × 10^7 cells/mL.

3. Anaesthetize mice by injection of Avertin intraperitoneally at 15 μL/g body weight (*see* **Note 15**) and inoculate the mice subcutaneously (near the shoulder) using a 1-mL syringe with a 27-gage needle. Inject 3 × 10^6 cells per site (0.1 mL at 3 × 10^7 cells /mL) (*see* **Note 16**).

4. Individually ear-tag mice, preferably while still under anaesthesia.

5. Starting 8 d after inoculation, measure tumors daily in two dimensions ($L \times W$) with calipers until they reach treatment size (mean diameter 9 ± 1 mm, approx 350 mg).

6. Prodrug stock solutions should be prepared in advance of treatment, characterized (e.g., by spectrophotometry or high-performance liquid chromatography [HPLC]) to determine concentration and purity, and stored appropriately (usually frozen).

7. At the time of treatment, all mice with tumors falling within the required size range are randomized to treatment groups. Weigh mice using a damped animal balance and adjust injection volumes according to body weight. For screening dinitrobenzamide NTR

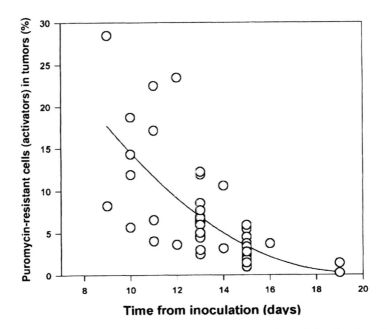

Fig. 6. EMT6-NTR[puro] cells in mixed tumors at various times following inoculation of CD-1 nude mice with 2 : 1 mixtures of EMT6-NTR[puro] (activator) and EMT6 (target) cells. Each symbol represents an individual tumor with a mean diameter in the range of 8–10 mm. The line is a second-order regression. The proportion of puromycin-resistant clonogens decreases progressively as a result of their dilution by faster-growing EMT6 cells.

prodrugs, animals are typically treated with single ip doses in dimethyl sulfoxide (DMSO) (1 µL/g body weight, using a Hamilton syringe) or, for more water-soluble compounds, in saline (optimally 10 µL/g using a 1-mL tuberculin syringe).

8. Eighteen hours after treatment, measure the tumor sizes again with calipers and cull the mice by cervical dislocation or terminal anaesthesia. Dissect the tumors under aseptic conditions by submersing the body briefly in 70% alcohol and removing the tumors in a sterile hood. Weigh dissected tumors and mince finely using crossed scalpels. Transfer up to 500 mg of the minced tumor into a pre-tared Falcon 2057 tube containing a magnetic spin bar and weigh.

9. Add chilled, filter-sterilized enzyme cocktail (pronase, 0.5 mg/mL; collagenase, 0.2 mg/mL; DNAase I, 0.2 mg/mL) in medium (αMEM + 5% FBS + Pen/Strep) at a rate of 1 mL/60 mg tumor and hold on ice until all samples are ready. Incubate samples in a 37°C water bath for 45 min over a magnetic stirrer.

10. After incubation, stand the tubes without stirring for 2 min to allow undissociated lumps to settle; then, sample 2 mL of the supernatant into 8 mL medium. Collect cells by low-speed centrifugation resuspending pellets in 10 mL of medium. Check under the phase-contrast microscope that a good single-cell suspension has been achieved and determine the cell density either with a hemocytometer or electronic particle counter (*see* **Note 17**). Dilute cell suspensions to 1.5×10^5 cells/mL and make 10-fold serial dilutions down to $1.5 \times 10_2$/mL.

11. Plate 1 mL of appropriate dilutions (depending on expected plating efficiencies) into P-60 tissue culture dishes containing 4 mL of nonselective medium (αMEM + 5% FBS +

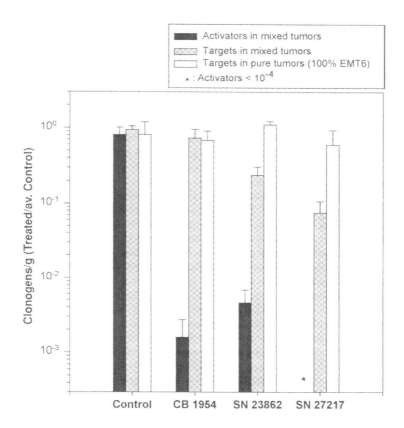

Fig. 7. Use of mixed EMT6-NTR^{puro} (activators)/EMT6^{wt} (targets) tumors (filled bars) and tumors grown from EMT6^{wt} targets only (open bars) to compare bystander effects and overall therapeutic utility in vivo of NTR prodrugs. Tumors were excised 18 h after single ip injections of prodrugs at the maximum tolerated dose (CB 1954 and SN 23862 at 0.2 mmol/kg, SN 27217 at 1.33 mmol/kg). In this experiment, the proportion of EMT6-NTR^{puro} activators in the un-treated mixed tumors at the time of assay was $4.8 \pm 2.2\%$(SD). The results show significant bystander killing by SN 23862 and SN 27217 (p-values for killing of targets in mixed tumors < 0.05 relative to targets in pure tumors) despite the very low proportion of activators.

Pen/Strep). Repeat plating in selective medium containing 3.75 μM puromycin (3 μM final concentration) to determine the number of clonogenic EMT6-NTR^{puro} cells in each sample. Target cells (EMT6) can usually be determined accurately as the difference be-tween total and activators, because the target cell is usually much less than activator kill in this model (*see* **Fig. 7**); if this is not the case, cells can be plated in medium containing SN 26634 (*see* **Fig. 1** for structure) to eliminate remaining activator cells (*see* **Note 8**).

12. Incubate plates in 5% CO_2 incubator at 37°C for 8 d and plates containing selective media for 9 d. Stain with 2% methylene blue in 50% EtOH. Count the dilutions providing between 10 and 100 colonies/dish, including colonies larger than 50 cells (*see* **Note 9**).

13. Use a spreadsheet to calculate plating efficiency (PE = colonies/cells plated), and number of clonogens (PE × total cells from **step 10**) per gram of tumor, for activators and for

targets (*see* **Note 18**). Also, calculate the ratio of clonogens for treated/control and plot the geometric mean and geometric standard error as illustrated in **Fig. 7** (*see* **Note 19**).

14. Estimate the fraction of activator cells in control tumors at the time of treatment, from the PE of activators and targets as in the MCL experiments (**Subheading 3.4.**). In this tumor model, despite stable expression of NTR in EMT6-NTR[puro] cells in the absence of puromycin in vitro (*see* **Table 1**, footnote d), the proportion of puromycin-resistant activators in the tumors at the time of assay is much lower than the proportion at inoculation. As shown in **Fig. 6**, this problem becomes more severe with time following inoculation; for this reason, it is preferable to use tumors over a narrow time window following inoculation. The loss of puromycin-resistant cells with tumor growth appears to be the result of their dilution by the faster-growing wild-type cells. (Following inoculation with pure cell populations at 10^6 cells/site, EMT6 tumors reach treatment size at a median time of 15 d vs 20 d for EMT6-NTR[puro] tumors).

15. Statistical analysis: Evaluate the significance of drug effects in the activator and target populations separately, using the log-transformed data (which then generally satisfies normality and equal variance tests), by one-way analysis of variance (ANOVA). Use Dunnett's test to determine p-values for pairwise comparisons with controls (i.e., to establish whether there is statistically significant of killing of activators or targets for each compound), or the Tukey test to compare prodrugs against each other.

16. A typical experiment using this assay to compare NTR prodrugs is illustrated in *Fig. 7*. This shows marked activity of CB 1954 against EMT6-NTR[puro] activator cells in mixed tumors comprising only $4.8 \pm 2.2\%$(SD) activators at the time of treatment, but this is not accompanied by statistically significant bystander killing of targets relative to either untreated mixed tumors or prodrug-treated tumors comprising EMT6 targets only (*see* **Note 20**). Killing of activators by the corresponding nitrogen mustard SN 23862 is slightly (but not significantly) less than by CB 1954, but killing of targets is now statistically significant with respect to either untreated mixed tumors or treated target-only tumors. This demonstrates a greater bystander effect for SN 23862 than CB 1954 in this model, as also demonstrated in WiDr/WiDr-NTR[neo] mixed tumors *(16)*. The same experiment also suggests that a dibromo mustard analog of SN 23862, SN 27217, provides greater bystander (target) cell killing at the MTD (i.e., has greater overall therapeutic utility) than either of the other NTR prodrugs in this model, although the difference in target cell kill by SN 23862 and SN 27217 did not quite reach statistical significance ($p>0.05$) in this experiment.

This protocol can be adapted for use with human tumor xenografts such as WiDr/WiDr-NTR[neo] mixed tumors in nude mice. The latter cell lines provide the important advantage of similar growth rates as tumors, with the ratio of activators to targets at the time of treatment is essentially the same as the ratio at inoculation *(16)*. However, the WiDr model is slightly less convenient for rapid screening in requiring inoculation of 10^7 rather than 10^6 cells, with a longer time required for the clonogenic assay (staining 14 vs 8 d after plating), higher FBS concentration (10% vs 5%), and lower plating efficiency from control tumors (5% vs 30%). The other difference from the EMT6 protocol is that preparation of single-cell suspensions from WiDr tumors requires higher enzyme concentrations (2.5 mg/mL pronase; 1 mL/mL collagenase, and 0.2 mg/mL DNAase I).

4. Notes

1. The uniformity of the collagen layer can be checked by staining representative inserts with 150 μL of 0.1% trypan blue in saline. After 2 min, wash off excess stain with 0.5 mL

saline two times and then dry. If this demonstrates nonuniform collagen deposition, the formation of uniform MCLs may be compromised. An alternative coating method, which appears to provide greater uniformity, is to precipitate collagen by neutralization of the acidic solutions as follows. Adjust the pH of normal saline to approx 8.0 using a small volume of dilute NaOH, and add 0.4 mL of this to the wells of a 24-well tray. Place inserts in the wells, ensuring that no air bubbles are trapped under the Teflon membranes. Dilute the collagen solution (3 mg/mL in 0.01 N HCl) into 3 parts 60% ethanol, and add 50-μL aliquots to each insert. Agitate the tray horizontally to spread the collagen solution over the surface. Leave overnight at room temperature with lid on and then aspirate the saline/NaOH and leave the inserts to dry. (Do not remove any liquid from the inside of the insert.) Wash salt deposits out of the inserts by dipping in Milli-Q water and allow to dry in a laminar-flow hood. Sterilize by dipping in 70 % ethanol and allow to dry again.

2. Fungizone (amphotericin B) should be used with caution; at concentrations of 1 μg/mL, it inhibits growth of some human tumor cell lines as MCLs, giving patchy structures.

3. Alternatively, inserts can be floated on the surface of the culture medium reservoir overnight to allow attachment, then submerged under the grill. We have not seen consistent differences between these methods.

4. Thicknesses determined by measurement of histological sections probably suffer from systematic errors resulting from shrinkage during fixation; we have not evaluated the magnitude of this effect. It is useful to measure the thickness of the Teflon support membrane and the MCL at the same position, each at approx 100 positions, and to use the apparent support thickness to correct for any nonorthogonality of the plane of sectioning (assuming a true thickness of the support of 30 μm, which is the minimum value observed). This may also partially correct for shrinkage artifacts, although it is not known whether the extent of shrinkage is the same for the support and for the cellular layer.

5. This marker diffusion method is relatively tedious to apply in the context of bystander measurements. It is more convenient in the context of measurement of prodrug transport through MCL when the radiolabeled flux markers can be used as internal standards for comparison with the prodrug. In most cases, the absolute thickness of individual MCLs is also more important in prodrug transport studies than in bystander studies. Provided that the prodrug in question penetrates MCLs efficiently [which can be investigated separately as described elsewhere *(41)*] and "edge effects" (e.g., washout of bystander metabolites into the medium from the surface of the MCL) are unimportant, strict uniformity in thickness is not essential in experiments of this type.

6. It should be noted that a patchy appearance under phase contrast may not necessarily reflect thickness variation in a straightforward manner; although not investigated rigorously, we suspect that areas in which central necrosis has developed have lower light transmittance, independent of thickness.

7. Multicellular layers under normal growth conditions become hypoxic in the center because of oxygen diffusion limitations *(38,40)*. Dinitrobenzamide prodrugs of the type illustrated in **Fig. 1** can be activated by endogenous reductases under hypoxic conditions *(53)*, as well as by NTR. This complication can be avoided by changing to a hyperoxic gas phase of 5% CO_2/95% O_2 (carbogen) at the start of prodrug exposure, which effectively reoxygenates the central hypoxic zone *(40)*. Conversely, activation by endogenous reductases under hypoxia can be investigated by examining sensitivity under anoxic, normoxic, and hyperoxic conditions of MCLs containing target cells only. Such activation would be therapeutically useful if it complemented activation by GDEPT vectors that failed to reach hypoxic zones efficiently.

8. In the absence of a specific selectable marker on the target cells, it is feasible to use a prodrug that is activated by the enzyme system of interest but has a negligible bystander effect at the low cell densities of the clonogenic assay. For example, for WiDr and EMT6 targets, the NTR prodrug SN 26634 (*see* **Fig. 1**), a hydrophilic analog of CB 1954, is highly selective for killing of NTR-expressing activators vs wild-type targets at 3 μM. SN 26634 has a lower bystander efficiency than CB 1954 in WiDr or V79 MCLs. For example, using an experimental design identical to **Fig. 5**, the Ac/Tc ratio is 0.14 ± 0.02 (mean ± sem for 3 expts) for CB 1954 and 0.025 ± 0.005 (2 expts) for SN 26634. In the same experiments, the BEE values were 0.52 ± 0.04 for CB 1954 and 0.16 ± 0.07 for SN 26634. SN 26634 does not cause any detectable bystander killing at 3 μM under the clonogenic assay conditions (up to 1.5×10^5 cells plated per P-60 dish), even with a large excess of activators over targets; data not shown.

9. The macroscopic appearance of a 50 cell colony should be confirmed, in each experiment, by checking several colonies near the threshold size using an inverting microscope. It is not necessary to examine every colony under the microscope; if growth conditions have been optimized, there should be few colonies near the 50-cell threshold and most surviving clonogens should form unambiguous colonies comprising thousands of cells.

10. The difference method is satisfactory except when the bystander effect is very large, in which case the activator and total surviving fractions are similar and the difference is therefore subject to large statistical errors. In such cases, specific selection for targets is necessary for accurate quantitation.

11. More importantly, this estimate of the proportion of activators in MCLs depends on the assumption that expression of the PAE and antibiotic resistance marker are closely correlated. This is most likely to be the case with bicistronic expression cassettes in which a single transcript with internal ribosome entry site codes for both the selection marker and PAE. This assumption needs to be validated by confirming PAE expression levels in antibiotic-resistant cells selected from MCLs.

12. This discussion assumes that differences in C_{10} reflect differences in exposure to the agent(s) responsible for the bystander effect; that is, that the intrinsic sensitivities of activators and targets to the bystander metabolite(s) are identical. With strictly isogenic cell line pairs, this is likely to be a reasonable first-order approximation. However, isolation of stable transfectants represents a stochastic clonal selection that can result in selection of a subline with altered drug sensitivity (even if plasmid integration and/or PAE expression does not itself affect sensitivity). The assumption of equivalent sensitivity of activators and targets should be tested using the authentic metabolite when this is known. In the case of CB 1954/NTR, the 4-hydroxylamine is considered responsible for the bystander effect in low-cell-density cultures (*32*), but recent studies in this laboratory indicate that other metabolites are also important mediators of bystander effects in MCL. This makes it difficult to address the intrinsic sensitivity question directly. The closest we have come to date is to compare bystander killing of V79[oua] with that of an empty vector control line T78-1 (*51*), analogous to V79-NTR[puro] but lacking the NTR gene. The C_{10} value for T78-1 in MCL cocultures comprising 3% V79-NTR[puro] was 480 μM (cf. 173 μM for V79[oua]). If the intrinsic sensitivity of V79-NTR[puro] were equal to that of T78-1 (which is, again, uncertain because of stochastic clonal effects), this would imply a 2.8-fold-higher sensitivity for V79[oua] targets relative to V79-NTR[puro] activators. Under this circumstance, a perfect bystander effect would provide an Ac/Tc ratio of 2.8 rather than unity.

13. The T/Tc ratio is only an in vitro therapeutic ratio. Ultimately, utility will also depend on in vivo pharmacokinetics and host toxicity. In this respect, the most important parameter

is the surviving fraction for targets in mixed tumors (related to the in vivo equivalent of Tc) at well-tolerated prodrug doses in vivo.

14. The reliance on immunodeficient hosts is a significant limitation in this field, as it compromises the ability to assess the role of immunological mechanisms in bystander killing.

15. Inoculation under anaesthesia is recommended to minimize animal stress and to ensure accurate placement of tumors; the position along the anterior–posterior axis influences angiogenesis and growth rates *(52,53)*.

16. EMT6 is a relatively immunogenic tumor, eliciting a specific T-cell response in its Balb/c host *(54)*. It grows significantly faster, with less ulceration, in nude mice than in immunocompetent Balb/c mice. However, the latter could be used to examine the contribution of immunological effects to GDEPT activity.

17. Hemocytometers are commonly used to count cells from dissociated tumors. Discrimination of tumor cells from erythrocytes under the microscope is straightforward (and can be facilitated by lysing erythrocytes with 1% acetic acid if required), but discrimination from nucleated host cells is more problematic. We prefer to use an electronic particle counter, such as a Coulter counter, as this provides an objective threshold (which is more important than absolute discrimination of host and tumor cells) and speeds enumeration of cells. Particle counters can be calibrated for this purpose using cultured tumor cells of the same type, adjusting the threshold so that it is just below the minimum tumor cell volume.

18. If tumors show significant regression between treatment and dissection, it is preferable to calculate clonogens per gram of tumor based on the estimated tumor weight at the time of treatment. Alternatively, if the tumors are closely size-matched at treatment, the results can be expressed as clonogens per tumor.

19. Given the limited dynamic range of clonogenic assays, it is not uncommon to fail to detect any activator clonogens after treatment with effective prodrugs. When the number of clonogens in a subset of tumors is below the sensitivity limit of the assay, it is recommended that these be represented as a value slightly below the sensitivity limit for the purpose of calculation of geometric mean and standard error and for statistical analysis.

20. The small magnitude of the CB 1954 bystander effect in this model is consistent with the low number of activators in the tumors at the time of treatment; significant bystander killing by CB 1954 is readily achieved in WiDr tumors containing 50% WiDr-NTR^{neo} cells using the same methodology *(16)*.

References

1. Culver, K. W., Ram, Z., Wallbridge, S., Ishii, H., Oldfield, E. H., and Blaese, R. M. (1992) In vivo gene transfer with retroviral vector-producer cells for treatment of experimental brain tumors. *Science* **256**, 1550–1552.

2. Mesnil, M. and Yamasaki, H. (2000) Bystander effect in herpes simplex virus-thymidine kinase/ganciclovir cancer gene therapy: role of gap-junctional intercellular communication. *Cancer Res.* **60**, 3989–3999.

3. Huber, B. E., Austin, E. A., Good, S. S., Knick, V. C., Tibbels, S., and Richards, C. A. (1993) In vivo antitumor activity of 5-fluorocytosine on human colorectal carcinoma cells genetically modified to express cytosine deaminase. *Cancer Res.* **53**, 4619–4626.

4. Kievit, E., Nyati, M. K., Ng, E., Stegman, L. D., Parsels, J., Ross, B. D., Rehemtulla, A., and Lawrence, T. S. (2000) Yeast cytosine deaminase improves radiosensitization and bystander effect by 5-fluorocytosine of human colorectal cancer xenografts. *Cancer Res.* **60**, 6649–6655.

5. Waxman, D. J., Chen, L., Hecht, J. E., and Jounaidi, Y. (1999) Cytochrome P450-based cancer gene therapy: recent advances and future prospects. *Drug Metab. Rev.* **31,** 503–522.

6. Springer, C. J., Antoniw, P., Bagshawe, K. D., Searle, F., Bisset, G. M., and Jarman, M. (1990) Novel prodrugs which are activated to cytotoxic alkylating agents by carboxypeptidase G2. *J. Med. Chem.* **33,** 677–681.

7. Marais, R., Spooner, R. A., Light, Y., Martin, J., and Springer, C. J. (1996) Gene-directed enzyme prodrug therapy with a mustard prodrug/carboxypeptidase G2 combination. *Cancer Res.* **56,** 4735–4742.

8. Anlezark, G. M., Melton, R. G., Sherwood, R. F., Coles, B., Friedlos, F., and Knox, R. J. (1992) The bioactivation of 5-(aziridin-1-yl)-2,4-dinitrobenzamide (CB1954)—I. Purification and properties of a nitroreductase enzyme from *Escherichia coli*—a potential enzyme for antibody-directed enzyme prodrug therapy (ADEPT). *Biochem. Pharmacol.* **44,** 2289–2295.

9. Anlezark, G. M., Melton, R. G., Sherwood, R. F., et al. (1995) Bioactivation of dinitrobenzamide mustards by an *E. coli* B nitroreductase. *Biochem. Pharmacol.* **50,** 609–618.

10. Grove, J. I., Searle, P. F., Weedon, S. J., Green, N. K., McNeish, I. A., and Kerr, D. J. (1999) Virus-directed enzyme prodrug therapy using CB 1954. *Anti-Cancer Drug Des.* **14,** 461–472.

11. Bridgewater, J. A., Springer, C. J., Knox, R. J., Minton, N. P., Michael, N. P., and Collins, M. K. (1995) Expression of the bacterial nitroreductase enzyme in mammalian cells renders them selectively sensitive to killing by the prodrug CB1954. *Eur. J. Cancer* **31A,** 2362–2370.

12. Green, N. K., Youngs, D. J., Neoptolemos, J. P., et al. (1997) Sensitization of colorectal and pancreatic cancer cell lines to the prodrug 5-(aziridin-1-yl)-2,4-dinitrobenzamide (CB1954) by retroviral transduction and expression of the *E. coli* nitroreductase gene. *Cancer Gene Ther.* **4,** 229–238.

13. Friedlos, F., Court, S., Ford, M., Denny, W. A., and Springer, C. (1998) Gene-directed enzyme prodrug therapy: quantitative bystander cytotoxicity and DNA damage induced by CB1954 in cells expressing bacterial nitroreductase. Gene Ther. 5, 105-112.

14. McNeish, I. A., Green, N. K., Gilligan, M. G., et al. (1998) Virus directed enzyme prodrug therapy for ovarian and pancreatic cancer using retrovirally delivered E. coli nitroreductase and CB1954. *Gene Ther.* **5,** 1061–1069.

15. Djeha, A. H., Hulme, A., Dexter, M. T., et al. (2000) Expression of *Escherichia coli* B nitroreductase in established human tumor xenografts in mice results in potent antitumoral and bystander effects upon systemic administration of the prodrug CB1954. *Cancer Gene Ther.* **7,** 721–731.

16. Wilson, W. R., Pullen, S. M., Hogg, A., et al. (2002) Quantitation of bystander effects in nitroreductase suicide gene therapy using three-dimensional cell cultures. *Cancer Res.* **62,** 1425–1432.

17. Chung-Faye, G., Palmer, D., Anderson, D., et al. (2001) Virus-directed, enzyme prodrug therapy with nitroimidazole reductase: a phase I and pharmacokinetic study of its prodrug, CB1954. *Clin. Cancer Res.* **7,** 2662–2668.

18. Freeman, S. M., Abboud, C. N., Whartenby, K. A., et al. (1993) The "bystander effect": tumor regression when a fraction of the tumor mass is genetically modified. *Cancer Res.* **53,** 5274–5283.

19. Sawant, S. G., Randers-Pehrson, G., Metting, N. F., and Hall, E. J. (2001) Adaptive response and the bystander effect induced by radiation in C3H 10T(1/2) cells in culture. *Radiat. Res.* **156,** 177–180.

20. Kanwar, J. R., Kanwar, R. K., Pandey, S., Ching, L. M., and Krissansen, G. W. (2001) Vascular attack by 5,6-dimethylxanthenone-4-acetic acid combined with B7.1 (CD80)-mediated immunotherapy overcomes immune resistance and leads to the eradication of large tumors and multiple tumor foci. *Cancer Res.* **61**, 1948–1956.
21. Ali, S. A., McLean, C. S., Boursnell, M. E., et al. (2000) Preclinical evaluation of "whole" cell vaccines for prophylaxis and therapy using a disabled infectious single cycle-herpes simplex virus vector to transduce cytokine genes. *Cancer Res.* **60**, 1663–1670.
22. Freeman, S. M. (2000) Suicide gene therapy. *Adv. Exp. Med. Biol.* **465**, 411–422.
23. Fife, K., Bower, M., Cooper, R. G., et al. (1998) Endothelial cell transfection with cationic liposomes and herpes simplex-thymidine kinase mediated killing. *Gene Ther.* **5**, 614–620.
24. Jager, U., Zhao, Y., and Porter, C. D. (1999) Endothelial cell-specific transcriptional targeting from a hybrid long terminal repeat retrovirus vector containing human prepro-endothelin-1 promoter sequences. *J. Virol.* **73**, 9702–9709.
25. Ram, Z., Walbridge, S., Shawker, T., Culver, K. W., Blaese, R. M., and Oldfield, E. H. (1994) The effect of thymidine kinase transduction and ganciclovir therapy on tumor vasculature and growth of 9L gliomas in rats. *J. Neurosurg.* **81**, 256–260.
26. Trinh, Q. T., Austin, E. A., Murray, D. M., Knick, V. C., and Huber, B. E. (1995) Enzyme/prodrug gene therapy: comparison of cytosine deaminase/5-fluorocytosine versus thymidine kinase/ganciclovir enzyme/prodrug systems in a human colorectal carcinoma cell line. *Cancer Res.* **55**, 4808–4812.
27. Denning, C. and Pitts, J. D. (1997) Bystander effects of different enzyme–prodrug systems for cancer gene therapy depend on different pathways for intercellular transfer of toxic metabolites, a factor that will govern clinical choice of appropriate regimes. *Hum. Gene Ther.* **8**, 1825–1835.
28. Nishihara, E., Nagayama, Y., Narimatsu, M., Namba, H., Watanabe, M., Niwa, M., and Yamashita, S. (1998) Treatment of thyroid carcinoma cells with four different suicide gene/prodrug combinations in vitro. *Anticancer Res.* **18**, 1521–1526.
29. Chen, L. and Waxman, D. J. (1995) Intratumoral activation and enhanced chemotherapeutic effect of oxazaphosphorines following cytochrome P-450 gene transfer: development of a combined chemotherapy/cancer gene therapy strategy. *Cancer Res.* **55**, 581–589.
30. Hughes, B. W., Wells, A. H., Bebok, Z., et al. (1995) Bystander killing of melanoma cells using the human tyrosinase promoter to express the *Escherichia coli* purine nucleoside phosphorylase gene. *Cancer Res.* **55**, 3339–3345.
31. Patterson, A. V., Zhang, H., Moghaddam, A., et al. (1995) Increased sensitivity to the prodrug 5'-deoxy-5-fluorouridine and modulation of 5-fluoro-2'-deoxyuridine sensitivity in MCF-7 cells transfected with thymidine phosphorylase. *Br. J. Cancer* **72**, 669–675.
32. Bridgewater, J. A., Knox, R. J., Pitts, J. D., Collins, M. K., and Springer, C. J. (1997) The bystander effect of the nitroreductase/CB1954 enzyme/prodrug system is due to a cell-permeable metabolite. *Hum. Gene Ther.* **8**, 709–717.
33. Sutherland, R. M. (1988) Cell and environment interactions in tumor microregions: the multicell spheroid model. *Science* **240**, 177–184.
34. O'Connor, K. C. (1999) Three-dimensional cultures of prostatic cells: tissue models for the development of novel anti-cancer therapies. *Pharm. Res.* **16**, 486–493.
35. Roskelley, C. D. and Bissell, M. J. (1995) Dynamic reciprocity revisited: a continuous, bidirectional flow of information between cells and the extracellular matrix regulates mammary epithelial cell function. *Biochem. Cell Biol.* **73**, 391–397.
36. Cukierman, E., Pankov, R., Stevens, D. R., and Yamada, K. M. (2001) Taking cell–matrix adhesions to the third dimension. *Science* **294**, 1708–1712.

37. Durand, R. E. and Olive, P. L. (2001) Resistance of tumor cells to chemo- and radiotherapy modulated by the three-dimensional architecture of solid tumors and spheroids. *Methods Cell Biol.* **64**, 211–233.

38. Cowan, D. S., Hicks, K. O., and Wilson, W. R. (1996) Multicellular membranes as an in vitro model for extravascular diffusion in tumours. *Br. J. Cancer* **27(Suppl)**, S28–S31.

39. Hicks, K. O., Ohms, S. J., van Zijl, P. L., Denny, W. A., Hunter, P. J., and Wilson, W. R. (1997) An experimental and mathematical model for the extravascular transport of a DNA intercalator in tumours. *Br. J. Cancer* **76**, 894–903.

40. Hicks, K. O., Fleming, Y., Siim, B. G., Koch, C. J., and Wilson, W. R. (1998) Extravascular diffusion of tirapazamine: effect of metabolic consumption assessed using the multicellular layer model. *Int. J. Radiat. Oncol. Biol. Phys.* **42**, 641–649.

41. Hicks, K. O., Pruijn, F. B., Baguley, B. C., and Wilson, W. R. (2001) Extravascular transport of the DNA intercalator and topoisomerase poison *N*-[2-(dimethylamino)ethyl]acridine-4-carboxamide (DACA): diffusion and metabolism in multicellular layers of tumor cells. *J. Pharmacol. Exp. Ther.* **297**, 1088–1098.

42. Baguley, B.C., Hicks, K.O., and Wilson, W.R. (2002) Tumour cell cultures in drug development, in *Anticancer Drug Development* (Baguley, B. C. and Kerr, D.J., eds.), Academic, San Diego, CA, pp. 269–284.

43. Minchinton, A. I., Wendt, K. R., Clow, K. A., and Fryer, K. H. (1997) Multilayers of cells growing on a permeable support. An in vitro tumour model. *Acta Oncol.* **36**, 13–16.

44. Phillips, R. M., Loadman, P. M., and Cronin, B. P. (1998) Evaluation of a novel in vitro assay for assessing drug penetration into avascular regions of tumors. *Br. J. Cancer* **77**, 2112–2119.

45. Topp, E. M., Kitos, P. A., Vijaykumar, V., DeSilva, B. S., and Hendrickson, T. L. (1998) Antibody transport in cultured tumor cell layers. *J. Control. Release* **53**, 15–23.

46. Kyle, A. H. and Minchinton, A. I. (1999) Measurement of delivery and metabolism of tirapazamine to tumour tissue using the multilayered cell culture model. *Cancer Chemother. Pharmacol.* **43**, 213–220.

47. Chen, T. R. (1977) In situ detection of mycoplasma contamination in cell cultures by fluorescent Hoechst 33258 stain. *Exp. Cell Res.* **104**, 255–262.

48. Kyle, A. H., Chan, C. T., and Minchinton, A. I. (1999) Characterization of three-dimensional tissue cultures using electrical impedance spectroscopy. *Biophys. J.* **76**, 2640–2648.

49. Thanou, M., Nihot, M. T., Jansen, M., Verhoef, J. C., and Junginger, H. E. (2001) Mono-*N*-carboxymethyl chitosan (MCC), a polyampholytic chitosan derivative, enhances the intestinal absorption of low molecular weight heparin across intestinal epithelia in vitro and in vivo. *J. Pharm. Sci.* **90**, 38–46.

50. Siim, B. G., Denny, W. A., and Wilson, W. R. (1997) Nitro reduction as an electronic switch for bioreductive drug activation. Oncol. Res. 9, 357–369.

51. Friedlos, F., Denny, W. A., Palmer, B. D., and Springer, C. J. (1997) Mustard prodrugs for activation by *Escherichia coli* nitroreductase in gene-directed enzyme prodrug therapy. *J. Med. Chem.* **40**, 1270–1275.

52. Kyriazis, A. A. and Kyriazis, A. P. (1980) Preferential sites of growth of human tumors in nude mice following subcutaneous transplantation. *Cancer Res.* **40**, 4509–4511.

53. Dipersio, L. P. (1981) Regional growth differences of human tumour xenografts in nude mice. *Lab. Anim.* **15**, 179–180.

54. Wilson, K. M. and Lord, E. M. (1987) Specific (EMT6) and non-specific (WEHI-164) cytolytic activity by host cells infiltrating tumour spheroids. *Br. J. Cancer* **55**, 141–146.

55. Hobbs, S., Jitrapakdee, S., and Wallace, J. C. (1998) Development of a bicistronic vector driven by the human polypeptide chain elongation factor 1alpha promoter for creation of stable mammalian cell lines that express very high levels of recombinant proteins. *Biochem. Biophys. Res. Commun.* **252,** 368–372.
56. Skehan, P., Storeng, R., Scudiero, D., et al. (1990) New colorimetric cytotoxicity assay for anticancer-drug screening. *J. Natl. Cancer Inst.* **82,** 1107–1112.

22

Suicide Gene Therapy in Liver Tumors

Long R. Jiao, Roman Havlik, Joanna Nicholls, Steen Lindkaer Jensen, and Nagy A. Habib

1. Introduction

Charaterization of a variety of genomic defects in malignant cells *(1)* has led to attempts to treat cancer by gene therapy. Gene therapy is a therapeutic approach in which therapeutic nucleic acids are transferred into the affected organs. Although the ideal concept would be the replacement of the abnormal gene by a copy of the functional gene, currently there have not been reliable and safe techniques to allow the site-specific integration of DNA into the human genome *(2)*. Thus, almost all gene therapies are developed by simply transferring the therapeutic gene into somatic cells without replacing the abnormal gene. The goal is to identify and correct genetic abnormalities interfering with the cell cycle and to correct them in all cells. Technically, there are two methods amenable for gene transfer: reintroduction of in vitro transferred gene into the body and direct transfer of gene into the target cells in vivo.

Cancer is a genetic disease characterized by failure to maintain the fidelity of DNA because of germ-line and/or somatic gene changes *(3)*. Genes involved in carcinogenesis are often usefully categorized as either oncogenes contributing to the development of cancer or tumor suppressor genes suppressing the development and maintenance of the cancer phenotype. Therefore, gene therapy is developed by targeting these two genes. Current strategies undergoing development for gene therapy involve in restoring tumor suppressor gene function, downregulating oncogeneic expression, stimulating immune response, introducing genes that either increase drug sensitivity or confer multidrug resistance, and modulating tumor angiogenesis genetically *(4–13)*. In this chapter, principles and methods of suicide gene therapy are reviewed together with the results of its clinical trials. Protocols required for application of human study are discussed in details by using Ad-*TK* gene therapy for liver tumors as an example.

From: *Methods in Molecular Medicine, Vol. 90, Suicide Gene Therapy: Methods and Reviews*
Edited by: C. J. Springer © Humana Press Inc., Totowa, NJ

2. Principles

Suicide gene therapy consists of the intracellular delivery of a gene encoded for an enzyme that can transform a nontoxic prodrug into a toxic substance *(14)*. These suicide genes are not present in human cells, so an elective delivery of these genes into cancer cells followed by the administration of a prodrug can lead to a conversion of the drug into cytotoxic substances in the transduced cells. The delivery and transcription of a tumor-specific suicide gene in vivo are crucial for suicide gene therapy to be effective. Currently, two strategies are being investigated to selectively transduce tumor cells: tumor-specific vectors and control of suicide gene transcription in tissues or tumors with a tumor-specific promoter. Promoters such as carcinoembryonic antigen (CEA), or α-fetoprotein (AFP) for liver tumors, limit gene expression to CEA- or AFP-positive cells only. The most commonly used suicide genes are cytosine deaminase *(CD)* and the herpes simplex virus-thymidine kinase *(HSV-TK)*.

2.1. Thymidine Kinase *Gene*

Acyclovir and ganciclovir are used for the treatment of herpes simplex virus (HSV) infections. These drugs are phosphorylated to the active form by the enzyme thymidine kinase *(TK)* encoded for part of the HSV genome. The *HSV-TK* gene is expressed after herpetic viral *TK* transcription, leading to activation of the drug and cell death. To achieve expression of *HSV-TK*, which is specific only to hepatocellular carcinoma (HCC) cells, an AFP promoter has been constructed. The promoter ensures that only cells expressing AFP are able to transcribe and express the *HSV-TK* gene.

The first *HSV-TK* suicide gene system was introduced by Moolten *(15,16)*. Under the control of an AFP promoter, an adenoviral vector was used to bring the *HSV-TK* gene into various HCC cell lines *(5)*. Following ganciclovir (GCV) administration, cell death occurred in hepatoma cells producing AFP, leaving non-AFP-producing cell lines unaffected. Phosphorylated GCV is thought to cause cell death by the inhibition of DNA polymerase and by causing chain termination during DNA synthesis in dividing cells, which then leads to apoptosis *(16)*. A bystander effect has been described, both in vitro and in vivo, where neighboring *HSV-TK*-negative cells have died when in contact with *HSV-TK*-positive cells after GCV treatment *(17)*. This increases the effectiveness of suicide gene therapy, and only a part of a tumor mass needs to be transfected by a suicide gene for tumor destruction. A glucocorticoid-responsive element exists upstream of the AFP gene in hepatoma cells, which explains the increase in AFP observed after the addition of dexamethasone into the culture medium of such cells *(18)*. It is possible that the potency of the TK/GCV suicide system could be enhanced by the addition of dexamethasone to a HepG2 cell line *(19)*.

A retrovirus vector (LNAF0.3TK) carrying the *HSV-TK* gene regulated only by a human AFP promoter has also been reported to provide GCV-mediated cytotoxicity in high-AFP-producing human hepatoma cells, but not in low-AFP-producing cells. The retrovirus has been further improved so that the *HSV-TK* gene expression is under the control of a human AFP enhancer directly linked to its promoter [LNAF0.3(E+)TK]. The vector also sensitized both low- and intermediate-AFP-producing hepatoma cells to GCV treatment, and did not affect cell growth in nonhepatoma cells *(20)*. In animal models, GCV treatment has led to more pronounced growth inhibition in the LNAF0.3(E+)TK infected cells than in the LNAF0.3TK infected cells *(20)*. These results indicate that an AFP enhancer directly linked to its promoter can further enhance tumoricidal activity in gene therapy for hepatocellular carcinoma.

Most in vivo studies have used subcutaneously grown human HCC tumor xenografts in mice followed by transfection with an AFP-*HSV-TK* gene in an adenoviral vector. Tumor selectivity was confirmed by the regression of HuH-7 established tumors in athymic mice, whereas normal tissues remained unaffected *(7)*. The bystander effect enabled tumor regression even when only 10% of the tumor mass expressed *HSV-TK (17)*. A similar therapeutic response has been seen in rats with colorectal liver metastases, where following direct intratumoral injections of *HSV-TK*-producing packaging cells, a 60-fold reduction in tumor mass was noted following GCV treatment when compared with controls *(21)*. Kuriyama et al. described cancer gene therapy with the GCV-*HSV-TK* system that induced efficient antitumor effects and protective immunity in immunocompetent mice, but not in nude mice. This indicates that a T-cell-mediated immune response may be a critical factor for *HSV-TK* gene therapy to be successful *(22)*.

Unfortunately, severe hepatic dysfunction has been described following adenovirus-mediated transfer of the *HSV-TK* gene and GCV administration in a rat model of colorectal liver metastases *(23)*. Hepatic expression of *HSV-TK* was demonstrated, both in tumor-bearing and in tumor-free liver tissue. The hepatic *HSV-TK* expression provoked severe liver dysfunction and mortality upon GCV administration, and, in addition, normal, nonmitotic tissues were affected by the adenovirus-mediated *HSV-TK* transfer and subsequent GCV administration *(23)*.

2.2. Cytosine Deaminase Gene

Cytosine deaminase is a nontoxic gene present in some fungi and bacteria. The gene plays a role in the conversion of cytosine to uracil. Cells containing this gene can convert 5-fluorocytosine (5-FC) into the cytotoxic chemotherapeutic reagent 5-fluorouracil (5-FU). The *Escherichia coli CD* gene is currently being used as a suicide gene so that genetically modified cells "commit suicide" in the presence of 5-FC.

The *CD* gene has been used with an AFP promoter to kill AFP-positive HCC cell lines in the presence of 5-FC *(6)*. A bystander effect occurred irrespective of cell-to-cell contact with transduced cells. On cell lysis, 5-FU is released into the medium and is thus likely to be responsible for the bystander effect, and, indeed, the 5-FU levels in the medium correlated well with the degree of cytotoxicity *(24)*. AFP-positive HCC tumors that have been established subcutaneously in vivo have been shown to regress significantly after adenoviral-mediated insertion of the *CD* gene (with an AFP promoter) and subsequent 5-FC administration, and in one study, nontumor tissue was unaffected *(6)*. Block et al. demonstrated regression of multiple hepatic metastases by systemic application of a recombinant replication-deficient adenovirus encoding for the *CD* gene under the control of the cytomegalovirus promoter (Ad.CMV-*CD*) *(25)*. Injection of Ad.CMV-*CD* into the tail vein of tumor-bearing mice resulted in delayed tumor growth with a significant reduction in hepatic metastases. Gnant et al. *(8)* published results with a recombinant *TK*-deleted vaccinia virus encoding *CD*, where tumor-bearing mice were treated with this recombinant vaccinia virus and 5-FC. It was found that tumor-specific gene delivery was achieved irrespective of the administration route, with gene expression in tumors increasing by up to 100,000-fold when compared with normal tissues. Treatment using a CD-expressing virus and systemic 5-FC resulted in significant survival benefit in all treatment groups when compared with controls *(8)*.

Sung et al. have recently published the result of a phase I clinical trial using intratumoral injection of escalating doses of adenovirus-mediated suicide gene followed by intravenous GCV at a fixed dose in patients with colorectal liver metastases *(13)*. The aim was to assess the safety and maximal tolerated dosage of Adv.RSV-*TK*. The vector was infected into a metastatic tumor in the liver under local anaethesia and ultrasound guidance. A total of 16 patients were entered into the trial who received five dose-level cohorts of Adv.RSV-*TK*, from 1.0×10^{10} to 1.0×10^{13} virus particles per patient. The response rate was assessed by World Health Organization (WHO) criteria with follow-up imaging studies. The assessment of toxicity was carried out according to Common Toxicity Criteria v. 2.0 from the National Cancer Institute (Bethesda, MD). One patient was withdrawn from the study because of clinical deterioration from disease and died. Stable disease (defined as $< 25\%$ change in the size of the tumor measured on computed tomography [CT] or magnetic resonance imaging [MRI]) was seen in 11 patients. One patient had a biopsy of the injected tumor at 11 wk following treatment that revealed extensive necrosis of the tumor on histology, whereas five others had a biopsy taken at the later date but showed no evidence of necrosis. Adv.RSV-*TK* DNA was not detected in any of these six biopsed specimen. Low transient toxicities were present in patients including grade 1 elevations in serum aminotransferase in three patients, grade 2–3 fevers in five patients, grade 3 thrombocytopenia in one patient, and grade 2 leucopenia in three patients. One patient is alive at 40.5 mo, but the remaining 15 died between 0.2 and 36.5 mo (median: 11.3 mo). The authors concluded that adv.RSV-*TK* could be safely administered by percutaneous intratumoral injection in patients with hepatic metastases at doses up to 1.0×10^{13} virus particles per patient and could provide the basis for future clinical trials. However, the trial did not demonstrate any tumor reponse following intratumoural injection of adv.RSV-*TK*.

A phase I clinical trial using a replication-deficient adenovirus to deliver the *CD* gene to metastatic colonic cancer of the liver has been initiated *(12)*. The patients are being treated with a direct intratumoral injection of the CD vector in combination with oral 5-FU.

3. Protocol

3.1. Introduction

To safeguard the development of human gene therapy for clinical application, various countries have now established regulatory bodies for gene therapy to ensure safety and benefit for humankind. In the United States, federal guidelines for research involving recombinant DNA molecules were issued in 1976. The guidelines require that institutions establish an institutional biosafety committee to monitor the use of recombinant DNA in the laboratory, in micro-organisms, in animals, and in humans. There are a number of approvals that are required for a proposed human clinical gene therapy trial to be approved and allow patient accrual. In the United Kingdom, the Gene Therapy Advisory Committee (GTAC) together with the Medicines Control Agency (MCA) are established to evaluate proposals for human gene therapy. The creation of the European Medicines Evaluation Agency (EMEA) has standardized approaches across European countires. In the United States, guidelines have been drawn up by the Recombinant DNA Advisory Committee (RAC) of the National Institutes of Health to facilitate documentation, review, and discussion on human gene therapy. In addition, each of the vector delivery systems used in human gene transfer trials is considered a biologic and requires the filing of an investigation new drug application for each specific vector.

3.2. A Therapeutic Clinical Protocol for Liver Cancer Using Ad TK Gene

3.2.1. Aims

1. To assess the safety of direct intratumoural injection of Ad-*TK* followed by GCV administration
2. To assess the efficacy of intratumoral injection of Ad-*TK* followed by GCV administration, and to compare this treatment with standard treatment of percutaneous ethanol injection alone in groups of patients with irresectable hepatocellular carcinoma.
3. To study the biological efficacy, including the efficiency and stability of gene transfer by analysis of tumor tissue following therapy. The clinical evidence of antitumor efficacy will also be noted.
4. To seek to identify dose level by injecting Ad-*TK* at differing dose levels in successive cohorts of patients.

3.2.2. Background

Live, wild-type (nonrecombinant) adenoviruses have been used clinically as vaccines for the prophylaxis of adenoviral upper respiratory infections, a disease of low morbidity but high incidence. These vaccines, which were at one time given routinely to military recruits, are well tolerated and are considered nononcogenic. Recombinant versions of the adenovirus have entered clinical trials both as injections and as oral vaccines *(26)*. Thus far, they appear to be without significant toxicity. Recently, clinical trials using recombinant, replication-defective adenoviral vectors for gene therapy have been initiated. In these studies, recombinant adenoviral vectors carrying the gene for cystic fibrosis transmembrane conductance regulator (CFTR) are given via intra-airway administration to patients with cystic fibrosis.

Tursz at the Gustave Roussy Institut, Paris, initiated a phase I study to evaluate the feasibility, safety, and clinical effects of the intratumor administration of a recombinant-deficient adenovirus containing the marker gene encoding the *E. coli* enzyme β-galactosidase (Ad-β-Gal) in untreated patients with advanced lung cancer *(27)*. The first dose level was 10^7, the second was 10^8, and the third was 10^9 pfu (plaque-forming units) (three patients per dose level). All patients received concomitant chemotherapy. β-Gal express (X-Gal) staining was observed in three out of six tumor biopsies. The microbiological and immunological follow-up of patients who were carriers of wild-type adenovirus before injection. Only viral cultures of bronchoalveolar (BAL) specimens taken immediately after Ad-β-Gal injection were positive in all patients. All body-fluid specimens were positive at polymerase chain reaction (PCR) analysis within the first 10 d after injection, as were blood samples drawn 30 min after injection in three patients at the second dose level. BAL samples remained positive at 1 mo in two patients and at 3 mo in one patient after Ad-β-Gal injection. No antibody (Ab) response to β-Gal was noted in patients, but four had a significant rise in their antiadenovirus Ab titers. All 363 samples (throat and stools) taken by the 54 medical staff before and after injection of patients were negative for wild-type adenovirus and Ad-β-Gal. Sera tests (CF) in 202 staff were also negative for antiadenovirus Ab titers. This study shows that a marker gene can be safely transferred into human tumor cells with a recombinant adenoviral vector.

3.2.3. Design

3.2.3.1. STUDY DESIGN

The study seeks to determine the safety, biological efficacy, and effect of the Ad-*TK*-GCV dose in the locoregional gene therapy of primary malignant tumors of the liver. The study design consists of an open-label, nonrandomized, dose-escalation phase I/II trial. The Ad-*TK* will be administered by direct intratumoral injection under CT scan or ultrasound control. The study will include sampling on one occasion of normal and malignant tissue from the livers of patients following Ad-*TK*-GCV treatment. This will greatly facilitate assessments of clinical safety and biological efficacy, including efficiency and stability of gene transfer. Furthermore, sampling of treated tissues will require minimal additional morbidity for study patients.

3.2.3.2. ROUTE

The replication-deficient adenovirus encoding for *HSV-TK* (Ad-*TK*) will be administered in 10 cm^3 of normal (0.9%) saline directly into the tumor under ultrasound or CT guidance. Dose escalation will occur until the maximum tolerated level or dose level 1×10^{11} pfu is achieved. Thereafter, a further 10 patients will receive the maximum tolerated level. The GCV will be administered intravenously at 5 mg/kg/d, twice a day for 14 d. The first dose will be given 7 d after Ad-*TK* administration.

3.2.3.3. RISK ASSESSMENT

This procedure will be used only in patients over the age of 35 yr in whom conventional treatments have failed or are inapplicable. The risks to the patients are the nforeseen effects of expression of the vector within the tumor, the transmission of other biologically active products with the vector construct, and the clinical risks associated with the percutaneous biopsy of a tumor. The risks seem to be negligible, as 27 patients were treated in the United States with 10^{13}-pfu doses (100 times more than the maximum proposed dose in this study) and showed no serious side effects. The only abnormalities observed at the 10^{13}-pfu dose level were low-grade fevers and transient elevation in liver function tests. Recently, however, a death was reported in a 17-yr-old man in Pennsylvania (USA), following the administration of 10^{13} pfu adenovirus. The cause of death was reported to be the result of acute respiratory distress syndrome (ARDS). To the best of our knowledge, the risk appears to be negligible for doses of adenovirus up to 10^{11} pfu.

The risk of bleeding after percutaneous biopsy of the tumor is less than 1%. A generally accepted mortality rate in standard textbooks is between 0.1% and 0.01% *(28,29)*.

3.2.3.4. INCLUSION CRITERIA

Patients must fulfill all of the following criteria in order to be eligible for study admission: histological diagnosis of primary liver tumor; at least 35 yr and less than 75 yr of age(women of childbearing potential may be included, but must use a reliable and appropriate contraceptive method, not including abstinence, for at least 1 mo before study start, for the duration of the study, and for three mo afterward. Results of a negative pregnancy test at study start must be available. Postmenopausal women must be amenorrheal for at least 12 mo before the study start. Men of childbearing potential should practice a barrier method of contraception for the duration of the study, have a life expectancy of at least 3 mo, and have adequate performance status (Karnofsky score $\geq$ 70%). The required values for initial laboratory data are as follows:

White blood cells (WBC)	$\geq$ 3,000/μL
Platelet count (Pt)	$\geq$ 100,000/μL
Hematocrit (HCT)	$\geq$ 25% (may be transfused prior to enrollment)
Prothromin (PT)	75%
Prothromin time (PTT)	Within normal range
Creatinine (Cr)	< 1.8 mg/dL or CrCl > 50 cm^3/min
Total Bilirubin (Bil)	< 2 mg/dL
Aspartate Transferase (AST)	< 5 × Upper limit of normal value
Alanine Transferase (ALT)	< 5 × Upper limit of normal value

Preserved cardio-pulmonary function:
SaO$_2$ $\geq$ 90% on room air
FEV$_1$ $\geq$ 70% or predicted value

3.2.3.5. EXCLUSION CRITERIA

Patients with any of the following will be excluded from study admission: pregnant or lactating women; women with either a positive pregnancy test at screen or baseline, or who have not had a pregnancy test; women of childbearing potential who are not using a reliable and appropriate contraceptive method; postmenopausal women who have been amenorrheal for less than 12 mo; uncontrolled serious bacterial, viral, fungal, or parasitic infection; patients who are human immunodeficiency virus (HIV) positive; systemic corticosteroid therapy or other immunosuppressive therapy administered within the last 3 mo; Karnofsky score less than 70%; participation in another investigation therapy study within the last 6 wk; any underlying medical condition that in the Principal Investigators' opinion, will make participation in the study hazardous or obscure the interpretation of adverse events.

3.2.3.6. PRESTUDY EVALUATION AND REQUIREMENTS

The following must be performed within 2 wk prior to study admission: complete medical history; physical examination; toxicity evaluation; performance status; height and weight and body surface area; laboratory screening (*eligibility criteria) for full blood count with differential, platelet count*, serum electrolytes (sodium, potassium, chloride, bicarbonate), urea, creatinine*, glucose, uric acid, albumin, liver function tests, including total protein, calcium, phosphorus, magnesium, aspartate transaminase (AST*), alanine transaminase (ALT*), total bilirubin*, alkaline phosphatase, lactate dehydrogenase (LDH), PT*, partial thomboplastin time (PTT*); urinalysis; α-fetoprotein; electrocardiogram (12-lead); chest X-ray (PA and lateral views); abdomen and pelvis CT or MRI scan.

3.3. Informing and Seeking Consent From Possible Subjects of Research

3.3.1. Patient Information Leaflet

This should contain a title like "Gene Therapy of Tumors of the Liver Using Ad-*TK* Intratumourally Followed by Ganciclovir Administration: A Phase I/II Study." Include the following sections and text in the leaflet.

PURPOSE AND BACKGROUND

You are being invited to take part in a research study because the cancer in your liver, unfortunately, cannot be removed surgically or treated in any other way.

The purpose of the study is to find out which of two treatments may be better for treating your type of liver cancer. The first is a gene therapy treatment that comprises two different drugs, Ad-*TK* (a gene therapy product) that will be given by direct injection into the tumor and ganciclovir (a drug that kills certain types of viruses) that will be injected into a vein in your arm. The second treatment is a treatment that is used commonly for liver cancer, which is the injection of ethanol (a type of alcohol) directly into the tumor. This is a randomized study and so you will only receive one of the treatments described above. Before you decide whether or not to take part in this study it is important for you to understand why the research is being done and what it will involve. Please take time to read the following information carefully and discuss it with friends and relatives if you wish. Ask us if there is anything that is not clear or you would like more information. Take time to decide whether or not you wish to take part.

Thank you for reading this.

STUDY PROCEDURES

Two weeks before you have one of the treatments, the following procedures will need to be undertaken:

1. You will have various blood samples taken from a vein in your arm.
2. You will have a physical examination.
3. You will be asked about your medical history.
4. You will have a chest X-ray and an electrocardiogram (ECG) of your heart.
5. You will have a special scan of your liver to show the doctors where the tumor is in your liver and so they can measure its size.

If you agree to take part in the study, you will be allocated to one of two treatment groups:

> Group 1: Treatment of your liver tumor with gene therapy (Ad-*TK*) followed by a 2-wk course of ganciclovir
>
> Group 2: Treatment of your liver tumor with ethanol injection

AD-*TK*-GANCICLOVIR

Ad-*TK* will be given by injecting it directly into the tumor under ultrasound or CT scan control in the X-ray department. One week after the Ad-*TK* injection, you will be given ganciclovir into a vein in our arm, twice a day, for 2 wk. Afterward, you will have to rest for a few hours before going home.

You will also have one liver biopsy performed during the period of the study to see if the drugs have affected the cancer. Blood samples will be taken on each occasion you come to the clinic.

On Day 60 (month 2) of your treatment schedule, you will undergo a CT scan or a MRI scan to measure the size of your tumor. This will help to tell us whether the treatment has been effective.

ETHANOL INJECTION

You will be given an injection of ethanol directly into the tumor in the liver under ultrasound or CT guidance in the x Ray department. Afterwards you will have to rest for a few hours before going home.

Blood samples will be taken on each occasion you come to the clinic.

On Day 60 (month 2) of your treatment schedule you will undergo a CT scan or a MRI scan to measure the size of your tumour. This will help to tell us whether the treatment has been effective.

FOLLOW-UP PROCEDURES

If you decide to take part in this study, your doctor would like to see you every 3 months in the clinic to follow your progress.

Your doctor would like to track your progress after the study has finished and would also like to keep you informed of any new treatment information about the drugs you had while participating in this study. In order for this to happen, you must tell your doctor if you move.

If the treatment has made a difference to the tumor, you will be invited to participate in a further study to receive a further course of treatment.

STUDY DURATION

This study will last for about 60 days (2 months), but the doctors would like to continue to see you every 3 months thereafter.

POSSIBLE RISKS AND DISCOMFORTS

There is a small risk of bleeding from the injection site in the liver after treatment with either the gene therapy drug or the ethanol. Also, a small bruise and some soreness may be left for a short time at the spot where the doctors inject the drug through the skin.

There is a small chance that the liver may bleed after the liver biopsy. If this happens, you will have to stay in hospital until the bleeding settles.

Normally, there may be slight pain in your arm when blood is taken. A small bruise may be left for a short time at the spot where the blood was taken.

As this is a new treatment, the risks associated with it are largely unknown. However, experiments suggest that the likelihood of serious side effect is extremely small. If you decide to participate and you experience a reaction to the drug, the doctors will provide you with every medical support.

We do ask that you or your partner take reliable and appropriate contraceptive precautions for 1 month prior to the treatment and for 3 months afterward to prevent a pregnancy. This is because we do not know the effect the drug might have on an unborn child.

It is important for you to know that recently a death occurred in the United States following an adenovirus injection given in the same way in which you will receive it. The patient was suffering from metabolic liver disease and was given a dose far higher than any that you will receive in this study.

REASONS WHY YOU MAY BE TAKEN OUT OF THE STUDY

Your doctor may take you out of the study if your disease becomes worse, if new relevant scientific developments occur, for administrative reasons, or if your doctor feels that taking part in this study is no longer in your best interest. You may, of course, wish to withdraw yourself from the study.

POSSIBLE BENEFITS

It is not possible to tell if there will be any personal benefit from taking part in this study. The information obtained may be used scientifically and might be helpful to others.

NEW FINDINGS

Sometimes during the course of a research project, new information becomes available. If this happens, your doctor will tell you or your legally accepted representative about it and discuss with you whether you want to continue in the study. If you decide to withdraw, your care will not be affected. If you decide to continue, you may be asked to sign an updated consent form.

Also, on receiving new information, your doctor might consider it to be in your best interests to withdraw you from the study. The reasons will be explained to you and your care will continue.

CONFIDENTIALITY

If you consent to take part in the research, your medical records may be inspected for the purposes of analyzing the results. Your name, however, will not be disclosed outside of the hospital. Any information that leaves the hospital will have your name and address removed so that you cannot be recognized from it.

You will not be identified in any report or publication that arises from this study.

ALTERNATIVE TREATMENT

You may choose not to take part in this study. You may choose to have no further tests and receive supportive care only. You doctor will discuss these choices with you.

OTHER INFORMATION

If you have any questions about taking part in this study or your future participation please contact Dr._____ on_____.

Thank you for considering helping us with this important trial.

3.3.2. Consent Form

"Gene Therapy of Tumours of the Liver Using Ad-*TK* Intratumourally Followed by Ganciclovir Administration: A Phase I/II Study"

Name of Researcher:_____

Please initial box

I confirm that I have read and understand the information sheet ☐
for the above study and have had the opportunity to ask questions.

I understand that my participation is voluntary and that I am
free to withdraw at any time without giving any reason without
my medical care or legal rights being affected.

I understand that sections of any of my medical notes may be ☐
looked at by responsible individuals or by individuals from
regulatory authorities where it is relevant. I give ☐
permission for these individuals to have access to my records.

I agree to take part in the above study. ☐

Name of patient	Date	Signature
Name of person taking consent	Date	Signature
Name of witness	Date	Signature

3.4. Clinical and Technical Procedures

3.4.1. Treatment Plan

3.4.1.1. ROUTE

The Ad-*TK* will be given intratumorally under ultrasound or CT scan guidance. GCV will be then administered intravenously twice per day for 14 d, starting at d 7 after Ad-*TK* injection.

3.4.1.2. DOSE

Dosages will be calculated based on functional units of Ad-*TK*. The dose of ganciclovir will be 5 mg/kg/d.

Dose Levels for Ad-*TK*:

Level 1:	1.0×10^8 units
Level 2:	1.0×10^9 units
Level 3:	1.0×10^{10} units
Level 4:	1.0×10^{11} units

The first three patients enrolled in the study will receive Ad-*TK* at Dose Level 1. If no dose-limiting toxicity (DLT) is observed after a period of at least 7 d of posttreatment monitoring, the next three patients will receive Ad-*TK* at Dose Level 2, and so on. If DLT is observed, the appropriate dose escalation decision rule will be followed.

3.4.1.3. DOSE ESCALATION

The dose level will be escalated to the next level according to the following rules.

# of Patients With DLT at Current Dose Level	Dose Escalation Decision Rule
0 out of 3	Enter next three patients at the next dose level.
1 out of 3	Enter up to three additional patients at current dose level. If none or one out of the three of the second group experiences DLT, then enter three patients at the next dose level. As soon as two of the second group experience DLT, then the MTD has been reached at the previous (lower) level and dose escalation will stop.
2 out of 3	Enter up to three additional patients at current dose level. If none experience DLT, then enter three patients at the next dose level. As soon as any patient of the second group experiences DLT, the MTD has been reached at the previous (lower) level and dose escalation will stop.
3 out of 3	The MTD has been reached at the previous (lower) level and dose escalation will stop.

3.4.1.4. ETHANOL INJECTION GROUP

Patients randomized for ethanol injection will be given 50 cm^3 of ethanol intratumorally under an ultrasound or CT scan guidance.

3.4.2. Schema

Once a patient has been enrolled in the study she/he will be randomized to receive either Ad-*TK*-GCV or ethanol. Patients will be treated in the radiology department or the clinic on an outpatient basis.

3.4.3. Flow Sheet

Ad-*TK*/GCV group

Day –14	Prestudy investigations and assessment
Day 1	Adenoviral injection and liver biopsy
Days 7–21	Intravenous GCV administration
Day 30	Liver biopsy
Day 60	CT scan and evaluation

Ethanol group

Day –14	Prestudy investigations and assessment
Day 1	Ethanol injection and liver biopsy
Day 60	CT scan and evaluation

3.5. Study Evaluation

3.5.1. Immediate Monitoring

Immediately following Ad-*TK* application, vital signs (body temperature, respiratory rate, heart rate, blood pressure) will be performed every 15 min during the first hour after the injection. These evaluations will be performed on d 1, 15, 30, and 60 and will include clinical evaluations (complete history, physical examination, toxicity evaluation, performance status, height and weight, body surface area), as well as blood tests (CBC with differential, platelet count, serum electrolytes [sodium, potassium, chloride, bicarbonate], BUN, creatinine, glucose, uric acid, albumin, total protein, calcium, phosphorus, and magnesium, AST, ALT, total bilirubin, alkaline phosphatase, LDH, PT, PTT), and urinalysis. Other studies will also be undertaken that will include pharmacokinetics and immune responses. Serum will be stored in case of future investigations.

Patients will undergo percutaneous Tru-cut liver biopsy of the liver tumor and normal liver as guided by ultrasound or CT scan.

3.5.2. Follow-Up Evaluation

Patients will be considered to be *actively on study* from the time of study admission until poststudy evaluation on d 60. Patients will be considered *associated with the study* after poststudy evaluation and will undergo regular follow-up evaluations thereafter.

The following evaluations will be performed on an outpatient basis on day 60 (poststudy evaluation), then every 3 mo for 1 yr, then annually. These evaluations will be the same as in **Subheading 3.5.1.** Abdomen and pelvis CT or MRI scan will be performed on d 60. If tumor response is noted, the abdominal scan will be repeated.

One of the main objectives of this study is to assess the biological efficacy of Ad-*TK*, including efficiency and stability. The molecular and cellular effects of Ad-*TK* treatment on malignant tissue will be assayed. Malignant tissue from the Ad-*TK*-treated liver will be obtained with Tru-cut biopsy.

3.5.3. Potential Toxicity, Dose Modification, and Management

Toxicity will be assessed using the National Cancer Institute criteria. Toxicity will be formally evaluated on d 1, 15, 30, 60 and then every 3 mo for 1 yr, then annually. All toxic events will be managed with full and optimal supportive care, including transfer to the intensive care unit (ICU) if appropriate.

3.5.4. Adverse Drug Reaction (ADR) Reports

The terms "adverse event," "adverse experience," and "adverse reaction" include any adverse event whether or not it is considered to be drug related. This includes any side effect, injury, toxicity, or sensitivity reaction.

An adverse event is considered *serious* if any of the following occur: It is fatal or life-threatening; it is severely or permanently disabling; it requires new or prolonged inpatient hospitalization; it involves the exacerbation of a congenital anomaly or the development of cancer; it results in an overdose. An adverse event is considered *unexpected* if it is not identified in nature, severity, or frequency in the current investigator brochure.

3.5.5. Adverse Event Reporting Requirements

Patients will be instructed to report any adverse event to the investigators. All adverse events occurring during participation in the study will be documented. All adverse events will be reported to both the local ethical committee and the GTAC, with a description of the severity, duration, and outcome of the event, and the investigator's opinion regarding the relationship, if any, between the event and the study treatment.

3.5.6. Response Criteria

The tumor response to either treatment regimen is one of the primary objectives of this study. Observations of antitumor activity will be collected and analyzed. Standard criteria will be formally employed to classify the antitumor responses observed in patients with *measurable disease* in the liver. Measurable disease will consist of bidimensionally measurable liver lesions with perpendicular diameters of ≥ 1 cm $\times \geq 1$ cm.

3.5.7. Removal From Study

Patients may withdraw or be removed from the study for any of the following reasons:

* Patient's request to withdraw
* Patient unwilling or unable to comply with study requirements
* Clinical need for concomitant or ancillary therapy not permitted in the study
* Any unacceptable treatment-related toxicity precluding further participation in the study
* Unrelated intercurrent illness that, in the judgment of the principal investigator, will affect assessments of clinical status to a significant degree

A patient removed from the study prior to any of the scheduled response evaluations will not be considered inevaluable for response.

3.5.8. Pharmacokinetic Analysis

The study will explore the relationships among pharmacokinetic parameters, toxicity, and biological efficacy.

3.5.9. Analysis of Gene Transfer Efficiency

The study will explore the relationship between dose of Ad-*TK* and efficiency of transduction (gene transfer).

3.5.10. Analysis of Clinical Efficacy

Evaluation of clinical efficacy is one of the primary objectives of this study. Treatment effect will be estimated as the proportion of patients with an objective response (complete or partial) following Ad-*TK*-GCV as compared with objective response to alcohol therapy. Chi-square tests and logistic regression will be used to analyze which variables are significant predictors of response.

3.5.11. Survival Analysis

The Kaplan–Meier method will be used to estimate progression-free survival.

3.6. Public Health Consideration

3.6.1. Precautions, Testing, and Measures to Mitigate Any Risks to the Public Health

It is expected that the construct will not spread to other persons. Tursz et al. studied 10 patients treated with recombinant adenoviral vectors in lung cancer patients and found no cross-contamination to the medical and nursing staff *(27)*. In the French study, there was no shedding of the virus beyond the third day, and we intend to keep the patients overnight in separate rooms with barrier nursing. We will analyze the urine and sputum of the medical and nursing staff during this period.

3.6.2. Exclusion of Risks to Offspring

In order to minimize the risk of cross-infection to offspring, only patients above the age of 40 will be included. It is unlikely that cancer patients above this age will remain reproductively active. Nevertheless, patients will be warned of the risk and will be advised to take contraceptive measures.

4. Another System of Gene Therapy in Patients With Liver Tumors: E1B-Deleted Adenovirus Gene Therapy

For this type of anticancer therapy, viruses need to be rigidly tumor-cell-specific. *dl*1520 originally produced by Barker and Berk in 1987 *(30)* has the ability to target and destroy tumor cells only and led to it being termed the "smart bomb" cancer virus *(31)*. After viral internalization, intracellular adenoviral replication augments an administered dose to the level required to kill the tumor host cells only, leaving neighboring normal tissues intact. *dl*1520 is an adenovirus hybrid of serotypes 2 and 5 with a genome deletion in the E1B region, causing loss of expression of viral 55-kDa protein (E1B 55K). E1B 55K has been shown to bind to the mammalian tumor cell suppressor protein *p53* and block *p53*-mediated transcriptional activation *(32)*. *p53* has many functions including arrest of the G_1 phase of cell proliferation via the cyclin-dependent kinase inhibitor p21/WAF1/Cip1, or apoptosis through induction of genes such as *bax* *(33)*. Studies have shown that *dl*1520 appears to replicate independently of *p53* status in many tumor cell lines *(33–36)*.

Phase I trials of direct intratumoral injection of *dl*1520 in more than 22 patients with recurrent head and neck cancer with *p53* mutations have already shown necrosis in a significant number of tumors, without evidence of damage to normal tissue *(37)*. Habib et al. *(11)* have reported the results of a phase I and a phase II clinical study, in which patients with primary and secondary liver tumors were treated with E1B 55-kDa deleted *dl*1520. The adenovirus was given via three different routes: intratumoral, intra-arterial, and intravenous. The study has confirmed that *dl*1520 was well tolerated when given as either monotherapy or in combination with chemotherapy. Furthermore, ultrastructural examination of tissue showed the presence of adenovirus in cell cytoplasm around the nucleus and revealed two dissimilar end points of cell death after virus infection: a preapoptotic sequence and necrosis *(11)*. Reid et al. have recently published their results of a phase I study in patients with colorectal liver metastases by using intra-arterial administration of a replication-selective adenovirus (*dl*1520) *(38)*. In this study, *dl*1520 was infused into the hepatic artery at doses of 2×10^8 to 2×10^{12} particles for two cycles (d 1 and 8) with subsequent cycles of *dl*1520 administered in combination with intravenous 5-FU and leucovorin. They have successfully demonstrated intravascular administration of *dl*1520 virus and have shown that hepatic artery infusion of the attenuated adenovirus *dl*1520 was well tolerated at doses resulting in infection, replication, and chemotherapy-associated antitumoral activity.

Acknowledgment

We are grateful to the Pedersen Family Charitable Foundation for supporting our research endeavors.

References

1. Bishop, J. M. (1987) The molecular genetics of cancer. *Science* **235**, 305–311.
2. Lantsov, V. A. (1994) Ideal gene therapy: approaches and horizons. *Mol. Biol.* **28**, 321–327.
3. Soloman, E., Borrow, J., and Goddard, A. D. (1991) Chromosome aberratons and cancer. *Science* **254**, 1153–1160.
4. Xu, G. W., Sun, Z. T., Forrester, K., et al. (1996) Tissue-specific growth suppression and chemosensitivity promotion in human hepatocellular carcinoma cells by tetroviral-mediated transfer of the wild-type p53 gene. *Hepatology* **24**, 1264–1268.
5. Kanai, F., Shiratori, Y., Yoshida, Y., et al. (1996)Gene therapy for alpha-fetoprotein-producing human hepatoma cells by adenovirus-mediated transfer of the herpes simplex virus. *Hepatology* **23**, 1359–1367.
6. Kanai, F., Lan, K. H., Shiratori, Y., et al. (1997) In vivo gene therapy for alpha-fetoprotein producing hepatocellular carcinoma by adenovirus-mediated transfer of cytosine deaminase gene. *Cancer Res.* **57**, 461–465.
7. Ukei, T., Nakata, K., and Mawatari, F. (1998) Retro-virus-mediated gene therapy for human hepatocellular carcinoma transplanted in athymic mice. *Int. J. Mol. Med.* **1**, 671–675.
8. Gnant, M. F., Puhlmann, M., Bartlett, D. L., et al. (1999) Regional versus systemic delivery of recombinant vaccinia virus as suicide gene therapy for murine liver metastases. *Ann. Surg.* **230**, 350–360.
9. Mitry, R. R., Sarraf, C. E., Wu, C. G., et al. (1997) Wild-type p 53 induces apoptosis in Hep 3 B through up-regulation of bax expression. *Lab. Invest.* **77**, 369–378.
10. Habib, N. A., Ding, S. F., El-Masry, R., et al. (1996) Preliminary report: the short-term effects of direct p53 DNA injection in primary hepatocellular carcinomas. *Cancer Detect. Prev.* **20**, 103–107.
11. Habib, N. A., Sarraf, C. E., Mitry, R. R., et al. (2001) E1B-deleted adenovirus (dl1520) gene therapy for patients with primary and secondary liver tumours. *Hum. Gene Ther.* **12**, 219–226.
12. Crystal, R. G., Hirschowitz, E., Lieberman, M., et al. (1997) Phase I study of direct administration of a replication deficient adenovirus vector containing *E. coli* cytosine

deaminase gene to metastatic colon carcinoma of the liver in association with the oral administration of the pro-drug 5-fluorocytosine. *Hum. Gene Ther.* **8**, 985–1001.

13. Sung, M. W., Yeh, H. C., Thung, S. N., et al. (2001) Intratumoral adenovirus-mediated suicide gene transfer for hepatic metastases from colorectal adenocarcinoma:results of a phase I clinical trial. *Mol. Ther.* **4**, 182–191.

14. Hubber, B. E., Richards, C. A., and Krenitsky, T. A. (1991) Retroviral-mediated gene therapy for the treatment of hepatocellular carcinoma: an innovative approach for cancer therapy. *Proc. Natl. Acad. Sci. USA* **88**, 8039–8043.

15. Moolten, F. L. (1986) Tumour chemosensitivity conferred by inserted herpes thymidine kinase genes: paradigm for a prospective cancer control strategy. *Cancer Res.* **46**, 5276–5281.

16. Moolten, F. L. and Wells, J. M. (1990) Curability of tumours bearing herpes thymidine kinase genes transferred by retroviral vectors. *J. Natl. Cancer Inst.* **82**, 297–300.

17. Freeman, S., Abboud, C., Whartenby, K. et al. (1993) The "bystander effect"; tumour regression when a fraction of the tumour mass is genetically modified. *Cancer Res.* **53**, 5274–5283.

18. Nakabayashi, H., Watanebe, K., Saito, A., et al. (1989) Transcriptional regulation of alpha-fetoprotein expression by dexamethsone in human hepatoma cells. *J. Biol. Chem.* **264**, 271.

19. Ido A., Nakata K., Kato Y., et al. (1995) Gene therapy for hepatoma cells using a retrovirus vector carrying herpes simplex virus thymidine kinase gene under the control of human alpha-fetoprotein gene promoter. *Cancer Res.* **55**, 3105–3109.

20. Mawatari, F., Tsuruta, S., Ido, A., et al. (1998) Retrovirus-mediated gene therapy for hepatocellular carcinoma:selective and enhanced suicide gene expression regulated by human alpha-fetoprotein enhancer directly linked to its promoter. *Cancer Gene Ther* **5**, 301–306.

21. Caruso, M., Panis, Y., Gagandeep, S., et al. (1993) Regression of established macroscopic liver metastases after in situ transduction of a suicide gene. *Proc. Natl. Acad. Sci. USA* **90**, 7024–7028.

22. Kuriyama, S., Kikukawa, M., Masui, K., et al. (1999) Cancer gene therapy with *HSV-TK/*GCV system depends on T cell mediated immune responses and causes apoptotic death of tumour cells in vivo. *Int. J. Cancer* **83**, 374–380.

23. Van der Eb, M. M., Cramer, S. J., Vergouwe, Y., et al. (1998) Severe hepatic dysfunction after adenovirus-mediated transfer of the herpes simplex virus thymidine kinase gene and ganciclovir administration. *Gene Ther.* **5**, 4451–4458.

24. Kuriyama, S., Kikukawa, M., Masui, K., et al. (1998) Bystander effect caused by cytosine deaminase gene and 5-fluorocytosine in vitro is substantially mediated by generated 5-fluorouracil. *Anticancer Res.* **18**, 3399–3409.

25. Block, A., Freund, C. T., Chen, S. H., et al. (2000) Gene therapy of metastatic comon carcinoma: regression of multiple hepatic metastases by adenoviral expression of bacterial cytosine deaminase. *Cancer Gene Ther.* **7**, 438–445.

26. Knowles, M. R., Hohneker, K. W., Zhou, Z., et al. (1995) A controlled study of adenoviral-vector-mediated gene transfer in the nasal epithelium of patients with cystic fibrosis. *N. Engl. J. Med.* **333**, 823–831.

27. Tursz, T., Cesne, A. L., Baldeyrou, P., et al. (1996) Phase I study of a recombinant adenovirus-mediated gene transfer ilung cancer patients. *J. Natl. Cancer Inst.* **88**, 1857–1863.

28. Piccinino, F., Sagnelli, E., Pasquale, G., and Giusti, G. (1986) Complications following percutaneous liver biopsy. *J. Hepatol.* **2**, 165–173.

29. Perrault, J., McGill, D. B., Ott, B., and Taylor, W. F. (1978) Liver biopsy: complications in 1000 inpatients and outpatients. *Gastroenterology* **74**, 103–106.

30. Barker D. D. and Berk A. J. (1987) Adenovirus proteins from both E1B reading frames are required for the transformation of rodent cells by viral infection and DNA transfection. *Virology* **156,** 107–121.
31. Lowe, S. W. (1997) Progress of the smart bomb cancer virus. *Nature Med.* **4,** 1012–1013.
32. Rothmann, T., Hengstermann, A., Whitaker, N. J., et al. (1998) Replication of ONYX-015, a potential anticancer adenovirus, is independent of p53 status in tumour cells. *J. Virol.* **72,** 9470–9478.
33. Goodrum, F. D. and Ornelles D. A. (1998) p53 Status does not determine outcome of E1B 55-kilodalton mutant adenovirus lytic infection. *J. Virol.* **72,** 9479–9490.
34. Harada, J. N. and Berk, A. J. (1999) p53-Independent and -dependent requirments for E1B-55K in adenovirus type 5 replication. *J. Virol.* **72,** 5333–5344.
35. Vollmer, C. M., Ribas, A., Butterfield, L. H., et al. (1999) p53 selective and nonselective replication of an E1B-deleted adenovirus in hepatocellular carcinoma. *Cancer Res.* **59,** 4369–4374.
36. Heise, C., Sampson-Johannes, A., Williams, A., et al. (1997) ONYX-015, an E1B gene-attenuated adenovirus, causes tumour-specific cytolysis and antitumoural efficacy that can be augmented by standard chemotherapeutic agents. *Nature Med.* **3,** 639–644.
37. Ganly, I. (1999) Phase II trial of intratumoural infection with an E1B deleted adenovirus in patients with recurrent refractory head and neck cancer. *Hum. Gene Ther.* **10,** 844.
38. Reid, T., Galanis, E., Abbruzzese, J., et al. (2001) Intra-arterial administration of a replication-selective adenovirus (dl1520) in patients with colorectal carcinoma metastatic to the liver: a phase I trial. *Gene Ther.* **8,** 1618–1626.

23

Clinical Trials With GDEPT

Cytosine Deaminase and 5-Fluorocytosine

Nicola L. Brown and Nicholas R. Lemoine

1. Introduction

One of the major goals for cancer therapies is to target toxic agents to tumor cells in a selective and specific manner, avoiding damage to normal tissues. One approach is to use "suicide" gene therapy or GDEPT (gene-directed enzyme–prodrug therapy) where the gene delivered encodes an enzyme that can activate a nontoxic prodrug into a cytotoxin. Expression of the "suicide" gene can be made selective by taking advantage of transcriptional differences between normal and neoplastic cells. Several combinations have been described for GDEPT, one of these being the cytosine deaminase/5-fluorocytosine system. Cytosine deaminase (CD) is a nonmammalian enzyme that catalyses the hydrolytic deamination of cytosine to uracil. Therefore, it is capable of converting the nontoxic prodrug 5-fluorocytosine (5-FC) to 5-fluorouracil (5-FU), which inhibits RNA and DNA synthesis during the S-phase of the cell cycle *(1)*. This system has been used both in vitro and in preclinical studies showing antitumor activity against many tumor types *(2–4)*. However, its use in clinical studies to date is rather limited. A recent phase I clinical trial has tested the safety and efficacy of the CD/5-FC system under the transcriptional control of the erbB-2 promoter to treat breast cancer *(5)*. This chapter describes the use of immunocytochemistry to determine the erbB-2 status of each patient and to determine CD protein expression following intratumoural gene delivery. *In situ* hybridization with a ^{35}S-labeled riboprobe was used to assess CD RNA expression and, finally, thin-layer chromatography was utilized to determine CD enzyme activity.

Immunocytochemistry allows the immunolocalization of the antigen of interest using a secondary antibody conjugated with an enzyme, typically either peroxidase or alkaline phosphatase. In the case of peroxidase, enzyme activity is detected using

From: *Methods in Molecular Medicine, Vol. 90, Suicide Gene Therapy: Methods and Reviews*
Edited by: C. J. Springer © Humana Press Inc., Totowa, NJ

diaminobenzidine (DAB) as the electron acceptor and hydrogen peroxidase as the substrate that results in a brown precipitate. In the case of alkaline phosphatase, bromochloroindolyl phosphate/nitroblue tetrazolium (BCIP/NBT) is the usual substrate giving a black/purple precipitate. *In situ* hybridization allows the visualization of defined nucleic acid sequences in cellular preparations by hybridization of a complementary probe. It is frequently carried out with nonradioactive probes, but the use of radiolabeled probes allows sensitive detection provided by long exposure to autoradiographic film. In this chapter, the transcription of a radiolabeled riboprobe from a cloned cDNA fragment of the CD gene is described using T7 or SP6 polymerase.

2. Materials

2.1. Immunocytochemistry to Determine erbB-2 Status

1. Polylysine or Vectabond-coated slides.
2. 0.3% H_2O_2 (Light sensitive; store at 4°C).
3. Diaminobenzidene (DAB). Store at 4°C. Make fresh. Highly toxic.
4. Primary and secondary antibodies. In this case, two primary rabbit antibodies to the human erbB-2 receptor were used (Dako, High Wycombe, UK; Signet, Cambridge, UK) and the enzyme system was peroxidase conjugated to goat antirabbit antibody.
5. Cover slips and Hydromount.

2.2. Immunocytochemistry to Detect CD Protein Expression

1. Cultured cells grown on sterile glass slides or cryostat sections of snap frozen tissue.
2. 0.05 M NH_4Cl/PBS (phosphate-buffered saline).
3. 3% Paraformaldehyde/PBS (*see* **Subheading 2.3.1.**, **item 10**).
4. Cold absolute methanol (–20°C).
5. 0.1% Triton-X-100/PBS
6. Primary and secondary antibodies [e.g., primary monoclonal antibody 16D8F2 (*6*)].
7. Cover slips and Hydromount.

2.3. In Situ Hybridization for Detection of CD mRNA

2.3.1. Preparation of Slides

1. Paraffin-embedded tissue sections.
2. 10% Decon-90.
3. 2% (v/v) 3-Aminopropylethoxysilane (TESPA) in acetone. Make up fresh solution only. TESPA can be stored at 4°C for up to 3 mo.
4. DEPC (diethylpyrocarbonate)-treated Milli-Q water. (Mix Milli-Q water with 0.1% [v/v] DEPC overnight and autoclave to destroy remaining DEPC.)
5. 70% Alcohol.
6. Xylene and 0.1% DEPC (make fresh).
7. 100%, 80%, 60%, 30% ethanol, each containing 0.1% DEPC.
8. Proteinase K (stock solution: 20 mg/mL in water. Store at –20°C).
9. 2X PBS with 0.2% (w/v) glycine.
10. 4% Paraformaldehyde in PBS (Paraformaldehyde solution should be made up fresh for each experiment. Carefully dissolve 4 g paraformaldehyde in 100 mL of PBS at approx 70°C in a fume hood. If necessary, add a drop of 1 M NaOH to clear the solution. Cool on ice to room temperature. Make fresh each time or freeze aliquots at –20°C.)
11. 0.1 M Triethanolamine with 0.25% acetic anhydride.

12. Plastic storage boxes for slides should be soaked in 5% H_2O_2 (caution: caustic) overnight to destroy any RNA-degrading enzymes present.

2.3.2. In Vitro Transcription of a ^{35}S-Labeled cRNA Probe

1. Riboprobe® Systems Kit (Promega, UK).
2. 800 Ci/mmol ^{35}S-UTP (Amersham, Arlington Heights, IL).
3. Chromaspin-30 column (Clontech, Palo Alto, CA).

2.3.3. Hybridization

1. Hybridization buffer (10% 10X salts buffer in Denhardt's solution; 50% formamide; 3% rRNA; 20% dextran sulfate; 1% of 1 M dithiothreitol (DTT); made up to volume with DEPC-treated Milli-Q water).
2. 10X Salts buffer: 3 M NaCl; 100 mM Na_2HPO_4; 100 mM Tris-HCl, pH 8.0; 50 mM EDTA. Dissolve Na_2HPO_4 in small amounts using Milli-Q water and adjust to pH 6.8. Add NaCl, then Tris-HCl and EDTA, and mix. Make up to the final volume with Milli-Q water (do not add DEPC). Do not autoclave or filter. Store at room temperature.
3. 50X Denhardt's solution (5 g Ficoll, 5 g polyvinyl pyrrolidone, 5 g BSA [bovine serum albumin]).
4. Box containing blotting paper saturated with 1X salts and 50% formamide.
5. TNE buffer: 0.5 M NaCl; 10 mM Tris-HCl, pH 7.5; 1 mM EDTA, pH 8.0.
6. 100 µg/m: RNase in TNE buffer.
7. 20X SSC: 0.3 M NaCl; 0.3 M sodium citrate, pH 7.0.
8. Graded ethanols from 30% to absolute, each containing 0.3 M ammonium acetate.

2.3.4. Autoradiography and Slide Development

1. Melt 25 mL Ilford K5 emulsion in 2.4 mL of 5 M ammonium acetate. Dilute with 25 mL Milli-Q water warmed to 45°C.
2. X-ray film (Kodak BIOMAX or X-OMAT).
3. Developer and fixative for autoradiography.
4. Toluidine blue (or Mayer's hematoxylin and eosin) for staining.

2.4. Thin-Layer Chromatography for Measuring CD Enzyme Activity

1. Hank's-balanced salt solution (HBSS) (Life Technologies, Scotland).
2. A minimum of 1×10^6 cells.
3. Lysis buffer: 100 mM Tris-HCl, pH7.8, 1 mM EDTA, 1 mM DTT.
4. Cytosine label mix: 0.97 mCi [12.2 Ci/mmol] ^{3}H-cytosine in 100 mM Tris-HCl, pH 7.8.
5. Fluorescent thin-layer chromatograpy (TLC) sheets (Merk, plates 1.05735).
6. Radioactive cytosine and uracil standards (0.4 mg/mL).
7. Chromatography chamber containing butan-1-ol and water (86 : 14 v/v). The TLC should be performed in a fume cupboard, as butan-1-ol fumes are an irritant.
8. Liquid scintillation analyzer (TriCarb 1500).

3. Methods

3.1. Immunohistochemistry to Establish erbB-2 Status

This may be performed on fresh biopsy tissue or paraffin-embedded tissue. The use of alternative primary antibodies should give similar results.

1. Mount 4 µm biopsy tissue onto polysine-coated or Vectabond-coated (not polylysine) slides.
2. Block endogenous peroxidases by incubating slides in 0.3% H_2O_2 for 15 min.

3. Block in normal goat serum at 1/20 dilution for 30 min to reduce nonspecific binding of the primary antibody (*Note*: The blocking agent should always be the normal serum from the animal species in which the secondary antibody was generated.)
4. Incubate with the primary antibody (rabbit antihuman erbB2) diluted according to the manufacturer's instructions at 4°C overnight.
5. Wash four times for 10 min at room temperature in PBS.
6. Incubate for 30 min at room temperature with the appropriate biotinylated secondary antibody. Label with peroxidase–streptavidin at 1 : 500 dilution for 30 min at room temperature.
7. Wash four times for 10 min in PBS.
8. Incubate slides in DAB solution for 10 min. Positive reactivity is visible as brown staining.
9. Wash four times for 10 min in PBS.
10. Mount a cover slip in Hydromount.

3.2. Immunocytochemistry to Detect CD Protein in Cells and Tissue

See **Note 1**.

1. Fix cultured cells grown on slides or cryostat tissue sections at room temperature in 3% paraformaldehyde/PBS for 5 min and then in 0.05 M NH_4Cl/PBS.
2. Incubate in cold absolute methanol at –20°C for 10 min, followed by permeabilization in 0.1% Triton-X-100/PBS at room temperature for 5 min.
3. Incubate in the primary monoclonal antibody, 16D8F2 *(6)*, at the recommended dilution for 30 min at room temperature.
4. Wash four times for 10 min in PBS at room temperature.
5. Incubate in the secondary antibody for 30 min at room temperature.
6. Wash four times for 10 min in PBS at room temperature.
7. Label with peroxidase–streptavidin at the recommended dilution (see manufacturer's instructions) for 30 min at room temperature.
8. Wash four times for 10 min in PBS at room temperature.
9. Incubate slides with DAB solution for 10 min. Positive immunoreactivity is visible as brown staining.
10. Wash four times for 10 min in PBS.
11. Mount a cover slip in Hydromount.

The degree of CD expression by this method is typically designated according to the proportion of tumor cells expressing the CD protein: (+++) indicates over 70% of the tumor cells are positive, (++) 50–70% are positive, and (+) less than 50% positive.

3.3. In Situ Hybridization for CD mRNA Expression

Cytosine deaminase mRNA expression in paraffin-embedded clinical trial biopsy tissue can be determined using *in situ* hybridization *(7)*.

3.3.1. Preparation of Slides

1. Wash microscope slides and cover slips overnight in 10% Decon-90, followed by washing in hot running water for 60 min, and, finally, rinse in Milli-Q water prior to baking in aluminum foil at 180°C for 4 h.
2. Immerse slides for 12 s in 2% (v/v) TESPA in acetone; rinse twice in acetone and twice in DEPC-treated water prior to drying in an oven at 40°C. Slides can be stored dust-free for up to 6 wk.

3. Cut 4-μm sections from paraffin-embedded tissue using a microtome (*see* **Note 2**) and float on DEPC-treated Milli-Q water. Make sure disposable microtome blades are used or the blade is cleaned thoroughly with alcohol prior to use. Collect the sections on the TESPA-coated slides and bake overnight at 40°C. Cover slips should be washed in 70% alcohol and oven-baked at 40°C for 4 h.

4. Dewax the sections using fresh xylene and 0.1% DEPC for 8 min, and rehydrate through sequential 100%, 80%, 60%, and finally, 30% ethanol containing 0.1% DEPC.

5. Permeabilize tissues using proteinase K at a final concentration of 20 μg/mL in PBS for 10 min. Rinse 2X in PBS containing 0.2% (w/v) glycine for 5 min.

6. Rinse twice in PBS and fix sections in 4% paraformaldehyde in PBS for 20 min.

7. Rinse twice in PBS.

8. Acetylate sections with 0.1 *M* triethanolamine and 0.25% acetic anhydride. Mix well for 10 min.

9. Wash slides three times with PBS for 5 min and dehydrate through graded alcohol from 30% to 100% containing 0.1% DEPC.

10. Air-dry sections prior to hybridization.

3.3.2. In Vitro Transcription of a ³⁵S-Labeled CD cRNA Probe

1. The CD cDNA should be directionally cloned into pGEM-4 vector (Promega) using the *Eco*RI and *Hind*III sites. The template is then prepared for in vitro transcription of the riboprobe by linearizing the vector with *Eco*RI for production of the sense strand (negative control) under control of the T7 promoter, and *Hind*III for production of the antisense strand under the control of the SP6 promoter. Also, β-actin cDNA cloned into pBluescript is linearized with *Dra*I and transcribed under the control of the SP6 promoter.

2. Linearize 1 μg of each vector, phenol/chloroform extract and ethanol precipitate the digestion products.

3. Add 1 μg of linearized vector to the in vitro transcription mix: 1X transcription buffer (Promega); 1.5 U/mL RNAsin (Promega); DTT (5.6 m*M* plus 5.6 m*M* ³⁵S-UTP); 6.25 μ*M* each of ATP, GTP, CTP; 10 U/μg template of RNA polymerase plus 3.5 μL (800 Ci/ mmol) 35S-UTP (Amersham, Arlington Heights, IL). Incubate at 37°C for 60 min.

4. Destroy the template by adding 1 μL of DNase I (RNase-free) to the reaction tube and incubating for 15 min.

5. Dilute the reaction mix in 25 μL of 10 m*M* DTT and 1.5 μL of ribosomal RNA (10 μg/mL used as a carrier).

6. To assess total ³⁵S content, take 1 μL into 50 μL water and add 3 mL scintillant fluid.

7. Equilibrate a Chromaspin-30 column (Clontech, Palo Alto, CA).

8. Add the bulk of the reaction mixture to the column and spin at 700*g* for 3 min at 15°C and collect the eluate.

9. Add 4 μL of 100 m*M* DTT, mix well, and count as in **step 6**. Calculate the percentage incorporation of ³⁵S (which should be 40–80%).

10. The riboprobe eluate should then be assessed for quality on a 6% polyacrylamide sequencing gel and then stored at –20°C until required (*see* **Note 3**).

3.3.3. Hybridization

1. Heat the hybridization buffer containing the riboprobe to 80°C for 1 min.

2. Pipet 20 μL of this hybridization buffer onto each of the slides (final concentration should be 1.5 ng cRNA/slide or 0.5×10^6 to 2×10^6 cpm/slide).

3. Place slides in a humidified box containing blotting paper saturated with 1X salts and 50% formamide. Seal the box with tape and hybridize overnight at 55°C.

4. After hybridization, place the slides in 50% formamide at 55°C for 4 h and then wash slides 10 times for 5 min with TNE buffer.
5. Incubate slides in 100 µg/mL RNase A in TNE buffer solution at 37°C for 1 h.
6. Wash slides in 2X SSC and 0.5% SSC, each for 30 min at 65°C.
7. To ensure that labeled hybrids remain in place, pass the slides through graded alcohols (all including 0.3 M ammonium acetate) increasing from 30% to absolute alcohol.
8. Air-dry slides overnight prior to autoradiography.

3.3.4. Autoradiography and Slide Development

1. Dip the slides into the emulsion to cover the tissue. Allow to cool and dry in total darkness by placing slides on a metal plate overlying ice.
2. Once dry, place slides in a plastic rack and expose for the appropriate time at 4°C in the dark (usually 2–12 wk depending on the abundance of the mRNA).
3. Develop the slides in Kodak D-19 developer at 18°C for 4 min and fix in 30% sodium thiosulphate.
4. Sections are stained with toluidine blue (or Mayer's haematoxylin and eosin) and mounted.

3.4. Measurement of Cytosine Deaminase Activity Using Thin-Layer Chromatography

This method was modified from that described by Anderson and co-workers *(8)*.

1. Wash at least 1×10^6 cells in HBSS and resuspend in 200 µL of lysis buffer.
2. Freeze–thaw lysates by immersion in liquid nitrogen and centrifuge at 15,800g for 10 min.
3. Take 10-µL aliquot of cleared lysates and mix with 10-µL of "cytosine label mix." Incubate for 1 h at 37°C and then spot 5–10 µL into fluorescent TLC sheets.
4. Spot radioactive standard samples of cytosine and uracil (0.4 mg/mL) at either end of the TLC plate. Because these standards absorb ultraviolet (UV) light, their positions on the TLC plate can be estimated using a hand-held UV source ($\lambda^2 = 240$ nm).
5. Place the TLC plates in a chromatography chamber containing butan-1-ol and water; seal the chamber with a cling film and run for 4 h (*see* **Note 4**).
6. To calculate the rate of uracil formation, cut out the bands corresponding to the radioactive products (i.e., at the level of the nonradioactive uracil control) and place in scintillation tubes containing 5 mL of liquid scintillation analyzer (TriCarb 1500). Measure the radioactivity using a scintillation counter.
7. The conversion of cytosine to uracil expressed as a percentage can be calculated as

$$\% \text{ conversion to uracil} = \frac{\text{dpm uracil band}}{\text{total dpm in uracil and cytosine bands}} \times 100\%$$

4. Notes

1. Ideally immunohistochemitry should be performed on cell lines either transfected or untransfected with the CD gene to provide both positive and negative controls and to evaluate the specificity of the antibody prior to investigating cryostat-cut sections of snap-frozen tissue.

2. An important parameter in obtaining a homogenous signal with *in situ* hybridization is the thickness of the tissue. Twelve to 15 μm gives a much better homogeneity compared with 8–10 μm and more intense hybridization signals.

3. For 100% incorporation of ^{35}S-cytosine into the riboprobe, the total number of counts would be 3.2×10^8, which is equivalent to 243 ng RNA. The expected dpm (disintegration per minute) is 10×10^6 dpm/mL. One million dpm is approximately equivalent to a 0.7 ng cRNA probe. The specific activity of the RNA transcript will be $(1.3-1.7) \times 10^9$ dpm/μg RNA using the ^{35}S as the only source of UTP.

4. To ensure uniform movement of all bands, it is important to ensure that the TLC plate is surrounded by a butan-1-ol atmosphere within the chromatography chamber. This can be achieved either with a heavy glass lid with Vaseline smeared on the rim of the chamber or by using several layers of a Cling film.

References

1. Springer, C. J. and Niculescu-Duvaz, I. (1996) Gene-directed enzyme prodrug therapy (GDEPT): choice of prodrugs. *Adv. Drug Delivery Rev.* **22,** 351–364.

2. Huber, B., Austin, E., Good, S., Knick, V., and Richards, C. (1993) In vivo antitumour activity of 5-fluorocytosine on human colorectal carcinoma cells lines genetically modified to express CD. *Cancer Res.* **53,** 4619–4625.

3. Mullen, C. A., Coale, M. M., Lowe, R. M., and Blaese, R. M. (1994) Tumours expressing the cytosine deaminase suicide gene can be eliminated in vivo with 5-fluorocytosine and induce protective immunity to wild type tumour. *Cancer Res.* **54,** 1503–1506.

4. Ohwada, A., Hiroshowitz, E. A., and Crystal, R. G. (1996) Regional delivery of an adenovirus vector containing the *Escherichia coli* cytosine deaminase gene to provide local activation of 5-fluorocytosine to suppress the growth of colon carcinoma metastatic to liver. *Hum. Gene Ther.* **7,** 1567–1576.

5. Pandha, H.S., Martin, L-A., Rigg, A., et al. (1999) Genetic prodrug activation therapy for breast cancer: a phase I clinical trial of erbB-2-directed suicide gene expression. *J. Clin. Oncol.* **17,** 2180–2189.

6. Haak, K., Moebius, U., Knebel Doeberitz, M., and Gebert, J. (1997) Detection of cytosine deaminase in genetically modified tumour cells by specific antibodies. *Hum. Gene. Ther.* **8,** 1395–1401.

7. Senior, P. V., Byrne S., Brammer W. J., and Beck F. (1990) Expression of the IGF-II/mannose-6-phosphate receptor mRNA and protein in the developing rat. *Development* **109,** 67–73.

8. Anderson, L., Kilstrup, M., and Neuhard, J. (1989) Pyrimidine, purine and nitrogen control of cytosine deaminase synthesis in *E. coli. Arch. Microbiol.* **153,** 115–118.

24

The Nitroreductase/CB1954 Enzyme–Prodrug System

Nicola K. Green, David J. Kerr, Vivien Mautner, Peter A. Harris, and Peter F. Searle

1. Introduction
1.1. The CB1954/Ntr Enzyme–Prodrug System

The prodrug CB1954 (5-[aziridin-1-yl]-2,4-dinitrobenzamide) is a weak monofunctional alkylating agent originally synthesized at the Chester Beatty Laboratories in the late 1960s (1). The antitumor activity of CB1954 was determined by screening a panel of aziridines for cytotoxicity against the rat Walker 256 carcinoma. It is highly selective and effective against Walker tumor cells in vivo and in vitro with a therapeutic index of 70 (2). Based on the efficacy against the Walker carcinoma, a small clinical trial using CB1954 was initiated at the Royal Marsden Hospital in 1970. The results of this study are unpublished; however, a dose-limiting toxicity was reached (the major side effect being diarrhea) without any evidence of tumor regression (Wiltshaw, unpublished data). Recently, a clinical trial to determine the maximum tolerated dose (MTD) of CB1954 by intravenous and intraperitoneal routes has been performed in Birmingham. This study concluded that the MTD for CB1954 is 24 mg/m^2 by iv administration and 37.5 mg/m^2 by the ip route. Toxicity included diarrhea and elevation of liver transaminases (3).

The enzyme responsible for CB1954 activation in Walker cells was purified and identified as DT-diaphorase [NAD(P)H dehydrogenase (quinone); E.C. 1.6.99.2], which is thought to be involved in the detoxification of quinones in a two electron transfer step that avoids the generation of toxic superoxide radicals. This enzyme was shown to catalyze the aerobic reduction of CB1954 to the cytotoxic derivative, 5-(aziridin-1-yl)-4-hydroxylamino 2-nitrobenzamide using either NADH or NADPH as an electron donor (4). A further activation step then occurs in the presence of thioesters such as coenzyme A to produce a DNA-reactive species (5) (see **Fig. 1**). Subsequently, a nitroreductase enzyme (Ntr) was purified from *Escherichia coli* B that was sensitive

From: *Methods in Molecular Medicine, Vol. 90, Suicide Gene Therapy: Methods and Reviews*
Edited by: C. J. Springer © Humana Press Inc., Totowa, NJ

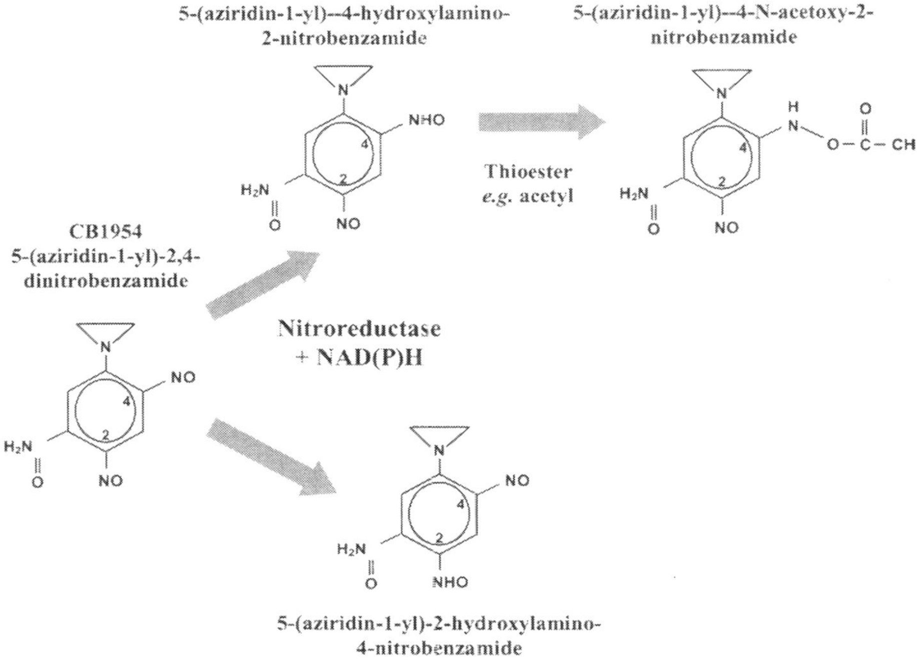

Fig. 1. The activation of CB1954.

to CB1954 *(6)*. Ntr was shown to reduce either, but not both, of the nitro groups of CB1954, forming the corresponding hydroxylamines at equal rates. The reduction of CB1954 by Ntr is about 100-fold faster than by the rat DT-diaphorase enzyme, although only the 4-hydroxylamino derivative, not the 2-hydroxylamino derivative, is able to form DNA crosslinks *(4)*. DT-Diaphorase is present in human tissues at levels comparable to those found in rats. Analysis of the DNA sequences indicate that the rat and human genes are 83% identical and the encoded proteins are 85% identical. Despite this similarity, CB1954 is much more cytotoxic to rat cell lines than human cell lines, with a 500- to 5000-fold higher dose being required to give similar cytotoxicity in human cells compared to rat cells *(7)*. Kinetic analysis of the rat and human DT-diaphorase enzymes revealed that human DT-diaphorase had a K_{cat} of 0.64/min for CB1954 compared to 4.1/min for the rat enzyme. The rat and human enzymes show similar activity toward an alternative substrate menadione, confirming that CB1954 is poorly activated by the human enzyme.

Chen et al. *(9)* demonstrated that the mouse DT-diaphorase has enzyme activity similar to the human enzyme but has more sequence homology to the rat enzyme. Site-directed mutagenesis was used to identify amino acids responsible for CB1954 activation. Tyrosine 104 is essential for CB1954 reductase activity in the rat enzyme and is substituted by glutamine in the mouse and human enzymes, explaining the insensitivity of mouse and human tumors to CB1954 *(8,9)*. The inability of human and mouse DT-diaphorase to activate CB1954 allows the use of *E. coli* Ntr in a virally directed enzyme prodrug (VDEPT) approach for human cancer and the use of mice for experimental studies.

1.2. In Vitro Ntr/CB1954 VDEPT Efficacy

The in vitro efficacy of Ntr/CB1954 in a VDEPT system was first described using retroviral delivery of the Ntr gene into NIH3T3 cells. After retroviral transduction, pooled NIH3T3 cells were 100-fold more sensitive to CB1954 and a single-cell clone was generated that was over 1000-fold more sensitive than the parental cells *(10)*. We have constructed a retroviral vector based on the LNCX vector *(11)* in which nitroreductase expression is directed from the highly active cytomegalovirus (CMV) promoter and enhancer sequence *(12)*. This vector was used to transduce human colorectal and pancreatic cancer cell lines. Clones sensitive to CB1954 were identified and characterized in dose–response experiments that demonstrated a 17- to 500-fold sensitization to CB1954 upon Ntr expression and demonstrated a significant bystander effect in vitro *(12)*. Western blotting using an antibody against Ntr showed that the increased susceptibility to the prodrug was associated with higher levels of Ntr present suggesting that the enzyme is limiting. We have demonstrated a clear correlation between the level of Ntr activity and sensitivity to CB1954 in SKOV3 ovarian carcinoma cell clones transduced with Ntr-expressing retrovirus and demonstrated regression of Ntr-expressing tumors following treatment with CB1954 *(13)*. Retroviral delivery of Ntr results in the integration of the gene into chromosomal DNA giving the possibility for long-term expression in the transduced cells and their descendants. This could be appropriate for ex vivo transduction of a cell population to incorporate a "suicide gene" before adoptive transfer. "Standard" retroviral vectors (i.e., excluding lentiviral vectors) can only successfully transduce replicating cells. Retroviral particles have a short half-life (typically 4 h at 37°C), and titres are often fairly low ($<10^6$ colony-forming units (cfu)/mL. The titer can be increased by centrifugation, and with a retrovirus concentrated to 3×10^7 cfu/mL we have transduced 80–90% of a target cell population in a single 12-h exposure.

Adenoviruses are relatively stable, can be produced in titers up to 10^{12} (pfu/mL), and can infect a wide range of both replicating and nonreplicating cells. Replication-defective adenoviruses can be used to achieve short-term, high-level expression of Ntr, allowing killing of infected cells by treatment with CB1954. To improve the delivery of the Ntr "suicide gene" to tumor cells, a replication-defective adenoviral vector expressing Ntr under the transcriptional control of the CMV promoter was constructed. When this adenovirus was used to infect SKOV3 ovarian cancer cells at a MOI (multiplicity of infection) of 50 pfu/cell, cells were sensitized 2000-fold to CB1954 *(14)*. Maximal levels of Ntr expression occurred at 48 h and were maintained for at least 6 d. A 1000-fold increase in sensitivity to CB1954 was also observed in SKOV3 cells cultured at low serum concentration to inhibit proliferation, indicating that this system is not DNA-replication dependent. The Ntr–CB1954 enzyme–prodrug system may be particularly useful clinically in ovarian cancer as chemotherapeutic treatment with platinum-containing drugs like cisplatin often gives short-lived results because of the formation of drug-resistant clones. We have demonstrated that both cisplatin-resistant ovarian cancer cells and early-passage ovarian carcinoma cells from patients with recurrent disease can be efficiently sensitized to CB1954 by retroviral and adenoviral delivery of the Ntr gene *(13,14)*. This chapter describes the construction and analysis of the retroviral and adenoviral vectors encoding Ntr, outlines their use in experimental tumor models, and includes a summary of the clinical trial protocol that was designed to offer proof that the adenovirus can infect and lead to Ntr expression in colorectal cancer metastases.

2. Materials

All chemicals were obtained from Sigma-Aldrich (Poole, Dorset, UK) unless stated otherwise.

1. The 293 cells (human embryo kidney cells transformed with sheared human Ad5 DNA; ECACC Ref. No. 85120602) *(15)* and FLY RD18 cells (derived from HT1080 human fibrosarcoma cells and transfected with Moloney murine leukemia virus cores with envelope glycoproteins of cat endogenous virus RD114) *(16)* were obtained from the European Collection of Animal Cell Cultures (Porton Down, Wiltshire, UK). SKOV3 (human ovarian carcinoma) cells were obtained from Dr. Martin Ford (Glaxo-Wellcome, Stevenage Herts. UK) and SUIT2 (human pancreatic adenocarcinoma) cells were obtained from Dr. Nick Lemoine (Hammersmith Hospital, London, UK).
2. Cell Culture Medium
   a. Dulbecco's modified Eagle's medium (DMEM) with 4500 mg/L D-glucose, 25 mM HEPES, and sodium bicarbonate (Sigma; cat. no. D6171); store at 4°C.
   b. L-Glutamine, 200 mM solution (Sigma; cat. no. G7513); aliquot and store at –20°C.
   c. Penicillin/streptomycin solution; 10,000 units penicillin and 10 mg streptomycin per milliliter. (Sigma; cat. no. P4333); aliquot and store at –20°C
   d. Heat-inactivated fetal bovine serum (Selborne Biological Services [Australia] Ltd. Mountford, Longford, Tasmania), 0.1-µL filtered batch no. GT-FBS-0401.
3. Complete growth medium: DMEM containing 10% heat-inactivated FCS, 25 mM HEPES, 2 mM glutamine, 100 U/mL penicillin, and 100 µg/mL streptomycin.
4. Adenoviral infection medium: DMEM containing 2% FCS, 2 mM glutamine, 100 U/mL penicillin and 100 µg/mL streptomycin.
5. Dulbecco's phosphate-buffered saline (complete) (PBS)
   a. Solution A: Dissolve 1 PBS tablet (Oxoid, Basingstoke, Hampshire, UK; cat. no. BR14a) per 10 mL H$_2$O.
   b. Solution B: 1 g/L CaCl$_2$·2H$_2$O.
   c. Solution C: 1 g/L MgCl$_2$·6H$_2$O.

   For complete PBS, use 8 parts solution A, 1 part solution B, and 1 part solution C.
6. Trypsin/versene: 1 volume trypsin: *4 volumes versene.*
   a. Trypsin: 0.25% in Tris-buffered saline (TBS); store in sterile 5-mL aliquots at –20°C.
   b. Versene: 0.6 mM EDTA in PBSa (**item 5a**), 0.002% phenol red, store in sterile 20-mL aliquots at 4°C.
7. TBS: 140 mM NaCl, 30 mM KCl, 28 mM Na$_2$HPO$_4$, 25 mM Tris-HCl, 1 mg/mL glucose, pH 7.0; filter sterilize and store at 4°C.

8. Solutions for calcium phosphate transfection
   a. 2.5 M CaCl$_2$: 183.7 g CaCl$_2$·2H$_2$O in H$_2$O, filter-sterilize and store in aliquots at –20°C.
   b. 2X HEPES-buffered saline (HeBS): 16.4 g NaCl, 11.9 g HEPES, 0.21 g Na$_2$HPO$_4$, 800 mL H$_2$O, pH to 7.05 using 5 M NaOH, made up to 1 L with H$_2$O; filter-sterilize and store in aliquots at –20°C.
   An exact pH is very important for efficient transfections. The optimal pH range is 7.05–7.12.
9. G418: G418 sulfate, cell culture tested (Calbiochem; cat. number 345810). Dissolve in deionized H$_2$O at 1.25 mg/mL; filter-sterilize and store in aliquots at –20°C.
10. Polybrene: Hexadimethrine bromide (Sigma; cat. no. H9268). Dissolve in deionized H$_2$O at 6 mg/mL; filter-sterilize and store in aliquots at 4°C.
11. CB1954: A gift from Cobra Therapeutics Ltd, Keele, Staffordshire, UK. For in vitro studies a 50 mM stock is made up in N-methylpyrrolidine : polyethylene glycol (NMP : PEG) 2 volumes NMP : 7 volumes PEG. For in vivo studies, we used a clinical batch at 17.8 mg/mL in NMP : PEG that is then diluted in NMP : PEG to 16 mg/mL and stored in aliquots at –20°C. Immediately prior to use the CB1954 is diluted to 4 mg/mL in sterile PBSa. The vehicle used in the in vivo studies was 1 volume NMP : PEG to 3 volumes PBSa.
12. Dulbecco's PBSa: Dissolve 1 PBS tablet (Oxoid; cat. no. BR14a) per 10 mL H$_2$O.
13. CsCl gradient solutions:
    CsCl ρ=1.45; 20.5 g CsCl, 2.9 mL 0.5 M Tris-HCl, pH 7.2, 28.5 mL H$_2$O
    CsCl ρ=1.32; 32.0 g CsCl, 6.8 mL of 0.5 M Tris-HCl, pH 7.9, 61.2 mL H$_2$O
    Filter solutions through Whatman No. 1 paper and store at room temperature.
14. 40% glycerol: 40 g glycerol, 2.0 mL of 0.5 M Tris-HCl, pH 7.9, 0.5 mL of 0.2 M EDTA (pH 8.0), H$_2$O to 100 mL. Make up using sterile reagents and store at room temperature.
15. PBS–glycerol: Complete PBS (**item 5**) containing 10% glycerol.
16. Pico Green DNA Assay Kit (Molecular Probes Inc., Eugene, OR; cat. no. P7589).
17. Noble agar (Difco Laboratories, Detroit, MI; cat. no. 0142-17-0): 1.4% made up in H$_2$O and autoclaved. Melt in microwave and put in 42°C water bath before use (at least 45 min—must not be too hot).
18. 2X Dulbecco's modified Eagle's medium (DME): 100 mL 2X DME, 4 mL FCS, 4 mL 200 mM glutamine, 1mL of 570 mM sodium bicarbonate, 1 mL of 1 M MgCl$_2$. Warm up to 37°C before use.
19. MTS assay: CellTitre96—cell proliferation assay (Promega UK; cat. no. G5430).
20. Urea buffer: 9 M urea, 50 mM Tris-HCl pH 7.5, 150 mM β–mercaptoethanol. Make up urea/tris. Store at room temperature; add β-mercaptoethanol prior to use.
21. Bio-Rad protein assay (Bio-Rad Protein Assay Dye Reagent Concentrate; cat. no. 500-0006).
22. Immobilon P transfer membrane (Millipore UK Ltd, cat. no. IPVH00010).
23. Antibodies: Primary antibodies: Sheep polyclonal to Ntr, a kind gift from Dr. Hakim Djeha, Cobra Therapeutics Ltd, Keele, Staffs; rabbit polyclonal to Ntr (108A/108B), a kind gift from Dr Martin Ford, Glaxo-Wellcome, UK; rabbit polyclonal to Ntr (655), a kind gift from Dr Roger Melton, CAMR, Porton Down, UK.
    a. 2°: Goat antirabbit IgG, horseradish peroxidase (HRP) coupled (Sigma; cat. no. A9169).
    b. 2°: Donkey antisheep IgG, HRP coupled (Sigma; cat. no. A3415).
24. ECL Western blotting detection reagents (Amersham Pharmacia Biotech; cat. no. RPN 2109).

3. Methods

3.1. Cell Culture

All cell lines are maintained in complete growth medium. Adenoviral infections are performed in medium containing 2% FCS (adenoviral infection medium). Cells are routinely grown in 75-cm^2 tissue culture flasks and passaged 1 : 6 twice weekly while still subconfluent.

3.2. Retroviral Delivery of Nitroreductase

3.2.1. Construction of a Retroviral Plasmid Expressing Nitroreductase

Construction of the plasmid has been described in detail *(12)*. Briefly, pNTR130, a plasmid containing the *E. coli* B nitroreductase gene (*see* **Note 1**) was modified to convert the sequence upstream of the initation codon to match the Kozak consensus *(17)* and introduce a *Hin*dIII restriction site into the DNA sequence. Subsequent *Hin*dIII digestion released the modified nitroreductase gene as an 833-bp fragment that was cloned into the *Hin*dIII site downstream of the cytomegalovirus (CMV) promoter in pxLNCX to generate pxLNC-*Ntr*. This original plasmid contained the bacterial transcription termination sequences. The greater efficiency of sensitizing transduced cells to CB1954 was later obtained using a modified version that lacked these additional bacterial sequences *(13)*.

3.3.2. Production of Retroviral Packaging Cell Lines Expressing Nitroreductase and Infection of Target Cells

1. FLY RD18 cells (*see* **Note 2**) are plated at 5 × 10^5 cells per 6-cm plate.
2. The next day, the cells are transfected using calcium phosphate with 10 μg DNA pxLNC-*Ntr*. The DNA is diluted into 175 μL sterile H$_2$O; then 25 μL 2.5M CaCl$_2$ was added. Then, 200 μL 2X HeBS is put into a sterile 15-mL conical tube and the DNA/CaCl$_2$ solution is added dropwise, and air bubbled through the solution. The solution is left for 20 min to allow the formation of a precipitate. Four hundred microliters of precipitate is added to 4 mL of medium in a 6-cm plate. The cells are incubated overnight, washed with PBS, and 10 mL complete medium added.
3. Twenty-four hours after transfection, the cells are replated into two 10-cm plates; the next day, 500 μg/mL G418 is added to the culture medium and cells grown in the presence of G418 for 10 d to select a pool of transduced cells.
4. Once G418-resistant clones are visible on the transfection plates, the culture medium is removed and plates washed in PBS. Cloning rings are placed over the clones and cells harvested using trypsin.
5. Each clone is grown in one well of a six-well plate until confluent, and then transferred to a 25-cm^2 flask. Once the cells are 70–80% confluent, fresh medium is added and the cells incubated overnight. The next day, the conditioned medium containing retroviral particles (retroviral supernatant) is harvested, filtered through a 0.45-μm filter and stored at −20°C.
6. The titer of the retroviral supernatants is assessed using a colony-forming assay. SKOV3 cells are plated at 1 × 10^5 cells per well in 6 well plates. The retroviral supernatants are diluted (10^{-2}–10^{-5} dilutions) in DMEM and polybrene is added to a final concentration of 6 μg/mL. The cells are transduced with 2 mL of the supernatants for 16 h, then split into

10-cm dishes, and grown in complete medium containing 1 mg/mL G418. Cells should be fed with G418-containing medium every 3 d until colonies are present. The plates are washed with PBS, and then fixed and stained with 0.3% crystal violet in 70% methanol and colonies counted. Titers are typically 10^6 cfu/mL. It has been reported that growing FLY RD18 cells in serum-free medium can lead to an increase in viral titres (*18*).

3.2.3. Concentration of Retroviral Supernatants

This is a modified version of the method of Bowles et al. (*19*).

1. Retroviral producer cells are plated in 40X 10-cm plates at 1×10^6 cells per plate.
2. When the cells are 90 % confluent (1–2 d), 5 mL of fresh complete growth medium is added per plate and the cells left for 12 h.
3. The medium is removed from the cells, collected into 250-mL centrifuge pots, and centrifuged at 6000g at 4°C for 16 h (using a Sorvall RC 5B plus centrifuge).
4. The supernatant is discarded, the cell pellet resuspended in 2.5 mL of medium and passed three times through a 25-gage needle, filtered through a 0.45-μm filter, and then used to transduce cells as described in **Subheading 3.2.4.**
5. Retroviral supernatant that is not used immediately should be aliquoted and stored at −70°C.

3.2.4. Transduction of Cancer Cell Lines

1. 1×10^6 SUIT2 or SKOV3 cells are plated onto a 10-cm plate. The next day, the culture medium is removed and replaced with 4 mL of filtered concentrated retroviral supernatant containing 6 μg/mL polybrene and incubated for 16 h.
   We have shown that following transduction with concentrated retroviral supernatants, 80–90% of the target cells express Ntr, and this population could be assessed directly in dose–response experiments (*see* **Subheading 3.2.5.**). Alternatively, the cells can be selected using G418, which allows the generation of individual clones, or calculate the transduction efficiency.
2. The supernatant is removed, cells split into 2X 10-cm plates, and fresh culture medium added.
3. Forty-eight hours after retroviral transduction, 500 μg/mL of G418 is added to select clones containing the retroviral vectors. The cells are fed with medium containing G418 every 3 d until clones are visible (usually 7–10 d).
4. Once G418-resistant clones are visible on the transduction plates, the culture medium is removed and plates washed in PBS. Cloning rings are placed over the clones and cells removed with trypsin. Each clone is grown in 1 well of a 24-well plate until confluent and then transferred into a 25-cm² flask. Clones are then assayed for Ntr expression.

3.2.5. Analysis of Nitroreductase Gene Expression Using CB1954 Cytotoxicity Assays

1. Nitroreductase–expressing clones and parental cell lines are plated at 5×10^3 cells/well in 96-well plates (*see* **Note 3**).
2. The next day, cells are exposed to varying concentrations of CB1954 (0–1000 μM diluted in 200 μL complete culture medium, n=6 for each treatment) for 3 d.
3. Cell survival is determined using the MTS assay (soluble MTT; Promega). Twenty-five microliters of diluted MTS solution is added per well and plates incubated at 37°C for 3–4 h.
4. Plates are read at 490 nm in a plate reader. Results are normalized so that cell survival in the absence of prodrug is 100%.

3.3. Adenoviral Delivery of Nitroreductase

3.3.1. Construction of an Adenoviral Vector Expressing Nitroreductase

Construction of the adenoviral vector Ad CMV-Ntr has been described in detail elsewhere *(14)*. The virus was generated by ligation of plasmids containing the left- and right-hand regions of the Ad5 genome in 293 cells (*see* **Note 4**). The left-hand plasmid (pPS976C4) contains nucleotides 1–10,589 of the Ad5 sequence and the right-hand plasmid (pPS972C10) contains nucleotides 10,589–35,935 *(20)*. The full-length construct was an E1,E3-deleted, replication-deficient viral genome containing CMV-Ntr in the E1 region. The viral construct was checked by restriction digest analysis and polymerase chain reaction (PCR). Virus was purified by two rounds of plaque purification and bulked up in 293 cells.

3.3.2. Bulk Preparation of Adenoviral Vectors

1. 293 cells (*see* **Note 5**) are plated into the required number of large (150-cm^2) flasks (we normally use 20–30 flasks per preparation).
2. When the cells are approx 80–90% confluent, the medium is removed and the cells infected with adenovirus in 5 mL of adenovirus infection medium. Virus at an original titer of 10^7–10^8 pfu/mL) is added at a 1 : 1000 dilution, (i.e., 5 µL/flask. Cells are incubated at 37°C for 90 min and then 20 mL of infection medium added to each flask.
3. Cells are monitored daily for evidence of a cytopathic effect (CPE).
4. When cells show a CPE, the medium turns acidic and the cells round up to give a characteristic "bunches of grapes" appearance; at this point, the cells are harvested and transferred to 250-mL centrifuge pots and spun at 700g for 10 min.
5. The supernatant is discarded into waste pots and autoclaved before disposal.
6. The cell pellet is resuspended in 1 mL infection media per flask and lysed by freezing and thawing three times (freeze in liquid N_2 and thaw at 37°C).
7. At this point, the pellet can be stored at –20°C.

3.3.3. Virus Banding

1. The cell pellet is allowed to thaw (if it had been stored at –20°C) and placed on ice.
2. Then, 1/100 volume of *N*-butanol is added to the virus and it is incubated on ice for 60 min, then spun at 2K for 10 min, and the supernatant transferred to a fresh tube.
3. The virus is layered onto a CsCl gradient, which is set up as follows: Take a SW40 tube and add 3 mL CsCl ρ=1.32 (using a 10-mL pipet), then underlay with 2 mL CsCl ρ=1.45 (using a 2-mL syringe and a 21-gage needle), then add 2 mL 40% glycerol on top of the 1.32 CsCl layer.
   Approximately 8 mL virus can be put onto each gradient, tubes are balanced by topping up the tubes with DMEM.
4. The gradients are spun in a SW40/Beckman Ultracentrifuge at 25K for 90 min at 4°C; the virus should form a discrete band (*see* **Fig. 2**)
5. The virus is harvested by puncturing the tube below the level of the virus band with a 21-gage needle and collecting drops into an 50-mL Falcon tube. As the band approached the needle, the drops are collected in a small tube or plastic bijoux until all of the virus has been harvested (usually 0.5–1.0 mL)

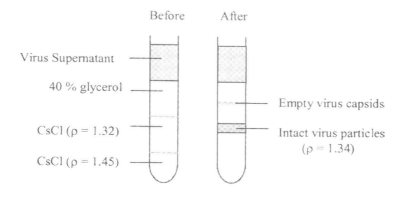

Fig. 2. Diagram showing virus-banding gradients before and after centrifugation.

3.3.4. Dialysis of Banded Virus

The virus is dialyzed to remove excess CsCl.

1. A Pierce "slide-a-lyser" dialysis cassette (molecular weight cuff-off [MWCO] 10,000) is prewetted in dialysis buffer: complete PBS (containing Mg and Ca)/10% glycerol (PBS-G).
2. The virus is taken up in a 2-mL syringe with a 21-gage needle and injected into the dialysis cassette, the air is withdrawn, and the cassette put into a float and immersed in dialysis buffer.
3. The beaker containing the dialysis buffer is placed on a stirrer and the virus is dialyzed overnight at 4°C.
4. The next morning, the buffer is replaced with fresh dialysis buffer and the virus dialyzed for 1 h. This procedure is repeated twice.
5. The virus is removed from the cassette by inserting a needle connected to a 2-mL syringe into an unused port and slowly withdrawing the virus.
6. The virus is aliquoted and stored at –70°C.

3.3.5. Determination of Viral Particle Numbers by the Pico Green DNA Assay

1. An aliquot of adenovirus is heat inactivated at 56°C for 30 min before continuing.
2. λ DNA and 20X TE are provided in the Pico Green Assay kit; the TE is diluted using deionized water and DNA standards are prepared by diluting the λ DNA to give standards of 1, 0.3, 0.1, 0.03, and 0.01 μg/mL.
3. A 10-μL aliquot of heat-inactivated banded virus is diluted to 100 μL with TE.
4. Pico Green is diluted 1 in 200 with TE (use a plastic container and keep in the dark).
5. One hundred-microliter samples of virus and DNA standards are plated into a black 96 well plate in duplicate. One hundred microliters of Pico Green reagent is added to each well and the plate covered and incubated for 2–5 min in the dark; the fluorescence is read at 480 nm excitation/520 nm emission on a plate reader.

6. A standard curve is constructed to determine the concentration of DNA. Becasue 10_µL of virus is used, the values are multiplied by 10 to calculate the DNA concentration in micrograms per milliliter. For Ad CMV–β-Gal virus 1 µg DNA = 2.7×10^{10} particles; the particle number is equal to the concentration of DNA in µg/mL $\times 2.7 \times 10^{10}$.

3.3.6. Determination of Viral Infectivity by Plaque Assay

1. 293 cells are plated at 5×10^5 cells per well in six-well plates, (two plates of cells are required for every virus being titred), and incubated overnight.
2. The next day the cells are examined; they should be 85–90% confluent.
3. Virus dilutions are made up as follows;

   −2 dilution = 20 µL banded virus + 1980 µL infection medium;
   −4 dilution = 20 µL of −2 dilution + 1980 µL infection medium;
   −6 dilution= 50 µL of −4 dilution + 4950 µL infection medium;
   −7 dilution= 500 µL of −6 dilution + 4500 µL infection medium;
   then further 1 : 10 dilutions up to a −10 dilution.

4. The medium is removed from wells and 500 µL of virus added per well. The virus should be added slowly down the side of the well to prevent detachment of the cell monolayer, then the plates tilted to ensure that the liquid covers all the cells. For each titration, the following wells are set up;

   1 Control well =500_l infection medium-no virus
   1 Well of −6 dilution;
   1 Well of −7 dilution;
   1 Well of −8 dilution;
   3 Wells of −9 dilution;
   3 Wells of −10 dilution.

5. The cells are incubated at 37°C for 90 min, and the plates rocked gently every 15 min to ensure even spread of virus across the plate and to prevent the cells from drying out.
   2X DME/nobles agar is prepared as described in **Subheading 2.**
   2X DME (at 37°C) and nobles agar (at 42°C) are mixed 1 : 1 in a prewarmed falcon tube (or tissue culture flask if using larger volumes). Twenty-five milliliters of DME/agar is required per six-well plate.
6. The infection medium is removed from each well and replaced with 4 mL of DME/agar (add 2 mL to every well, then top up with another 2 mL). Ensure that the DME/agar is added slowly down the sides of each well to prevent detachment of the cell monolayer; leave for 10 min until the agar has set.
7. Incubate at 37°C, 5% CO_2; check daily and feed with 3–4 mL DME + agar every 4 d.
8. Plaques should start to appear around d 5–7; count plaques at day 10.

To calculate the viral titer:
If you have two, three, and four plaques on the three wells of the −10 dilution

$$\frac{2+3+4}{3} = (3 \times \text{dilution factor} -10) \times 2 \text{ (as infected in 500 µL)} = 6 \times 10^{10} \text{ pfu/mL}$$

3.4. Analysis of Nitroreductase Gene Expression

3.4.1. CB1954 Cytotoxicity Assays Following Infection With Adenoviruses Expressing Nitroreductase

1. Cells are plated at 2.5×10^5 cells/plate in 6-cm plates.
2. The next day, a cell count is performed and the exact number of cells per plate determined.
3. The cells are infected with Ad-CMV-Ntr at a range of MOIs, which is the number of plaque-forming units per cell. We normally used between 10 and 350 pfu/cell, depending on the susceptibility of the target cell to adenoviral infection. Virus is diluted in Ad infection medium and the cells infected in 300 μL/plate for 90 min. The plates are tilted every 15 min to prevent the cells from drying out. After 90 min, 4 mL of Ad infection medium is added and the plates are incubated overnight
4. The next day the cells are trypinised and replated into 96-well plates at 1×10^4 cells/well.
5. After 24 h, the cells are exposed to varying concentrations of CB1954 (0–1000 μM diluted in 200 μL Ad infection medium, n=6 for each treatment) for 3 d.
6. Cell survival is determined using the MTS assay (soluble MTT; Promega). Twenty-five microliters of diluted MTS solution is added per well and plates are incubated at 37°C for 3–4 h.
7. Plates are read at 490 nm in a plate reader. Results are normalized so that cell survival in the absence of prodrug is 100%.

3.4.2. Examination of Ntr Protein Expression by Western Blotting

1. Cells expressing nitroreductase are grown in 25-cm^2 flasks until confluent, washed and harvested by trypsinisation.
2. Cell pellets are resuspended in 200 μL of urea buffer and sonicated for 10 s on setting 2 using a W380 ultrasonic processor (Life Science Labs, Luton, Bedfordshire, UK).
3. Protein concentration is measured using the Bio-Rad protein assay.
4. Protein samples are denatured at 90°C for 5 min and put on ice to cool. Twenty micrograms of protein per track is separated on a 15% sodium dodecyl sulfate (SDS) polyacylamide gel and transferred to a Immobilon P membrane by semidry electroblotting (80 mA for 15 min using a LKB Novablot electrophoretic transfer apparatus).
5. Blots are blocked in 20% nonfat milk, washed, and incubated with primary rabbit or sheep antibodies raised against purified Ntr protein (1 : 1500 dilution, 4°C for 16 h) and 2° horseradish peroxidase coupled antirabbit IgG or donkey antisheep IgG depending upon the 1° antibody used (1 : 10,000 dilution, room temperature for 90 min).
6. Antibody binding is visualized by enhanced chemiluminescence (ECL) using the Amersham Western blotting detection reagents.

3.5. In Vivo Tumor Models

Xenografts were grown in adult female BALB/c nude mice (aged 10–12 wk) obtained from the Biomedical Services Unit, University of Birmingham. Procedures were performed in accordance with the guidelines produced by the UK Co-ordinating Committee on Cancer Research (UKCCCR) and were performed with the authority of Home Office Project and Personal Licences.

3.5.1. Subcutaneous Tumors Stably Expressing Nitroreductase

Cell lines stably expressing Ntr can be produced by transfection or retroviral transduction. We have used SKOV-Ntr or SUIT-Ntr clones that were generated by retroviral transduction (*see* **Subheading 3.2.4.**).

1. Cells are grown in 150-cm^2 tissue culture flasks until confluent, harvested by trypsinization, and then washed and resuspended in PBS at 2.5×10^7 cells/mL.
2. Adult female BALB/c nude mice are lightly anaesthetized using Halothane (3% in 2 L/min O$_2$).
3. 5×10^6 cells (in 200 μL) are implanted subcutaneously (s.c.) into the right flank of the mice. Animals are weighed and monitored daily.
4. When tumors first appeared, usually 7–10 days after implantation, the mice are treated with two subsequent daily ip injections of 40 mg/kg CB1954 or vehicle (NMP : PEG in PBS). The mice are retreated with CB 1954 7 days after the first injection of CB1954.
5. Animals are monitored daily, tumor sizes are measured twice weekly with calipers and tumor volumes are calculated as,

   $V = (4/3\ \pi \times \text{length}/2 \times \text{width}/2 \times \text{height})/2.$
6. Animals are culled when tumor volumes exceeded 1000 mm^3 or if they display any clinical signs of illness.
7. Tumor volumes and survival times are calculated and analyzed statistically (Graph-Pad Prism) using ANOVA and Kaplan-Meier survival curves to compare the treatment groups.

3.6. Adenoviral Delivery of Nitroreductase

3.6.1. Direct Intratumoral Injection of Adenoviruses

SKOV3 and SUIT2 cells are grown in 150-cm^2 tissue culture flasks until confluent, harvested by trypsinization, and then washed and resuspended in PBS at 2.5×10^7 cells/mL.

1. Female BALB/c nude mice are lightly anaesthetized using Halothane (3% in 2 L/min O$_2$).
2. Then 5×10^6 cells (in 200 μL) are implanted subcutaneously into the right flank of the mice. Animals are weighed and monitored daily.
3. When the tumors are approx 60–80 mm^3, the mice are anaesthetised and 50 μL of banded virus (containing 5×10^8 to 2×10^9 plaque–forming units) is injected into the tumors using a 0.5-mL insulin syringe (Becton-Dickinson).
4. Two days later, the mice are treated with two subsequent daily ip injections of 40 mg/kg CB1954 or vehicle.
5. Animals are monitored daily, tumor sizes are measured twice weekly with calipers, and tumor volumes are calculated as follows:

   $V = (4/3\ \pi \times \text{length}/2 \times \text{width}/2 \times \text{height})/2.$
6. Animals are sacrificed when tumor volumes exceeded 1000 mm^3 or if they display any clinical signs of illness.
7. Tumor volumes and survival times are calculated and analyzed statistically to compare the treatment groups.

3.6.2. Intraperitoneal Delivery of Nitroreductase-Expressing Adenoviruses

1. SUIT2 cells are grown in 150-cm^3 tissue culture flasks until confluent, harvested by trypsinization, and then washed and resuspended in PBS at 7.5×10^6 cells/mL.

2. Female BALB/C nude mice are lightly anaesthetized using Halothane (3% in 2 L/min O_2).
3. Then 3×10^6 cells (in 400 μL) are implanted intraperitoneally. Animals are weighed and monitored daily.
4. Two days after the cells are implanted, virus is administered by i.p. injection. The dose used is $1–3 \times 10^{10}$ viral particles diluted into 400 μL PBS–glycerol.
5. Two days later, the mice are treated with two subsequent daily ip injections of 40 mg/kg CB1954 or vehicle.
6. Animals are monitored and weighed daily, tumor burden being apparent by an increase in body weight and abdominal distension.
7. Animals are sacrificed if they demonstrate a >15% increase in body weight or if they display any clinical signs of illness.
8. Survival times are calculated and analyzed statistically to compare the treatment groups.

3.7. Clinical Trial Protocol

All clinical trials must comply with the appropriate legal and ethical requirements. In the United Kingdom, trials require the approval of the local Research and Ethics Committee, the Gene Therapy Advisory Committee (GTAC), the Medicines Control Agency (MCA), and the Health and Safety Executive (HSE).

We present here "A Study of Gene Directed Enzyme Prodrug Therapy in Primary and Metastatic Liver Cancer: Intratumoral administration of CTL 102, a replication-deficient adenovirus encoding the Nitroreductase Gene, With Intravenous Administration of the Prodrug CB 1954."

3.7.1. Objectives

1. To determine the safety and tolerability of direct intratumoral administration of escalating doses of a replication-deficient adenovirus carrying the nitroreductase (Ntr) gene under the control of the CMV promoter to patients with primary and secondary hepatic tumors, some of whom will undergo surgical resection of the tumor. Patients with inoperable disease will be treated 2 d following viral inoculation with an intravenous infusion of the prodrug CB1954.
2. To show gene expression of Ntr in resected specimens.
3. To determine evidence of prodrug activation following appropriately timed sequential administration of CTL 102 and CB 1954.
4. To show some evidence of efficacy in patients with inoperable disease.

3.7.2. Study Design

This is an open-label, nonrandomized, multicenter, sequential group study. Groups of three patients will be dosed with CTL 102 in increasing steps at 10^8, 10^9, 10^{10}, 10^{11}, and 5×10^{11} particles/tumor. In patients with inoperable disease, this will be followed 2 days later by a fixed dose of CB1954 (24 mg/m^2). Dose escalations will be dependent on tolerability. In this way, dosing of CTL 102 will be titrated up to the maximum tolerated dose (MTD). Initially, patients with operable disease will be recruited to the study, and only when it is possible to demonstrate expression of the *ntr* gene using immunocytochemical methods will patients with inoperable disease join the study.

The MTD will be defined as being reached if one-third or more of patients show evidence of significant treatment-related toxicity at that particular dose. Thus, if one out of three patients shows evidence of significant treatment-related toxicity, a further three patients will be treated. If one of these additional three patients shows evidence of significant treatment-related toxicity, then the MTD will have been reached, and the study terminates. If less than one-third of patients (i.e., less than either one out of three or two out of six) shows evidence of significant treatment-related toxicity, or there is no treatment-related toxicity at that dose, then the virus dose will be increased to the next level.

3.7.3. Treatment Procedures

3.7.3.1. VIRUS PREPARATION

1. Virus will be supplied in predispensed aliquots by ML Laboratories, stored in a specified area of the hospital pharmacy under the supervision of the Principal Pharmacist, and prepared for administration in a designated clean room and sterile hood in the pharmacy sterile lab, which meets appropriate health and safety criteria (e.g. HSE) for handling recombinant virus.
2. Patients will be injected with the virus using ultrasound guidance in an appropriately approved (HSE) facility for gene therapy. Reverse-barrier nursing will apply while the patient is in the unit to minimize risk of inadvertent spread of virus. Patients will remain in the gene therapy unit until viral shedding has ceased. All clinical waste contaminated with virus will be autoclaved before disposal. Samples sent to the laboratory will be discussed in advance with the laboratory directors and will be clearly labelled.
3. Materials to be analyzed for the presence of virus or for expression of Ntr will be handled in the Gene Therapy containment laboratory (level 2+ containment) until virus inactivation has been achieved by conventional methods. Staff with prior experience of working with viruses will perform the work. All materials for analysis will be transported by hand in a shatter-resistant, closed container.
4. Because of blood sample requirements for virus and CB1954 kinetics a peripheral venous cannula of at least 21G will be inserted and flushed with heparinized saline by research nursing staff who are qualified to undertake the procedure. The cannula is to be used for blood sample withdrawal and, therefore, the ability to withdraw blood should be checked and the cannula kept patent with heparinized saline flushes for up to 72 h. If central venous access is already available, this may be used, but a central venous cannula will not be inserted solely for the purposes of this study.

3.7.3.2. TUMOR INJECTION

Direct injection of the virus under ultrasound guidance will be performed in a room approved for gene therapy studies, by a hepato-biliary radiologist experienced in percutaneous procedures, in the designated radiology procedures room under aseptic conditions using lignocaine local anaesthetic and iodine antisepsis, unless allergies contraindicate. The liver is imaged by ultrasound and a 22-gage needle is advanced percutaneously into only one previously selected tumor nodule. After radiological confirmation, the adenovirus (in a volume of 0.25 mL) is injected directly into the tumor nodule.

3.7.3.3. PRODRUG ADMINISTRATION

An intravenous line will be established using a 500-mL bag of normal saline. A port on the iv line will be established and an infusion of CB1954 in buffered saline and organic solvents connected. CB1954 will be administered over a period of 15 min. The total dose administered will be 24 mg/m^2.

3.7.3.4. BLOOD SAMPLES FOR ANTI-AD AND ANTI-NTR ANTIBODIES

Five-milliliter blood samples will be collected for the measurement of anti-Ad and anti-NTR antibodies. These measurements will be conducted at the following time-points:

baseline, d 14 and 28, and 2 and 3 mo.

A group-specific enzyme-linked immunosorbent (ELISA) assay will indicate seroconversion; in this case, a virus neutralization test will indicate if the response is specific to Ad5.

3.7.3.5. SAMPLES FOR VIRUS SHEDDING

Virus shedding will be determined by measurement of plasma, urine and feces. Samples of each will be measured at baseline. Plasma, urine, and feces are measured daily until negative results indicate viral clearance. For fecal samples, about 0.1 g is required. For urine samples about 5ml should be collected into plain tubes at each daily assessment point. For plasma measurements about 2ml blood should be collected (approx 1 mL plasma) into citrate tubes at each daily assessment point.

3.7.3.6. BLOOD SAMPLES FOR VIRUS KINETICS

Five-milliliter blood samples are taken at the following times: baseline, 0.5, 1, 2, 4, 8, 24, 48, and 72 h postdose.

3.7.3.7. BLOOD SAMPLES FOR CB 1954 PHARMACOKINETICS

Inoperable patients will receive a 15-min infusion of CB1954 at a dose of 24 mg/m^2, 48 h after virus inoculation. The plasma–concentration time profile of CB1954 will be monitored by collection of peripheral venous samples. Blood samples are taken into heparin tubes at the end of the CB1954 infusion (time 0) and then at subsequent intervals of 0.1, 0.25, 0.5, 1, 2, 4, and 6 h postdose. The blood is centrifuged at 1400*g* for 10 min, to separate cells from plasma and stored at –20°C in freezer in a the HSE designated laboratories until analyzed. The CB1954 concentration will be estimated using a sensitive and specific high-performance liquid chromatography (HPLC) assay with a coefficient of variation of <5%.

3.7.3.8. SURGICAL RESECTION

Two to five days after virus injection, after detectable virus shedding has ceased, the patient will undergo partial hepatectomy as planned, according to the usual surgical protocol. No extra procedures will be performed. A portion of the resected liver will then be subject to histological and immunocytochemical analysis.

3.7.3.9. HISTOLOGICAL EXAMINATION

The resected liver will be fixed and stained for the presence of adenovirus using a monoclonal antibody to Ad5 hexon (major capsid protein) and for nitroreductase with an available polyclonal antiserum. The proportions of different cell types (principally tumor cells, hepatocytes, and lymphocytes) will also be assessed from this material, using immunocytochemical stains (e.g., epithelial membrane antigen [EMA], pancytokeratins).

Estimates of apoptotic cell deaths will be made using accepted morphologic criteria, in tumor and normal hepatic tissue.

3.7.4. Adverse Events

All treatment-related adverse events occurring during the course of the study should be documented on the Case Record Form and reported without delay by Cobra Therapeutics Ltd to appropriate regulatory authorities. An adverse event is any adverse change from the patient's pretreatment condition.

3.7.4.1. DOSE-LIMITING TOXICITY

Common toxicity criteria will be used for monitoring and reporting purposes. Two toxicity scores will be allocated; the first will include any adverse events within the 48 h following virus administration and will be considered acute viral toxicity and the second will include any subsequent toxicity and will be attributed to the combination of virus and prodrug. Either of these toxicities will be considered dose limiting, as follows:

Dose-limting toxicity (DLT) will be defined as grade 2 renal, hepatic, or neurological toxicity, grade 3 mucositis or diarrhea, or grade 4 hematological toxicity that lasts more than 1 wk or is associated with fever.

If DLT is documented in one of the three patients at a particular dose level, a further three patients will be treated at the same level. If no further problems arise in those patients, the dose will be escalated and recruitment commenced at the next dose level.

3.7.4.2. MAXIMUM TOLERATED DOSE

The maximum tolerated dose is defined as the dose at which one-third or more of the patient cohort develop dose-limiting toxicity (i.e., if two or more out of six patients develop DLT. Note: If one patient out of the intended cohort of three patients develops DLT a further three patients will be treated at that level).

Follow-up Evaluation

Follow-up assessments will be made as necessary to establish normalization or other explanation of any abnormal physical signs, symptoms, or laboratory tests that are thought, by the investigator, to be attributable to study medication. Patients will be followed monthly for the first 3 mo. Patients will also be followed every 3 mo, up to 12 mo, for safety assessments of clinical examination and toxicity if the 3 mo assessment indicates that this is necessary. These patients will be then followed at least annually during their lifetime. Subsequent follow-up assessments will be by local investigators' protocol.

4. Notes

1. The nitroreductase gene can also be readily obtained by PCR from *E. coli* genomic DNA; the sequence in *E. coli* K12 and derived strains (e.g., DH5α) are identical to the original published sequence from *E. coli* B, but some differences have been noted in *E. coli* BL21 *(22)*.
2. One of the major problems with using retroviruses is the potential to generate replication-competent retroviruses (RCR). Original producer cells contained only two retroviral plas-

mids, the first encoding the *gag, pol,* and *env* genes but lacking the packaging signal Ψ and the second plasmid containing the viral long terminal repeats (LTRs), the transgene of interest, and Ψ. However, frequent recombination can lead to the generation of RCR, to overcome this problem, so-called second- [called PA317 *(22)*] and third (Ψ CRIP *(23)* and gp + env AM12 *(24)* generation packaging cell lines have been developed. In these improved cells, the *gag-pol* and *env* genes are encoded on separate plasmids that are introduced sequentially into the packaging cells to prevent recombination during transfection. Although this reduces the chances of generating RCR, a report has shown that RCR have been detected using gp + env AM12 cells *(25)*. We have used the FLY RD18 retroviral packaging cells *(16)* because they have several advantages over the third-generation packaging cell lines described here. The RD18 cells are based on the human fibrosarcoma cell line HT1080 rather than 3T3 murine fibroblasts, use the env gene from the cat virus RD114 and contain the 5' LTR from the Friend rather than Moloney strain of MLV. There have been no reports of RCR arising from the RD18 cells and the virus is resistant to inactivation by human complement *(16)*.

3. If experiments are to assess the bystander effect, cells should be plated at a higher cell density. We have found that 5×10^4 cells/p well in a 96-well plate gives optimal results *(12)*.

4. Other methods for the construction of adenoviral vectors are readily available. A recently developed *(25)*, commercially available method is the "AdEasy system" (Stratagene, cat. no. 240009). The AdEasy adenoviral vector system simplifies the production of recombinant adenoviruses. The construction of a recombinant adenoviral vector using the AdEasy system is a two-step process in which the desired expression cassette is first subcloned into a shuttle vector, and subsequently transferred into the adenoviral genome by means of homologous recombination in *E.coli.*

5. We have also used 911 packaging cells, which are Human Embryonic Retinoblasts transformed with plasmids containing the E1 sequences of Ad 5 *(27)*. These cells are only available under licence from Leiden University Medical Center, Holland.

6. **Safety Considerations:**
The ability of retroviruses to insert their genomes stably into the DNA of replicating host cells makes them attractive gene transfer vectors. The genetically modified retroviral vectors typically retain the LTRs and packaging signal and can accommodate up to around 8 kb of foreign DNA, but all remaining viral functions are provided *in trans* in specially constructed packaging cell lines. In the event of accidental human inoculation with the retroviral Ntr-expression vectors, it is possible that the nucleic acid sequences would become integrated into the chromosomal DNA of a host cell. The potential target cell population is very small (e.g., a low proportion of cells in the basal layer of the epidermis) and it would require a fairly large volume of virus-containing fluid to be delivered (e.g., to a wounded area of the skin), before proviral integration into a host cell would be a likely outcome. The constructs are replication defective and so will be incapable of further spread within the host. Virus stocks and producer cells should be tested for the presence of RCR (e.g., by ability to mobilize a defective provirus carrying a G418-resistance gene) and any contaminated stocks discarded. Expression of Ntr is not expected to be harmful to the cell, although there may be a remote possibility of inducing autoimmunity in the unlikely event that a large number of cells in the body were accidentally transduced by the virus.

Ad5 infects humans and is classified as an ACDP group 2 pathogen. In healthy adults it does not normally cause overt disease, and most adults will have been exposed to one of the common subgroup C viruses (includes Ad5) by adolescence. Ad5 primarily infects the respiratory tract, although it is shed via the gut and can probably replicate therein. The vectors used in this work are replication defective by virtue of E1 deletion, and so are regarded as safer than the wild-type virus. Any exposure to recombinant virus would be likely to elicit an immune response to the incoming virus, and as the major capsid protein (hexon) is the major neutralizing antigen, this would be primarily a type 5 response. Many individuals have pre-existing immunity to Ad5 and a secondary immune response to the recombinant virus would be expected. All viral manipulations are designed to prevent aerosol generation. Work with large-scale virus preparations and high concentrations of virus should be conducted in a class II cabinet. All liquid waste should be autoclaved and contaminated material should be soaked in 1% Virkon, for at least 30 min before disposal.

References

1. Khan, A. H. and Ross, W. C. J. (1969/1970) Tumor growth inhibitory nitrophenyllaziridines and related compounds: structure activity relationships. *Chem. Biol. Interact.* **1**, 27–47.
2. Cobb, L. M., Connors, T. A., Elson, L. A., et al. (1969). 2,4-dinitro-5-ethyleneiminobenzamide (CB1954): a potent and selective inhibitor of the growth of the Walker carcinoma 256. *Biochem. Pharmacol.*, **18**, 1519-1527.
3. Chung-Faye, G. A., Palmer, D., Anderson, D., et al. (2001) Virus directed, enzyme prodrug therapy with Nitroimidazole Reductase: A phase I and pharmacokinetic study of its prodrug, CB1954. *Clin. Cancer Res.*, in press.
4. Knox, R. J., Boland, M., Friedlos, F., Coles, B., Southan, C., and Roberts, J. J. (1988) The nitroreductase enzyme in Walker cells that activates 5-(aziridin-1-yl)-2,4-dinitrobenzamide (CB 1954) to 5-(aziridin-1-yl)-4-hydroxylamino-2-nitrobenzamide is a form of NAD(P)H dehydrogenase (quinone) (EC 1.6.99.2). *Biochem. Pharmacol.*, **37**, 4661-4669.
5. Knox, R. J., Friedlos, F., Marchbank, T. and Roberts, J. J. (1991) Bioactivation of CB1954: reaction of the active 4-hydroxylamino derivative with thioesters to form the ultimate DNA-DNA interstrand crosslinking species. *Biochem. Pharmacol.* **42**, 1691-1697.
6. Anlezark, G.M., Melton, R.G., Sherwood, R.F., Coles, B., Friedlos, F. and Knox R.J. (1992). The bioactivation of 5-(aziridin-1-yl)-2,4-dinitrobenzamide (CB1954) I: Purification and properties of a nitroreductase enzyme from Escherichia coli - a potential enzyme for antibody-directed enzyme prodrug therapy (ADEPT). *Biochem. Pharmacol.*, **44**, 2289-2295.
7. Boland, M.P., Knox, R.J., and Roberts, J.J. (1991) The differences in kinetics of rat and human DT-diaphorase result in a differential sensitivity of derived cell lines to CB1954 (5-(aziridin-1-yl)-2,4-dinitrobenzamide). *Biochem. Pharmacol.* **41**, 867-875.
8. Chen, S., Know, R., Lewis, A.D., et al. (1995). Catalytic properties of NAD(P)H: quinone acceptor oxidoreductase: study involving mouse, rat human and mouse-rat chimeric enzymes. *Mol. Pharmacol.*, **47**, 934-939.
9. Chen, S., Knox, R., Wu, K., et al. (1997). Molecular basis of the catalytic differences among DT-diaphorase of human, rat and mouse. *J. Biol. Chem.*, **272**, 1437-1439.
10. Bridgwater, J. A., Springer, C. J., Knox, R. J., et al. (1995) Expression of the bacterial nitroreductase enzyme in mammalian cells renders them selectively sensitive to killing by the prodrug CB1954. *Eur. J. Cancer* **31a**, 2362-2370.
11. Miller, A. D. and Rosman, G. J. (1989) Improved retroviral vectors for gene transfer and expression. *BioTechniques* **7**, 980-988.
12. Green, N. K., Youngs, D. J., Neoptolemos, J. P., et al. (1997). Sensitization of colorectal and pancreatic cancer cell lines to the prodrug 5-(aziridin-1-yl)-2,4-dinitrobenzamide

(CB1954) by retroviral transduction and expression of the *E. coli* nitroreductase gene. *Cancer Gene Ther.* **4**, 229-238.

13. McNeish, I. A., Green, N. K., Gilligan, M. G., et al. Virus directed enzyme prodrug therapy for ovarian and pancreatic cancer using retrovirally delivered E.coli nitroreductase and CB1954. *Gene Ther.* **5**, 1061-1069.
14. Weedon, S. W., Green, N. K., McNeish, I. A., et al. (2000). Sensitisation of human carcinoma cells to the prodrug CB1954 by adenovirus vector-mediated expression of *E. coli* nitroreductase. *Int. J. Cancer* **86**, 848-854.
15. Graham, F. L., Smiley, J., Russell, W. C., and Nairn R. (1977) Characteristics of a human cell line transformed by DNA from human adenovirus type 5. *J. Gen. Virol.*, **36(1)**, 59-74;
16. Cosset, F. L., Takeuchi, Y., Battini, J. L., Weiss, R. A., and Collins, M.K. (1995) High-titer packaging cells producing recombinant retroviruses resistant to human serum. *J. Virol*, **69(12)**, 7430-7436.
17. Kozak, M. (1986) Point mutations define a sequence flanking the AUG initiator codon that modulates translation by eukaryotic ribosomes. *Cell* **44**, 283-292.
18. Gerin, P. A., Gilligan, M. G., Searle, P. F., and Al-Rubeai, M. (1999). Improved titers of retroviral vectors from the human FLY RD18 packaging cell line in serum- and protein-free medium. *Hum. Gene Ther.* **10(12)**, 1965-1974.
19. Bowles, N. E., Eisensmith, R. C., Mohuiddin, R., Pyron, M., and Woo, S.L. (1996) A simple and efficient method for the concentration and purification of recombinant retrovirus for increased hepatocyte transduction in vivo. *Hum. Gene Ther.* **7(14)**, 1735-1742.
20. Gilligan, M. G., Knox, P., Weedon, S., et al. (1998) Adenoviral delivery of B7-1 (CD80) increases the immunogenicity of human ovarian and cervical carcinoma cells. *Gene Ther.*, **5(7)**, 965-974.
21. Grove, J. I., Searle, P. F., Weedon, S. J, Green, N. K, McNeish, I. A., and Kerr, D. J. (1999). Virus-directed enzyme prodrug therapy using CB1954. *Anticancer Drug Design,* **14(6)**, 461-472.
22. Miller, A. D. and Buttimore, C. (1986) Redesign of retrovirus packaging lines to avoid recombination leading to helper virus production. *Mol. Cell. Biol.*, **6**, 2895-2909.
23. Danos. O. and Mulligan, R. C. (1998) Safe and efficient generation of recombinant retroviruses with amphotrophic and ecotropic host ranges. *Proc. Natl. Acad. Sci. USA*, **86**, 6460-6464.
24. Markowitz, D., Goff, S., and Bank A. (1998) Construction and use of a safe and efficient amphotrophic packaging cell line. *Virology* **167**, 400-406.
25. Tong-Chuan, H., Zhou, S., Da Costa, L. T., Yu, J., Kinzler, K. W., and Vogelstein, B. (1998). A simplified system for generating recombinant adenoviruses. *Proc. Natl. Acad. Sci. USA*, **95**, 2509-2514.
26. Fallaux, F. J., Kranenburg, O., Cramer, S. J., et al. (1996). Characterization of 911: a new helper cell line for the titration and propagation of early region 1-deleted adenoviral vectors. *Hum. Gene Ther.* **7(2)**, 215-222.

25

Side Effects of Suicide Gene Therapy

Marjolijn M. van der Eb, Bertie de Leeuw, Alex J. van der Eb, and Rob C. Hoeben

1. Introduction

The efficacy of standard chemotherapy tends to be limited by an inability to achieve sufficiently high drug concentrations to tumor cells without inducing concomitant toxicity elsewhere. If the tumor itself were induced to produce the drug, the efficacy would be increased. This strategy can be achieved by installing in tumor cells a gene that can activate a harmless prodrug into a cytotoxic drug. The premise is that activation of prodrugs in or near the tumor would lead locally to a high concentration of the toxic drug.

An essential factor in such strategies is the tumor specificity that can be achieved. The tools of molecular biology offer various possibilities of activating prodrugs specifically at the site of neoplastic cells. First, either the gene transfer vector or the prodrug can be targeted or administered specifically to the tumor mass (local gene and local prodrug delivery). Second, the gene vector can be modified to transduce preferentially the neoplastic cells (targeted transduction). Third, the activity of the transgene can be regulated in such a way that the transgene is preferentially active in the transformed cells (transcriptional targeting). Fourth, genes can be chosen such that have intrinsic specificity for tumor cells (tumor-specific gene products). Finally, the activated prodrug can have selectivity for the neoplastic cells (e.g., drugs that specifically kill cycling cells [viz. nucleotide analogs like 5-fluorouracil {5-FU}]).

The suicide gene therapy approach in combination with its many options to achieve tumor specificity has attracted much attention in the past years. Many approaches have been evaluated, both in preclinical and clinical experiments. These experiments have highlighted the feasibility of the approach and have lead to many powerful enzyme–prodrug combinations. However, the hurdles, limitations, and side effects of the technology have also become apparent. Here, we will summarize the potential side effects of the cancer gene therapy and, in particular, the suicide gene therapy. Rather than

From: *Methods in Molecular Medicine, Vol. 90, Suicide Gene Therapy: Methods and Reviews*
Edited by: C. J. Springer © Humana Press Inc., Totowa, NJ

listing all side effects reported, we will provide a summary of general points that need consideration when formulating a suicide gene therapy protocol. The focus will be on those aspects specific to gene therapy.

2. Safety of the Gene Vector

The unique feature that differentiates gene therapy from other cancer treatments is the transfer of a protein coding gene into some of the patient's somatic cells. Highly efficient gene transfer techniques are required to facilitate the transfer of genes into significant numbers of cells. Although several nonviral gene delivery systems have been used in experimental gene therapy research, none of the nonviral systems can match the efficiencies that can be obtained with virus-derived vectors. Therefore, in most clinical gene therapy protocols, viral vectors are used.

Viral vectors for gene therapy are among the most complex therapeutics. If used for clinical gene therapy, the batches of viral vectors must be produced following the guidelines for Good Manufacturing Practice. The quality control and quality assurance aspects associated with the clinical-grade vector production make their in-house production difficult and costly and beyond the capabilities (and budgets) of most laboratories and academic institutions. In many instances, vectors have been prepared on contract, often by industry. A detailed description of critical parameters of vector production is beyond the scope of this chapter.

2.1. Vector-Related Toxicity

In order to transduce a significant number of cells, highly concentrated stocks of viral vectors are administered to patients. It should be realized, however, that high vector doses could have acute side effects. The administration of high doses of adenovirus vectors into the liver, lung, and muscle led to hepatitis, pneumonitis, and myositis, respectively, in recipient mice (1–5) as result of an acquired immune response. In addition, activation of the innate immune system was noted in mice and in nonhuman primates. This phenomenon was most likely the cause of a fatal incident in a recent trial aimed at ameliorating the effects of ornithine transcarbamilase deficiency (6,7). Although most prominent with adenovirus vectors, some vector-related toxicity has also been observed after the administration of retrovirus packaging lines, herpesvirus, and poxvirus vectors (8–11), reviewed by Walther and Stein (12).

2.2. The Occurrence of Replication-Competent Viruses and Vector Shedding

A particular concern related to the use of replication-deficient viral vectors is the occurrence of replication-competent viruses (RCVs) in the vector stocks. RCVs may lead to a stronger antivector immune response, tissue destruction, and vector mobilization and spread. RCV can be generated during the production of the vector viruses in helper cell lines. The emergence of replication-competent retroviruses (13,14), adenoviruses (15) and wild-type adeno-associated virus (AAV) (16,17) during vector production is well documented. In most cases, the RCV is generated by homologous recombination(s) between the helper elements present in the cell line and the vector.

The risk and potential side effects are obviously strongly dependent on the nature of the RCV. New production systems, in which sequence homology between the vector and the helper cell line is minimized or completely eliminated, have reduced the magnitude of the problem. However, continuous screening of vector batches appears justified, especially when vector mutants with an altered host range are employed.

It should be borne in mind, however, that even in the cases where batches of vector are used that are free of RCVs, mobilization and potential shedding of the vector might occur in patients during a viremia with the wild-type virus from which the vector is derived. For instance, adenoviral vectors may be mobilized if a patient is infected by wild-type adenovirus. For this to occur, a wild-type virus should infect a cell that carries the vector. The mobilizing adenovirus can be one of several serotypes. In cell culture experiments, Rademaker and colleagues demonstrated that adenovirus serotype 5 (subgroup C)-derived vectors can be mobilized by serotypes of subgroup A, B, C, and E, albeit with varying efficiencies (18). Similarly, AAV vectors could be mobilized when wild-type AAV and adenoviruses or herpesviruses that could provide helper functions were present (19). Although it is unclear whether some shedding of vector viruses poses a real safety hazard for the patient or people in his vicinity, several groups are devising vectors that are less efficiently mobilized by wild-type viruses (20–23).

Depending on the route of administration of the vector viruses the patients may shed vectors for a considerable period of time after vector administration. Shedding is not dependent on the presence of corresponding RCVs in the vector batch used, although RCVs may facilitate shedding of vector viruses. In many clinical trials, sputum, urine, and feces are monitored for the presence of vector viruses.

As a result of prior exposure to the virus, some patients may have circulating antibodies that have the capacity to neutralize the vector viruses. Antibodies directed against AAV, adenovirus, herpesviruses, and vaccinia virus occur in a significant fraction of the healthy population. Although intuitively one would assume that neutralizing antibodies reduce vector shedding, hardly any data are published that formally demonstrate this hypothesis. Especially in cases where cells die by apoptosis, the vector may spread via apoptotic vesicles (24). In many countries, the protocols are required to include procedures to reduce the shedding of vector viruses after treatment. This may involve the patients being hospitalized after receiving the vector, although more recently in an increasing number of trials, the patients are released from the hospital on the day of treatment.

2.3. Pre-Existing Immunity

Administration of viral vectors to patients results in a humoral immune response against the viral proteins of the vector. The immunity will reduce the efficiency of subsequent vector administrations, especially if the vectors are delivered intravenously or intraperitoneally. The neutralizing antibodies have less impact on the efficiency upon intratumoral administration of the vector (25). A significant fraction of the population carries neutralizing antibodies against vector viruses prior to inoculation, most prominently against adenoviruses, adeno-associated viruses, herpesviruses, and vaccinia viruses (26). The pre-existing immunity may affect the gene transfer efficiency, and as a consequence, the efficacy of the treatment *(27)*. Several approaches have been taken to reduce the impact of pre-existing immunity. In adenoviruses, the hexon capsid protein is the main determinant of immunity. Adenovirus vectors have been developed in which the hexon protein of the vector virus has been replaced by the hexon of another serotype to which no pre-existing immunity exists, allowing readministration of the vector *(28–30)*. Also, adenovirus vectors are being developed based entirely on serotype 35, a serotype to which pre-existing immunity is only rarely observed *(31)*. Similar approaches have been followed with AAV vectors *(32)*. Such strategies may circumvent the variability in gene transfer efficiencies as a result of pre-existing immunity.

2.4. Mutation Induction

Vector systems are usually divided into those where the vector genome inserts itself into the host genome and those with vectors genomes that remain extrachromosomal. Integrated vectors are the system of choice if persistent expression is required. However, their insertion results in an alteration of the chromosomal DNA and therefore may lead to insertional mutagenesis. Although the risk of insertional mutagenesis is a recognized disadvantage, many gene therapy protocols embrace the use of integrating vectors. Recently, the clinical relevance of the risk of insertional mutagenesis became evident in an otherwise successful trial for treatment of patients with X-SCID. Two of the patients developed leukemia as result of insertional activation of the *LMO-2* gene.

The absence of integration is often used as a safety argument to promote the use of nonintegrating vectors, such as adenovirus-derived vectors or plasmid vectors. This argument should be used with caution *(33)*. Adenovirus DNA can recombine with chromosomal DNA, and as a result, vector sequences can become integrated into the host-cell genome. Recently, Harui and co-workers demonstrated that the frequency of adenovirus integration into chromosomal DNA was around 10^{-3}–10^{-5} event per infected cell *(34)*. However, these frequencies have been determined in established cell lines, and it is not clear whether it is justified to extrapolate these frequencies to the in vivo situation and to estimate the risk. It would be very interesting to know the frequency with which the adenovirus vectors integrate into the host-cell genome of diploid cells. In a study with E1-containing, but replication-defective adenovirus vectors in cultures of rat diploid kidney cells, Fallaux et al. *(15)* reported the frequent occurrence of transformed foci. This indicates that in diploid cells too parts of the viral genome, including the E1 region, can become integrated into the host-cell genome as a result of illegitimate recombination, a process in which the E1 proteins may participate.

In rodents, particularly, in hamsters, adenoviruses can also become integrated into the host-cell genome, as is evidenced by the occurrence of E1-containing tumors upon injection of subgroup-A adenoviruses. If one assumes the integration frequencies in vivo to be equivalent to those observed in cell lines, then one would predict from the vector amounts used for in vivo gene therapy (up to 10^{13} vector particles per dose) that a significant number of cells (even millions) may acquire genome-integrated vector fragments. Thus, it is not strictly accurate to categorize adenovirus vectors as being nonintegrating, when considering the risk of insertional mutagenesis. It should be noted that the insertion of vector sequences is not provoked by a function of the replication strategy of the adenovirus but, rather, is the result of illegitimate recombination. It seems justified, therefore, to assume that the use of other vector systems that introduce naked DNA (e.g., plasmids) into nuclei will also be accompanied by the integration of vector sequences into the host-cell genome. This being the case, the use of "nonintegrating" vectors will be associated with a small but finite risk of insertional mutagenesis and perturbation of (proto)oncogenes and tumor-suppressor genes, similar to the situation with retroviruses. However annoying this may appear at first sight, it should be seen in its proper perspective. In healthy human cells, chromosomal DNA is not static but subject to mutation and recombination. Also, human cells are modified, at a fairly high frequency, by transposable elements *(35)*. Hence, it will be extremely difficult to estimate and assess the increased risk (if any) of gene therapy for insertional mutagenesis. As long as the potential benefit outweighs the risk, one should not hesitate to choose gene therapy for the treatment of severe disorders, but it is essential to ensure a proper follow-up of all patients who participate in clinical trials.

The situation is different if there would be a risk of insertion of vector sequences into nonsomatic cells (viz. the germ-line cells). Germ-line transmission of vector sequences is clearly undesirable. However, one should realise that DNA is not static and also germ-line cells are modified at significant frequencies by transposable elements. Recently, it has been suggested to allow the frequency with which transposable elements modify the germ line be the maximally acceptable level of vector integration *(35)*. Yet, it goes without saying that if there is a chance that the vector transduces germ-line cells, the patients should be advised to use effective contraceptive treatment for some time after the treatment.

3. Safety of the Transgene Product

Not only can (components of) the vector affect the recipient cell, but also expression of the transgene may affect cell function, even in the absence of the prodrug. In experiments in rat liver, it was noted that expression of the herpes simplex virus–thymidine kinase *(HSV-TK)* gene moderately skewed the nucleotide profile, with increased concentrations of thymidine nucleotides *(36)*. It is not unreasonable to expect that expression of other prodrug-converting enzymes may influence aspects of the cellular metabolism. In addition, the products of the suicide genes may in many cases be foreign for the recipients and may lead to humoral and cellular immune responses. Indeed, in a graft-vs-leukemia protocol, with *HSV-TK* transduced T-cells, a cytotoxic T lymphocyte (CTL)-response was noted against the *TK* transgene product in 8 out of 24 recipients *(37,38)*. This thwarted the possibility to eliminate the T-cells in case graft-vs-host disease (GvHD) develops. Recently, a "human" suicide gene–prodrug combination based on the Fas-mediated cell death has been developed to overcome this problem *(38)*.

4. Safety of the Prodrug

In almost all cases, the prodrug is a small-molecule drug. Obviously, this prodrug should be evaluated thoroughly before its clinical application, and in this respect, its should not be treated differently from other experimental drugs. The production of the prodrug should be performed under the applicable guidelines and the basic toxicity and pharmacokinetics profiles should be determined. One should also consider that in particular cases, the prodrugs could be activated in vivo. For instance, if the activating enzyme is derived from bacteria (e.g., cytosine deaminase, nitroreductase), one should evaluate the prodrug activation by bacteria, for example, in the gastrointestinal tract.

If the prodrug is also indicated for other treatments (e.g., ganciclovir is used for treatment of cytomegalovirus infections), such data should be made available. However, the use of these compounds as a prodrug in a suicide gene strategy has a drawback: It disqualifies the drug for use in its standard indications. This aspect is most pertinent in those cases where the cells that have been modified to express the prodrug-activating enzyme are anticipated to persist for long periods of time. This occurs in strategies where suicide genes are transferred to allow eradication of donor T-cells in case GvHD develops. If *HSV-TK* is used as the activating enzyme, the use in these patients of ganciclovir (GCV) for indications other than the experimental gene therapy is no longer an option.

5. Safety of the Enzyme–Prodrug Combination

The safety of the enzyme–prodrug combinations should be evaluated in appropriate animal models, in which the efficacy should also be evaluated. In addition, the potential effects of expression of the suicide gene outside the target tissue should be monitored, in combination with the effects of dissemination of the activated prodrug from the target tissue. A notorious problem in this respect is the fact that adenovirus vectors have a strong tendency to transduce the liver upon intravascular administration. Because intratumoral administration has a significant risk of systemic leakage, liver transduction is often seen upon intratumoral administration of adenovirus vectors in small-animal experiments. Therefore, liver functions should be monitored in patients treated with adenovirus vectors carrying suicide genes.

6. Liver Toxicity With HSV-TK Adenoviruses: An Example

The potential of the suicide gene principle using the *HSV-TK* gene has been tested extensively. Currently, phosphorylated GCV is presumed to act via the inhibition of nuclear DNA synthesis during the S-phase thus affecting only proliferating cells *(39–41)*. We and others provided evidence that the thymidine kinase and GCV mechanism can interfere not only with proliferating cells but also with metabolically active, but normally nonproliferating cells *(42,43)*. We initiated a study on the safety and feasibility of this approach for the treatment of multiple irresectable hepatic metastases. The hepatotropic properties of recombinant adenoviral vectors, independent of the vascular administration site, can be exploited for in vivo liver-directed gene therapy. The efficacy of the suicide gene approach was confirmed by establishing complete eradication of colorectal tumor cells both in vitro and after ex vivo transduction of CC531 tumors in a rat model. In accordance with the experiments performed by others *(44,45)*, we detected no adverse effects of either ex vivo transduction of injected tumor cells or intratumoral administration of adenoviral vectors *(41)*. However, if tumor-bearing rats were injected systemically (viz., into the portal vein) with adenovirus containing the *HSV-TK* gene and subsequently treated with GCV, we could not inhibit the growth of the tumor. This suggested that either the virus dose applied was insufficient or that the tumor structure prevented efficient transduction of the tumor cells *(46)*. More importantly, TK expression in combination with GCV treatment, both in tumor-bearing and healthy rats, proved to be deleterious for the quiescent hepatocytes. This resulted in widespread disruption of the tissue structure of the liver parenchyma and severe hepatic dysfunction. Microscopic examination of liver sections showed abnormal parenchymal cells and an influx of T-cells, macrophages and monocytes, and islands of extramedullar hematopoiesis *(41)*. Extramedullar hematopoiesis has been associated with the presence of activated macrophages, which are abundantly present in the livers of TK + GCV-treated animals, creating a favorable microenvironment for hepatic hematopoiesis *(47,48)*. The induction of focal hematopoiesis in the adult rat liver has also been claimed to be a secondary effect to severe anemia *(49)*.

It has been shown by us *(50)* and by others *(1,51)* that over 90% of systemically (or portally) administered adenoviral vectors will home to, and be expressed in, the liver. Consequently, intraportally injected Ad-CMV-TK will primarily transduce the liver, thus rendering the majority of the parenchymal cells TK positive. Because our data suggest that the combination of the *HSV-TK* gene and GCV is responsible for the liver dysfunction detected in the rats, one could speculate that a minor proliferative stimulus of the liver parenchyma could be responsible for triggering a cascade of destructive events in the liver. The involvement of growing tumor tissue inside the liver parenchyma, inducing some proliferation in the adjacent liver tissue, can be excluded because non-tumor-bearing rats also show destruction of the liver parenchyma. Two factors may contribute to the sensitivity of the normally nonmitotic hepatocytes. First, adenovirus injection may trigger some hepatocytes to proliferate *(52)*. In addition, the fact that proliferation in our experiments was only marginally enhanced at death *(41)*, Brand et al. *(42)* showed significant mortality in mice upon GCV treatment started as long as 51 d after Ad-CMV-TK injection, arguing against this hypothesis. Additionally, experiments in adult transgenic mice showing GCV-induced ablation of nonproliferating thyrocytes expressing *HSV-TK* by Wallace et al. *(53)* corroborate the findings. Second, the rapid onset of toxicity and the fact that only few immune cells were found in the liver after injection of adenovirus-encoding marker genes argues against an immunological basis of the toxicity *(41)*.

Alternatively, the toxicity caused by *HSV-TK* and GCV may be brought about not only by interfering with cellular DNA synthesis but also by inhibition of mitochondrial DNA (mtDNA) synthesis in the parenchymal cells. Hepatocytes are known to be nonproliferating, but metabolically very active cells: One single hepatocyte can harbor up to 2000 mitochondria, providing the energy needed for its function. Phosphorylated nucleoside analogs appear to be transported into the mitochondria and to exert their inhibitory effect on mtDNA synthesis *(54–57)*. Mitochondria are selective in their membrane permeability, however, it has been shown *(58,59)* that other antiviral nucleotide analogs can be efficiently incorporated into mitochondrial DNA and inhibit mtDNA polymerase *(55–57)*. In humans, multisystem toxicity resulting from nucleoside analogs, affecting slowly proliferating but metabolically active tissues (liver, pancreas, muscle, neuronal tissue), has been described for zidovudine, didanosine and zalcitabine, fialuridine, stavudine, and lamivudine *(60–63)*. Recently, a clinical trial using fialuridine for the treatment of hepatitis B viral infection failed because of high liver toxicity attributed to generalized mitochondrial injury, which cost the lives of 13 of the 15 patients treated *(64)*. In line with such a mechanism, light microscopy of livers of Ad-CMV-TK-GCV-treated rats showed marked accumulation of macrovesicular and microvesicular fat, depletion of glycogen, iron precipitation, and scant hepatocellular necrosis and apoptosis. Electron microscopy revealed hypodense matrices and aberrant cristae of the mitochondria specifically in the Ad-CMV-TK-GCV-treated group, providing further evidence for mitochondrial defects. The finding that GCV nucleotides account for up to 30% of the mitochondrial nucleotide pools, already 3 d after initiation of GCV treatment further supported this observation *(36)*. In addition, a significant decrease in the mitochondrial membrane potential was observed in Ad-CMV-TK transduced rats that received GCV.

Irrespective of the underlying mechanism, the occurrence of hepatic failure emphasizes the importance of restricting the expression of the *HSV-TK* gene to the tumor. Even with extrahepatic administration, upon systemic leakage, adenoviral vectors will transduce the liver, as has been observed in experimental animal models. Already a patient receiving an adenovirus carrying the *HSV-TK* gene in a trial for prostate cancer developed grade 3 hepatotoxicity, and as a result, GCV administration had to be terminated *(65)*. Leakage of the vector and inadvertent transduction of the liver could well explain the toxicity data.

7. Epilogue

A plethora of methods is currently being evaluated for cancer gene therapy in preclinical and in clinical studies. Still, there are hurdles that need to be taken. Especially, the efficiency of gene transfer needs to be increased. Despite the high titers that can be obtained with the current viral vector systems, it proved to be difficult to achieve efficient gene transfer throughout the tumor *(66)*. The development of (conditionally) replicating vectors (viz. vectors that replicate selectively in tumor cells) will stimulate the spread of the vectors within the tumor *(67–71)*. Although it remains to be determined whether this suffices for transduction in the entire tumor *(72)*, the conditionally replicating viruses are a powerful addition to the arsenal of tools that make the future of cancer gene therapy an exciting one.

References

1. Li, Q., Kay, M. A., Finegold, M., Stratford-Perricaudet, L. D., and Woo, S. L. (1993) Assessment of recombinant adenoviral vectors for hepatic gene therapy. *Hum. Gene Ther.* **4,** 403–409.
2. O'Neal, W. K. , Zhou, H., Morral, N., et al. (1998) Toxicological comparison of E2a-deleted and first-generation adenoviral vectors expressing alpha1-antitrypsin after systemic delivery. *Hum. Gene Ther.* **9,** 1587–1598.

3. Wilmott, R. W., Amin, R. S., Perez, C. R., et al. (1996) Safety of adenovirus-mediated transfer of the human cystic fibrosis transmembrane conductance regulator cDNA to the lungs of nonhuman primates. *Hum. Gene Ther.* **7**, 301–318.
4. Yang, Y., Su, Q., Grewal, I. S., et al. (1996) Transient subversion of CD40 ligand function diminishes immune responses to adenovirus vectors in mouse liver and lung tissues. *J. Virol.* **70**, 6370–6377.
5. Hermens, W. T. and Verhaagen, J. (1997) Adenoviral vector-mediated gene expression in the nervous system of immunocompetent Wistar and T cell-deficient nude rats: preferential survival of transduced astroglial cells in nude rats. *Hum. Gene Ther.* **8**, 1049–1063.
6. Schnell, M. A., Zhang, Y., Tazelaar, J., et al. (2001) Activation of innate immunity in nonhuman primates following intraportal administration of adenoviral vectors. *Mol. Ther.* **3**, 708–722.
7. Zhang, Y., Chirmule, N., Gao, G., et al. (2001) Acute cytokine response to systemic adenoviral vectors in mice is mediated by dendritic cells and macrophages. *Mol. Ther.* **3**, 697–707.
8. Krisky, D. M., Wolfe, D., Goins, W. F., et al. (1998) Deletion of multiple immediate–early genes from herpes simplex virus reduces cytotoxicity and permits long-term gene expression in neurons. *Gene Ther.* **5**, 1593–1603.
9. Link, C. J., Jr., Seregina, T., Levy, J. P., Martin, M., Ackermann, M., and Moorman, D. W. (2000) Murine retroviral vector producer cells survival and toxicity in the dog liver. *In Vivo* **14**, 643–649.
10. Link, C. J., Jr., Moorman, D. W., Ackerman, M., Levy, J. P., and Seregina, T. (2000) Murine retroviral vector producer cells survival and toxicity in the peritoneal cavity of dogs. *In Vivo* **14**, 635–641.
11. Rampling, R., Cruickshank, G., Papanastassiou, V., et al. (2000) Toxicity evaluation of replication-competent herpes simplex virus (ICP 34.5 null mutant 1716) in patients with recurrent malignant glioma. *Gene Ther.* **7**, 859–866.
12. Walther, W. and Stein, U. (2000) Viral vectors for gene transfer: a review of their use in the treatment of human diseases. *Drugs* **60**, 249–271.
13. Garrett, E., Miller, A. R., Goldman, J. M., Apperley, J. F., and Melo, J. V. (2000) Characterization of recombination events leading to the production of an ecotropic replication-competent retrovirus in a GP+envAM12-derived producer cell line. *Virology* **266**, 170–179.
14. Otto, E., Jones-Trower, A., Vanin, E. F., et al. (1994) Characterization of a replication-competent retrovirus resulting from recombination of packaging and vector sequences. *Hum. Gene Ther.* **5**, 567–575.
15. Fallaux, F. J., Van der Eb, A. J., and Hoeben, R. C. (1999) Who's afraid of replication-competent adenoviruses? *Gene Ther.* **6**, 709–712.
16. Wang, X. S., Khuntirat, B., Qing, K., et al. (1998) Characterization of wild-type adeno-associated virus type 2-like particles generated during recombinant viral vector production and strategies for their elimination. *J. Virol.* **72**, 5472–5480.
17. Allen, J. M., Debelak, D. J., Reynolds, T. C., and Miller, A. D. (1997) Identification and elimination of replication-competent adeno-associated virus (AAV) that can arise by nonhomologous recombination during AAV vector production. *J. Virol.* **71**, 6816–6822.
18. Rademaker, H. J., Abou El Hassan, M., and Hoeben, R. C. (2002) Mobilization of E1-deleted adenovirus type 5-derived vectors by wild-type viruses of other serotypes. *J. Gen. Virol.* **83**, 1311–1314.
19. Afione, S. A., Conrad, C. K., Kearns, W. G., et al. (1996) In vivo model of adeno-associated virus vector persistence and rescue. *J. Virol.* **70**, 3235–3241.

20. Imler, J. L., Bout, A., Dreyer, D., et al. (1995) Trans-complementation of E1-deleted adenovirus: a new vector to reduce the possibility of codissemination of wild-type and recombinant adenoviruses. *Hum. Gene Ther.* **6,** 711–721.

21. Yu, S. F., von Ruden, T., Kantoff, P. W., et al. (1986) Self-inactivating retroviral vectors designed for transfer of whole genes into mammalian cells. *Proc. Natl. Acad. Sci. USA* **83,** 3194–3198.

22. Naviaux, R. K., Costanzi, E., Haas, M., and Verma, I. M. (1996) The pCL vector system: rapid production of helper-free, high-titer, recombinant retroviruses. *J. Virol.* **70,** 5701–5705.

23. Olsen, J. C. and Swanstrom, R. (1985) A new pathway in the generation of defective retrovirus DNA. *J. Virol.* **56,** 779–789.

24. Mi,J., Li,Z.Y., Ni,S., Steinwaerder,D., and Lieber,A. (2001) Induced apoptosis supports spread of adenovirus vectors in tumors. *Hum. Gene Ther.* **12,** 1343–1352.

25. Bramson, J. L., Hitt, M., Gauldie, J., and Graham, F. L. (1997) Pre-existing immunity to adenovirus does not prevent tumor regression following intratumoral administration of a vector expressing IL-12 but inhibits virus dissemination. *Gene Ther.* **4,** 1069–1076.

26. Chirmule, N., Propert, K., Magosin, S., Qian, Y., Qian, R., and Wilson, J. (1999) Immune responses to adenovirus and adeno-associated virus in humans. *Gene Ther.* **6,** 1574–583.

27. Elshami, A. A., Kucharczuk, J. C., Sterman, D. H., et al. (1995) The role of immunosuppression in the efficacy of cancer gene therapy using adenovirus transfer of the herpes simplex thymidine kinase gene. *Ann. Surg.* **222,** 298–307.

28. Mastrangeli, A., Harvey, B. G., Yao, J., et al. (1996) "Sero-switch" adenovirus-mediated in vivo gene transfer: circumvention of anti-adenovirus humoral immune defenses against repeat adenovirus vector administration by changing the adenovirus serotype. *Hum. Gene Ther.* **7,** 79–87.

29. Roy, S., Shirley, P. S., McClelland, A., and Kaleko, M. (1998) Circumvention of immunity to the adenovirus major coat protein hexon. *J. Virol.* **72,** 6875–6879.

30. Parks, R., Evelegh, C., and Graham, F. (1999) Use of helper-dependent adenoviral vectors of alternative serotypes permits repeat vector administration. *Gene Ther.* **6,** 1565–1573.

31. Goossens, P. H., Vogels, R., Pieterman, E., et al. (2001) The influence of synovial fluid on adenovirus-mediated gene transfer to the synovial tissue. *Arthritis Rheum.* **44,** 48–52.

32. Rutledge, E. A., Halbert, C. L., and Russell, D. W. (1998) Infectious clones and vectors derived from adeno-associated virus (AAV) serotypes other than AAV type 2. *J. Virol.* **72,** 309–319.

33. Schagen, F. H., Rademaker, H. J., Fallaux, F. J., and Hoeben, R. C. (2000) Insertion vectors for gene therapy. *Gene Ther.* **7,** 271–272.

34. Harui, A., Suzuki, S., Kochanek, S., and Mitani, K. (1999) Frequency and stability of chromosomal integration of adenovirus vectors. *J. Virol.* **73,** 6141–6146.

35. Kazazian, H. H., Jr. (1999) An estimated frequency of endogenous insertional mutations in humans. *Nature Genet.* **22,** 130.

36. Van der Eb, M. M., Geutskens, S. B., Van Kuilenburg, A. B. P., et al. (2003) Ganciclovir nucleotides accumulate in mitochondria of rat liver cells expressing the herpes simplex virus thymidine kinase gene. *J. Gene Med.* (in press).

37. Bordignon, C., Bonini, C., Verzeletti, S., et al. (1995) Transfer of the *HSV-TK* gene into donor peripheral blood lymphocytes for in vivo modulation of donor anti-tumor immunity after allogeneic bone marrow transplantation. *Hum. Gene Ther.* **6,** 813–819.

38. Thomis, D. C., Marktel, S., Bonini, C., et al. (2001) A Fas-based suicide switch in human T cells for the treatment of graft-versus-host disease. *Blood* **97,** 1249–1257.

39. Culver, K. W., Ram, Z., Wallbridge, S., Ishii, H., Oldfield, E. H., and Blaese, R. M. (1992) In vivo gene transfer with retroviral vector-producer cells for treatment of experimental brain tumors. *Science* **256,** 1550–1552.

40. Moolten, F. L. (1986) Tumor chemosensitivity conferred by inserted herpes thymidine kinase genes: paradigm for a prospective cancer control strategy. *Cancer Res.* **46,** 5276–5281.

41. Van der Eb, M. M., Cramer, S. J., Vergouwe, Y., et al. (1998) Severe hepatic dysfunction after adenovirus-mediated transfer of the herpes simplex virus thymidine kinase gene and ganciclovir administration. *Gene Ther.* **5,** 451–458.

42. Brand, K., Arnold, W., Bartels, T., et al. (1997) Liver-associated toxicity of the *HSV-TK/* GCV approach and adenoviral vectors. *Cancer Gene Ther.* **4,** 9–16.

43. Bustos, M., Sangro, B., Alzuguren, P., et al. (2000) Liver damage using suicide genes. A model for oval cell activation. *Am. J. Pathol.* **157,** 549–559.

44. Chen, S. H., Chen, X. H., Wang, Y., et al. (1995) Combination gene therapy for liver metastasis of colon carcinoma in vivo. *Proc. Natl. Acad. Sci. USA* **92,** 2577–2581.

45. Eck, S. L., Alavi, J. B., Alavi, A., et al. (1996) Treatment of advanced CNS malignancies with the recombinant adenovirus H5.010RSVTK: a phase I trial. *Hum. Gene Ther.* **7,** 1465–1482.

46. Ackerman, N. B., Lien, W. M., Kondi, E. S., and Silverman, N. A. (1969) The blood supply of experimental liver metastases. I. The distribution of hepatic artery and portal vein blood to "small" and "large" tumors. *Surgery* **66,** 1067–1072.

47. Deimann, W. and Strobel, E. S. (1991) Activated macrophages induce hemopoietic islands in the adult rat liver. *Blood Cells* **17,** 97–101.

48. Ploemacher, R. E., Van Soest, P. L., and Vos, O. (1977) Kinetics of erythropoiesis in the liver induced in adult mice by phenylhydrazine. *Scand. J. Haematol.* **19,** 424–434.

49. Piacentini, G., Baronciani, L., Rapa, S., Benedetti, C., and Ninfali, P. (1990) Hepatic hematopoiesis in phenylhydrazine-induced hemolytic anemia. *Boll. Soc. Ital. Biol. Sper.* **66,** 725–728.

50. de Roos, W. K., Fallaux, F. J., Marinelli, A. W., et al. (1997) Isolated-organ perfusion for local gene delivery: efficient adenovirus-mediated gene transfer into the liver. *Gene Ther.* **4,** 55–62.

51. Smith, T. A., Mehaffey, M. G., Kayda, D. B., et al. (1993) Adenovirus mediated expression of therapeutic plasma levels of human factor IX in mice. *Nature Genet.* **5,** 397–402.

52. Lieber, A., Vrancken Peeters, M. J., et al. (1995) Adenovirus-mediated urokinase gene transfer induces liver regeneration and allows for efficient retrovirus transduction of hepatocytes in vivo. *Proc. Natl. Acad. Sci. USA* **92,** 6210–6214.

53. Wallace, H., Clarke, A. R., Harrison, D. J., Hooper, M. L., and Bishop, J. O. (1996) Ganciclovir-induced ablation non-proliferating thyrocytes expressing herpesvirus thymidine kinase occurs by p53-independent apoptosis. *Oncogene* **13,** 55–61.

54. Chen, C. H. and Cheng, Y. C. (1992) The role of cytoplasmic deoxycytidine kinase in the mitochondrial effects of the anti-human immunodeficiency virus compound, 2',3'-dideoxycytidine. *J. Biol. Chem.* **267,** 2856–2859.

55. Lewis, W., Gonzalez, B., Chomyn, A., and Papoian, T. (1992) Zidovudine induces molecular, biochemical, and ultrastructural changes in rat skeletal muscle mitochondria. *J. Clin. Invest.* **89,** 1354–1360.

56. Lewis, W. and Perrino, F. W. (1996) Severe toxicity of fialuridine (FIAU). *N. Engl. J. Med.* **334,** 1136–1138.

490   *van der Eb et al.*

57. Lewis, W., Levine, E. S., Griniuviene, B., etal. (1996) Fialuridine and its metabolites inhibit DNA polymerase gamma at sites of multiple adjacent analog incorporation, decrease mtDNA abundance, and cause mitochondrial structural defects in cultured hepatoblasts. *Proc. Natl. Acad. Sci. USA* **93,** 3592–3597.
58. Colacino, J. M., Malcolm, S. K., and Jaskunas, S. R. (1994) Effect of fialuridine on replication of mitochondrial DNA in CEM cells and in human hepatoblastoma cells in culture. *Antimicrob. Agents Chemother.* **38,** 1997–2002.
59. Cui, L., Yoon, S., Schinazi, R. F., and Sommadossi, J. P. (1995) Cellular and molecular events leading to mitochondrial toxicity of 1-(2-deoxy-2-fluoro-1-beta-D-arabinofuranosyl)-5-iodouracil in human liver cells. *J. Clin. Invest.* **95,** 555–563.
60. Bakker, H. D., Scholte, H. R., Dingemans, K. P., Spelbrink, J. N., Wijburg, F. A., and Van den, B. C. (1996) Depletion of mitochondrial deoxyribonucleic acid in a family with fatal neonatal liver disease. *J. Pediatr.* **128,** 683–687.
61. Dalakas, M. C., Illa, I., Pezeshkpour, G. H., Laukaitis, J. P., Cohen, B., and Griffin, J. L. (1990) Mitochondrial myopathy caused by long-term zidovudine therapy. *N. Engl. J. Med.* **322,** 1098–1105.
62. Freiman, J. P., Helfert, K. E., Hamrell, M. R., and Stein, D. S. (1993) Hepatomegaly with severe steatosis in HIV-seropositive patients. *AIDS* **7,** 379–385.
63. Gopinath, R., Hutcheon, M., Cheema-Dhadli, S., and Halperin, M. (1992) Chronic lactic acidosis in a patient with acquired immunodeficiency syndrome and mitochondrial myopathy: biochemical studies. *J. Am. Soc. Nephrol.* **3,** 1212–1219.
64. McKenzie, R., Fried, M. W., Sallie, R., et al. (1995) Hepatic failure and lactic acidosis due to fialuridine (FIAU), an investigational nucleoside analogue for chronic hepatitis B. *N. Engl. J. Med.* **333,** 1099–1105.
65. Herman, J. R., Adler, H. L., Aguilar-Cordova, E., et al. (1999) In situ gene therapy for adenocarcinoma of the prostate: a phase I clinical trial. *Hum. Gene Ther.* **10,** 1239–1249.
66. Kuppen, P. J., Van der Eb, M. M., Jonges, L. E., et al. (2001) Tumor structure and extracellular matrix as a possible barrier for therapeutic approaches using immune cells or adenoviruses in colorectal cancer. *Histochem. Cell Biol.* **115,** 67–72.
67. Curiel, D. T. and Rancourt, C. (1997) Conditionally replicative adenoviruses for cancer therapy. *Adv. Drug Delivery Rev.* **27,** 67–81.
68. Khuri, F. R., Nemunaitis, J., Ganly, I., et al. (2000) a controlled trial of intratumoral ONYX-015, a selectively-replicating adenovirus, in combination with cisplatin and 5-fluorouracil in patients with recurrent head and neck cancer. *Nature Med.* **6,** 879–885.
69. Miyatake, S., Iyer, A., Martuza, R. L., and Rabkin, S. D. (1997) Transcriptional targeting of herpes simplex virus for cell-specific replication. *J. Virol.* **71,** 5124–5132.
70. Oyama, M., Ohigashi, T., Hoshi, M., Murai, M., Uyemura, K., and Yazaki, T. (2001) Treatment of human renal cell carcinoma by a conditionally replicating herpes vector G207. *J. Urol.* **165,** 1274–1278.
71. Lambright, E. S., Amin, K., Wiewrodt, R., et al. (2001) Inclusion of the herpes simplex thymidine kinase gene in a replicating adenovirus does not augment antitumor efficacy. *Gene Ther.* **8,** 946–953.
72. Harrison, D., Sauthoff, H., Heitner, S., Jagirdar, J., Rom, W. N., and Hay, J. G. (2001) Wild-type adenovirus decreases tumor xenograft growth, but despite viral persistence complete tumor responses are rarely achieved: deletion of the viral E1B-19-kd gene increases the viral oncolytic effect. *Hum. Gene Ther.* **12,** 1323–1332.

26

Antibody-Directed Enzyme–Prodrug Therapy

R. Barbara Pedley, Surinder K. Sharma, Robert E. Hawkins, and Kerry A. Chester

1. Introduction

Over a century ago, Paul Ehrlich proposed the magic bullet theory of targeting therapeutic agents to specific tissues in order to increase their efficacy and reduce systemic toxicity. Because of their selectivity and the rapid development of hybridoma technology in the 1980s, monoclonal antibodies either alone or linked to a wide range of therapeutic agents such as radionuclides, drugs, toxins, enzymes, and growth factors have been used for diagnosis and therapy of diseases, particularly cancer. However, inherent problems with the monoclonal antibodies themselves, coupled with the heterogeneous structure and pathophysiology of solid tumours, reduce effective delivery following systemic administration. The more recent development of phage technology and antibody engineering is now addressing these problems by allowing the creation of antibodies with required characteristics for specific purposes. Antibody-directed enzyme–prodrug therapy (ADEPT) is a complex two-phase system in which an enzyme is targeted to the tumor site by an antibody, where it selectively activates a relatively nontoxic prodrug to a potent cytotoxic agent. This system has progressed from the monoclonal antibody approach to that of genetically engineered fusion proteins, in order to provide optimized molecules for clinical trials. This chapter will start by giving a brief overview of the field, concentrating on the developments in our own department using anti-CEA antibodies and the bacterial enzyme carboxypeptidase G2. This will be followed by a description of the major materials and methods involved in fusion protein production.

1.1. Antibody-Directed Cancer Therapy

Antibodies raised against tumor-associated antigens, such as carcinoembryonic antigen (CEA) in colorectal carcimomas, have significantly improved the selective delivery of anticancer agents (1,2). One of the most widely employed systems is

From: *Methods in Molecular Medicine, Vol. 90, Suicide Gene Therapy: Methods and Reviews*
Edited by: C. J. Springer © Humana Press Inc., Totowa, NJ

radioimmunotherapy (RIT), in which a therapeutic radionuclide such as ^{90}Y or ^{131}I is targeted to the tumor. This system has produced significant therapeutic effects in model systems and in clinical trials (3–7), but the tumors frequently regrow.

There are several reasons for the failure of antibody-directed therapies to produce cures in cancer patients, the major one being low tumor uptake because of poor target specificity and lower than optimal affinity. A further problem is the heterogeneity of tumor pathophysiology (8), particularly with regard to the distribution of blood vessels and target antigen. In comparison with drug molecules, antibodies frequently do not penetrate far from the tumor vasculature, binding to antigen close to their exit from the circulation. This is compounded by the irregular nature of the tumor blood supply, producing a heterogeneous pattern of both antibody distribution and therapeutic efficacy throughout the tumor (9). Frequently, the outer, well-perfused tumor region retains most of the antibody and receives a therapeutic radiation dose, whereas the less well-perfused inner region, containing more radio- and chemo-resistant hypoxic cells, remains relatively untreated and will continue to survive and grow (3,10). The development of phage technology and antibody engineering is providing a way of addressing these obstacles by optimizing antibodies for the delivery of therapy (11,12).

1.2. ADEPT

Antibody-directed enzyme–prodrug therapy is a two-phase system that was developed in an attempt to overcome some of the above problems associated with antibody targeting (13). In this approach a nontoxic, generally exogenous enzyme is conjugated to an antitumour antibody, adminstered systemically, and allowed to localize within the tumor and clear from normal tissues (for reviews, *see* refs. *14–17*). When there is a high tumor-to-plasma ratio of enzyme, a relatively nontoxic prodrug is given, which is catalyzed by the prelocalized enzyme to produce a potent cytotoxic agent selectively within the tumor (*see* **Fig. 1**). There are several advantages to this system: (1) There is a bystander effect because the active drug is a small molecule that can readily diffuse through the tumor to reach both antigen-positive and antigen-negative tumor cells, (2) there is an amplification step because one enzyme molecule can activate many prodrug molecules, and (3) systemic toxicity is reduced because the active drug is generated selectively within the tumor. The problems of this approach are the necessity for prolonged retention of the antibody–enzyme conjugate within the tumor and the potential immunogenicity of the conjugate when repeated therapy is employed. Antibody engineering is again allowing us to address these problems (18) and will be discussed, with the relevant practical procedures, later in the chapter.

1.3. ADEPT Employing Chemical Conjugates

1.3.1. Model Systems

Many different ADEPT systems have been developed (14–17), but the original studies employed enzymes chemically conjugated to monoclonal antibodies for tumor targeting. Both bacterial and mammalian enzymes have been evaluated as potential candidates for ADEPT (19–21). One such system employs carboxypeptidase G2 (CPG2), a well-characterized, homodimeric, bacterial enzyme with no mammalian

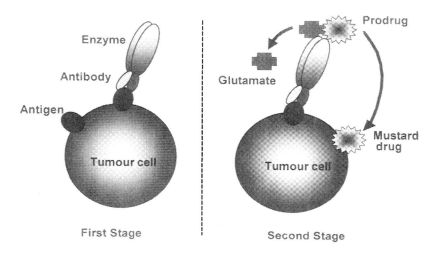

Fig. 1. ADEPT: in the first stage an antibody targets an enzyme to antigen on the tumor cell; in the second stage a prodrug is converted to an active drug by targeted enzyme at the tumor site.

equivalent *(22)*. This cleaves glutamic acid from a variety of prodrugs, releasing potent nitrogen mustard drugs within the tumor. Using CPG2 conjugated to a range of antibody F(ab')$_2$ fragments, this system has produced therapeutic efficacy in several xenograft systems in nude mice *(23–25)*.

Our initial work focused on the use of CPG2 conjugated to a F(ab)$_2$ fragment of the anti-CEA antibody A5B7 (A5B7 F(ab')$_2$-CP), and the prodrug 4-[(2-chloroethyl)(2-mesyloxyethyl) amino]benzoyl-L-glutamic acid (CMDA) in CEA-expressing colorectal xenograft models. A major problem was the relatively slow clearance of conjugate from blood and normal tissues, which necessitated one of two approaches. The first was to wait for a prolonged period of time before administering the prodrug. By giving CMDA at 96 h after conjugate administration, we avoided toxicity but still retained sufficient enzyme in the tumor to achieve positive tumor-to-blood ratios of enzyme *(see* **Fig. 2**) and significant tumor growth inhibition in therapy studies *(26,27)*. The combined administration of the antivascular agent (DMXAA) significantly enhanced the effect of ADEPT alone *(23)*. The second approach was to administer a clearing antibody to reduce circulating conjugate, allowing the prodrug to be administered while higher levels of enzyme remain in the tumor, with the potential for improved therapy. The galactosylated monoclonal antibody was directed at the active site of CPG2, which inactivated the conjugate, accelerated clearance via liver receptors, and enhanced therapy *(28)*.

The CMDA also suffered from the problem of a relatively long chemical and biological half-life, giving rise to the possibility of leakage of activated drug from the tumor and an increased risk of systemic toxicity. However, a second nitrogen mustard prodrug, 4-[N,N-bis(2-iodoethyl)amino] phenoxycarbonyl L-glutamic acid (ZD2767P) has also shown significant antitumour activity with A5B7 F(ab')$_2$-CP. The active drug

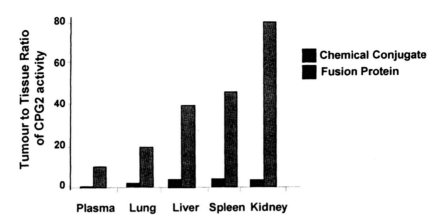

Fig. 2. Biodistribution of ADEPT: tumor to normal tissue ratios for the *E. coli*-produced fusion protein MFE::CPG2 and the chemical conjugate A5B7 F(ab')$_2$-CP, 24 h after injection.

has the advantages of a very short half-life, which reduces tumor leakage, and increased potency *(29,30)*. The primary mode of action of nitrogen mustards is the production of DNA interstrand crosslinks (ISC). A modified comet assay was therefore employed to test the therapeutic efficacy of ZD2767 in LS174T xenografts *(31)*. A clear dose–response was seen between the level of ISC, tumor growth inhibition, and ZD2767 concentration.

1.3.2. Clinical Trials

The effective treatment of colorectal xenografts using A5B7 F(ab')$_2$-CP, CMDA prodrug, and a clearing antibody led to two clinical trials *(32,33)*. The conjugate localized selectively in the tumor, and therapeutic levels of CPG2 were achieved. However, the patients rapidly developed human antimouse (HAMA) and anti-CPG2 (HACA) antibody responses. Repeat doses of ADEPT required concomitant immunosuppression with cyclosporin A, but produced partial remissions. Active drug could be detected in the plasma, indicating that successful conversion from the prodrug had taken place, but also that undesirable leakback from the tumor might be occurring *(34)*. Therefore, CMDA was replaced in a third clinical trial by ZD2767. Tumor biopsies and peripheral lymphocytes were taken where possible and analyzed for ISC by comet assay, in order to assess therapeutic efficacy *(31)*. A significant level of ISC was detected in one biopsy, which also showed evidence of both conjugate localization and clinical response.

1.4. ADEPT Employing Engineered Antibodies

Although chemical conjugates have produced therapeutic effects in ADEPT, there were several associated problems. Circulatory clearance was slow, it was difficult to obtain a reproducible product, and both the antibody and enzyme arms of the conjugate were immunogenic. Because CPG2 naturally forms a noncovalent dimer, it was proposed that a genetic fusion protein composed of a single-chain antibody (sFv) and

CPG2 would give a dimeric molecule for improved ADEPT. Recombinant fusion proteins can be reproducibly expressed in clinically useful quantities and have the potential to be tailored to control pharmacokinetics and overcome hurdles such as tumor distribution and immunogenicity *(12)*.

1.4.1. Single-Chain Fv Antibody Production (Method 1)

Recombinant antibody fragments have many advantages over the chemically modified fragments originally employed for ADEPT: (1) There is no requirement for complex manipulation after production, (2) they are readily defined at the molecular level and selected or genetically engineered to give the required antigen-binding characteristics, and (3) they can be produced in bacteria or yeast, which is comparatively rapid and inexpensive and avoids the problem of contamination inherent with mammalian or viral DNA. The sFvs consist of the variable heavy and light (VH and VL) chains tethered by a flexible linker, and at 27 kDa, they are the smallest antibody fragments to retain full antigen-binding capacity. Recombinant sFvs can be displayed as functional antibody fragments on the surface of bacteriophage, therefore allowing both the generation and selection of antigen binders with the desired characteristics *(35)*. The phage approach is much more efficient than the screening approach used in hybridoma technology, increasing the selection of antibodies with the desired characteristics from 10^2–10^3 clones to 10^{10} or more clones (*see* **Fig. 3**). A further advantage of the phage system is that it permits the selection of stable antibodies as cloned DNA, which can be expressed in many ways. This facilitates the attachment of enzymes for ADEPT. We employed phage technology *(11)* to produce the sFv antibody MFE-23, which had a 10-fold higher affinity for CEA than A5B7 and was the first sFv to be reported in clinical trials. These trials (imaging and radioimmunoguided surgery) revealed efficient tumor penetration and antigen binding, with no evidence of anti-MFE-23 antibody formation in patients *(36–38)*.

However, effective targeted therapy relies on efficient antibody retention in the tumor following clearance from normal tissues. We have shown that increasing the valency increased both the total amount of antibody retained in the tumor and the selective residence time in viable tumor regions *(39,40)*. Therefore, multivalent molecules have a distinct therapeutic advantage. This knowledge led to the creation of multivalent fusion proteins, composed of recombinant antibody fragments and CPG2, for ADEPT *(18)*.

1.4.2. Fusion Protein Production

Several different antibody–enzyme fusion proteins have been employed in ADEPT studies (e.g., **ref.** *41–43*). Successful production of the sFv arm of an antibody–enzyme fusion protein may be readily achieved with phage technology, as described earlier. If good quality antigen is available for immunization, selection, and characterization, the method is generally applicable. Fusion of the selected sFv with the enzyme, however, is specific for each case and, therefore, specific methods are not supplied here. However, it is generally advisable to establish that the enzyme will be functionally active in the expression system of choice before embarking on fusion protein con-

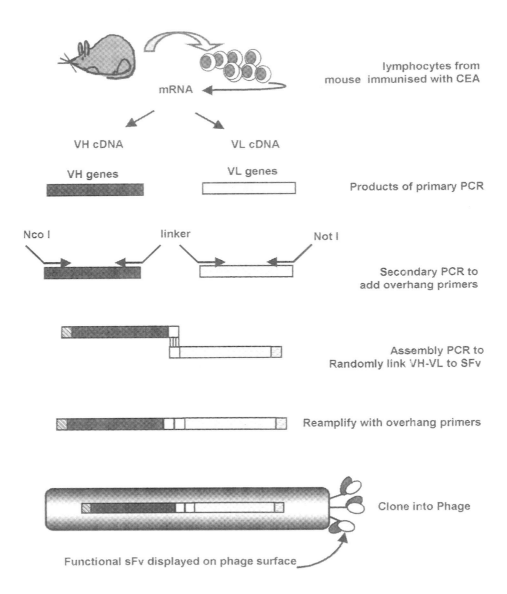

mRNA

lymphocytes from
mouse immunised with CEA

VH cDNA   VL cDNA

VH genes   VL genes   Products of primary PCR

Nco I   linker   Not I

Secondary PCR to
add overhang primers

Assembly PCR to
Randomly link VH-VL to SFv

Reamplify with overhang primers

Clone into Phage

Functional sFv displayed on phage surface

Fig. 3. Preparation of MFE-23: construction of a sFv library using the two-fragment assembly method.

struction. It is also useful to compare a variety of gene constructs (e.g., with the enzyme at the N-terminus and the C-terminus of the sFv and joined without/with various linkers) to get the format that gives the most desirable sFv–enzyme fusion protein. Factors such as yield and stability of the fusion protein should be considered.

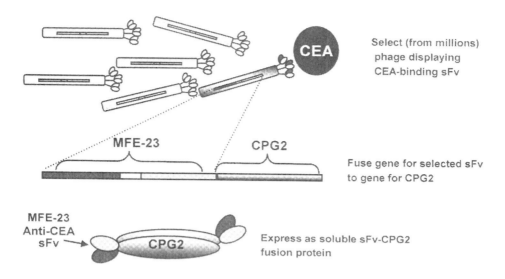

Fig. 4. Preparation of MFE-CPG2 fusion protein: the gene for MFE-23 was genetically fused to the gene for CPG2. The resultant fusion protein was dimeric owing to the natural dimer formation of the CPG2 enzyme.

1.4.2.1. BACTERIAL PRODUCTION OF MFE-CP FUSION PROTEIN

We constructed MFE-CP by fusing the gene for MFE-23 to the gene for CPG2 (*see* **Fig. 4**). The fusion protein was initially expressed in *Escherichia coli* and purified using CEA-affinity chromatography (**44**). Efficacy of MFE-CP delivery to tumors in vivo was assessed by measuring CPG2 catalytic activity in blood and excised tissue (Method 2) after intravenous injection of purified fusion protein into nude mice bearing LS174T xenografts (**45**). Recombinant MFE-CP cleared rapidly from the circulation and normal tissues without a clearing agent, giving CPG2 tumor-to-plasma ratios of 1.5 : 1 at 6 h and 10 : 1 at 24 h. The superiority of the recombinant fusion protein over the chemical conjugate is illustrated in **Fig. 2**. In addition, there was substantially more enzyme delivered to the tumor by the fusion protein than the chemical conjugate (21% vs 3.2% injected activity/g tissue at 24 h). These results established the potential of recombinant fusion protein to give improved clinical efficiency for ADEPT.

1.4.2.2. YEAST PRODUCTION OF MFE-CP

In order to produce sufficient MFE-CP to support a clinical trial, a yeast (*Pichia pastoris*) expression system was used. Yields improved over 100-fold using this system and the resulting product was glycosylated. Biodistribution studies of enzyme activity in nude mice bearing the LS174T xenograft showed that glycosylated fusion protein was retained in the tumor but cleared rapidly from plasma, resulting in a tumor-to-plasma ratio of 250 : 1 at 6 h after injection when the prodrug was given. This produced tumor growth delays with minimal toxicity in mice *(46)*. Therefore, in addition to the higher yields obtained with a yeast expression system, the rapid clearance from normal tissues combined with selective enzyme activity retention in tumors gave the yeast-derived product even better localization characteristics than the bacterial product. This product is currently (July 2003) in clinical trials.

2. Materials

2.1. sFv Preparation

2.1.1. Chemicals

All chemicals are of AnalaR grade and purchased from BDH, Merck Ltd. (Poole, Dorset, UK) or Sigma-Aldrich Company Ltd. (Poole, Dorset, UK), unless otherwise stated.

1. Ampicillin and kanamycin (Roche Molecular Biochemicals, East Sussex, UK).
2. Yeast extract, Bacto-agar, and Bacto-tryptone (Becton Dickenson., Oxford UK).
3. Mineral oil (Applied Biosystems Ltd, Chesire, UK).
4. Dynabeads M-280 (product no. 112.05) [Dynal (UK) Ltd., Mersyside, UK].
5. NuSieve GTG agarose gels (Flowgen, Maidstone, UK).

2.1.2. Kits

1. RNAgents Total RNA Isolation System (Promega, Southampton, UK).
2. Wizard PCR Preps DNA Purification System (Promega, Southampton, UK).
3. GeneAmp kit (Applied Biosystems Ltd).
4. DNA Ligation System (Amersham Life Science, Bucks., UK).
5. ECL Protein Biotinylation Kit (Amersham Life Science, Bucks., UK).

2.1.3. Equipment

1. Hi-Set mini horizontal electrophoresis unit (Anachem Ltd., Bedfordshire, UK).
2. Transilluminator UVP (Genetic Research Instrumentation Ltd, Dunmow, Essex, UK).
3. Mineralight® UV lamp (UVP, Milton Keynes, UK).
4. Polytron® PT 10/35 homogenizer (Kinematica, Luzern, Switzerland).
5. Electroporator (Gene Pulser, Bio-Rad Laboratories Ltd., Herts., UK).
6. Gene Pulsar 0.2-cm disposable cuvet (Bio-Rad Laboratories Ltd).
7. Bio-assay dish (NUNC, Tissue Culture Services Ltd., Bucks, UK).
8. Microfuge (Centra MP 4R, Thermo Quest Scientific Group Ltd., Baisingstoke, UK).
9. Microfuge tubes (Sure Lock, Fisher Scientific Ltd., Leics, UK).
10. Magnetic Particle Concentrator (Dynal Product No. 120.04).

2.1.4. Enzymes and Antibodies

1. "Klenow" fragment of *E. coli* DNA polymerase I, reverse transcriptase, RNAsin, and restriction enzymes (Roche Molecular Biochemicals).
2. Amplitaq® DNA polymerase (Applied Biosystems).
3. 9E10 Anti c-myc antibody (Sigma-Aldrich Company Ltd. Poole, Dorset, UK).
4. Sheep anti-mouse horseradish peroxidase (HRP) antibody (Amersham Life Science).

2.1.5 Bacterial Strain

E. coli strain TG1: K12, Δ(*lac-pro*), *sup*E, *thi*, *hsd*D5/F'(*tra*D36, *pro*A⁺B⁺, *lac*I^q, *lac*ZΔM15) *(47)*.

2.1.6. Plasmids and Phage

The phagemid vector pHEN is a derivative of pUC119 *(47)*. The bacterial expression vector pUC119his is also based on pUC119. The multiple-cloning site has been replaced with an expression cassette containing the pelB leader sequence and the C-terminal tag His_6 *(48)*. VCS M13 helper phage is supplied by Stratagene Ltd., Cambridge UK.

2.1.7. Solutions

1. Tris-borate (TBE) buffer stock (10X): 108 g Tris-base, 55 g boric acid, 9.3 g EDTA (pH 8.0). Add dH_2O to 1 L.
2. Tris-acetate (TAE) buffer stock (50X): 242 g Tris base, 57.1 mL glacial acetic acid, 100 mL 0.5 M EDTA (pH 8.0). Add dH_2O to 1 L.
3. 1 M Tris-HCl: 121.1 g/L Tris, adjust to pH 7.4 using HCl.
4. DNA agarose gel loading buffer (10X): 2.7 mL glycerol, 0.3 mL TBE buffer (10X), 1% sodium dodecyl sulfate (SDS), 1 mL of 0.5 M EDTA. Store at 4°C.
5. TE buffer: 10 mM Tris-HCl, 1 mM EDTA. Adjust to pH 8.0 with HCl.
6. Ethidium bromide (10 mg/mL): 1 g ethidium bromide. Add dH_2O to 100 mL. Wrap container in aluminum foil. Store at room temperature.
7. PEG/NaCl: 20% polyethylene glycol 6000, 2.5 M NaCl. Store at 4°C.
8. 3 M Sodium acetate, pH 6: 27.22 g sodium acetate·$3H_2O$, 5.75 mL acetic acid, 75.4 g dH_2O. Store at 4°C.
9. Ampicillin stock 25 mg/mL; working concentration 100 µg/mL: 0.25 mg ampicilin. Add sterile dH_2O to 10 mL. 0.2 µm filter sterilize.
10. Kanamycin stock 25 mg/mL; working concentration 50 µg/mL: 0.25 mg kanamycin. Add sterile dH_2O to 10 mL. 0.2 µm filter sterilize.
11. 2X TY medium: 16 g Bacto-tryptone, 10 g yeast extract, 5 g NaCl. Add dH_2O to 1 L. Sterilize by autoclaving.
12. 2X TY/A/G: 2X TY medium with 1% sterile glucose and 100 µg/mL ampicillin.
13. 2X TY agar: Add 15 g/L Bacto-agar to 2X TY medium. Sterilize by autoclaving. Sufficient for 40 plates.
14. PBS: Dulbecco's phosphate-buffered saline (Sigma; D-5773).
15. BPBS: 3% bovine serum albumin (BSA), 0.05% Tween-20, 0.02% sodium azide.
16. 100 mM Triethylamine: 140 µL triethylamine in 10 mL dH_2O. Must be freshly prepared.

2.1.8. Primers for Murine V-Gene Amplification

2.1.8.1. PRIMARY PCR: VL AMPLIFICATION

VKAbak	GAT GTT TTG ATG ACC CAA ACT CCA
VKCbak	GAC ATT GTG CTR ACC CAG TCT CCA
VKDbak	GAC ATC CAG ATG CAN CAG TCT CCA
VKEbak	CAA ATT GTT CTC ACC CAG TCT CC
VKFbak	GAA AAT GTG CTC ACC CAG TCT CC
VK2FOR1	CCG TTT GAT TTC CAG CTT GGT GCC
VK2FOR2	CCG TTT TAT TTC CAG CTT GGT CCC
VK2FOR3	CCG TTT TAT TTC CAA CTT TGT CCC
VK2FOR4	CCG TTT CAG CTC CAG CTT GGT CCC

(Forward primers were used simultaneously as a VK2FOR mix.)

2.1.8.2. PRIMARY PCR: VH AMPLIFICATION

VH1FOR-2   TGA GGA GAC GGT GAC CGT GGT CCC TTG GCC CC
VH1BACK   AGG TSM ARC TGC AGS AGT CWG G

2.1.8.3. SECONDARY PCR: VL AMPLIFICATION

ScVKAbak   GGC GGA GGT GGC TCT GGC GGT GGC GGA TCG — — — — — —
ScVKCbak   ("   ) — — — — — —
ScVKDbak   ("   ) — — — — — —
ScVKEbak   ("   ) — — — — — —
ScVKFbak   ("   ) — — — — — —

(Dashes represent the first 18 bases of each corresponding VKbak primary PCR primer.)

NotVK2FOR1 GAT ATG AGA TAC TGC GGC CGC — — — — — —
NotVK2FOR2 ("   ) — — — — — —
NotVK2FOR3 ("   ) — — — — — —
NotVK2FOR4 ("   ) — — — — — —

(Dashes represent the first 18 bases of each corresponding VK2FOR primary PCR primer.)

2.1.8.4. SECONDARY PCR: VH AMPLIFICATION

NcoVHBAK   TAC TCG CGG CCC AAC CGG CCA TGG CCC AGG TSM ARC TGC AGS AGT C
ScVHFOR   AGA GCC ACC TCC GCC TGA ACC GCC TCC ACC TGA GGA GAC GGT GAC CG

For assembly PCR and amplification, the outer primers are NcoVHBAK and VK2FOR mix.

2.1.8.5. DEGENERATE BASES

R = A + G	Y = C + T
M = A + C	K = T + G
S = C + G	W = A + T
H = A + T + C	B = T + C + G
D = A + T + G	V = A + C + G
N = A + C + G + T	

2.2. Estimation of CPG2 Levels
Using the Methotrexate HPLC Assay

For the determination of CPG2 levels in plasma and tissues using methotrexate as a substrate and HPLC as the means of analysis.

1. Automated HPLC system (ThermoFinnigan, Hemel Hempstead, UK). HPLC parameters: ultraviolet (UV) wavelength-320 nm; flow rate-1 mL/min; injection volume-60 μL; run time-10 min.
2. 25 cm ODS HPLC column with guard column.
3. Carboxypetidase G2 (CPG2) standard stock solution (50 units/mL).
4. 10 mM Methotrexate solution (4.54 mg/mL in dimethyl sulfoxide [DMSO]).
5. HPLC-grade methanol/Hipersolve (BDH, Merck Ltd., Poole, Dorset, UK).

6. Ammonium formate (0.06 *M*) (BDH, Merck Ltd., Poole, Dorset, UK).
7. Assay buffer: PBS + 0.2 m*M* ZnCl$_2$ (Sigma-Aldrich Company Ltd., Poole, Dorset, UK).
8. HPLC mobile phase: 55% ammonium formate + 45% methanol.
9. Reaction "stop" solution: 90% ice-cold methanol + 10% ammonium formate stock CPG2 solution 50 units/mL; take 20 μL of CPG2 and add to 980 μL assay solution.

3. Methods

3.1. SFv Preparation (see Notes 1–5)

3.1.1. General Methods

3.1.1.1. ANALYTICAL AGAROSE GEL ELECTROPHORESIS

1. Dissolve 0.5 g Agarose MP (Roche) in 50 mL TBE buffer.
2. Melt in a microwave.
3. Add 5 μL of ethidium bromide stock.
4. Pour into a Hi-Set mini horizontal electrophoresis unit.
5. Add appropriate well formers.
6. Allow to set.
7. Submerge in 50 mL of TBE buffer.
8. Add 2 μL of DNA loading buffer to 20 μL of DNA sample.
9. Load into wells.
10. Carry out electrophoretic separation at a constant voltage of 50 mV until sufficient separation is observed (15–30 min).
11. Estimate DNA fragment size by coelectrophoresis of DNA standard molecular weight marker ∅X174 and/or λ DNA (Roche).
12. Visualize DNA using an ultraviolet light transilluminator.

3.1.1.2 PURIFICATION AGAROSE GEL ELECTROPHORESIS

As for analytical gels (*see* **Subheading 3.1.1.1.**) with the following exceptions:

1. Prepare 2% NuSieve GTG agarose gels in 50 mL TAE buffer.
2. Run at 30 mV submerged in 1X TAE buffer.
3. Visualize the desired bands with long-wave UV light.

3.1.2. SFv Library

3.1.2.1. TO OBTAIN SPLENIC LYMPHOCYTES FROM IMMUNIZED MOUSE

1. Immunize Balb/c mice with 40 μg of heat-treated CEA *(49)*.
2. Boost with 40 μg of heat-treated CEA at approximately monthly intervals.
3. Bleed 10 d after each boost and test the serum (using enzyme-linked immunosorbent assay [ELISA]) for polyclonal antibodies to CEA.
4. When antibody response is established (usually 1–3 boosts), give final boost.
5. Sacrifice mice 4 d after final boost and remove spleen.
6. Trim contaminating tissue and place spleen in a 100-mm tissue culture dish containing 10 mL sterile PBS.
7. Release spleen cells by teasing apart with two needles and disrupt cell clumps by pipetting.
8. Transfer cells and medium into a sterile centrifuge tube, wash in sterile PBS, and split into 5X 2-mL aliquots.
9. Use immediately for RNA extraction or store in liquid nitrogen.

3.1.2.2. Extraction and Precipitation of Total RNA

3.1.2.2.1. REMOVAL OF RNASE

1. Wear latex gloves at all times to minimize RNase contamination.
2. Use disposable sterile plasticware where possible.
3. Incubate sterile plugged plastic tips at 100°C for 8 h prior to use.
4. Nondisposable glassware and plasticware must be rendered RNase free by treatment with diethyl pyrocarbonate (DEPC) as follows:
   a. Add 0.1% DEPC to plasticware and 50-mL dH$_2$O aliquots overnight at room temperature.
   b. Autoclave to deactivate remaining DEPC.
   c. Prepare solutions in preautoclaved DEPC-treated dH$_2$O.

3.1.2.2.2. RNA PREPARATION

Use RNAgents Total RNA Isolation System (*see* **Subheading 2.1.2.**) as follows:

1. Resuspend one aliquot of spleen cells in 6 mL of denaturing solution (guanidinium thiocyanate).
2. Place on ice for 5 min.
3. Homogenize using a Polytron PT 10/35 cleaned with DEPC-treated H$_2$O and absolute alcohol.
4. Place homogenized sample on ice.
5. Add 0.6 mL of 2 *M* sodium acetatem pH 4 (*see* **Subheading 2.1.**) and mix by inversion.
6. Add 6 mL of phenol : chloroform : isoamyl alcohol mixture (provided with kit).
7. Shake vigorously for 10 s.
8. Chill on ice for 15 min.
9. Transfer mixture to a DEPC-treated centrifuge tube.
10. Centrifuge at 10,000g and 4°C for 20 min.
11. Transfer (top) aqueous RNA-containing phase in to a fresh DEPC-treated tube.
12. Precipitate RNA by adding an equal volume of isopropanol and incubate at –20°C overnight.
13. Pellet RNA by centrifugation at 10,000g for 30 min.
14. Decant supernatant and the resuspend pellet in 5 mL of denaturing solution.
15. Add an equal volume of isopropanol.
16. Mix by inversion.
17. Place at –20°C for a minimum of 4 h.
18. Pellet by centrifugation at 8250g and 4°C for 15 min.
19. Wash with 5 mL of ice-cold 75% ethanol.
20. Air-dry RNA pellet and resuspend in RNAse-free dH$_2$O.
21. Quantify yield of RNA by measuring the optical density (OD) at 260 nm. (1.0 A$_{260}$ = 40 µg/mL RNA).

3.1.2.3. Preparation of cDNA

The VH and VL reactions are performed separately from this stage until PCR assembly (*see* **Fig. 3**). VH genes are obtained by priming the reverse transcriptase reaction with VH1FOR2 (*see* **Subheading 2.1.** for sequences of primer). VL genes are obtained by priming with the VK2FOR mix of four primers (*see* **Subheading 2.1.** for sequences of primer).

1. Prepare the following reaction mix: 5 µL of 10 mM dNTP mix, 10 µL reverse transcriptase buffer (10X), 10 µL 0.1 M DTT (dithiothreitol), 10 µL forward (FOR) primer (10 pmol/µL), 4 µL RNAsin (40 units/µL), and 19 µL dH$_2$O.
2. Microcentrifuge solution containing 10 µg of RNA at 1800g for 15 min.
3. Resuspend resulting pellet in 10 µL of DEPC-treated dH$_2$O.
4. Heat at 65°C for 3 min.
5. Chill on ice.
6. Add to the reaction mix along with 2 µL of reverse transcriptase (to give a total reaction mix of 100 µL).
7. Incubate at 42°C for 1 h.
8. Boil for 3 min.
9. Chill on ice.
10. Spin in a microfuge (1800g) to pellet any debris.
11. Transfer the supernatant (containing cDNA) to a new tube.
12. Use 5 µL of cDNA solution to prime a 100-µL PCR reaction.

3.1.2.4. PCR TO CREATE sFv

The library is constructed using the Two Fragment Assembly Method developed by Hawkins *(50)*. Prepare the PCR reaction buffer using the GeneAmp kit (*see* **Subheading 2.1.2.**) with the following:

1. Reaction kit buffer (10 mM Tris-HCl, pH 8.3, 50 mM KCl, 1.5 mM MgCl$_2$).
2. 0.001% (w/v) Gelatin.
3. All four deoxynucleoside triphosphates (dNTPs; diluted from their original individual stock concentrations of 10 mM to 1.25 mM in sterile dH$_2$O as a mixture, and used at a working concentration of 0.2 mM).
4. Oligonucleotide primers at a final concentration of 0.2 µM.

3.1.2.4.1. Primary PCR

VH genes are amplified (from cDNA made with VH1FOR-2) using VH1FOR-2 forward primer and VH1BACK back primer. VL genes are amplified (from cDNA made with VK2FORmix) using VK2FORmix forward primer and equimolar mix of VKAbak, VKCbak, VKDbak, VKFbak, and VKFbak back primer (*see* **Subheading 2.1.** for sequences of primers).

1. Mix the following in microcentrifuge tubes in a final volume of 100 µL:
   85 µL of PCR reaction buffer;
   5 µL template (cDNA);
   5 µL forward primer (10 pmol/µL);
   5 µL back primer (10 pmol/µL).
2. Add 0.5 µL (2.5 units) of Amplitaq DNA polymerase.
3. Overlay with 4X drops of mineral oil to prevent evaporation of the reaction mixture during the heating cycles.
4. PCR (30 cycles) using the following program:
   94°C for 1 min (linearisation of DNA);
   55°C for 2 min (annealing of primers);
   72°C for 2 min (elongation).

5. Hold for 5 min at 65°C.
6. Cool to 4°C.
7. On completion of PCR, carefully remove samples from beneath the oil and transfer to a fresh microcentrifuge tube.
8. Check the success of amplification by analyzing samples on a 1.5% standard agarose gel with TBE buffer (*see* **Subheading 3.1.1.1.**).
9. Extract amplified DNA using the Wizard purification protocol (*see* **Subheading 2.1.**).
10. Use extracted DNA for secondary PCR.

3.1.2.4.2. Secondary PCR

During secondary PCR, the VH and VL genes are extended to include restriction sites and overhangs to make a 3X(Gly$_4$Ser) linker. This is achieved for VH using ScVHFOR forward primer and NcoVHBACK back primer. VL genes are amplified using an equimolar mix of NotVK2FOR1–4 (forward primer) and equimolar mix of ScVKAbak, ScVKCbak, ScVKDbak, and ScVKFbak, and ScVKFbak (back primer) (*see* **Subheading 2.1.** for sequences of primers).

1. Mix the following in a final volume of 100 µL:

   85 µL PCR reaction buffer;
   5 µL template (1° PCR);
   5 µL forward primer (10 pmol/µL);
   5 µL back primer (10 pmol/µL).
2. Add 1.0 µL (5 units) of Amplitaq DNA polymerase.
3. Overlay with 4X drops of mineral oil.
4. PCR (10 cycles) using the following program:
   94°C for 1 min;
   50°C for 2 min;
   72°C for 2 min.
5. On completion of the PCR, carefully remove samples from beneath the oil and transfer to a fresh microcentrifuge tube.
6. Check the success of amplification by analyzing samples on a 1.5% standard agarose gel with TBE buffer (*see* **Subheading 3.1.1.1.**).
7. End polish by adding 10 µL of NTP and 1 µL of Klenow per 100 µL of PCR products; incubate for 15 min at room temperature.
8. Purify DNA from a 2% low-melting-point (TAE) gel.

3.1.2.4.3. Assembly PCR

1. For PCR assembly of the sFv repertoires, approx 1 µg of heavy-chain product and 1 µg of a kappa-chain product are combined in a PCR reaction as follows:
   1 µg VH secondary PCR product;
   1 µg VL secondary PCR product;
   10 µL of 10X PCR buffer;
   10 µL dNTPs.
2. Make to 100-µL final volume with dH$_2$O.
3. Add 1 µL Taq polymerase (5 units).
4. Overly with 4X drops of mineral oil.
5. PCR (10 cycles) using the following:
   94°C for 1 min;
   50°C for 1 min.

6. Hold at 74°C for 1 min (to join the fragments).
7. Hold for 2 min at 94°C.
8. Add 18 μL of the following PCR/primer mix with 1 μL *Taq* polymerase (5 units):
     35 μL NotVK2FOR mix primer;
     35 μL NcoVHBAK primer;
     10.5 μL 10X PCR mix;
     10.5 μL dNTP mix and 14 μL dH$_2$O.
9. PCR (20 cycles) using the following:
     94°C for 1 min;
     60°C for 1 min;
     74°C for 1 min.
10. Cool to 4°C.
11. Remove aqueous phase from under the oil and analyze 10 μL on a 1.5% TBE gel.
12. Purify assembled DNA product.
13. The assembled sFv's are now ready to cut and clone.

3.1.2.5. SFv Preparation for Cloning

The assembled sFv DNA are cloned using *Nco*I/*Not*I or with *Sfi*I/*Not*I . (Cloning is easier with *Nco*I/*Not*I, as they use the same buffer and temperature, but *Sfi*I/*Not*I is sometimes used to ensure that sFv's with an *Nco*I site in the V-regions are not lost).

1. Cut with *Not*I in the following mix:
     200 μL assembly PCR products (containing 1–5 μg of DNA).
     50 μL of 10X Roche buffer *M*.
     20 μL *Not*I;
     230 μL dH$_2$O.
2. Leave for 3 h at 37°C
3. Add 20 μL *Nco*I.
4. Leave 2 h at 37°C.
5. Gel purify from a low-melting-point TAE agarose gel using the Wizard method.
6. Store at –20°C.

3.1.2.6. Vector Preparation

1. Digest pHEN with *Nco*I and *Not*I in the following mix:
     80 μL (approx 20 μg) pHEN DNA.
     20 μL of 10X Roche buffer *M*.
     10 μL *Not*I;
     100 μL dH$_2$O.
2. Leave for 3 h at 37°C.
3. Add 10 μL *Nco*I.
4. Leave 2 h at 37°C.
5. Gel purify from a low-melting-point TAE agarose gel.
6. Store at –20°C.

3.1.2.7. Ligation Reactions

1. As a general rule, a 3 : 1 molar ratio of insert to vector should lead to a satisfactory ligation.

2. Ligate *NcoI/NotI* restricted sFv DNA into *NcoI/NotI* restricted pHEN using the Amersham DNA Ligation System (*see* **Subheading 2.1.**) according to the manufacturer's instructions.

3.1.2.8. TRANSFORMATION OF ELECTRO-COMPETENT BACTERIAL CELLS WITH pHEN LIGATED sFv

3.1.2.8.1. PREPARATION OF BACTERIAL CELLS

1. Streak TG1 *E. coli* cells to single colonies onto a minimal agar plate.
2. Incubate at 37°C overnight.
3. Innoculate a single colony into 10 mL of 2X TY medium.
4. Incubate culture at 37°C, 250 rpm for 16 h.
5. Inoculate 1 L (2X 500 mL in 2X 2-L flasks) of 2X TY with 1/100 dilution of overnight culture.
6. Incubate at 37°C, 250 rpm until OD_{600} = 0.5–1.0.
7. Chill on ice.
8. Centrifuge for 15 min at 4000*g*.
9. Wash pellet in 1 L of ice-cold pyrogen-free H_2O.
10. Centrifuge for 15 min at 4000*g*.
11. Wash with 500 mL ice-cold pyrogen-free H_2O.
12. Centrifuge for 15 min at 4000*g*.
13. Wash with 20 mL of ice-cold 10% glycerol in H_2O.
14. Centrifuge for 15 min at 4000*g*.
15. Resuspend in 3 mL of ice-cold 10% glycerol.
16. Aliquot cells in 200-μL fractions.
17. Place in ice if to be used immediately for electroporation (*see* **Subheading 3.1.2.8.2.**) freeze and store at –80°C for later use.
18. Check the competency of the cells by transforming with a known quantity of plasmid DNA. The competency should be at least 10^7/μg of DNA.

3.1.2.8.2. ELECTROPORATION TO GENERATE SFV LIBRARY

1. Put 40 μL of TG1 electro-competent cells (*see* **Subheading 3.1.2.8.1.**) on ice.
2. Or if frozen, the TG1 electro-competent cells are thawed on ice.
3. Set electroporator to 2.5 kV, capacitance at 25 μF, resistance at 200 Ω.
4. In a chilled tube, mix 40 mL of cells with 1–2 μL of DNA thoroughly by pipetting.
5. Incubate on ice for 1 min prior to electroporation.
6. Transfer the mixture of cells and DNA to an ice-cold sterile disposable cuvette.
7. Place the cuvet in the prechilled slide chamber.
8. Push into electroporator.
9. Pulse once at the stated settings (the time constant should be between 4 and 5 ms).
10. Immediately resuspend electroporated cells into 1 mL of 2X TY + 0.1% glucose.
11. Incubate at 37°C, for 30 min.
12. Centrifuge at 17,860*g* for 5 min.
13. Remove supernatant and resuspend cells in 100 μL of 2X TY media.
14. Mix the individual 100-μL aliquots.
15. Make triplicate serial dilutions (to 1×10^6).
16. Plate 100 μL of each dilution onto 2X TY/A/G agar plates and incubate at 37°C overnight to estimate library size.
17. Plate remaining electroporation mix onto a 29 × 29-cm bioassay dish containing 2X TY/ A/G agar.
18. Incubate overnight at 37°C.
19. Scrape the bacterial lawn from the plate using 25 mL of 2X TY/A/G.
20. Add 15% glycerol and store at –80°C.
21. This is the sFv library glycerol stock.

3.1.2.8.3. PREPARATION OF FILAMENTOUS PHAGE FROM PHAGEMID-TRANSFORMED *E. COLI*

1. Innoculate 50 mL of 2X TY/A/G with 750 µL of scFv library-transformed *E. coli* TG1 (*see* **Subheading 3.1.2.8.**).
2. Grow 1 h at 37°C in an incubator/shaker at 300 rpm.
3. Add 50 µL of VCS M13 helper phage (*see* **Subheading 2.1.6.**).
4. Grow 1 h at 37°C in an incubator/shaker at 300 rpm.
5. Centrifuge at 2772*g* for 15 min, to pellet cells.
6. Discard supernatant.
7. Resuspend pellet in 50 mL of fresh 2X TY/A supplemented with 50 µg/mL kanamycin (NO GLUCOSE).
8. Incubate overnight at 37°C in an incubator/shaker at 300 rpm.
9. Remove cells from the liquid culture by centrifugation at 2772*g* for 20 min at 4°C.
10. Transfer 45 mL of supernatant to a clean tube.
11. Add 9 mL of 20% PEG 6000 in 2.5 *M* NaCl.
12. Leave 4°C for 1 h to precipitate.
13. Centrifuge at 2772*g* for 10 min at 4°C.
14. Discard supernatant.
15. Resuspend pellet (containing phage) in 1.5 mL of sterile dH$_2$O.
16. Microfuge at 10,500*g* for 5 min—to pellet any remaining bacterial cells.
17. Transfer 1.25 mL supernatant (containing phage) to microfuge tubes.
18. Add 0.25 mL of 20% PEG 6000 in 2.5 *M* NaCl to the tube.
19. Leave 4°C for 1 h to precipitate.
20. Microfuge at 12,000 rpm for 10 min to pellet phage.
21. Discard supernatant.
22. Resuspend the phage pellets in 500 µL of sterile dH$_2$O.
23. Use immediately for selection and titre as detailed in **Subheading 3.1.3.** and store remainder at –20°C.

3.1.3 Selection of Phage Antibodies Using Biotinylated Antigens

3.1.3.1. SELECTION OF CEA-REACTIVE PHAGE

This method was developed *(51)* to capture phage whose sFv bind to antigen when it is present at low concentrations. It is generally very successful and may be adapted to select for other desired binding conditions (e.g., low pH or different temperatures). However, it does require more antigen (0.5–1 mg/sFv library) than the "panning" (coated tube) method, which can usually be completed with 100 µg/sFv library.

   1. Prepare selection solutions as follows:

Reagent added	Test tube	Control tube
Phage prepared as in **Subheading 3.1.2.8.3.**	200 µL	200 µL dH$_2$O volume equivalent to biotinylated CEA
Biotinylated CEA, prepared using Amersham kit according to the manufacturer's instructions	Amount calculated to give desired final concentration of biotinylated CEA: 100 n*M* for selection I, 50 n*M* for selection II, 20 n*M* for selection III, and 5 n*M* for selection IV	
BPBS	To final volume of 1 mL	To final volume of 1 mL

2. Incubate at room temperature for 1 h.
3. During this hour, block the magnetic Dynabeads as follows.
4. Take 75 µL of beads per reaction.
5. Microfuge at 10,500g for 3 min.
6. Tip off solution and resuspend beads in 75 µL of BPBS.
7. Rotate for 1 h at room temperature.
8. Add the 75 µL of blocked bead suspension to the test and control tubes.
9. Leave at room temperature for 5 min.
10. Place the tubes on the magnetic particle concentrator.
11. Allow beads to concentrate by magnetic force.
12. Remove supernatant without disturbing beads.
13. Remove tubes from magnetic particle concentrator.
14. Add 1 mL of BPBS to beads in tube and mix quickly.
15. Wash 10 times by repeating **steps 10–14** for each wash.
16. Resuspend beads in 1 mL of 100 mM triethylamine.
17. Allow tubes to stand for 5 min at room temperature away from magnetic particle concentrator.
18. Return tubes to magnetic particle concentrator.
19. Allow beads to concentrate by magnetic force.
20. Remove eluent without disturbing beads and transfer to a clean tube.
21. Neutralize eluent with 500 µL of 1 M Tris-HCl, pH 7.4 (gives final volume of 1.5 mL).
22. Take 1 mL neutralized eluent.
23. Add 4 mL of 2X TY.
24. Add 5ml of TG1 culture (prepared earlier; in **steps a–d**).
    a. Set up overnight culture of TG1 in 2X TY on the day prior to selection of scFv phage library with biotinylated CEA.
    b. Set up 1/100 dilution of this overnight culture in 2X TY on day of selection.
    c. Grow at 37°C in an incubator/shaker at 250 rpm until cells reach OD$_{600}$ of 0.6 (approx 1 h 45 min).
    d. Store cells on ice until required for infection with phage.
25. Incubate at 37°C with shaking at 250 rpm for 30 min.
26. Remove 500 µL to estimate the "phage titer" in cfu (colony forming units)/mL as follows:
    a. Prepare serial dilutions (1/10, 1/100, and 1/1000 for neutralized eluant and 1/1000, 1/10,000, and 1/100,000 for PEG-precipitated phage).
    b. Plate onto 2X TY agar with 1% glucose and 100 µg/mL ampicillin.
    c. Incubate plates at 37°C overnight.
    d. The following day, the cfus are counted to determine the titer of the phage for Test and Control selections.
    e. Colonies are also used to test for individual sFv binding characteristics (*see* **Subheading 3.1.3.2.**).
27. The Test bacterial culture contains the sFv's selected as reactive with biotinylated CEA. This is used to generate culture for the next round of selection.
28. Centrifuge culture from TEST SELECTION ONLY at 2772g for 10 min at 4°C.
29. Discard the supernatant.
30. Resuspend the pellet in 1 mL of 2X TY/A/G.
31. Spread on to a a 29 × 29-cm bioassay dish containing 2X TY/A/G agar.
32. Incubate overnight at 37°C.
33. The following day scrape the bacterial culture into 2X TY/A/G (takes 25 mL).

34. Add 15% glycerol.
35. Aliquot into 500-μL amounts and store at –80°C.
36. Repeat the selection process (**steps 1–34**) until satisfactory sFv's are obtained.

3.1.3.2 TESTING SUCCESS OF THE sFV LIBRARY BY ELISA

This is achieved during selection of CEA-reactive phage by testing antigen binding of individual sFv by ELISA on colonies taken from the titer plates obtained at each round (*see* **Subheading 3.1.3.1.**). ELISA may be performed directly on phage to detect phage-bound sFv using anti-phage (M13) antibody to detect CEA binding, but we have found that the method (below) that uses soluble sFv is more reliable. The scFv's are cloned adjacent to the *lacZ* site, which enables induction of expression by the lactose analogue isopropyl β-D-thiogalactoside (IPTG). All in-frame sFv's expressed in pHEN have a c-terminal human myc tag *(47)* readily detected by the 9E10 monoclonal antibody (originally made by Gerrard Evan, now commercially available). Antigen-reactive colonies should be obtained from the second to third round of selection.

Other tests for the sFv library should include DNA sequencing of randomly selected clones to confirm that sFv's are present and the linker is correct. *Bst*1 finger printing is also useful to assess the diversity of the library *(52)*.

3.1.3.2.1. INDUCTION OF SOLUBLE SFVS

1. Using a sterile disposable loop, select a single bacterial TG1 colony from the agar plate. Transfer into 1 mL of 2X TY/A/G.
2. Incubate overnight at 37°C with shaking.
3. Pellet cells by centrifugation.
4. Wash once in 2X TY medium.
5. Resuspend in 2X TY/A/G with 1 mM IPTG (to induce sFv expression).
6. Grow for a further 16 h at 30°C.
7. Pellet cells by centrifugation.
8. Supernatant (containing the secreted sFv) is used directly in ELISA or stored at 4°C with sodium azide (0.02%).

3.1.3.2.2. ELISA

1. Coat 96-well plates with CEA at 2 μg/mL in PBS, 100 μL/well.
2. Leave at room temperature for 1 h.
3. Wash 2X with PBS (*see* **Subheading 2.1.**).
4. Quench with 150 μL of 3% BSA in PBS+sodium azide (0.02%).
5. Cover with sealing film and parafilm.
6. Store at 4°C overnight.
7. Wash 2X with PBS.
8. Incubate with induced supernatant and controls (2X TY as negative and any known positives) at 100 μL/well.
9. Leave at room temperature for 1 h.
10. Wash 3X with PBS 0.05% Tween-20, 4X with dH$_2$O.
11. Incubate with 1/1000 (in PBS) 9E10 anti-myc (*see* **Subheading 2.1.**) 100 μL/well for 1 h at room temperature.
12. Wash 3X with PBS+0.05% Tween-20, 4X with dH$_2$0.
13. Incubate with 1/500 (in PBS) sheep anti mouse-HRP (*see* **Subheading 2.1.**) at 100 μL/well for 1 h at room temperature.

14. Wash 3X with PBS+ 0.05% Tween-20, 4X with dH_2O.
15. Prepare OPD (Sigma) substrate according to manufacturer's instructions.
16. Add 100 μL of substrate to each well.
17. Leave for 3–5 min, to allow color to develop.
18. Stop the reaction with 4 *M* HCl.
19. Read at 490 n*M* wavelength.

3.2. Estimation of CPG2 Levels Using the Methotrexate HPLC Assay (see Notes 6–11)

3.2.1. Construction of a CPG2 Calibration Curve in Assay Buffer

1. From the stock 50 units/mL CPG2 solution, take 20 μL of CPG2 and add to 980 μL assay buffer (PBS+0.2 m*M* $ZnCl_2$) to make 1-unit/mL solution of CPG2.
2. Prepare the following concentrations of CPG2 in assay buffer using the 1-U/mL solution: 0.0, 0.1, 0.2, 0.4, 0.6, 0.8 U/mL. Keep solutions on ice at all times.
3. Aliquot 0.5 mL stop solution into each of seven Eppendorf tubes and place on ice.
4. Add 600 μL of assay buffer to each of seven labeled tubes and equilibrate to 30°C in a water bath.
5. Add 6.0 μL of MTX solution (10 m*M*) to each tube and mix well.
6. Start reaction by adding 6.0 μL of the CPG2 solution prepared in **step 2**.
7. Allow reaction to occur for 30 min.
8. Stop reaction by transferring 0.5 mL of the reaction mixture into 0.5 mL of the stop solution.
9. Mix well and spin in microfuge at 10,500 rpm for 5 min at room temperature.
10. Transfer to appropriate HPLC vials and analyze.

3.2.2. CPG2 Assay for Experimental Samples

1. For tissue samples, prepare 10% homogenates in assay buffer and equilibrate to 30°C in a water bath. For serum samples, prepare appropriate dilution (depending on expected enzyme concentration) in assay buffer and equilibrate to 30°C in a water bath.
2. Start reaction by adding 6.0 μL of MTX solution (10 m*M*) to 600 μL of tissue homogenate and mix well.
3. Allow reaction to occur for 30 min at 30°C in a water bath.
4. Stop reaction by transferring 0.5 mL of the reaction mixture into 0.5 mL of the stop solution.
6. Mix well and spin in microfuge at 14,000 rpm for 5 min at room temperature.
7. Remove supernatant, transfer to HPLC vials and analyze.
8. Calculate the CPG2 U/g present in the tissue, using the CPG2 calibration curve plotted from the metabolite area vs CPG2 concentration.

4. Notes

1. Some of the materials and equipment described are potentially hazardous to health if not properly handled. For example, ethidium bromide is toxic and exposure to ultraviolet light is harmful. Risk assessments should be completed for all equipment, chemicals, and biological agents prior to starting the project and adequate precautions taken to protect workers and environment.
2. It is essential to ensure there is an adequate supply of good quality antigen. People often fail to address this and it should be done at onset of the project. Antigen will be required for immunization, selection, and characterization of scFvs.

3. Do not take shortcuts with RNA procedures. Buy a reputable kit and follow the manufacturer's instructions carefully. Do not forget that RNAse is everywhere, including the tissues you are extracting, and it is not removed by autoclaving. You will not get a good library with degraded RNA.

4. One of the main factors in determining library size is the competency (number of transformants/μg DNA) of the bacterial cells. It is worth spending some time to get this stage right. We and others have found electro-competent *E. coli* TG1 strain (*supE thi-1* Δ(*lac-proAB*) Δ(*mcrB-hsdSM*)5 (r_K^- m_K^-) [*F' traD36 proAB lacIqZ* Δ *M15*]) to be successful but have observed a large (up to 100-fold) variation in competency between batches. One way to address this is to check the competency before use and only attempt to make your library with the most competent batches. However, because it takes overnight to assess competency, this inevitably means freezing the cells before use. In our experience, this usually results in an approximately 10-fold loss of competency. A good compromise is to make the library in stages and use fresh cells each time. In any case, it is important to establish the conditions that give the maximum number of transformants/ μg of DNA, for example, by trying different ratios of your ligated library DNA and competent cells. Do this with test transformations, using only small aliquots of your ligated library to prevent waste of valuable material.

5. It is possible to buy ready-made competent cells from companies such as Stratagene. Beware that the competencies quoted (up to 10^9 transformants/μg DNA) are for plasmid DNA and you will be unlikely to achieve such high transformation efficiencies/μg DNA in your ligation mix. Check out the best cells for your library with the manufacturer and make sure that the cell strain is compatible with your vector—for example, that it has the F' pilus for phage entry and does not have inappropriate antibiotic resistance.

6. The temperature in the water bath should be at 30°C for a 30-min incubation.

7. The reaction in the CPG2 assay may be speeded up by incubating standards and samples at 36°C for 5 min only.

8. Stop solution should be ice cold.

9. Stock solution of CPG2 (50 units/mL) should be single-use aliquots and stored at –70°C.

10. Methotrexate should be stored in the dark.

11. All solvents should be filtered before use for HPLC.

References

1. Pedley, R. B. (1996) Pharmacokinetics of monoclonal antibodies: implications for their use in cancer therapy. *Clin. Immunother.* **6,** 54–67.
2. Glennie, M. J. and Johnson, P. W. M. (2000) Clinical trials of antibody therapy. *Immunol. Today* **21,** 403–410.
3. Pedley, R. B., Boden, J. A., Boden, R., et al. (1996) Ablation of colorectal xenografts with combined radioimmunotherapy and tumour blood flow modifying agents. *Cancer Res.* **56,** 3293–3300.
4. Pedley, R. B., Hill, S. A., Boxer, G. M., et al. (2001) Eradication of colorectal xenografts by combined radioimmunotherapy and cambretastatin A-4 3-*O*-Phosphate. *Cancer Res.* **61,** 4716–4722.
5. Press, O. W., Eary, J. F., Applebaum, F. R., et al. (1993) Radiolabeled antibody therapy of B-cell lymphoma with autologous bone marrow support. *N. Engl. J. Med.* **329,** 1219–1224.
6. Lane, D. M., Eagle, K. F., Begent, R. H. J., et al. (1994) Radioimmunotherapy of metastatic colorectal tumours with iodine-131-labelled antibody to carcinoembryonic antigen: phase I/II study with comparative biodistribution of intact and F(ab')$_2$ antibodies. *Br. J. Cancer* **70,** 521–525.

7. Napier, M. P. and Begent, R. H. J. (1998) Radioimmunotherapy of gastrointestinal cancer, in *Cancer Radioimmunotherapy*. Riva, T., (ed.). Harwood Academia, Boston, pp. 333–388.

8. Jain, R. K. (1998) The next frontier of molecular medicine: delivery of therapeutics. *Nature Med.* **4,** 655–657.

9. Flynn, A. A., Boxer, G. M., Begent, R. H. J., and Pedley, R. B. (2001) Relationship between tumour morphology, antigen and antibody distribution, measured by fusion of digital phosphor and photographic images. *Cancer Immunol. Immunother.* **50,** 77–81.

10. Flynn, A. A., Green, A. J., Boxer, G. M., Casey, J., Pedley, R. B., and Begent, R. H. J. (1999) A novel technique, using radioluminography, for the measurement of uniformity of radiolabeled antibody distribution on a colorectal cancer xenograft model. *Int. J. Radiat. Oncol. Biol. Phys.* **43,** 183–189.

11. Chester, K. A., Bhatia, J., Boxer, G., et al. (2000) Clinical applications of phage-derived sFvs and sFv fusion proteins. *Dis. Markers* **16,** 53–62.

12 Chester, K. A., Mayer, A., Bhatia, J., et al. (2000) Recombinant anti-carcinoembryonic antigen antibodies for targeting cancer. *Cancer Chemther. Pharmacol.* **46(Suppl.),** S8–S12.

13. Bagshawe, K. D. (1989) Towards generating cytotoxic agents at cancer sites. *Br. J. Cancer* **60,** 275–281.

14. Melton, R. G. and Knox, R. J., eds. (1999) *Enzyme-Prodrug Strategies for Cancer Therapy*, Kluwer Academic/Plenum, New York.

15. Blakey, D. A. (1997) Enzyme prodrug therapy of cancer. *Expert Opin. Ther. Patents* **7,** 965–977.

16. Niculescu-Duvaz I. and Springer, C.J. (1995) Antibody-directed enzyme prodrug therapy (ADEPT): a targeting strategy in cancer chemotherapy. *Curr. Med. Chem.* **2,** 687–706.

17. Bagshawe K. D. (1995) Antibody-directed enzyme prodrug therapy: a review. *Drug Dev. Res.* **34,** 220–230.

18. Chester, K. A., Melton, R. G., and Hawkins, R. E. (1999) Phage technology for producing antibody-enzyme fusion proteins, in *Enzyme-Prodrug Strategies for Cancer Therapy* (Melton, R. G. and Knox, R. J., eds.), Kluwer Academic/Plenum, New York, pp. 179–193.

19. Bosslet, K., Czech, J., and Hoffmann, D. (1994) Tumor-selective prodrug activation by fusion protein-mediated catalysis. *Cancer Res.* **54,** 2151–2159.

20. Senter, P. D., Saulnier, M. G., Schreiber, G. J., Hirschberg, D. L., Brown, J. P., and Hellstrom, K. E. (1988) Anti-tumor effects of antibody-alkaline phosphatase conjugates in combination with etoposide phosphate. *Proc. Natl. Acad. Sci. USA* **85,** 4842–4846.

21. Vrudhula, V. M., Svenssen, H. P., Kennedy, K. A., Senter, P. D., and Wallace, P. M. (1993) Antitumor activities of a cephalosporin prodrug in combination with monoclonal antibody β-lactamase conjugates. *Bioconjug. Chem.* **4,** 334–340.

22. Sherwood, F. R., Melton, R. G., Alwan, S. M., and Hughes P. (1985) Purification and properties of carboxypeptidase G2 from Pseudomonas sp. strain RS-16; use of a novel triazine dye affinity method. *Eur. J. Biochem.* **148,** 447–453.

23. Pedley, R. B., Sharma, S. K, Boxer, G. M., et al. (1999) Enhancement of Antibody-directed Enzyme Prodrug Therapy in colorectal xenografts by an antivascular agent. *Cancer Res.* **59,** 3998–4003.

24. Eccles, S. A., Court, W. J., Box, G. A., Dean, C. J., Melton, R. G., and Springer, C. J. (1994) Regression of established breast carcinoma xenografts with antibody-directed enzyme prodrug therapy against c-erbB2. *Cancer Res.* **54,** 5171–5177.

25. Springer, C. J., Bagshawe, K. D., Sharma, S. K., et al. (1991). Ablation of human chorio-carcinoma xenografts in nude mice by antibody-directed enzyme prodrug therapy (ADEPT) with three novel compounds. *Eur. J. Cancer* **11**, 1361–1366.

26. Stribbling, S. M., Martin, M., Pedley, R. B., Boden, J, A., Sharma, S. K., and Springer, C. J. (1997). Biodistribution of an antibody-enzyme conjugate for antibody-directed enzyme prodrug therapy in nude mice bearing human colon adenocarcinoma xenografts. *Cancer Chemother. Pharmacol.* **40**, 277–284.

27. Blakey, D. C., Valcaccia, B. E., East, S., et al. (1993) Anti-tumour effects of an antibody–carboxypeptidase G2 conjugate in combination with a benzoic acid mustard prodrug. *Cell. Biophys.* **22**, 1–8.

28. Sharma, S. K., Bagshawe, K. D., Burke, P. J., et al. (1994) Galactosylated antibodies and antibody–enzyme conjugates in antibody-directed enzyme prodrug therapy. *Cancer* **73**, 1114–1120.

29. Springer, C. J., Dowell, R., Burke, P. J., et al. (1995) Optimization of alkylating agent prodrugs derived from phenol and aniline mustards: a new clinical candidate prodrug (ZD2767) for ADEPT. *J. Med. Chem.* **38**, 5051–5065.

30. Blakey, D. C., Burke, P. J., Davies, D. H., et al. (1996) ZD2767, an improved system for antibody-directed enzyme prodrug therapy that results in tumour regressions in colorectal tumour xenografts. *Cancer Res.* **56**, 3287–3292.

31. Webley, S. D., Francis, R. J., Pedley, R. B., et al. (2001) Measurement of the critical DNA lesions produced by antibody-directed enzyme prodrug therapy (ADEPT) in vitro, in vivo and in clinical material. *Br. J. Cancer* **84**, 1671–1676.

32. Bagshawe, K. D., Sharma, S. K., Springer, C. J., and Antoniw, P. (1995) Antibody directed enzyme prodrug therapy: a pilot-scale clinical trial. *Tumor Target.* **1**, 17–29.

33. Napier, M. P., Sharma, S. K., Springer, C. J., et al. (2000) Antibody-directed enzyme prodrug therapy: efficacy and mechanism of action in colorectal carcinoma. *Clin. Cancer Res.* **6**, 765–772.

34. Martin, J., Stribbling, S. M., Poon, G. K., et al. (1997) Antibody-directed enzyme prodrug therapy: pharmacokinetics and plasma levels of prodrug and drug in a phase I clinical trial. *Cancer Chemother. Pharmacol.* **40**, 189–201.

35. Winter, G., Griffiths, A. D., Hawkins, R. E., and Hoogenboom, H. R. (1994) Making antibodies by phage display technology. *Annu. Rev. Immunol.* **12**, 433–455.

36. Chester, K. A., Begent, R. H., Robson, L., et al. (1994). Phage libraries for generation of clinically useful antibodies. Lancet 343, 455–456.

37. Begent, R. H., Verhaar, M. J., Chester, K. A., et al. (1996) Clinical evidence of efficient tumor targeting based on single-chain Fv antibody selected from a combinatorial library. *Nature Med.* **2**, 979–984.

38. Mayer, A., Chester, K. A., Flynn, A. A., and Begent, R. H. (1999) Taking engineered anti-CEA antibodies to the clinic. *J. Immunol. Methods* **231**, 261–273.

39. Flynn, A. A., Pedley, R. B. Green, A. J., et al. (2001) Effectiveness of radiolabeled anti-bodies for radio-immunotherapy in a colorectal xenograft model: a comparative study us-ing the linear-quadratic formulation. *Int. J. Radiat. Biol.* **77**, 507–517.

40. Flynn, A. A., Green, A. J., Boxer, G. M., Pedley, R. B., and Begent, R. H. J. (1999) A comparison of image registration techniques for the correlation of radiolabelled antibody distribution with tumour morphology. *Phys. Med. Biol.* **44**, 151–159.

41. Bosslet, K., Czech, J., and Hoffmann, D. (1994) Tumor-selective prodrug activation by fusion protein-mediated catalysis. *Cancer Res.* **54**, 2151–2159.

42. Rodrigues, M. L., Presta, L. G., Kotts, C. E., et al. (1995) Development of a humanised disulphide stabilised anti-p185^{ER2} Fv-B-lactamase fusion protein for activation of a cephalosporin doxorubicin prodrug. *Cancer Res.* **55,** 63–70.

43. Siemers, N. O., Kerr, D. E., Yardold, S., et al. (1997) Construction, expression, and activities of L49-sFv-β-lactamase, a single-chain antibody fusion protein for anticancer prodrug activation. *Bioconjug. Chem.* **8,** 510–519.

44. Michael, N. P., Chester, K. A., Melton, R. G., et al. (1996) In vitro and in vivo characterization of a recombinant carboxypeptidase G2::anti-CEA scFv fusion protein. *Immunotechnology* **2,** 47–57.

45. Bhatia, J., Sharma, S. K., Chester, K. A., et al. (2000) Catalytic activity of an in vivo tumor targeted anti-CEA scFv::carboxypeptidase G2 fusion protein. *Int. J. Cancer* **85,** 571–577.

46. Sharma, S. K., Pedley, R. B., Bhatia, J., et al. (2001) Optimising antibody-directed enzyme prodrug therapy (ADEPT) in human colon cancer xenografts. *Proc. AACR* **21,** 136.

47. Hoogenboom, H. R., Griffiths, A. D., Johnson, K. S., Chiswell, D. J., Hudson, P., and Winter, G. (1991) Multi-subunit proteins on the surface of filamentous phage: methodologies for displaying antibody (Fab) heavy and light chains. *Nucleic Acids Res.* **19,** 4133–4137.

48. Casey, J. L., Keep, P. A., Chester, K. A., Robson, L., Hawkins, R. E., and Begent, R. H. J. (1995) Purification of bacterially expressed single chain Fv antibodies for clinical applications using metal chelate chromatography. *J. Immunol. Methods* **179,** 105–116.

49. Harwood, P. J., Britton, D. W., Southall, P. J., Boxer, G. M., Rawling, G., and Rogers, G. T. (1986) Mapping epitope characteristics on carcinoembryonic antigen. *Br. J. Cancer* **54,** 75–82.

50. Hawkins, R. E., Zhu, D., Ovecka, M., et al. (1994) Idiotypic vaccination against human B-cell lymphoma. Rescue of variable region gene sequences from biopsy material for assembly as single-chain Fv personal vaccines. *Blood* **83,** 3279–3288.

51. Hawkins, R. E., Russell, S. J., and Winter, G. (1992) Selection of phage antibodies by binding affinity: mimicking affinity maturation. *J. Mol. Biol.* **226(3),** 889–96.

52. Vaughan, T. J., et al. (1996) Human antibodies with sub-nanomolar affinities isolated from a large non-immunized phage display library. *Nature Biotechnol.* **14,** 309–314.

27

Bioreductive Prodrugs for Cancer Therapy

Beatrice Seddon, Lloyd R. Kelland, and Paul Workman

1. Introduction

This chapter will review a particular class of antitumor prodrugs that are designed to exploit the ability of solid cancers to carry out reductive metabolism. These so-called bioreductive prodrugs are constructed in such a way that metabolic reduction leads to the production of a cytotoxic species which can then damage and kill the malignant cells. Preferential killing of cancer cells can occur in one of two ways or via of the combination of the two. The first involves the fact that the bioreductive metabolism reaction, especially when catalyzed by one-electron reductases, is oxygen sensitive—only occurring in the absence of oxygen. Because many, if not most, solid cancers contain hypoxic tumor cells because of their insufficient and aberrant vasculature, bioreductive drug activation is therefore favored in the malignant tissue. The second mechanism by which tumor selectivity vs normal tissues can be obtained occurs when one or more bioreductive enzymes are overexpressed in the cancer. This is particularly common in the case of the two-electron reductase NQO1 or DT-diaphorase. In this case, bioreductive drug activation may be independent of tumor oxygenation status.

The two approaches can be described as hypoxia selective and enzyme directed, respectively. Both are covered in this chapter, but particular attention is paid to the hypoxia-based approach, not least because of the resurgence of interest in tumor hypoxia as a major driver of malignant progression and angiogenesis in cancer, as well as in the determination of clinical outcome. Accordingly, the biology and clinical significance of tumor hypoxia will be discussed and recent advances in the molecular basis of the tumor response to hypoxia will be reviewed. The main classes of bioreductive prodrugs will be described, methods of measuring tumor hypoxia and of predicting response to bioreductive prodrugs will be discussed, and prospects for the future will be considered.

From: *Methods in Molecular Medicine, Vol. 90, Suicide Gene Therapy: Methods and Reviews*
Edited by: C. J. Springer © Humana Press Inc., Totowa, NJ

2. Biology of Tumor Hypoxia

It has long been recognized that oxygen levels within tumors are lower than in normal tissues in both animals *(1)* and humans *(2)*. This phenomenon is termed tumor hypoxia and has a number of sources *(3)*. Classical histological studies of human squamous cell carcinoma of the bronchus revealed viable tumor regions consisting of solid cords that were surrounded by a vascular stroma, suggesting that oxygen and nutrients diffuse from stroma into tumor where they are progressively consumed by tumor cells *(4)*. Cells beyond an oxygen diffusion distance of around 180 μm from blood vessels are unable to survive and hence become necrotic. This indicates that cells bordering the necrosis might be chronically hypoxic yet viable and clonogenic, exhibiting chronic diffusion-limited hypoxia (*see* **Fig. 1a**). In addition, acute hypoxia occurs within tumors as a result of temporary reversible cessation of blood flow by closure or blockage of a blood vessel that can occur over a period of minutes *(5–7)*. These acutely hypoxic cells exhibit perfusion-limited hypoxia (*see* **Fig. 1b**). As tumors grow and outstrip their vasculature, the development of tumor hypoxia results in the stimulation of angiogenesis, developing disorganized vasculature that is markedly abnormal both structurally and functionally *(8)*. Vessels are tortuous and dilated with excessive branching and shunts, are lacking in functional smooth muscle, and frequently have an incomplete endothelial lining. The latter contributes to vessel leakiness, also caused by endothelial cells that are abnormal in shape and possessing fenestrae, leading to widened intercellular junctions *(8)*. These abnormalities result in chaotic blood flow, contributing further to the hypoxic and acidic regions in tumors, in addition to the more classical acute and chronic forms of tumor hypoxia.

3. Molecular Basis of Hypoxia

Although hypoxia has been known to be present within tumors for many years, it is only relatively recently that the molecular pathways governing oxygen homeostasis and the normal physiological response to the cellular stress of hypoxia have been elucidated. The key regulator of this pathway is the hypoxia-inducible transcription factor HIF, a heterodimer consisting of two basic helix–loop–helix subunits *(9–11)*. The HIF-1β subunit is a constitutively produced nuclear protein that is not specific to the hypoxia pathway, having originally been identified as participating in the xenobiotic response. However, the HIF-1α subunit is specifically upregulated by hypoxic stress. Under conditions of normal oxygenation, it is degraded rapidly by the ubiquitin–proteasome pathway via a ubiquitin E3 ligase complex which targets HIF-1α by binding of the von Hippel–Lindau protein (pVHL) in a manner analogous to the Mdm2-mediated degradation of p53 *(12)*. Conversely, under hypoxic conditions, ubiquitination of HIF-1α is dramatically reduced *(13)*. The HIF-1α subunit undergoes posttranscriptional stabilization, translocates to the nucleus, and dimerizes with HIF-1β. The resultant HIF heterodimer then activates the transcription of a range of genes that participate in the normal adaptive response of the cell to hypoxia (*see* **Fig. 2**). These genes include *VEGF* (angiogenesis), *erythropoietin* (red blood cell production), glycolytic enzymes (glucose metabolism and energy), and *carbonic anhydrase* (pH homeostasis) *(9)*. The HIF pathway is regulated by p53 via two distinct mechanisms.

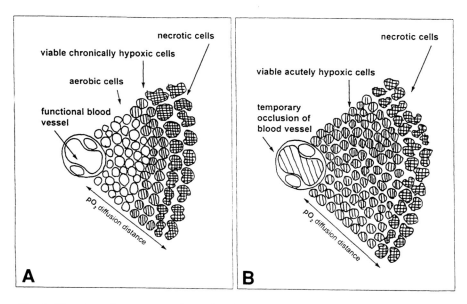

Fig. 1. Chronic and acute tumor hypoxia. (**A**) A cord of viable tumor cells around a functional central blood vessel, surrounded by necrotic tumor cells that are beyond the pO_2 diffusion distance (approx 180 μm). The rim of cells adjacent to the necrotic cells are chronically hypoxic (i.e., exhibiting diffusion-limited hypoxia). (**B**) A similar cord of tumor cells around a central blood vessel that has been temporarily occluded, rendering all viable cells within the rim of necrotic cells acutely hypoxic (i.e., exhibiting perfusion-limited hypoxia).

HIF-1α protein stability is negatively regulated in a Mdm-2-dependent manner *(14)*. In addition, HIF-induced transcription of hypoxia-responsive genes has recently been shown to be regulated by p53 binding to HIF-1α *(15,16)*. Microarray analysis is being used to profile, on a genomewide scale, the gene expression changes induced by hypoxia *(17,18)*.

Thus, in normal cells, HIF is central to oxygen homeostasis and the ability to adapt to changes in the microenvironment. However, there is evidence that the HIF pathway can be deregulated in cancerous cells. In vivo studies have shown decreased growth in tumors that are null for HIF-1α *(19,20)* or HIF-1β *(20)*, indicating that HIF acts as a positive regulator of tumor growth. This may be partly explained by the observations that tumors null for HIF-1β have low levels of ATP and are unable to upregulate glycolysis *(20)*. HIF-1α can be deregulated in response to inactivation of tumor suppressor genes (e.g., *p53, VHL*) *(21)*, activation of oncogenes (e.g., *v-src, H-ras*) *(21)*, and activation of growth factor pathways [e.g., HER2(neu)] *(22)*. Although as yet there has been no description of direct mutational activation of a HIF-1α molecule, immunohistochemical studies using monoclonal antibodies to HIF-1α have demonstrated high levels of immunoreactivity in human tumor specimens compared with very low levels in normal tissues *(23,24)*. Antibody binding to HIF-1α has been shown to correlate with VEGF expression *(25)*, tumor grade *(26)*, and intratumoral vessel density

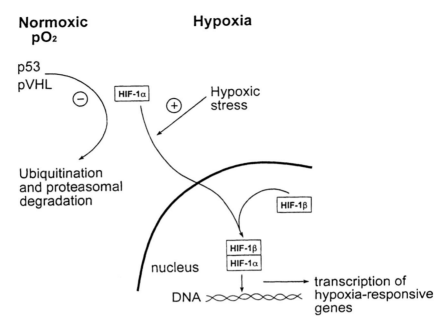

Fig. 2. Illustration of pathways for HIF-1α-induced transcription of hypoxia-responsive genes under hypoxic conditions, and regulation of HIF-1α under normoxic conditions.

(25,27–29). Furthermore, high HIF-1α expression correlates with response of primary oropharyngeal carcinoma to radiotherapy *(27)* and predicts for a worse clinical outcome compared with tumors with low or absent expression in a number of tumors *(25,27–30).*

Hypoxia induces *p53* gene expression *(31)* and mediates apoptosis in oncogenically transformed cells that possess wild-type *p53 (32).* However, cells lacking wild-type *p53* are unable to undergo hypoxia-induced apoptosis and are consequently conferred with a survival advantage *(32).* Thus, by selecting for mutant *p53,* hypoxia leads not only to deregulation of HIF-1α and stimulation of angiogenesis but also to genetic instability and enhanced tumor progression *(21).* This hypothesis is supported by the demonstration of a link between tumor hypoxia and metastasis in a number of experimental systems *(33,34)* and by the clinical observations of the prognostic importance of hypoxia *(35–37)* and HIF-1α expression *(27,30)* in human tumors.

4. Effect of Hypoxia on Anticancer Treatment Efficacy

Hypoxic cells are directly resistant to radiation compared with normally oxygenated cells *(38).* Radiosensitivity declines rapidly with oxygen tensions ranging from 30 to 0 mm Hg, whereas oxygen tensions greater than 30 mm Hg have no major impact on radiation response *(39).* Molecular oxygen present during irradiation acts to "fix" radiation-induced DNA damage, by a mechanism involving oxygen free radicals formed by the interaction of radiation with intracellular water. This results in an "oxygen enhancement" effect, such that radiation doses under hypoxic conditions may need to be up to three times greater than in the presence of oxygen in order to produce an equivalent biological effect on tumor *(38)*. As a consequence, hypoxia is an important source of radiotherapy treatment failure, having been associated in clinical studies with poor local tumor control following radiotherapy in carcinomas of the head and neck *(37,40)* and cervix *(41,42)*.

Hypoxia has also been associated with reduced cytotoxicity of a number of chemotherapeutic agents to tumors cells both in vitro *(43)* and in vivo *(44,45)*. However, there is no current published clinical evidence demonstrating hypoxia-induced chemoresistance in human tumors. Nonetheless, hypoxia would be expected to be associated with chemoresistance for a number of reasons. It is known to inhibit cell proliferation *(31,46)* by induction of *p27*, causing cell cycle arrest at the G1–S-phase transition in a pathway that is independent of *p53* *(47)*. Hypoxia would therefore be expected to decrease cytotoxicity of cell-cycle-specific agents. Furthermore, abnormal tumor vasculature and perfusion may impair the ability of chemotherapeutic agents to reach poorly perfused, hypoxic areas of tumor at therapeutically useful concentrations *(48)*. However, although the concept of hypoxia-induced chemoresistance and chemotherapy treatment failure appears intuitively likely, in humans, at least, it remains speculative.

5. Clinical Significance of Hypoxia

In recent years, a commercially available polarographic microelectrode (Eppendorf, Hamburg, Germany) has been used to make direct pO_2 measurements in human tumors *(49)*, providing extensive evidence of the presence therein of hypoxia. In addition, it has been shown that hypoxia in human tumors can be predictive of response to, and outcome following, tumor treatment *(50)*. In carcinoma of the cervix, tumor hypoxia has been related to lower rates of local control of the primary tumor in the pelvis following treatment *(42,51)* and predicts poor subsequent disease-free and overall survival *(36,42,51,52)*. It has been related to the incidence of pelvic and retroperitoneal lymph node metastases present at time of primary diagnosis *(36,53,54)*, and a recent study has shown that hypoxia is also an independent prognostic indicator of decreased progression-free survival in patients with negative pelvic lymph nodes *(52)*. Hypoxia in squamous cell head and neck carcinomas has been related to lower rates of local tumor control after radiotherapy *(37,40)*, and poorer disease-free and overall survival *(40)*. Similarly, in patients with sarcoma treated with a range of modalities, pretreatment tumor hypoxia has predicted reduced disease-free and overall survival *(35,55)*. These latter findings suggest that poor outcome does not merely reflect hypoxia-related intrinsic tumor radioresistance. The concept that hypoxia somehow relates to a more aggressive tumor biology and more malignant tumor phenotype is supported by the observation that hypoxic primary tumors are associated with a higher rate of subsequent development of distant metastases *(35,52)*. It is also consistent with the findings discussed earlier that at the molecular level, hypoxia causes genetic instability and enhances tumor progression (*see* **Subheading 3.**).

6. Hypoxia-Based Therapeutic Strategies

Attempts have been made to reduce the effects of tumor hypoxia in patients, with the aim of increasing efficacy of anticancer treatments. These have included inhalation of hyperbaric oxygen or high oxygen content gases such as carbogen during radiotherapy to reverse chronic hypoxia, nicotinamide to reverse acute hypoxia, oxygen-mimetic radiosensitizers to reduce hypoxia-induced radioresistance, and blood transfusions to improve hemoglobin content of blood *(56,57)*.

An alternative approach to reducing tumor hypoxia is to exploit it as a unique feature of the tumor microenvironment that differentiates it from most normal tissues, therefore providing an Achilles' heel and a potential therapeutic target. Hypoxia-targeted bioreductive drugs achieve this aim by virtue of intracellular chemical reduction by reductase enzymes to generate active cytotoxic species selectively under hypoxic conditions *(58–60)*. This hypoxia-driven generation of a cytotoxic species is a key feature of many bioreductive drugs and provides a therapeutic advantage against a subpopulation of hypoxic cells that are potentially resistant to conventional treatment modalities. Thus, a combined modality approach using hypoxic cytotoxins with radiotherapy, chemotherapy, or both may be optimal, and indeed clinical trials of tirapazamine, an aliphatic *N*-oxide, combined with radiotherapy and/or cisplatin have yielded promising early results *(61–64)*.

Thus, bioreductive drugs have future potential as a hypoxia-targeted therapy. Moreover, they conform to the model of an inactive prodrug metabolized by a specific enzyme to a pharmacologically active species, making them ideal candidates for incorporation into a GDEPT (gene-directed enzyme–prodrug therapy) approach.

7. Bioreductive Prodrugs

7.1. Introduction

Prodrugs are defined as inactive compounds that are converted in the body to species that are pharmacologically active *(65,66)*. Bioreductive drugs are prodrugs that are activated by metabolic reduction to cytotoxins *(58–60)*. They can be divided into two categories, dependent on the nature of activation. Oxygen-dependent hypoxia-targeted cytotoxins undergo rapid metabolism to a transient intermediate that can be converted back to the parent drug by reaction with molecular oxygen in a process termed futile recycling, thus restricting prodrug activation to hypoxic cells. The rates of such reactions are determined by the one-electron redox potential of the individual drug *(67)*. In contrast, enzyme-directed cytotoxins exhibit oxygen selectivity that is primarily dependent on the activating reductase enzyme *(68)*. One-electron reductases such as NADPH : cytochrome P450 reductase catalyze oxygen-dependent metabolism, producing a reduction product that is susceptible to futile recycling by oxygen. However, the two-electron reduction products produced by reductases such as DT-diaphorase (NQO1) are generally not so susceptible to futile recycling and, therefore, such metabolism is most commonly oxygen independent. It follows then that the reductase enzyme profile of a tumor could influence the therapeutic effectiveness of bioreductive drugs that can undergo both one- and two-electron reduction including agents such as mitomycin C and EO9.

The variable oxygen dependence of enzyme-directed cytotoxins is undoubtedly important, and the development of bioreductive drugs activated by DT-diaphorase continues to be of significant interest. Nevertheless, the activation of the great majority of bioreductive drugs is oxygen dependent, making the hypoxia-activated cytotoxins the more prominent group. For hypoxia-targeted cytotoxins to be useful as prodrugs, they should possess certain properties:

- Efficient distribution within tumors, including poorly vascularized hypoxic regions
- Conversion in hypoxic cells by endogenous enzymes to a cytotoxin, or to a species that releases a cytotoxin, by a process that is inhibited or reversed by the presence of oxygen
- Minimal activation in, and toxicity to, nonhypoxic cells

It is useful to think of prodrugs as modular, defining two functionally distinct elements: the *trigger* and the *effector (69)*. The *trigger* activates the prodrug and must be capable of rapid metabolism to a transient intermediate. The *effector* is activated by the trigger to become, or release, a cytotoxin. The cytotoxin should be of high potency and should have the ability to kill cells in a variety of pH environments and proliferative states. In the case of hypoxia-targeted prodrugs, it should be active against noncycling cells because hypoxia induces G1 arrest *(31,47)*. For this reason, effectors have frequently been DNA alkylating agents such as nitrogen mustards *(58,69)*. Furthermore, the cytotoxin should ideally be able to exert a substantial bystander effect, killing nearby cells within reasonable proximity. To achieve this, it should be sufficiently long-lived with a half-life measured in minutes *(70)* and should be capable of diffusing a limited distance beyond the site of activation. It is important, however, that diffusion out of the tumor and into the general circulation should not be possible, in order to prevent toxicity to normal tissues.

Bioreductive prodrugs can be classified in a number of ways, but it is conceptually helpful to do so by trigger (*see* **Table 1**).

7.2. Drugs Classified According to Type of Trigger

The chemical structures of some of the major bioreductive compounds are shown in **Fig. 3**. At present, the only clinically approved bioreductive agent is mitomycin C. However, a number of compounds are currently either under clinical investigation (e.g., tirapazamine, AQ4N) or about to enter the clinic (e.g., RH1).

7.2.1. Quinones

7.2.1.1. Mitomycin C

The prototype quinone-containing bioreductive drug is mitomycin C. Currently, its main use lies in the treatment of non-small-cell lung cancer *(71,72)*, superficial bladder cancer *(73)*, and squamous cell carcinoma of the anus given concurrently with radiotherapy *(74)*. The reductive activation of mitomycin C to produce DNA alkylation and selective kill under hypoxic conditions is complex. The drug is activated by one-electron reduction to a semiquinone radical mainly by NADPH : cytochrome P450 reductase (but also by xanthine oxidase and cytochrome-b_5 reductase) *(68,75,76)*. In addition, oxygen-insensitive two-electron reduction to a hydroquinone may occur, mainly by DT-diaphorase *(68,77)*. In vitro, DT-diaphorase activity across the NCI human tumor

Table 1
Bioreductive Prodrugs Classified According to Trigger

Trigger	Effector	Mechanism of action	Activating enzymes	Hypoxic selectivity ratio	Preclinical development	Clinical development
Quinones						
Mitomycin C	Aziridine ring Carbamate group	Bifunctional alkylating agent → DNA monoadducts and cross-links	1e⁻ and 2e⁻ reductases	1.5–3.0×		Routine use, in lung and bladder cancer, and with radiotherapy in head and neck and anus
Porfiromycin	Aziridine ring Carbamate group	Bifunctional alkylating agent → DNA monoadducts and cross-links	1e⁻ and 2e⁻ reductases	5–15×	Synergistic activity with radiation	Activity as single agent (phase I and II) and in combination with radiotherapy; phase III study ongoing.
Indoloquinone EO9	Aziridine ring	Hydroquinone fragments to alkylating agent → DNA cross links	1e⁻ and 2e⁻ reductases	50×	Preferential activity against tumors with high levels of DT-diaphorase	Phase I and II trials completed; no clinical activity, renal toxicity, short plasma half-life — clinical use systemically abandoned.
RH1	Aziridine rings (2)	Bifunctional alkylating agent → DNA monoadducts and cross-links	1e⁻ and 2e⁻ reductases		Preferential activity against tumors with high levels of DT-diaphorase	Due to enter clinical study.
Aromatic N-oxides						
Tirapazamine	Reactive nitroxyl free radical	Abstracts hydrogen from DNA → DNA double-strand breaks	1e reductases	15–200×		Phase II and III studies with radiotherapy and/or cisplatin ongoing
Aliphatic N-oxides						
AQ4N	AQ4 (stable DNA affinic agent)	Binds and blocks topoisomerase II → cell-cycle-specific cytotoxicity	Cytochrome P450, especially A3	10×		Phase I study opened 2001

(Continued on next page)

522

Table 1
Bioreductive Prodrugs Classified According to Trigger

Trigger	Effector	Mechanism of action	Activating enzymes	Hypoxic selectivity ratio	Preclinical development	Clinical development
Nitacrine N-oxide	Nitro group N→O group	Bifunctional alkylating agent → DNA monoadducts and cross-links		1000x	Rapidly metabolised in vivo → abandoned	
Nitroheterocyclics RSU 1069/ RB 6145	Nitro group Aziridine ring	Bifunctional alkylating agent → DNA monoadducts and cross links (RB 6145 is prodrug of RSU 1069)	1e⁻ reductases	10–100x	RB 6145 causes irreversible retinopathy in animals	RSU 1069 causes severe emesis—clinical use abandoned
CB 1954	Nitro groups (2) Aziridine ring	Bifunctional alkylating agent → DNA monoadducts and cross-links	DT-diaphorase, 1e⁻ reductase-	3.6x	Significant antitumor activity in vivo in rat tumors but not human tumors; now being developed as GDEPT approach with E. coli nitroreductase	Phase I studies completed; clinical responses when used as single agent; trials involving GDEPT or coadministration with cofactor for NQO2 planned
SN 23862	Nitro groups (2) Nitrogen mustard	Bifunctional alkylating agent → ∆NA monoadducts and cross-links	1e⁻ and 2e⁻ reductases	60x	Being developed as GDEPT approach with E. coli⁻ nitroreductase	
Transition metal complexes SN 24771	Nitrogen mustard	Bioreductively triggered release of active cytotoxin	1e⁻ reductases		Active in vitro but not in vivo → abandoned	

523

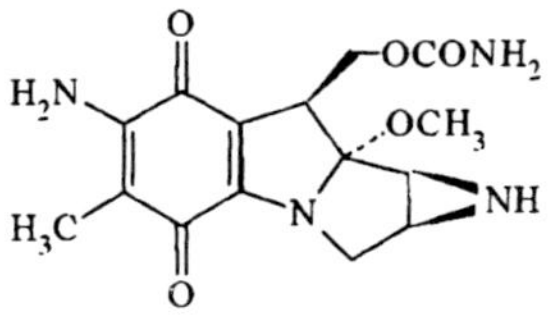

Mitomycin C

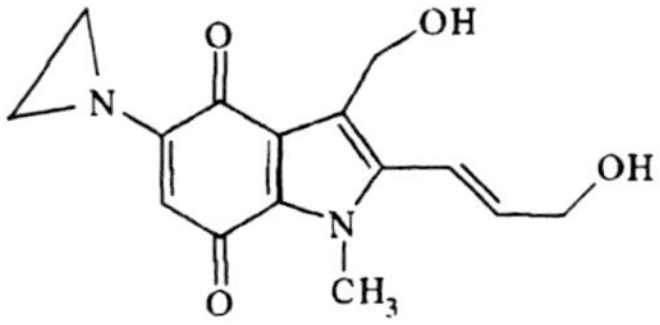

EO9

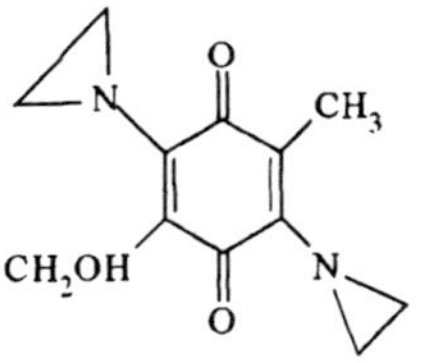

RH1

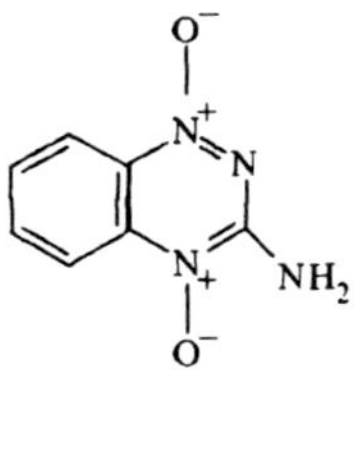

Tirapazamine

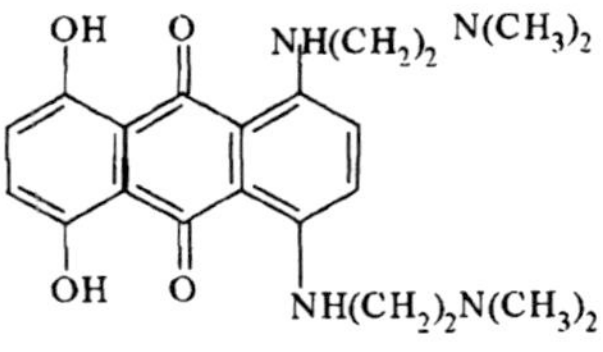

AQ4N

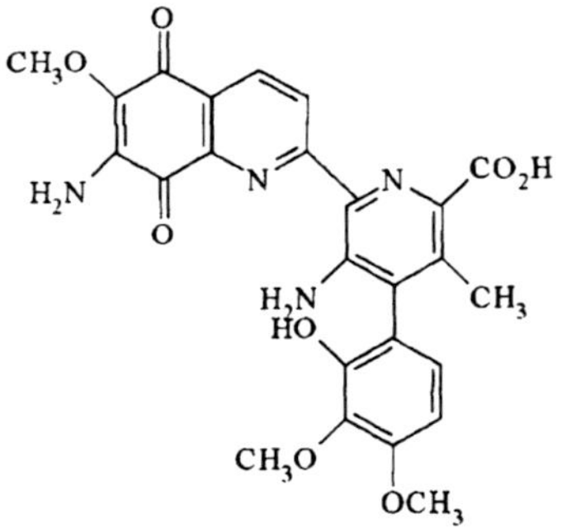

Streptonigrin

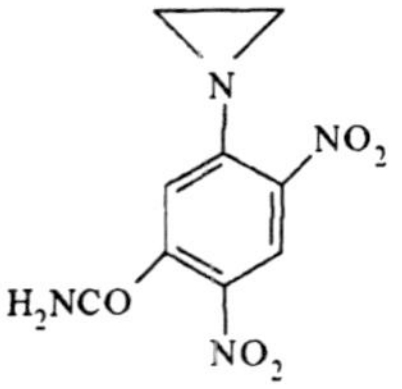

CB1954

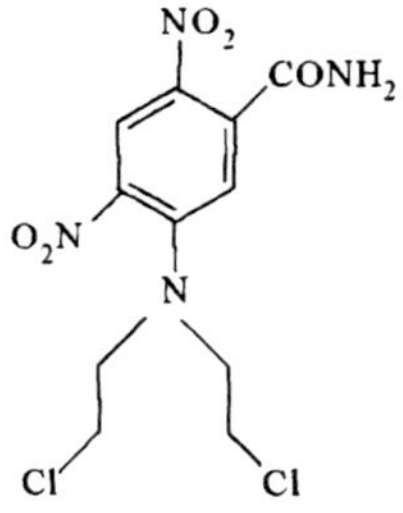

SN 23862

Fig. 3. Chemical structures of some bioreductive prodrugs.

cell panel has been shown to correlate with sensitivity to mitomycin C *(78)*. Furthermore, a recent clinical study has shown that expression of DT-diaphorase and NADPH: cytochrome P450 reductase in bladder tumor biopsies correlates with mitomycin C activity in corresponding patients *(79)*, although other studies (e.g., ref. *80*) have shown no correlation between response to mitomycin C in vivo and DT-diaphorase activity. Induction of DT-diaphorase in human tumor cells in vitro by dietary inducers has been shown to increase the cytotoxic activity of mitomycin C, offering a potential strategy to increase the efficacy of bioreductive antitumor agents *(81)*.

7.2.1.2. PORFIROMYCIN

Early quinone-containing compounds also shown to be activated by DT-diaphorase included diaziquone (AZQ), methylDZQ, streptonigrin, porfiromycin, and the indoloquinone EO9 *(60,68,77)*. Porfiromycin (a methyl analog of mitomycin C) has greater hypoxic selectivity than mitomycin C and has been shown in vivo to act synergistically with radiotherapy *(82)*. It has shown some activity as a single agent in phase I and II studies and has been evaluated in combination with radiotherapy for locally advanced poor prognosis squamous cell carcinoma of the head and neck, achieving a 5-yr actuarial survival of 32% *(83)*. As a result, a follow-on randomized phase III study in the same patient population has been initiated, comparing radiotherapy combined with porfiromycin or mitomycin C.

7.2.1.3. INDOLOQUINONE EO9

The indoloquinone EO9 (3-hydroxy-5-aziridinyl-1-methyl-2-(1*H*-indole-4,7-indione)-propenol) *(84,85)* (*see* **Fig. 3**) is structurally related to mitomycin C, but is a better substrate for DT-diaphorase. The role of DT-diaphorase and other reductases in the metabolism of EO9, together with the interplay with hypoxia, is complex in that whereas activation by DT-diaphorase is oxygen insensitive, EO9 is also activated selectively under hypoxic conditions, probably by NADPH : cytochrome P450 reductase *(78,84,86–91)*. Phase II clinical trials of single-agent EO9 have been performed in patients with non-small-cell lung cancer *(92)* and with breast, gastric, pancreatic, or colorectal cancer *(93)*, but have demonstrated disappointing antitumor activity. The dose-limiting toxicity was proteinuria and renal impairment. Furthermore, the drug was rapidly cleared from the circulation. In the light of randomized studies combining mitomycin C with radiation *(74)*, it is possible that some advantageous role for EO9 may have been seen if used concurrently with radiotherapy.

7.2.1.4. RH1

RH1 (2,5-diaziridinyl-3-(hydroxymethyl)-6-methyl-1,4-benzoquinone) (*see* **Fig. 3**) is a more water-soluble analog of the aziridinylbenzoquinone methylDZQ. It has exhibited antitumor activity in mice bearing H460 non-small-cell lung cancer xenografts *(94)* and has been shown to possess preferential activity against tumor cells with high levels of DT-diaphorase *(95)*. In comparison to EO9, RH1 possesses improved pharmacokinetic properties, with 10-fold slower elimination from plasma in mice *(94)*. It is due to enter clinical trials under the auspices of Cancer Research UK.

7.2.1.5. Novel Strategies for Identification of New Quinones

The role of DT-diaphorase in activating mitomycin C has led to a complementary bioreductive strategy aimed at exploiting differences in metabolizing enzymes between solid tumors and normal tissue. DT-diaphorase and the encoding gene NQO1 have received most attention in this enzyme-directed approach, following observations of relatively high expression in tumors (notably lung and colon) compared with corresponding normal tissues (96,97). To date, the concept of DT-diaphorase-mediated bioreductive drug activation has not been adequately tested in the clinic. Mitomycin C is activated by additional reductases and EO9 suffers from poor pharmacokinetic properties. The results of trials with RH1 are awaited with considerable interest. The selection of patients with high DT-diaphorase activity suitable for an enzyme-directed approach could be based on measurements of enzyme levels or NQO1 gene expression profiling performed on tumor biopsy specimens. Such selection is also important because 5–20% of the general population (dependent on ethnicity) are homozygous for a point mutation of the NQO1 gene that results in a lack of DT-diaphorase activity (98).

In recent years, isogenic cell line models differing only in DT-diaphorase status have been established by ourselves (99) and others (95,100), which should prove valuable in the search for improved prodrugs of this type. These models have shown the predicted DT-diaphorase-mediated potentiation of cell kill by streptonigrin (see Fig. 3) and EO9. In addition, the determination of the crystal structure of human DT-diaphorase provides another useful aid to the rational design of improved DT-diaphorase-activated bioreductive prodrugs (101). Furthermore, reductase expression across the National Cancer Institute human tumor cell panel has been measured and has confirmed correlations of DT-diaphorase activity with sensitivity to mitomycin C and EO9 (78). This information now allows, through molecular COMPARE and cluster analysis, the identification of new compounds that show a correlation (positive or negative) with reductase enzyme expression and offers potential for the identification of new prodrug leads. Our own studies using the BE colon carcinoma isogenic pair of cell lines differing only in DT-diaphorase status have shown that the potency of the quinone-containing ansamycin heat shock protein 90 inhibitor, 17-allylamino,17-demethoxygeldanamycin (17AAG), now in phase I trials, is markedly enhanced by DT-diaphorase (102).

7.3. Aromatic N-Oxides: Tirapazamine

Tirapazamine (3-amino-1,2,4-benzotriazine 1,4-dioxide, formerly known as SR 4233) (see Fig. 3) shows a 50- to 200-fold hypoxic : oxic cytotoxicity differential (103,104). This is in contrast to only a 1.5- to 3-fold differential for mitomycin C. Tirapazamine undergoes one-electron reduction under hypoxia to form a cytotoxic free radical that abstracts a hydrogen from nearby DNA, producing single- and double-strand breaks. Further reduction produces the inactive mono-N-oxide (SR 4317) and eventually the amino product (SR 4300). Under oxic conditions, rapid back-oxidation occurs to produce the parent molecule and the less cytotoxic superoxide radical (105). Although the enzymology of tirapazamine metabolism is not completely understood, key roles for cytochrome P450 and NADPH : cytochrome P450 reductase are apparent *(105–109)*, along with an as yet unidentified intranuclear reductase, which may explain the high proportion of DNA double-strand breaks formed *(110)*. DT-Diaphorase is able to metabolise tirapazamine, but not to an active free radical *(107,111)*.

Preclinical studies have shown substantial activity when tirapazamine was combined with either radiation or cisplatin *(112)*. The basis of the synergism with cisplatin, for which tirapazamine needs to be present at least 30 min before cisplatin, is not completely elucidated but appears to involve effects on the repair of platinum–DNA adducts *(113)*. Following phase I studies (e.g., ref. *114*), no single-agent phase II trials were performed but rather, based on the preclinical combination studies, tirapazamine was combined with cisplatin or radiation *(62)*. The results of a phase III randomized trial in patients with advanced previously untreated non-small-cell lung cancer (CATAPULT I) revealed that the addition of tirapazamine significantly enhanced the activity of cisplatin in this disease (median survival of 35 vs 28 wk; response rates of 27.5 vs 13.7%) *(62)*. A second, large randomized study in lung cancer, CATAPULT II, is currently comparing cisplatin and etoposide with cisplatin and tirapazamine. Toxicities associated with tirapazamine include reversible hearing loss, muscle cramps, and nausea and vomiting. Tirapazamine is now being evaluated in combination with cisplatin and radiotherapy, with phase I and II studies in carcinoma of the cervix *(64)* and head and neck *(63)* demonstrating impressive response rates, translating into very good rates of local control for the advanced tumors treated. The results are sufficiently encouraging that the triple combination is currently being evaluated in a phase II setting in parallel with cisplatin/5-fluorouracil-based chemoradiation in head and neck cancer *(63)*.

7.2.3. Aliphatic N-Oxides

7.2.3.1. AQ4N

AQ4N is the di-*N*-oxide of 1,4-bis[{2-(dimethylaminoethyl}-amino]5,8-dihydroxyanthracene-9,10-dione (AQ4) (*see* **Fig. 3**) and is bioreductively activated under hypoxic conditions to AQ4, a DNA intercalator and topoisomerase II inhibitor, by enzymes of the cytochrome P450 family, particularly CYP3A *(115,116)*. Preclinical studies have shown that AQ4N enhances the antitumor efficacy of radiation and cytotoxic agents (including cyclophosphamide, cisplatin, and thiotepa) *(117)*. A phase I study started in 2001 under the auspices of Cancer Research UK and BTG *(118)*.

7.2.3.2. NITRACRINE N-OXIDE

Nitracrine *N*-oxide is based on nitracrine (1-nitro-9-[*N*,*N*-(dimethylamino)propylamino] acridine) *(119)*, a DNA intercalator that forms a cytotoxic alkylating agent via bioreduction of the nitro substituent. The side-chain *N*-oxide analog (which thus has the potential to be bioreduced in two positions on the molecule) has shown exceptional (1000-fold) hypoxic selectivity in vitro but poor activity in vivo *(119)*. Structural modification to improve biodistribution properties in vivo are ongoing.

7.2.4. Nitroaromatics and Nitroheterocyclics

This class of bioreductive agents emerged as a result of studies of 2-nitroimidazoles as radiosensitizers (e.g., misonidazole) in which, in addition to radiosensitization, hypoxia-selective cytotoxicity was observed in the absence of radiation *(120,121)*. Bioreductive metabolism of such agents at the nitro group is well characterized *(122–124)*. In recent years, new hypoxia-selective cytotoxins have been developed that are more potent than the early radiosensitizers, by the introduction of alkylating groups such as aziridines or nitrogen mustards.

7.2.4.1. RSU 1069 AND RB 6145

One such compound, RSU 1069 (1[2-nitro-1-imidazolyl]-3-aziridinyl-2-propanol), introduced an aziridine group onto the N-1 side chain, exhibiting up to a 100-fold hypoxic : oxic cytotoxicity differential *(125–127)*. RSU 1069 entered clinical trials, but gastrointestinal toxicity limited its utility *(128)*. A prodrug of RSU 1069, RB 6145, was subsequently developed, but clinical trials were not initiated because of preclinical observations of retinopathy *(129)*.

7.2.4.2. CB 1954

CB 1954 (5-aziridin-1-yl-2,4-dinitrobenzamide; *see* **Fig. 3**), another interesting agent in this class, was shown to be highly active against the Walker 256 adenocarcinoma in rats *(130)*. On this basis and despite being ineffective in human tumor cell lines, it entered clinical trials in the 1970s in which it showed no antitumor activity *(131)*. An explanation for this paradox was sought, but the mechanism of action of CB 1954 was initially poorly understood *(132,133)*. However, subsequent studies showed that CB 1954 was bioreductively activated by DT-diaphorase *(134)*, explaining its only modest hypoxia selectivity *(135)*. Specifically, the 4-nitro group undergoes two-electron reduction [by *NQO1* and *NQO2* *(136)*] to the 4-hydroxylamine, which can then form a reactive thioester that crosslinks DNA along with the aziridine moiety *(131)*. Activation of CB 1954 by DT-diaphorase explains its marked effectiveness in Walker 256 cells, which express high levels of this enzyme *(134)*. However, human cell lines are considerably less sensitive to CB 1954 than would be predicted by their levels of DT-diaphorase, requiring 50- to 500-fold higher doses of CB 1954 to produce equivalent cytotoxicity to that observed in rat cell lines *(137)*. This is because of reduced activating ability of the human compared to rat enzyme *(137)* and provides an explanation for the lack of effect of this agent on human tumor cells *(131)*. CB 1954 remains of current clinical interest, either coadministered with the cofactor nicotinamide riboside (reduced) to facilitate bioreductive activation by the enzyme NQO2 *(136)* or for use in GDEPT approaches (*see* **Subheading 8.**).

7.2.4.3. SN 23862

The 2,4-dinitrobenzamide mustard SN 23862 (*see* **Fig. 3**) is the nitrogen mustard analog of CB 1954. It is considerably less efficient as a substrate for DT-diaphorase than CB 1954, which probably accounts for its markedly superior hypoxia-selective cytotoxicity *(135)*. Reduction of either or both nitro groups results in increased reactivity of the mustard and correspondingly increased cytotoxicity *(69,138,139)*. There is current interest in the use of SN 23862 as a GDEPT prodrug (*see* **Subheading 8.**).

7.2.5. Transition Metal Complexes

Agents with a cobalt-based metal ion bioreductive trigger have been designed, in which the one-electron reduction of Co(III) to Co(II) allows the release of nitrogen mustard ligands *(140)*. The process of reduction results in the conversion of the mustard from a stable inactive form to an active diffusible form *(69,135)*. The lead compound SN 24771 showed moderate hypoxic selectivity in vitro, but little activity against hypoxic cells in vivo *(141)*. It has not been developed further.

8. GDEPT Approaches

Gene-directed enzyme prodrug therapy (GDEPT) is a technique in which a gene encoding an enzyme with the ability to activate a prodrug is introduced into tumor cells and targeted for selective expression in tumor cells by being placed under the control of a tumor-specific promoter. The enzyme thus activates the administered prodrug selectively in tumor cells to a cytotoxic species. The selected enzyme must not be endogenous, so that the prodrug cannot be activated in enzyme-expressing normal tissues. The prodrug must be nontoxic to normal tissues, must penetrate tumor cells, should not act as a substrate for endogenous enzymes expressed in normal tissues, and must be a good substrate for the delivered enzyme to ensure effective activation. The active drug should be highly cytotoxic, should exert a bystander effect such that it diffuses to and kills adjacent tumor cells, and should have a short half-life to prevent systemic distribution and toxicity *(142,143)*. The transfection of prodrug-activating genes into tumor cells is analogous to the enzyme-directed approach discussed in **Subheading 7.1.**, in which the intrinsic reductase enzyme profile of a tumor can be exploited to influence the therapeutic effectiveness of bioreductive drugs. However, the GDEPT approach does not rely upon an intrinsically high expression of the reductase in the tumor but, rather, targets the reductase to the tumor by gene therapy.

Bioreductive prodrugs are ideal candidates for a GDEPT approach. CB 1954 (*see* **Subheading 7.2.4.2.**) has been most widely studied *(131,143)*. It is particularly suitable because it is a poor substrate for human DT-diaphorase such that it has little cytotoxicity in human tumor cells *(137)*. However, it is a highly efficient substrate for *Escherichia coli* nitroreductase (NTR), an oxygen-insensitive monomeric flavin mononucleotide nitroreductase which reduces CB 1954 92 times faster than DT-diaphorase *(144)*. NTR has been successfully transfected into human tumor cells, producing 50- to 500-fold increases in CB 1954 toxicity, with a marked bystander effect *(145)*. The CB 1954–NTR enzyme prodrug system is currently in phase I clinical trials in humans *(146)*.

SN 23862, a mustard analog of CB 1954 (*see* **Subheading 7.2.4.3.**), shows similar cytotoxic selectivity to transfected tumor cells as CB 1954, but is a better substrate for NTR and exhibits a greater bystander effect, suggesting that it may be superior to CB 1954 in a GDEPT context *(146)*. A series of nitrogen analogs of CB 1954 have been evaluated in vitro as potential prodrugs for NTR GDEPT systems and also appear to offer advantages over CB 1954 *(147)*. Furthermore, early evaluation of 4-nitro benzylcarbamates and nitroinidolines has shown reasonable cytotoxic selectivity for NTR-transfected cell lines in culture *(146)*.

9. Prediction of Response to Bioreductive Drugs

Hypoxia-targeted bioreductive drugs are active selectively against cells that are hypoxic but not those that are normally oxygenated. Therefore, it would be useful to be able to predict patients with hypoxic tumors who are likely to benefit from bioreductive-based therapeutic strategies. A number of methods for detection of hypoxic cells in tumors have been developed, although only a small number are in use in humans *(148)*. Although none of these are used as part of routine clinical practice, several techniques are currently in use as part of clinical research programs. pO_2 can be measured directly by insertion into tissue of oxygen-detecting probes, such as a polarographic needle microelectrode electrode (Eppendorf, Hamburg, Germany), producing parameters of pO_2 that have been proved to be of prognostic value (*see* **Subheading 5.**). A newly available luminescence-based fiber-optic sensor, the OxyLite (Oxford Optronix, Oxford, UK), also measures pO_2 directly, producing a time-resolved pO_2 trace, but, as yet, is unlicensed for use in humans *(149,150)*. The comet assay, performed on fine-needle aspirates, assesses DNA strand breaks in response to radiation and therefore provides a means to evaluate radiobiological hypoxia *(151–153)*. Magnetic resonance imaging techniques can utilize the paramagnetic properties of deoxyhemoglobin in order to produce blood oxygenation-level-dependent (BOLD) contrast *(154)*.

All of these methods give either direct or surrogate measures of tumor oxygenation and therefore provide an indirect estimate of the likelihood of response to a bioreductive drug. However, in order to produce a more representative estimate, the ideal would be to use an assay that directly assesses tumor metabolism of bioreductive drugs. The optimal approach would be to give a test dose of a bioreductive drug and to assess in vivo whether it has been effectively bioreduced, via direct detection of metabolized drug present in tumor. Several nitroimidazoles (*see* **Subheading 7.2.4.**) have been used in this manner as a surrogate measure of tumor hypoxia, detected by immunohistochemistry or a variety of scanning or imaging methods *(155)* (*see* **Table 2**). Pimonidazole and EF5 are detected in tumor biopsy specimens by immunohistochemistry. The prognostic value of pimonidazole is currently being evaluated prospectively in a number of tumor sites including carcinoma of the cervix *(156)*, whereas EF5 is still undergoing early evaluation *(157–159)*. However, immunohistochemical approaches are invasive, which has led to interest in detecting nitroimidazoles noninvasively by single photon-emission computerized tomography *(160)*, positron-emission tomography *(161)*, and magnetic resonance spectroscopy *(162,163)*. The most recent addition to these noninvasive hypoxia probes is SR-4554, a new fluorinated 2-nitroimidazole specifically designed for the purpose, which, following favorable preclinical evaluation *(164–166)*, has recently entered phase I study under the auspices of Cancer Research UK. Promising early results have been obtained, with demonstration of minimal toxicity, reproducible pharmacokinetics, and evidence of

Table 2
Nitroimidazole Hypoxia Markers Used Clinically

Detection method	Nitroimidazole	Marker label
Immunohistochemistry	Pimonidazole	Antibody
	EF5	Antibody
SPECT[a]	IAZA	^{131}I
PET[b]	Fluoromisonidazole	^{18}F
	EF5	^{18}F
MRS[c]	SR 4554	^{19}F

[a]Single-photon-emission computerized tomography.
[b]Positron-emission tomography.
[c]Magnetic resonance spectroscopy.

detection of SR-4554 in tumors *(167)*. The use of such markers to identify patients with hypoxic tumors likely to respond to bioreductive prodrug therapies represents a rational approach to patient selection.

10. Concluding Remarks and Future Prospects

The field of tumor hypoxia is a particularly interesting one at the moment because of the bringing together of the following themes:

* The well-established role of hypoxia in the resistance of tumors to radiation and cytotoxic drugs
* More recent data demonstrating the importance of hypoxia as a prognostic factor for clinical outcome
* The rapidly emerging understanding of the molecular basis for the control of gene expression and tumor angiogenesis, particularly the function of HIF-1α
* The role of hypoxia in selecting for cells with mutant p53, thereby contributing to drug resistance and tumor progression
* The ability to exploit hypoxia as an Achilles' heel of solid tumors by the design, development, and use of appropriate bioreductive prodrugs that selectively kill hypoxic tumor cells (or cells overexpressing bioreductive enzymes)
* The potential use of bioreductive drugs in ADEPT and GDEPT strategies
* The development of various other hypoxia-based therapies, including hypoxia-directed gene therapy, and drugs targeted to the HIF-1α pathways or to downstream angiogenesis signalling processes (e.g., through VEGF and its cognate receptor tyrosine kinases)
* The possibility of using bioreductive agents in combination with antiangiogenic or antivascular drugs (e.g., combretastatin, DMXAA)
* The development of various methods for measuring hypoxia in tumors, thereby providing a means to identify patients most suited to hypoxia-based therapies or to monitor the effects of antiangiogenic or antivascular treatments.

We have an increasingly detailed understanding of the physiology and molecular biology of tumor hypoxia. We also have increasingly sophisticated tools to monitor tumor hypoxia itself and the various factors responsible for and associated with it. In addition, we have a range of bioreductive prodrugs, in various flavors, for which proof of principle for anticancer activity, alone or in combination with other treatments, has been demonstrated. In the next few years, it will be important to bring these various strands together in order to thoroughly and critically evaluate the potential of bioreductive prodrugs to play a leading role in cancer treatment.

Acknowledgments

We would like to thank Dr. Margaret Ashcroft for advice and comments on the manuscript and Peter Seddon for preparation of figures. The authors' work is funded by Cancer Research UK (www.icr.ac.uk/cctherap/). BS was a Cancer Research UK Clinical Fellow and PW is a Cancer Research UK Life Fellow and Harrap Professor of Pharmacology and Therapeutics at the University of London and the Institute of Cancer Research.

References

1. Moulder, J. E. and Rockwell, S. (1987) Tumour hypoxia: its impact on cancer therapy. *Cancer Metastasis Rev.* **5,** 313–341.
2. Vaupel, P., Thews, O., Kelleher, D. K., and Höckel, M. (1998) Current status of knowledge and critical issues in tumour oxygenation. Results from 25 years research in tumour pathophysiology. *Adv. Exp. Med. Biol.* **454,** 591–602.
3. Brown, J. M. and Giacca, A. J. (1998) The unique physiology of solid tumours: opportunities (and problems) for cancer therapy. *Cancer Res.* **58,** 1408–1416.
4. Thomlinson, R. H. and Gray, L. H. (1955) The histological structure of some human lung cancers and the possible implications for radiotherapy. *Br. J. Cancer* **9,** 539–549.
5. Brown, J. M. (1979) Evidence for acutely hypoxic cells in mouse tumours, and a possible mechanism of reoxygenation. *Br. J. Radiol.* **52,** 650–656.
6. Chaplin, D. J., Durand, R. E., and Olive, P. L. (1986) Acute hypoxia in tumours: implications for modifiers of radiation effects. *Int. J. Radiat. Oncol. Biol. Phys.* **12,** 1279–1282.
7. Chaplin, D. J., Olive, P. L., and Durand, R. E. (1987) Intermittent blood flow in a murine tumour: radiobiological effects. *Cancer Res.* **47,** 597–601.
8. Carmeliet, P. and Jain, R. K. (2000) Angiogenesis in cancer and other diseases. *Nature* **407,** 249–257.
9. Maxwell, P. H., Pugh, C. W., and Ratcliffe, P. J. (2001) Activation of the HIF pathway in cancer. *Curr. Opin. Genet. Dev.* **11,** 293–299.
10. Semenza, G. L. (2001) HIF-1 and mechanisms of hypoxia-sensing. *Curr. Opin. Cell Biol.* **13,** 167–171.
11. Semenza, G. L. (2002) HIF-1 and tumour progression: pathophysiology and therapeutics. *Trends Mol. Med.* **8(Suppl.),** S62–S67.
12. Ivan M. and Kaelin, W. G., Jr. (2001) The von Hippel-Lindau tumour suppressor protein. *Curr. Opin. Genet. Dev.* **11,** 27–34.
13. Sutter, C. H., Laughner, E., and Semenza, G. L. (2000) Hypoxia-inducible factor 1alpha protein expression is controlled by oxygen-regulated ubiquitination that is disrupted by deletions and missense mutations. *Proc. Natl. Acad. Sci. USA* **97,** 4748–4753.
14. Ravi, R., Mookerjee, B., Bhujwalla, Z. M., et al. (2000) Regulation of tumour angiogenesis by p53-induced degradation of hypoxia-inducible factor 1α. *Genes Dev.* **14,** 34–44.
15. An, W. G., Kanekal, M., Simon, M. C., Maltepe, E., Blagosklonny, M. V., and Neckers, L. M. (1998) Stabilisation of wild-type p53 by hypoxia-inducible factor 1α. *Nature* **392,** 405–408.

16. Blagosklonny, M. V., An, W. G., Romanova, L. Y., Trepel, J., Fojo, T., and Neckers, L. M. (1998) p53 inhibits hypoxia-inducible factor-stimulated transcription. *J. Biol. Chem.* **273,** 11,995–11,998.
17. Scandurro, A. B., Weldon, C. W., Figureroa, Y.G., Alam, J., and Beckman, B. S. (2001) Gene microarray analysis reveals a novel hypoxia signal transduction pathway in human hepatocellular carcinoma cells. *Int. J. Oncol.* **19,** 129–135.
18. Harris, A. L. (2002) Hypoxia—a key regulatory factor in tumour growth. *Nature Rev. Cancer* **2,** 38–47.
19. Williams, K. J., Telfer, B. A., Airley, R. E., et al. (2002) A protective role for HIF-1 in response to redox manipulation and glucose deprivation: implications for tumourigenesis. *Oncogene* **21,** 282–290.
20. Griffiths, J. R., McSheehy, P. M. J., Robinson, S. P., et al. (2002) Metabolic changes detected by in vivo magnetic resonance studies of HEPA-1 wild-type tumours and tumours deficient in hypoxia-inducible factor-1 β (HIF-1β): evidence of an anabolic role for the HIF-1 pathway. *Cancer Res.* **62,** 688–695.
21. Semenza, G. L. (2000) Hypoxia, clonal selection, and the role of HIF-1 in tumour progression. *Crit. Rev. Biochem. Mol. Biol.* **35,** 71–103.
22. Laughner, E., Taghavi, P., Chiles, K., Mahon, P. C., and Semenza, G. L. (2001) HER2(neu) signalling increases the rate of hypoxia-inducible factor 1α (HIF-1α) synthesis: novel mechanism for HIF-1-mediated vascular endothelial growth factor expression. *Mol. Cell Biol.* **21,** 3995–4004.
23. Zhong, H., De Marzo, A. M., Laughner, E., et al. (1999) Over-expression of hypoxia-inducible factor 1α in common human cancers and their metastases. *Cancer Res.* **59,** 5830–5835.
24. Talks, K. L., Turley, H., Gatter, K. C., et al. (2000) The expression and distribution of the hypoxia-inducible factors HIF-1α and HIF-2α in normal human tissues, cancers, and tumour-associated macrophages. *Am. J. Path.* **157,** 411–421.
25. Giatromanolaki, A., Koukourakis, M. I., Sivridis, E., et al. (2001) Relation of hypoxia inducible factor 1 alpha and 2 alpha in operable non-small cell lung cancer to angiogenic/molecular profile of tumours and survival. *Br. J. Cancer* **85,** 881–890.
26. Zagzag, D., Zhong, H., Scalzitti, J. M., Laughner, E., Simons, J. W., and Semenza, G. L. (2000) Expression of hypoxia-inducible factor 1α in brain tumours. *Cancer* **88,** 2606–2618.
27. Aebersold, D. M., Burri, P., Beer, K. T., et al. (2001) Expression of hypoxia-inducible factor-1α: a novel predictive and prognostic parameter in the radiotherapy of oropharyngeal cancer. *Cancer Res.* **61,** 2911–2916.
28. Birner, P., Schindl, M., Obermair, A., Breitenecker, G., and Oberhuber, G. (2001) Expression of hypoxia-inducible factor 1α in epithelial ovarian tumours: its impact on prognosis and on response to chemotherapy. *Clin. Cancer Res.* **7,** 1661–1668.
29. Birner, P., Gatterbauer, B., Oberhuber, G., et al. (2001) Expression of hypoxia-inducible factor-1a in oligodendrogliomas: its impact on prognosis and on neoangiogensis. *Cancer* **92,** 165–171.
30. Birner, P., Schindl, M., Obermair, A., Plank, C., Breitenecker, G., and Oberhuber, G. (2000) Over-expression of hypoxia-inducible factor 1α is a marker for an unfavourable prognosis in early-stage invasive cervical cancer. *Cancer Res.* **60,** 4693–4696.
31. Graeber, T., Peterson, J. F., Tsai, M., Monica, K., Fornace, A. J., and Giacca, A. J. (1994) Hypoxia induces accumulation of p53 protein, but activation of G1-phase checkpoint by low-oxygen conditions is independent of p53 status. *Mol. Cell. Biol.* **14,** 6264–6277.

32. Graeber, T., Osmanian, C., Jacks, T., et al. (1996) Hypoxia-mediated selection of cells with diminished apoptotic potential in solid tumours. *Nature* **379**, 88–91.
33. Rofstad, E. K. (2000) Microenvironment-induced cancer metastasis. *Int. J. Radiat. Biol.* **76**, 589–605.
34. Cairns, R. A., Kalliomaki, T., and Hill, R. P. (2001) Acute (cyclic) hypoxia enhances spontaneous metastasis of KHT murine tumours. *Cancer Res.* **61**, 8903–8908.
35. Brizel, D. M., Scully, S. P., Harrelson, J. M., et al. (1996) Tumour oxygenation predicts for the likelihood of distant metastases in human soft tissue sarcoma. *Cancer Res.* **56**, 941–943.
36. Höckel, M., Schlenger, K., Aral, B., Mitze, M., Schaffer, U., and Vaupel, P. (1996) Association between tumour hypoxia and malignant progression in advanced cancer of the cervix. *Cancer Res.* **56**, 4509–4515.
37. Nordsmark, M. and Overgaard, J. (2000) A confirmatory prognostic study on oxygenation status and locoregional control in advanced head and neck squamous cell carcinoma treated by radiation therapy. *Radiother. Oncol.* **57**, 39–43.
38. Hall, E. J. (1994) The oxygen effect and reoxygenation, in *Radiobiology for the Radiologist*, 4th ed., Lippincott, Philadephia, pp. 133–152.
39. Gray, L. H., Conger, A. D., Ebert, M., Hornsey, S., and Scott, O. C. A. (1953) The concentration of oxygen dissolved in tissues at the time of irradiation as a factor in radiotherapy. *Br. J. Radiol.* **26**, 638–648.
40. Brizel, D. M., Dodge, R. K., Clough, R. W., and Dewhirst, M. W. (1999) Oxygenation of head and neck cancer: changes during radiotherapy and impact on treatment outcome. *Radiother. Oncol.* **53**, 113–117.
41. Fyles, A. W., Milosevic, M., Wong, R., et al. (1998) Oxygenation predicts radiation response and survival in patients with cervix cancer. *Radiother. Oncol.* **48**, 149–156.
42. Sundfør, K., Lyng, H., Tropé, C. G., and Rofstad, E. K. (2000) Treatment outcome in advanced squamous cell carcinoma of the uterine cervix: relationships to pre-treatment tumour oxygenation and vascularisation. *Radiother. Oncol.* **54**, 101–107.
43. Teicher, B. A., Lazo, J. S., and Sartorelli, A. C. (1981) Classification of antineoplastic agents by their selective toxicities toward oxygenated and hypoxic tumour cells. *Cancer Res.* **41**, 73–81.
44. Grau, C. and Overgaard, J. (1988) Effect of cancer chemotherapy on the hypoxic fraction of a solid tumour measured using a local tumour control assay. *Radiother Oncol.* **13**, 301–309.
45. Teicher, B. A., Holden, S. A., Al-Achi, A., and Herman, T. S. (1990) Classification of antineoplastic treatments by their differential toxicity toward putative oxygenated and hypoxic tumour subpopulations in vivo in the FSaIIC murine fibrosarcoma. *Cancer Res.* **50**, 3339–3344.
46. Durand, R. E. and Raleigh, J. A. (1998) Identification of non-proliferating but viable hypoxic tumour calls in vivo. *Cancer Res.* **58**, 3547–3550.
47. Gardener, L. B., Li, Q., Park, M. S., Flanagan, W. M., Semenza, G. L., and Dang, C. V. (2001) Hypoxia inhibits G1/S transition through regulation of p27 expression. *J. Biol. Chem.* **276**, 7919–7926.
48. Jain, R. K. (2001) Delivery of molecular and cellular medicine to solid tumours. *Adv. Drug Delivery Rev.* **46**, 149–168.
49. Vaupel, P., Schlenger, K., Knoop, C., and Hockel, M. (1991) Oxygenation of human tumours: evaluation of tissue oxygen distribution in breast cancers by computerised O_2 tension measurements. *Cancer Res.* **51**, 3316–3322.

50. Vaupel, P. and Höckel, M. (1999) Predictive power of the tumour oxygenation status. *Adv. Exp. Med. Biol.* **471**, 533–539.

51. Knocke, T., Weitmann, H., Feldmann, H., Selzer, E., and Pötter, R. (1999) Intratumoural pO_2-measurements as predictive assay in the treatment of carcinoma of the uterine cervix. *Radiother. Oncol.* **53**, 99–104.

52. Fyles, A. W., Milosevic, M., Hedley, D., et al. (2002) Tumour hypoxia has independent predictor impact only in patients with node-negative cervix cancer. *J. Clin. Oncol.* **20**, 680–687.

53. Sundfor, K., Lyng, H., and Rofstad, E. K. (1998) Tumour hypoxia and vascular density as predictors of metastasis in squamous cell carcinoma of the uterine cervix. *Br. J. Cancer* **78**, 822–827.

54. Pitson, G., Fyles, A. W., Milosevic, M., Wylie, J., Pintilie, M., and Hill, R. P. (2001) Tumour size and oxygenation are independent predictors of nodal disease in patients with cervix cancer. *Int. J. Radiat. Oncol. Biol. Phys.* **51**, 699–703.

55. Nordsmark, M., Alsner, J., Nielsen, O. S., Jensen, O. M., Horsman, M. R., and Overgaard, J. (2001) Hypoxia in human soft tissue sarcomas: adverse impact on survival and no association with p53 mutations. *Br. J. Cancer* **84**, 1070–1075.

56. Overgaard, J. and Horsman, M. R. (1996) Modification of hypoxia-induced radioresistance in tumours by use of oxygen and sensitizers. *Semin. Radiat. Oncol.* **6**, 10–21.

57. Saunders, M. I. and Dische, S. (1996) Clinical results of hypoxic cell radiosensitisation from hyperbaric oxygen to accelerated radiotherapy, carbogen and nicotinamide. *Br. J. Cancer* **74(Suppl. XXVII)**, S271–S278.

58. Rauth, A. M., Melo, T., and Misra, V. (1998) Bioreductive therapies: an overview of drugs and their mechanisms of action. *Int. J. Radiat. Oncol. Biol. Phys.* **42**, 755–762.

59. Workman, P. and Stratford, I. J. (1993) The experimental development of bioreductive drugs and their role in cancer therapy. *Cancer Metastasis Rev.* **12**, 73–82.

60. Stratford, I. J. and Workman, P. (1998) Bioreductive drugs into the next millennium. *Anti-Cancer Drug Des.* **13**, 519–528.

61. Lee, D. J., Trotti, A., Spencer, S., et al. (1998) Concurrent tirapazamine and radiotherapy for advanced head and neck carcinomas: a phase II study. *Int. J. Radiat. Oncol. Biol. Phys.* **42**, 811–815.

62. von Pawel, J., von-Roemeling, R., Gatzemeier, U., et al. (2000) Tirapazamine plus cisplatin versus cisplatin in advanced non-small-cell lung cancer: a report of the international CATAPULT I study group. Cisplatin and tirapazamine in subjects with advanced previously untreated non-small-cell lung tumours. *J. Clin. Oncol.* **18**, 1351–1359.

63. Rischin, D., Peters, L., Hicks, R., et al. (2001) Phase I trial of concurrent tirapazamine, cisplatin, and radiotherapy in patients with advanced head and neck cancer. *J. Clin. Oncol.* **19**, 535–542.

64. Craighead, P. S., Pearcey, R., and Stuart, G. (2000) A phase I/II evaluation of tirapazamine administered intravenously concurrent with cisplatin and radiotherapy in women with locally advanced cervical cancer. *Int. J. Radiat. Oncol. Biol. Phys.* **48**, 791–795.

65. Workman, P. and Double, J. A. (1978) Drug latentiation in cancer chemotherapy. *Biomedicine* **28**, 255–262.

66. Workman, P. (1979) Latent drugs for cancer chemotherapy. *Cancer Topics* **2**, 6.

67. Adams, G. E. (1992) Fallia Memorial Lecture: Redox, radiation, and reductive bioactivation. *Radiat. Res.* **132**, 129–139.

68. Workman, P. (1994) Enzyme-directed bioreductive drug development revisited: a commentary on recent progress and future prospects with emphasis on quinone anticancer

agents and quinone metabolising enzymes, particularly DT-diaphorase. *Oncol. Res.* **6,** 461–475.

69. Denny, W. A., Wilson, W. R., and Hay, M. P. (1996) Recent developments in the design of bioreductive drugs. *Br. J. Cancer* **74,** S32–S38.

70. Denny, W. A. and Wilson, W. R. (1993) Bioreducible mustards: a paradigm for hypoxia-selective prodrugs of diffusible cytotoxins (HPDCs). *Cancer Metastasis Rev.* **12,** 135–151.

71. Ellis, P. A., Smith, I. E., Hardy, J. R., et al. (1995) Symptom relief with MVP (mitomycin C, vinblastine and cisplatin) chemotherapy in advanced non-small-cell lung cancer. *Br. J. Cancer* **71,** 366–370.

72. Crinò, L., Scagliotti, G. V., Ricci, S., et al. (1999) Gemcitabine and cisplatin versus mitomycin, ifosfamide, and cisplatin in advanced non-small cell lung cancer: a randomised phase III study of the Italian Lung Cancer Project. *J. Clin. Oncol.* **17,** 3522–3530.

73. Malmström, P., Wijkström, H., Lundholm, C., et al., and Members of the Swedish–Norwegian Bladder Cancer Study Group. (1999) 5-Year follow-up of a randomised prospective study comparing mitomycin C and Bacillus Calmette–Guerin in patients with superficial bladder carcinoma. *J. Urol.* **161,** 1121.

74. UKCCCR Anal Cancer Trial Working Party (1996) Epidermoid anal cancer: results from the UKCCCR randomised trial of radiotherapy alone versus radiotherapy, 5-fluorouracil, and mitomycin. *Lancet* **348,** 1049–1054.

75. Cummings, J., Spanswick, V. J., Tomasz, M., and Smyth, J. F. (1998) Enzymology of mitomycin C metabolic activation in tumour tissue: implications for enzyme-directed bioreductive drug development. *Biochem. Pharmacol.* **56,** 405–414.

76. Hoban, P. R., Walton, M. I., Robson, C. N., et al. (1990) Decreased NADPH:cytochrome P-450 reductase activity and impaired drug activation in a mammalian cell line resistant to mitomycin C under aerobic but not hypoxic conditions. *Cancer Res.* **50,** 4692–4697.

77. Ross, D., Beall, H., Travers, R. D., Siegel, D., Phillips, R. M., and Gibson, N. (1994) Bioactivation of quinones by DT-diaphorase, molecular, biochemical and chemical studies. *Oncol. Res.* **6,** 493–500.

78. Fitzsimmons, S. A., Workman, P., Grever, M., et al. (1996) Reductase enzyme expression across the National Cancer Institute Tumour Cell Line Panel: correlation with sensitivity to mitomycin C and EO9. *J. Natl. Cancer Inst.* **88,** 259–269.

79. Gan, Y., Mo, Y., Kalns, J. E., et al. (2001) Expression of DT-diaphorase and cytochrome P450 reductase correlates with mitomycin C activity in human bladder tumours. *Clin. Cancer Res.* **7,** 1313–1319.

80. Phillips, R. M., Burger, A. M., Loadman, P. M., Jarrett, C. M., Swaine, D. J., and Fiebig, H.-H. (2000) Activity or drug metabolism by tumour homogenates: Implications for enzyme-directed bioreductive drug development. *Cancer Res.* **60,** 6384–6390.

81. Wang, X., Doherty, G. P., Leith, M. K., Curphey, T. J., and Begleiter, A. (1999) Enhanced cytotoxicity of mitomycin C in human tumour cells with inducers of DT-diaphorase. *Br. J. Cancer* **80,** 1223–1230.

82. Rockwell, S., Keyes, S. R., and Sartorelli, A. C. (1988) Preclinical studies of porfiromycin as an adjunct to radiotherapy. *Radiat. Res.* **116,** 100–113.

83. Haffty, B. G., Son, Y. H., Wilson, L. D., et al. (1997) Bioreductive alkylating agent porfiromycin in combination with radiation therapy for the management of squamous cell carcinoma of the head and neck. *Radiat. Oncol. Invest.* **5,** 235–245.

84. Walton, M. I., Smith, P. J., and Workman, P. (1991) The role of NAD(P)H : quinone reductase (EC 1.6.99.2, DT-diaphorase) in the reductive bioactivation of the novel indoloquinone antitumour agent EO9. *Cancer Commun.* **3,** 199–206.

85. Hendriks, H. R., Pizao, P. E., Berger, D. P., et al. (1993) EO9: a novel bioreductive alkylating indoloquinone with preferential solid tumour activity and lack of bone marrow toxicity in preclinical models. *Eur. J. Cancer* **29A**, 897–906.

86. Bailey, S. M., Suggett, N., Walton, M. I., and Workman, P. (1992) Structure–activity relationships for DT-diaphorase reduction of hypoxic cell directed agents: indoloquinones and diaziridinyl benzoquinones. *Int. J. Radiat. Oncol. Biol. Phys.* **22**, 649–653.

87. Walton, M. I., Sugget, N., and Workman, P. (1992) The role of human and rodent DT-diaphorase in the reductive metabolism of hypoxic cell cytotoxins. *Int. J. Radiat. Oncol. Biol. Phys.* **22**, 643–647.

88. Walton, M. I., Bibby, M. C., Double, J. A., Plumb, J. A., and Workman, P. (1992) DT-Diaphorase activity correlates with sensitivity to the indoloquinone EO9 in mouse and human colon carcinomas. *Eur. J. Cancer* **28A**, 1597–1600.

89 Plumb, J. A., Gerritsen, M., Milroy, R., Thomson, P., and Workman, P. (1994) Relative importance of DT-diaphorase and hypoxia in the bioactivation of EO9 by human lung tumour cell lines. *Int. J. Radiat. Oncol. Biol. Phys.* **29**, 295–299.

9C. Plumb, J. A. and Workman, P. (1994) Unusually marked hypoxic sensitization to indoloquinone EO9 and mitomycin C in a human colon-tumour cell line that lacks DT-diaphorase activity. *Int. J. Cancer* **56**, 134–139.

91. Plumb, J. A., Gerritsen, M., and Workman, P. (1994) DT-diaphorase protects cells from the hypoxic cytotoxicity of indoloquinone EO9. *Br. J. Cancer* **70**, 1136–1143.

S2. Pavlidis, N., Hanauske, A. R., Gamucci, T., et al. (1996) A randomised Phase II study of two schedules of the novel indoloquinone EO9 in non-small-cell lung cancer: a study of the EORTC Early Clinical Trials Group. *Ann. Oncol.* **7**, 529–531.

93. Dirix, L. Y., Tonnesen, F., Cassidy, J., et al. (1996) EO9 Phase II study in advanced breast, gastric, pancreatic and colorectal carcinoma by the EORTC early clinical studies group. *Eur. J. Cancer* **32A**, 2019–2022.

94. Loadman, P. M., Phillips, R. M., Lim, L. E., and Bibby, M. C. (2000) Pharmacological properties of a new aziridinylbenzoquinone, RH1 (2,5-diaziridinyl-3-(hydroxymethyl)-6-methyl-1,4-benzoquinone), in mice. *Biochem. Pharmacol.* **59**, 831–837.

95. Winski, S. L., Hargreaves, R. H., Butler, J., and Ross, D. (1998) A new screening system for NAD(P)H : quinone oxidoreductase (NQO1)-directed antitumour quinones: identification of a new aziridinylbenzoquinone, RH1, as a NQO1-directed antitumour agent. *Clin. Cancer Res.* **4**, 3083–3088.

96. Malkinson, A. M., Siegel, D., Forrest, G. L., et al. (1992) Elevated DT-diaphorase activity and messenger RNA content in human non-small cell lung carcinoma: relationship to the response of lung tumour xenografts to mitomycin C. *Cancer Res.* **52**, 4752–4757.

97. Smitskamp-Wilms, E., Giaccone, G., Pinedo, H. M., van der Laan, B. F., and Peters, G. J. (1995) DT-Diaphorase activity in normal and neoplastic human tissues; an indicator for sensitivity to bioreductive agents? *Br. J. Cancer* **72**, 917–922.

98. Kelsey, K. T., Ross, D., Traver, R. D., et al. (1997) Ethnic variation in the prevalence of a common NAD(P)H quinone oxidoreductase polymorphism and its implications for anti-cancer chemotherapy. *Br. J. Cancer* **76**, 852–854.

99. Sharp, S. Y., Kelland, L. R., Valenti, M. R., Brunton, L. A., Hobbs, S., and Workman, P. (2000) Establishment of an isogenic human colon tumour model for NQO1 gene expression: application to investigate the role of DT-diaphorase in bioreductive drug activation in vitro and in vivo. *Mol. Pharmacol.* **58**, 1146–1155.

100. Winski, S. L., Swann, E., Hargreaves, R. H., et al. (2001) Relationship between NAD(P)H:quinone oxidoreductase 1 (NQO1) levels in a series of stably transfected cell lines and susceptibility to antitumour quinones. *Biochem. Pharmacol.* **61**, 1509–1516.

101. Skelly, J. V., Sanderson, M. R., Duter, D. A., et al. (1999) Crystal structure of human DT-diaphorase: a model for interaction with the cytotoxic prodrug 5-(aziridin-1-yl)-2,4-dinitrobenzamide (CB1954). *J. Med. Chem.* **42**, 4325–4330.

102. Kelland, L. R., Sharp, S. Y., Rogers, P. M., Myers, T. G., and Workman, P. (1999) DT-Diaphorase expression and tumour cell sensitivity to 17-allylamino, 17-demethoxygeldanamycin, an inhibitor of heat shock protein 90. *J. Natl. Cancer Inst.* **91**, 1940–1949.

103. Brown, J. M. (1999) The hypoxic cell: a target for selective cancer therapy—Eighteenth Bruce F. Cain Memorial Award Lecture. *Cancer Res.* **59**, 5863–5870.

104. Denny, W. A. and Wilson, W. R. (2000) Tirapazamine: a bioreductive anticancer drug that exploits tumour hypoxia. *Expert Opin. Invest. Drugs* **9**, 2889–2901.

105. Patterson, A. V., Saunders, M. P., Chinje, E. C., Patterson, L. H., and Stratford, I. J. (1998) Enzymology of tirapazamine metabolism: a review. *Anti-Cancer Drug Des.* **13**, 541–573.

106. Walton, M. I., Wolf, C. R., and Workman, P. (1992) The role of cytochrome P450 and cytochrome P450 reductase in the reductive bioactivation of the novel benzotriazine di-N-oxide hypoxic cytotoxin 3-amino-1,2,4-benzotriazine-1,4-dioxide (SR 4233, WIN 59075) by mouse liver. *Biochem. Pharmacol.* **44**, 251–259.

107. Walton, M. I. and Workman, P. (1990) Enzymology of the reductive bioactivation of SR 4233. A novel benzotriazine di-N-oxide hypoxic cell cytotoxin. *Biochem. Pharmacol.* **39**, 1735–1742.

108. Fitzsimmons, S. A., Lewis, A. D., Riley, R. J., and Workman, P. (1994) Reduction of 3-amino-1,2,4-benzotriazine-1,4-di-N-oxide (tirapazamine, WIN 59075, SR 4233) to a DNA-damaging species: a direct role for NADPH : cytochrome P450 oxidoreductase. *Carcinogenesis* **15**, 1503–1510.

109. Riley, R. J., Hemingway, S. A., Graham, M. A., and Workman, P. (1993) Initial characterisation of the major mouse cytochrome P450 enzymes involved in the reductive metabolism of the hypoxic cytotoxin 3-amino-1,2,4-benzotriazine-1,4-di-N-oxide (tirapazamine, SR 4233, WIN 59075). *Biochem. Pharmacol.* **45**, 1065–1077.

110. Evans, J. W., Yodoh, K., Delahoussaye, Y. M., and Brown, J. M. (1998) Tirapazamine is metabolised to its DNA damaging radical by intranuclear enzymes. *Cancer Res.* **58**, 2098–2101.

111. Riley, R. J. and Workman, P. (1992) Enzymology of the reduction of the potent benzotriazine-di-N-oxide hypoxic cell cytotoxin SR 4233 (WIN 59075) by NAD(P)H : (quinone acceptor) oxidoreductase (EC 1.6.99.2) purified from Walker 256 rat tumour cells. *Biochem. Pharmacol.* **43**, 167–174.

112. Dorie, M. J. and Brown, J. M. (1993) Tumour-specific, schedule-dependent interaction between tirapazamine (SR 4233) and cisplatin. *Cancer Res.* **53**, 4633–4636.

113. Goldberg, Z., Evans, J., Birrell, G., and Brown, J. M. (2001) An investigation of the molecular basis for the synergistic interaction of tirapazamine and cisplatin. *Int. J. Radiat. Oncol. Biol. Phys.* **49**, 175–182.

114. Senan, S., Rampling, R., Graham, M. A., et al. (1997) Phase I and pharmacokinetic study of tirapazamine (SR 4233) administered every three weeks. *Clin. Cancer Res.* **3**, 31–38.

115. Patterson, L. H., McKeown, S. R., Robson, T., Gallagher, R., Raleigh, S. M., and Orr, S. (1999) Antitumour prodrug development using cytochrome P450 (CYP) mediated activation. *Anti-Cancer Drug Des.* **14**, 473–486.

116. Patterson, L. H. and McKeown, S. R. (2000) AQ4N: a new approach to hypoxia-activated cancer chemotherapy. *Br. J. Cancer* **83**, 1589–1593.

117. Patterson, L. H., McKeown, S. R., Ruparelia, K., et al. (2000) Enhancement of chemotherapy and radiotherapy of murine tumours by AQ4N, a bioreductively activated antitumour agent. *Br. J. Cancer* **82,** 1984–1990.

118. BTG initiates Phase I trial of AQ4N, an innovative cancer drug. (2001) Available at www.btgplc. com/news_content/mn_pharmaceutical_release. cfm?doc_id=587#top

119. Lee, H. H., Wilson, W. R., and Denny, W. A. (1999) Nitracrine N-oxides: effects of variations in the nature of the side chain N-oxide on hypoxia-selective cytotoxicity. *Anti-Cancer Drug Des.* **14,** 487–497.

120. Brown, J. M. (1982) The mechanisms of cytotoxicity and chemosensitization by misonidazole and other nitroimidazoles. *Int. J. Radiat. Oncol. Biol. Phys.* **8,** 675–682.

121. Adams, G. E. and Stratford, I. J. (1986) Hypoxia-mediated nitroheterocyclic drugs in the radio- and chemotherapy of cancer. an overview. *Biochem. Pharmacol.* **35,** 71–76.

122. Wardman, P. (1977) The use of nitroaromatic compounds as hypoxic cell radiosensitizers. *Curr. Topics Radiat. Res. Q.* **11,** 347–398.

123. Rauth, A. M. (1984) Pharmacology and toxicology of sensitizers: mechanism studies. *Int. J. Radiat. Oncol. Biol. Phys.* **10,** 1293–1300.

124. Bigalow, J. E., Varnes, M. E., Roizen-Towle, L., et al. (1986) Biochemistry of reduction of nitroheteocycles. *Biochem. Pharmacol.* **35,** 77–90.

125. Stratford, I. J., Walling, J. M., and Silver, A. R. (1986) The differential cytotoxicity of RSU 1069: cell survival studies indicating interaction with DNA as a possible mode of action. *Br. J. Cancer* **53,** 339–344.

126. Adams, G. E., Ahmed, I., Sheldon, P. W., and Stratford, I. J. (1984) RSU 1069, a 2-nitroimidazole containing an alkylating group: high efficiency as a radio- and chemosensitizer in vitro and in vivo. *Int. J. Radiat. Oncol. Biol. Phys.* **10,** 1653–1656.

127. Bremner, J. C. (1993) Assessing the bioreductive effectiveness of the nitroimidazole RSU 1069 and its prodrug RB 6145: with particular reference to in vivo methods of evaluation. *Cancer Metastasis Rev.* **12,** 177–193.

128. Horwich, A., Holliday, S. B., Deacon, J. M., and Peckham, M. J. (1986) A toxicity and pharmacokinetic study in man of the hypoxic-cell radiosensitizer RSU 1069. *Br. J. Radiol.* **59,** 1238–1240.

129. Parker, R. F., Vincent, P. W., and Elliot, W. L. (1996) Alkylating properties of nitroimidazole radiosensitizers is required for induction of murine retinal degeneration. *Vet. Pathol.* **33,** 625.

130. Cobb, L. M., Connors, T. A., Elson, L. A., et al. (1969) 2,4-dinitro-5-ethyleneiminobenzamide (CB 1954): a potent and selective inhibitor of the growth of the Walker carcinoma 256. *Biochem. Pharmacol.* **18,** 1519–1527.

131. Knox, R. J., Friedlos, F., and Boland, M. P. (1993) The bioactivation of CB 1954 and its use as a prodrug in antibody-directed enzyme prodrug therapy (ADEPT). *Cancer Metastasis Rev.* **12,** 195–212.

132. Workman, P., Morgan, J. E., Talbot, K., Wright, K. A., Donaldson, J., and Twentyman, P. R. (1986) CB 1954 revisited. II. Toxicity and antitumour activity. *Cancer Chemother. Pharmacol.* **16,** 9–14.

133. Workman, P., White, R. A., and Talbot, K. (1986) CB 1954 revisited. I. Disposition kinetics and metabolism. *Cancer Chemother. Pharmacol.* **16,** 1–8.

134. Knox, R. J., Boland, M. P., Friedlos, F., Coles, B., Southan, C., and Roberts, J. J. (1988) The nitroreductase enzyme in Walker cells that activates 5-(aziridin-1-yl)-2,4-dinitrobenzamide (CB 1954) to 5-(aziridin-1-yl)-4-hydroxylamino-2-nitrobenzamide is a form of NAD(P)H dehydrogenase (quinone) (EC 1.6.99.2). *Biochem. Pharmacol.* **37,** 4671–4677.

135. Denny, W. A. and Wilson, W. R. (1993) Bioreducible mustards: a paradigm for hypoxia-selective prodrugs of diffusible cytotoxins (HPDCs). *Cancer Metastasis Rev.* **12**, 135–151.
136. Knox, R. J., Jenkins, T. C., Hobbs, S. M., Chen, S., Melton, R. G., and Burke, P. J. (2000) Bioactivation of 5-(aziridin-1-yl)-2,4-dinitrobenzamide (CB 1954) by human NAD(P)H quinone oxidoreductase 2: a novel co-substrate-mediated antitumour prodrug therapy. *Cancer Res.* **60**, 4179–4186.
137. Boland, M. P., Knox, R. J., and Roberts, J. J. (1991) The differences in kinetics of rat and human DT diaphorase result in a differential sensitivity of derived cell lines to CB 1954 (5-(aziridin-1-yl)-2,4-dinitrobenzamide). *Biochem. Pharmacol.* **41**, 867–875.
138. Lee, H. H., Palmer, B. D., Wilson, W. R., and Denny, W. A. (1998) Synthesis and hypoxia-selective cytotoxicity of a 2-nitroimidazole mustard. *Bioorg. Med. Chem. Lett.* **8**, 1741–1744.
139. Siim, B. G., Denny, W. A., and Wilson, W. R. (1997) Nitro reduction as an electronic switch for bioreductive drug activation. *Oncol. Res.* **9**, 357–369.
140. Ware, D. C., Palmer, B. D., Wilson, W. R., and Denny, W. A. (1993) Hypoxia-selective antitumour agents. 7. Metal complexes of aliphatic mustards as a new class of hypoxia-selective cytotoxins. Synthesis and evaluation of cobalt(III) complexes of bidentate mustards. *J. Med. Chem.* **36**, 1839–1846.
141. Anderson, R. F., Denny, W. A., Ware, D. C., and Wilson, W. R. (1996) Pulse radiolysis studies on the hypoxia-selective toxicity of a colbalt-mustard complex. *Br. J. Cancer* **27(Suppl XXVII)**, S48–S51.
142. Niculescu-Duvaz, I., Friedlos, F., Niculescu-Duvaz, D., Davies, L., and Springer, C. J. (1999) Prodrugs for antibody- and gene-directed enzyme prodrug therapies (ADEPT and GDEPT). *Anticancer Drug Des.* **14**, 517–538.
143. Grove, J. I., Searle, P. F., Weedon, S. J., Green, N. K., McNeish, I. A., and Kerr, D. J. (1999) Virus-directed enzyme prodrug therapy using CB1954. *Anticancer Drug Des.* **14**, 461–472.
144. Anlezark, G. M., Melton, R. G., Sherwood, R. F., Coles, B., Friedlos, F., and Knox, R. J. (1992) The bioactivation of 5-(aziridin-1-yl)-2,4-dinitrobenzamide (CB1954)—I. Purification and properties of a nitroreductase enzyme from *Escherichia coli*—a potential enzyme for antibody-directed enzyme prodrug therapy (ADEPT). *Biochem. Pharmacol.* **44**, 2289–2295.
145. Green, N. K., Youngs, D. J., Neoptolemos, J. P., et al. (1997) Sensitization of colorectal and pancreatic cancer cell lines to the prodrug 5-(aziridin-1-yl)-2,4-dinitrobenzamide (CB 1954) by retroviral transduction and expression of the *E. coli* nitroreductase gene. *Cancer Gene Ther.* **4**, 229–238.
146. Denny, W. A. (2002) Nitroreductase-based GDEPT. *Curr. Pharm. Des.* **8**, 1349–1361.
147. Friedlos, F., Denny, W. A., Palmer, B. D., and Springer, C. J. (1997) Mustard prodrugs for activation by Escherichia coli nitroreductase in gene-directed enzyme prodrug therapy. *J. Med. Chem.* **40**, 1270–1275.
148. Raleigh, J. A., Dewhirst, M. W., and Thrall, D. E. (1996) Measuring tumour hypoxia. *Semin. Radiat. Oncol.* **6**, 37–45.
149. Young, W. K., Vojnovic, B., and Wardman, P. (1996) Measurement of oxygen tension in tumours by time-resolved fluorescence. *Br. J. Cancer* **74(Suppl. XXVII)**, S256–259.
150. Seddon, B. M., Honess, D. J., Vojnovic, B., Tozer, G., and Workman, P. (2001) Measurement of tumour oxygenation: *in vivo* comparison of a luminescence fibre-optic sensor and a polarographic electrode in the P22 tumour. *Radiat. Res.* **55**, 837–846.

151. Olive, P. L., Banath, J. P., and Durand, R. E. (1990) Heterogeneity in radiation-induced DNA damage and repair in tumour and normal cells measured using the "comet" assay. *Radiat. Res.* **122**, 86–94.

152. Aquino-Parsons, C., Luo, C., Vikse, C. M., and Olive, P. L. (1999) Comparison between the comet assay and the oxygen microelectrode for measurement for measurement of tumour hypoxia. *Radiother. Oncol.* **51**, 179–185.

153. Partridge, S. A., Aquino-Parsons, C., Luo, C., Green, A., and Olive, P. L. (2001) A pilot study comparing intratumoral oxygenation using the comet assay following 2.5% and 5% carbogen and 100% oxygen. *Int. J. Radiat. Oncol. Biol. Phys.* **49**, 575–580.

154. Robinson, S. P., Howe, F. A., Rodrigues, L. M., Stubbs, M., and Griffiths, J. R. (1998) Magnetic resonance imaging techniques for monitoring changes in tumour oxygenation and blood flow. *Semin. Radiat. Oncol.* **8**, 197–207.

155. Hodgkiss, R. J. (1998) Use of 2-nitroimidazoles as bioreductive markers for tumour hypoxia. *Anti-Cancer Drug Des.* **13**, 687–702.

156. Nordsmark, M., Loncaster, J., Chou, S. J., et al. (2001) Invasive oxygen measurements and pimonidazole labelling in human cervix carcinoma. *Int. J. Radiat. Oncol. Biol. Phys.* **49**, 581–586.

157. Evans, S. M., Hahn, S. M., Mageralli, D. P., et al. (2001) Hypoxia in human intraperitoneal and extremity sarcomas. *Int. J. Radiat. Oncol. Biol. Phys.* **49**, 587–596.

158. Evans, S. M., Hahn, S. M., Pook, D. R., et al. (2000) Detection of hypoxia in human squamous cell carcinoma by EF5 binding. *Cancer Res.* **60**, 2018–2024.

159. Koch, C. J., Hahn, S. M., Rockwell, K., Jr., Covey, J. M., McKenna, W. G., and Evans, S. M. (2001) Pharmacokinetics of EF5 [2-(2-nitro-1-*H*-imidazol-1-yl)-*N*-(2,2,3,3,3-pentafluoropropyl) acetamide] in human patients: implications for hypoxia measurements in vivo by 2-nitroimidazoles. *Cancer Chemother. Pharmacol.* **48**, 177–187.

160. Parliament, M. B., Chapman, J. D., Urtasun, R. C., et al. (1992) Non-invasive assessment of human tumour hypoxia with ^{123}I-iodoazomycin arabinoside: preliminary report of a clinical study. *Br. J. Cancer* **65**, 90–95.

161. Koh, W.-J., Rasey, J. S., Evans, M. L., et al. (1991) Imaging in hypoxia in human tumours with F-18 fluoromisonidazole. *Int. J. Radiat. Oncol. Biol. Phys.* **22**, 199–212.

162. Maxwell, R. J., Workman, P., and Griffiths, J. R. (1989) Demonstration of tumour-selective retention of fluorinated nitroimidazole probes by ^{19}F magnetic resonance spectroscopy in vivo. *Int. J. Radiat. Oncol. Biol. Phys.* **16**, 925–929.

163. Jin, G.-Y., Li, S.-J., Moulder, J. E., and Raleigh, J. A. (1990) Dynamic measurements of hexafluoromisonidazole (CCI-103F) retention in mouse tumours by ^{1}H/^{19}F magnetic resonance spectroscopy. *Int. J. Radiat. Biol.* **58**, 1025–1034.

164. Aboagye, E. O., Maxwell, R. J., Horsman, M. R., et al. (1998) The relationship between tumour oxygenation determined by oxygen electrode measurements and magnetic resonance spectroscopy of the fluorinated 2-nitroimidazole SR-4554. *Br. J. Cancer* **77**, 65–70.

165. Aboagye, E. O., Maxwell, R. J., Kelson, A. B., et al. (1997) Preclinical evaluation of the fluorinated 2-nitroimidazole *N*-(2-hydroxy-3,3,3-trifluoropropyl)-2-(2-nitro-1-imidazolyl) acetamide (SR-4554) as a probe for the measurement of tumour hypoxia. *Cancer Res.* **57**, 3314–3318.

166. Aboagye, E. O., Kelson, A. B., Tracy, M., and Workman, P. (1998) Preclinical development and current status of the fluorinated 2-nitroimidazole hypoxia probe *N*-(2-hydroxy-3,3,3-trifluoropropyl)-2-(2-nitro-1-imidazolyl) acetamide (SR-4554, CRC 94/17): a non-invasive diagnostic probe for the measurement of tumour hypoxia by magnetic resonance spectroscopy and imaging, and by positron emission tomography. *Anti-Cancer Drug Des.* **13**, 703–730.

167. Seddon, B. M., Payne, G. S., Simmons, L., et al. (2002) Phase I pharmacokinetic and magnetic resonance spectroscopic study of the non-invasive hypoxia probe SR-4554. *Proc. Am. Soc. Clin. Oncol.* **21,** 91b (abstract).

Index

Acyclovir, *see* Thymidine kinase
Adenovirus vectors,
  genomic mutation induction, 482, 483
  liver toxicity, 484–486
  liver tumor targeting, *see* Liver tumors
  nitroreductase delivery, *see*
    Nitroreductase
  nonreplicating vector generation and
    testing,
    approaches, 61
    E1/E3 deletion, 61
    materials, 63–65, 69
    plasmid construction, 65, 69
    promoter analysis using luciferase
      expression vector,
      in vitro analysis, 67, 68, 70
      in vivo analysis, 68, 70
    promoter for transgene expression,
      61, 63
    shuttle plasmid, 61, 62
    suicide gene therapy efficacy
      studies with thymidine kinase/
      ganciclovir,
      in vitro, 68, 70
      in vivo, 69, 70
    vector generation, 65–67, 69, 70
  preexisting immunity, 481, 482
  replication-competent virus
    emergence and safety, 480,
    481
  replication-selective oncolytic viruses
    as vectors,
    bioluminescence imaging in vivo,
      data analysis, 80
      luciferase-expressing virus
        construction, 76, 88
      materials, 73
      rationale, 72, 73

      small mammal imaging, 79, 80,
      88
      testing of viral constructs in vivo,
      78, 79
      verification of results ex vivo, 80
      viral construct design
        considerations, 76–78, 88
    colorectal cancer clinical trials,
      assessment criteria, 87, 88
      assignment to treatment arm and
        dose cohort, 86
      exclusion criteria, 84, 86
      inclusion criteria, 84, 88
      objectives, 83, 84, 88
      overview, 73
      phase I dose escalation scheme,
      86, 88
      phase II, 87
      rationale, 83, 88
    cytotoxic chemotherapy drug
      interaction studies,
      cell culture, 74, 87
      cell killing assay, 74, 75
      cisplatin, 74–76, 87
      data analysis, 75, 76
      drug preparation, 74, 87
      materials, 73
      paclitaxel, 74–76, 87
      rationale, 72
      sequencing studies, 75, 88
    overview, 39, 71
  toxicity, 480
ADEPT, *see* Antibody-directed enzyme
    prodrug therapy
Antibody-directed enzyme prodrug
    therapy (ADEPT),
  advantages over antibody-directed
    cancer therapy, 491, 492

antibody engineering rationale, 494, 495

carboxypeptidase G2 systems, *see* Carboxypeptidase G2

β-glucuronidase utilization, 306, 307

historical perspective, 491, 492

single-chain Fv antibody-carboxypeptidase G2 fusion protein production,

bacterial production, 497

overview, 495–497

yeast production, 497, 498

single-chain Fv antibody production,

agarose gel electrophoresis, 501

cDNA preparation, 502, 503

library characterization with enzyme-linked immunosorbent assay, 509, 510

ligation reactions, 505, 506

materials, 498–500

overview, 495

polymerase chain reaction, 503–505

restriction enzyme digestion, 505

selection of phage antibodies using biotinylated antigens, 507–l509

splenic lymphocyte RNA extraction, 501, 502

transformation, 506, 507

vector preparation, 505

AQ4N, bioreductive prodrug properties, 527

Bioluminescence imaging in vivo, *see* Adenovirus vectors

Bioreductive prodrugs, *see* Prodrugs

Breast cancer, cytosine deaminase/5-fluorocytosine system studies,

cytosine deaminase immunocytochemistry, 454, 456

cytosine deaminase *in situ* hybridization,

autoradiography, 456

hybridization, 455, 456

probe synthesis, 455, 457

slide preparation, 454, 455, 457

erbB-2 immunocytochemistry, 453, 454

materials, 452, 453

overview, 451, 452

thin-layer chromatography assay of cytosine deaminase, 456, 457

Bystander effects,

comparison of systems, 12–14

CYP2B1/cyclophosphamide system, 208, 209

enzyme subcellular targeting, *see* Carboxypeptidase G2; Nitroreductase

immune effect, 20, 21

immune responses, *see* Immune response, suicide gene therapy

improvement strategies, 19, 20

mechanisms, 18, 19, 404, 405

multicellular layer assays,

activator and target cell characteristics, 408

cell lines, 409

culture,

collagen-coated insert with polyethylene float preparation, 413, 414, 424, 425

seeding and growth, 414, 425

limitations, 405, 406

materials, 406, 408, 410–412

multicellular layer characterization,

cell number, 415

electrical impedance spectroscopy, 415

flux markers, 415, 425

hematoxylin and eosin staining, 417

histology of frozen sections, 416

histology of paraffin sections, 416, 417

principles, 405, 406
survival analysis, 417–420, 425–427
validation of differential plating
assays, 412
prodrug optimization, 188, 189
purine nucleoside phosphorylase/
prodrug systems, 223, 224,
240, 242
thymidine phosphorylase/5'-deoxy-5-
fluorouridine system, 263, 264,
272–274, 276
tumor xenograft assay, 420–424, 427

Carboxylesterase/CPT-11 system,
carboxylase selection,
computer prediction of substrate
specificity, 251–253
human enzymes, 250, 251
rabbit liver enzyme, 249, 250
characterization,
CPT-11 and metabolite extraction
from biological samples, 257
enzyme activity assay,
calculations, 260
fluorometric assay, 257, 260
high-performance liquid
chromatography of
metabolites, 257
spectrophotometric assay, 258
materials, 256, 257
clinical applications and prospects,
255, 256
comparison with other systems, 253–
255
CPT-11 activation, toxicity, and
metabolites, 248, 249
overview, 247, 248
tumor cell line studies, 253
Carboxypeptidase G2 (CPG2),
antibody-directed enzyme prodrug
therapy,
antibody engineering rationale, 494,
495
clinical trials, 494

fusion protein production of single-
chain Fv antibody-
carboxypeptidase G2
bacterial production, 497
overview, 495–497
yeast production, 497, 498
principles, 491–493
single-chain Fv antibody
production,
agarose gel electrophoresis,
501
cDNA preparation, 502, 503
library characterization with
enzyme-linked immunosorbent
assay, 509, 510
ligation reactions, 505, 506
materials, 498–500
overview, 495
polymerase chain reaction, 503–
505
restriction enzyme digestion,
505
selection of phage antibodies
using biotinylated antigens,
507–509
splenic lymphocyte RNA
extraction, 501, 502
transformation, 506, 507
vector preparation, 505
bystander effect modulation with
subcellular localization, 289,
290
characterization of prodrug system,
antitumor efficacy in mice, 296,
297
bystander cytotoxicity assay, 292,
298
cytotoxicity assay, 292, 298
cytotoxicity assay for prodrug
comparison,
cell dilution, 294
plate preparation, 293, 294
plate staining and scoring, 294,
295

prodrug dosing of cells, 293, 294
enzyme activity assays,
    cell extracts, 291, 292
    tissues, 295, 296
    materials, 291, 298
glycosylation site modification, 284–
    286, 297, 298
methotrexate high-performance liquid
    chromatography assay, 500,
    501, 510, 511
prodrugs, 283, 493
signal peptide,
    deletion, 283
    receptor tyrosine kinase sequence
        utilization, 283, 284
    structure, 283
    transfection, 283, 297
tumor killing assays with prodrugs,
    286, 287
Cationic liposomes, *see* Lipofection
CB1954,
    bioreductive prodrug properties, 528–
        530
    nitroreductase activation, *see*
        Nitroreductase
Clostridium, overview of vectors, 37
Colorectal cancer, adenovirus vector
    clinical trials,
    assessment criteria, 87, 88
    assignment to treatment arm and dose
        cohort, 86
    exclusion criteria, 84, 86
    inclusion criteria, 84, 88
    objectives, 83, 84, 88
    overview, 73
    phase I dose escalation scheme, 86, 88
    phase II, 87
    rationale, 83, 88
Combination suicide gene therapy, *see*
    Cytosine deaminase;
    Thymidine kinase
CPG2, *see* Carboxypeptidase G2
CPT-11, *see* Carboxylesterase/CPT-11
    system

Cyclophosphamide, *see* Cytochrome P450
CYP, *see* Cytochrome P450
Cytochrome P450 (CYP),
    anticancer drug metabolism,
        cyclophosphamide, 203–205
        ifosfamide, 203, 205
        overview, 203, 204
    carcinogen activation, 203
    clinical trials of prodrug systems, 217,
        218
    CYP2B1/cyclophosphamide system,
        antiangiogenic scheduling of
            cyclophosphamide, 215, 216
        bystander effects, 208, 209
        clinical utility, 206, 207
        coexpression with P450 reductase,
            213, 214
        gene delivery with encapsulated
            cells or macrophages, 216
        gene delivery with replicating
            viruses, 209–211
        prodrug delivery with polymers,
            212, 213
        suppression of liver prodrug
            activation, 214, 215
        synergy with other gene therapies,
            211, 212
    CYP4B1/4-ipomeanol system, 216, 217
    prospects for prodrug systems, 217
    types, 203
Cytofectin, *see* Lipofection
Cytosine deaminase/5-fluorocytosine
        system,
    breast cancer studies,
        overview, 451, 452
        materials, 452, 453
        erbB-2 immunocytochemistry, 453,
            454
        cytosine deaminase
            immunocytochemistry, 454,
            456
        cytosine deaminase *in situ*
            hybridization,
            autoradiography, 456

hybridization, 455, 456
probe synthesis, 455, 457
slide preparation, 454, 455, 457
thin-layer chromatography assay of
cytosine deaminase, 456, 457
bystander effect, 354
combination suicide gene therapy with
thymidine kinase,
bystander effect analysis, 349, 351
cytotoxicity assay, 349, 351
materials, 346–349
overview, 346
rationale, 345, 346
retrovirus generation, 348–351
transfection of retroviral plasmids
into packaging cells, 348, 350
tumor cell transduction, 349
immune responses, 361–363
liver tumor targeting,
adenovirus vector, 435, 436
bystander effects, 435
mechanisms, 451
optimization for prodrug activation,
331, 332
Cytotoxicity differential, prodrug
optimization, 184–187

5'-Deoxy-5-fluorouridine, *see*
Thymidine phosphorylase/5'-
deoxy-5-fluorouridine system

ELISA, *see* Enzyme-linked
immunosorbent assay
Enzyme-linked immunosorbent assay
(ELISA),
phage display antibody library
characterization, 509, 510
4-methylumbelliferyl β-D-glucuronide
staining with solid-phase
enzyme-linked immunosorbent
assay, 320, 323, 324
Enzyme random mutagenesis, *see*
Random sequence
mutagenesis

Enzyme subcellular targeting, *see*
Carboxypeptidase G2;
Nitroreductase
EO9, bioreductive prodrug properties, 525
ErbB-2, immunocytochemistry, 453, 454

Flow cytometry,
horseradish peroxidase/indole-3-acetic
acid system analysis of gene
expression,
CD2, 381
green fluorescent protein, 382, 384
radiation-responsive gene therapy
vector analysis of green
fluorescent protein reporter,
397
5-Fluorocytosine, *see* Cytosine
deaminase/5-fluorocytosine
system
5-Fluorouracil, *see* Uracil
phosphoribosyltransferase/5-
fluorouracil system

Ganciclovir, *see* Thymidine kinase
GDEPT, *see* Gene-directed enzyme
prodrug therapy
Gene-directed enzyme prodrug therapy
(GDEPT), see also specific
systems,
advantages, 2
bioreductive prodrug approaches, 529,
530
bystander effects, *see* Bystander
effects
challenges, 2
enzyme-prodrug systems,
classification, 3
prodrug types, 3, 4
requirements, 2, 3
summary of, 6–10
immune response, 20, 21
multiple gene transfection systems, 15
nomenclature, 1, 2
overview, 1, 2, 279, 280, 353, 434

potentiation and synergistic effects in
    efficiency improvement, 16, 17
prodrugs, see Prodrugs
prospects, 21, 22
quantitative parameters in comparative
    analysis, 4, 5
radiosensitization in efficiency
    improvement, 17, 18
vectors, see Vectors
GFP, see Green fluorescent protein
β-Glucuronidase,
    antibody-directed enzyme prodrug
        therapy, 306, 307
    deficiency and treatment of
        mucopolysaccharidosis type
        VII, 308–310
    endogenous expression, 303, 305
    function, 305
    gene-directed enzyme prodrug therapy,
        307, 308
    prodrug specificity, 303, 304
    structure, 305
    subcellular localization of forms,
        ELF-97 β-D-glucuronide staining,
            fixation, 317
            staining, 317, 318
        HMR 1826 staining, 320, 321, 323,
            324
        immunoprecipitation, gel
            electrophoresis, and
            radiography, 313
        materials, 310–312, 323
        4-methylumbelliferyl β-D-
            glucuronide staining,
            cell extract preparation, 319
            organ extract preparation, 319
            overview, 318, 319
            quantitative analysis, 319, 323
            solid-phase enzyme-linked
                immunosorbent assay, 320,
                323, 324
        naphthol AS-BI β-D-glucuronide
            staining,
            fixation, 315, 316

staining, 316, 317
    radioactive labeling and saponin
        extraction, 312, 313
    X-gluc staining,
        fixation, 313–315, 323
        staining, 315
    tumor targeting, 305, 306
Green fluorescent protein (GFP), imaging
    of transgene expression, 18,
    382, 384, 394, 395, 399

Hepatocellular carcinoma, see Liver
    tumors
Herpes simplex virus (HSV),
    replication-selective viruses as vectors,
        38, 39
    thymidine kinase, see Thymidine
        kinase
Horseradish peroxidase/indole-3-acetic
    acid system,
    clinical utility, 5
    hypoxia-induced system,
        alkaline comet assay of DNA
            fragmentation, 382, 383
        cell culture, 379, 383
        flow cytometry analysis of gene
            expression,
            CD2, 381
            green fluorescent protein, 382,
                384
        hypoxia-responsive promoters, 380
        hypoxic condition induction in
            vitro, 379, 380, 383, 384
        materials, 378, 379, 383
        prodrug activation assay, 383, 384
        transfection, 380, 381, 384
    overview, 5
HSV, see Herpes simplex virus
Hypoxia,
    bioreductive prodrugs in targeted
        therapy, 520, 521, 531, 532
    chemotherapy resistance of tumors,
        519
    gene control, 372, 516, 517

gene-directed enzyme prodrug therapy system selection, 377, 378
gene therapy targeting using hypoxia-responsive elements, 374–376
horseradish peroxidase/indole-3-acetic acid system induction,
  alkaline comet assay of DNA fragmentation, 382, 383
  cell culture, 379, 383
  flow cytometry analysis of gene expression,
    CD2, 381
    green fluorescent protein, 382, 384
  hypoxia-responsive promoters, 380
  hypoxic condition induction in vitro, 379, 380, 383, 384
  materials, 378, 379, 383
  prodrug activation assay, 383, 384
  transfection, 380, 381, 384
hypoxia-inducible factor-1
  activation, 372, 373, 516
  dysregulation in tumors, 517, 518
  responsive element binding, 373
  structure, 516
p53 induction, 518
radiation resistance of tumors, 518, 519
reporter gene selection for gene expression studies, 376, 377
tumor biology, 516
tumor environment and prognosis, 371, 372, 519

Immune response, suicide gene therapy,
  cytosine deaminase/5-fluorocytosine system, 361–363
  preexisting immunity to viral vectors, 481, 482
  prospects for immune modulation, 363, 364
  thymidine kinase, 483
  thymidine kinase/ganciclovir system,
    bystander effect contributions, 354, 355
    controversial mechanisms, 359–361
    mouse studies, 355, 356
    natural killer cell response, 359
    T-cell-mediated responses, 357, 358
    tumor immunity induction, 356, 357
Indole-3-acetic acid, *see* Horseradish peroxidase/indole-3-acetic acid system
4-Ipomeanol, *see* Cytochrome P450
Irinotecan, *see* Carboxylesterase/CPT-11 system

Lipofection,
  barriers to efficient transfection, 113
  cytofectin structures, 108–111
  LPDII system, 124–126
  neutral liposome systems, 123
  pH-sensitive systems, 124
  platform technologies, 120–123
  prospects, 127, 128
  structure-activity studies, 116–118
  systems and formulations, 107, 112
  ternary transfection systems, 118–120
  virosome system, 126, 127
Liver tumors,
  clinical trial protocol for nitroreductase/CB1954 system,
    biological sample collection, 473
    dose-limiting toxicity, 474
    histological examination, 473, 474
    maximum tolerated dose, 474
    objectives, 471
    prodrug administration, 472, 473
    study design, 471, 472
    surgical resection, 473
    tumor injection, 472
    virus preparation, 472
  cytosine deaminase/5-fluorocytosine system,
    adenovirus vector, 435, 436
    bystander effects, 435

promoters for gene therapy, 434, 435
thymidine kinase/ganciclovir system,
    adenovirus vectors, 435, 447, 448
    bystander effects, 434, 435
    clinical trial protocol,
        adverse event reporting, 445,
            446
        aims, 437
        clinical efficacy analysis, 446,
            447
        dosing, 443, 444
        ethanol injection group, 444
        exclusion criteria, 439
        follow-up, 445
        gene transfer efficiency analysis,
            446
        immediate monitoring, 445
        inclusion criteria, 439
        inform and consent, 440–443
        pharmacokinetic analysis, 446
        phase I trial, 437, 438
        prestudy evaluation and
            treatment, 440
        public health considerations, 447
        regulatory guidelines, 436, 437
        removal from study, 446
        response criteria, 446
        risk assessment, 438, 439
        route of administration, 438, 443
        study design, 438
        survival analysis, 447
        timeline, 444, 445
        toxicity assessment, 445
Loligomer,
    DNA complex preparation, 155
    DNA weight and charge ratio, 152,
        153
    endosomal escape enhancement, 153,
        154
    multivalent DNA targeting molecule
        advantages, 151, 152
    preparation, 154
    purification, 154, 155
    structure, 152

Magnetic resonance spectroscopy (MRS),
    imaging of transgene
        expression, 18
Methotrexate high-performance liquid
    chromatography assay,
        carboxypeptidase G2, 500, 501,
            510, 511
Midkine promoter, tumor expression and
    suicide gene therapy
        utilization, 39, 40
Mitomycin C, bioreductive prodrug
    properties, 521, 525
MPS VII, *see* Mucopolysaccharidosis
    type VII
MRS, *see* Magnetic resonance
    spectroscopy
Mucopolysaccharidosis type VII (MPS
    VII),
    cell-based therapy, 309
    enzyme replacement therapy, 309
    gene therapy, 309, 310
    β-glucuronidase deficiency, 308, 309
Multicellular layers, *see* Bystander effects

Nitracine N-oxide, bioreductive prodrug
    properties, 527
Nitroreductase (NR),
    adenovirus vector delivery,
        bulk preparation of vectors, 466,
            475
        CB1954 cytotoxicity assays, 469
        cell culture, 464
        clinical trial protocol for liver
            tumors
            biological sample collection,
                473
            dose-limiting toxicity, 474
            histological examination, 473,
                474
            maximum tolerated dose, 474
            objectives, 471
            prodrug administration, 472,
                473
            study design, 471, 472

surgical resection, 473
tumor injection, 472
virus preparation, 472
direct intratumoral injection, 470
intraperitoneal delivery, 470, 471
materials, 462, 463
overview, 461, 462
plaque assay of viral infectivity,
468
safety considerations, 475, 476
vector construction, 466, 475
viral particle number determination,
467, 468
virus banding, 466, 467
CB1954 as prodrug, 459–461
multicellular layer assays of bystander
effects in gene-directed
enzyme prodrug therapy,
activator and target cell
characteristics, 408
cell lines, 409
culture,
collagen-coated insert with
polyethylene float preparation,
413, 414, 424, 425
seeding and growth, 414, 425
limitations, 405, 406
materials, 406, 408, 410–412
multicellular layer characterization,
cell number, 415
electrical impedance
spectroscopy, 415
flux markers, 415, 425
hematoxylin and eosin staining,
417
histology of frozen sections, 416
histology of paraffin sections,
416, 417
principles, 405, 406
survival analysis, 417–420, 425–
427
validation of differential plating
assays, 412
prodrugs, 287, 403, 404

retroviral vector delivery,
cancer cell line transduction, 465
CB1954 cytotoxicity assays, 465,
475
cell culture, 464
materials, 462, 463
mouse xenograft expression, 469,
470
overview, 461
packaging cell line production and
infection of target cells, 464,
465, 475
plasmid construction, 464, 474
retroviral supernatant
concentration, 465
safety considerations, 475
structure, 287
subcellular localization, 287, 289,
290, 291
tumor xenograft assay of bystander
effects in gene-directed
enzyme prodrug therapy, 420–
424, 427
Western blot analysis of expression, 469
NR, *see* Nitroreductase

Osteocalcin promoter, tumor expression
and suicide gene therapy
utilization, 40

p53, hypoxia induction, 518
Peptide-based polymer vectors, *see*
Loligomer; Polycation vectors
PET, *see* Positron emission tomography
PNP, *see* Purine nucleoside
phosphorylase
Polycation vectors, *see also* Loligomer,
DNA complex preparation, 145, 146
DNA stabilization, 140
endosomal escape enhancement, 147–
149
local tissue administration, 146, 147
nuclear targeting, 149, 150
overview, 41

peptides in cell targeting, 140, 143,
    150–152
poly-L-lysine,
    charge ratio, 141
    hydrolysis, 140
    internalization of DNA complexes,
        141
    polyamidoamine dendrimers, 142, 143
    polyethyleneimine, 141
    prospects, 155
    receptor-specific ligand attachment, 147
    size considerations, 143, 145
    suppliers, 145
    virus mimicry properties, 139
Porfiromycin, bioreductive prodrug
        properties, 525
Positron emission tomography (PET),
        imaging of transgene
        expression, 18
Prodrugs, *see also specific systems,*
    activation reactions,
        α,β-elimination, 170
        hydrolytic functional group
            transformation, 166
        nucleotide phosphorylation, 166
        oxidation, 169
        reduction, 166, 167, 169
        ribosyl transfer, 169
    bioreductive prodrugs,
        AQ4N, 527
        CB1954, 528–530
        classification, 520–523
        clinical response prediction, 530,
            531
        definition, 520
        EO9, 525
        gene-directed enzyme prodrug
            therapy approaches, 529, 530
        hypoxia-targeted therapy, 520, 521,
            531, 532
        mitomycin C, 521, 525
        nitracine N-oxide, 527
        novel quinone identification, 526
        porfiromycin, 525

prospects, 531, 532
prospects, 531, 532
RB6145, 528
RH1, 525
RSU1069, 528
SN23862, 528–530
SN24771, 529
structures, 524
tirapazamine, 526, 527
tumor oxidation state effects, 515
design,
    advantages over using known
        drugs, 164, 165
    optimization approaches, 163, 164
    overview, 15, 16
direct prodrug features, 170–173
ideal criteria, 161–163
optimization,
    bystander effect, 188, 189
    cytotoxicity, 187, 188
    cytotoxicity differential, 184–187
    kinetics of activation,
        enzyme improvement, 190, 191
        parameters, 190
        prodrug design, 191, 192
    pharmacological properties, 192, 193
    physiochemical properties, 192, 193
    stability, 189, 190
prospects, 193
safety considerations, 483, 484
self-immolative prodrug,
    activation reactions,
        cyclization, 177, 178
        1,2-elimination, 177
        1,4-elimination, 175, 176
        1,6-elimination, 174, 175
    advantages, 173, 174
    definition, 173
    structural considerations in design,
        178–181, 183
    types and enzyme reactions, 182
types, 3, 4, 163, 164
Purine nucleoside phosphorylase (PNP),
        Escherichia coli enzyme/
        prodrug systems,

bystander effect activity, 223, 224,
240, 242
cell killing mechanism, 224, 232,
233
clinical studies,
in vitro tumor cell killing, 233
in vivo tumor cell killing using
retroviral gene delivery, 233
comparison with other systems, 231,
232
dosing, 234, 240
large tumor efficacy, 225
nonproliferating cell targeting, 224,
226–228, 242
optimization, 229–231
overview, 223
potency, 224
prodrug specificity, 225, 227, 228
treatment period, 224, 238, 240

Radiation therapy,
cancer treatment, 389
gene expression response, 389, 390
responsive gene therapy vectors,
construction and characterization,
cell culture, 394, 399
cell growth inhibition assay with
thymidine kinase/ganciclovir
system, 397, 400, 401
flow cytometry analysis of
green fluorescent protein, 397
green fluorescent protein reporter
gene cloning, 394, 395, 399
irradiation of cells, 397, 400
materials, 391–394
radiation-responsive gene
enhancer cloning, 395, 396,
399
transfection, 396, 397, 400
overview, 390
promoters,
sequences, 390
synthetic gene promoters, 390,
391

Random sequence mutagenesis,
competent cell preparation and
transformation, 338, 343
DNA shuffling, 339, 340, 343
double-stranded DNA preparation
from oligonucleotides, 335,
336, 342
error-prone polymerase chain reaction,
339, 343
extension, 336, 342
ligation, 337, 338, 343
materials, 333, 335, 341, 342
polymerase chain reaction of extended
products, 336, 337, 342
primer design, 341
primerless polymerase chain reaction
and reamplification of
products, 340, 343
principles, 332–334
rationale, 331, 332
restriction digestion, 337
selection of transformants, 338, 339
vector preparation, 337, 342, 343
RB6145, bioreductive prodrug properties,
528
Retroviral vectors,
characterization, 93
clinical utility, 93
combination suicide gene therapy, *see*
Cytosine deaminase/5-
fluorocytosine system;
Thymidine kinase
construction,
cell infection and vector
production, 101, 102
characterization, 102
concentrating of vectors, 102, 103,
105
helper virus screening, 102, 105
materials, 93, 94, 96
packaging cell systems, 95
plasmid design and construction,
96, 97, 104
producer cell generation,
preliminary screening, 99

titer determination with
selectable markers, 98, 99, 104
titer determination with Southern
blot, 99–101, 104
transfection and selection, 97, 98,
104
transient virus production, 101
design, 91, 92
nitroreductase delivery, *see*
Nitroreductase
packaging system, 92, 93
virus types, 91
RH1, bioreductive prodrug properties,
525
RSU1069, bioreductive prodrug
properties, 528

Salmonella,
advantages in tumor targeting, 47, 48
overview of vectors, 37
safety of vectors, 49
VNP2009 vector,
advantages, 48
construction,
materials, 49, 50
mutagenization and clone
selection, 50
transposon insertion and Bochner
selection, 50, 51, 57
YS1643 derivation, 51, 52
YS1644 clone selection, 52, 57
YS1645 derivation, 53
YS1646 derivation, 53, 57
prospects, 56
tumor inhibition assay, 55, 56
tumor targeting assay, 53, 55
Self-immolative prodrugs, *see* Prodrugs
Site-directed mutagenesis,
enzymes in gene-directed enzyme
prodrug therapy, 11
random mutagenesis, *see* Random
sequence mutagenesis
SN23862, bioreductive prodrug
properties, 528–530

SN24771, bioreductive prodrug
properties, 529
Southern blot, retroviral vector titering,
99–101, 104

Thymidine kinase (TK),
combination suicide gene therapy with
cytosine deaminase,
bystander effect analysis, 349, 351
cytotoxicity assay, 349, 351
materials, 346–349
overview, 346
rationale, 345, 346
retrovirus generation, 348–351
transfection of retroviral plasmids
into packaging cells, 348, 350
tumor cell transduction, 349
engineering for kinetic optimization,
282
fusion with other prodrug-activating
enzymes, 282
ganciclovir system,
assays with adenovirus vector,
in vitro, 68, 70
in vivo, 69, 70
immune responses,
bystander effect contributions,
354, 355
controversial mechanisms, 359–
361
mouse studies, 355, 356
natural killer cell response, 359
T-cell-mediated responses, 357,
358
tumor immunity induction, 356,
357
liver toxicity with adenoviral
vectors, 484–486
liver tumor targeting, *see* Liver
tumors
radiation-responsive gene therapy
vectors, *see* Radiation therapy
immune responses, 483
novel prodrug design, 16

potentiation and synergistic effects in
efficiency improvement, 16, 17
prodrugs, 353, 354
VP22 fusion protein, 281, 282
Thymidine phosphorylase/5'-deoxy-5-
fluorouridine system,
bystander effect, 263, 264
delivery and characterization,
cell sensitivity assay,
bystander effect analysis, 272–
274, 276
neutral red assay, 270, 271, 276
enzyme activity assay,
cell lysis, 267, 268, 274, 275
spectrophotometric assay, 268,
269, 275
materials, 265, 266, 274
prodrug metabolite determination,
cell treatment and cytosol
isolation, 269, 276
high-performance liquid
chromatography, 270, 274
stable transfection, 266, 267, 275
enzyme features and functions, 263
Tirapazamine, bioreductive prodrug
properties, 526, 527
TK, *see* Thymidine kinase
Tyrosinase/prodrug systems, overview, 5

Uracil phosphoribosyltransferase/5-
fluorouracil system, overview,
5, 11

Vascular endothelial growth factor
(VEGF) promoter,, 40
Vectors, *see also specific vectors*,
bacteria, 37
hypoxia-responsive gene therapy
vectors, *see* Hypoxia
nonviral vectors, 40, 41
radiation-responsive gene therapy
vectors, *see* Radiation therapy
safety and side effects of viral vectors,
genome mutation induction, 482, 483
preexisting immunity, 481, 482
replication-competent virus
emergence, 480, 481
vector shedding, 481
vector-related toxicity, 480
transfection efficiencies, comparison
of vectors, 29–36
viruses,
conditionally replicating virus
development, 486
Coxsackie and adenovirus receptor-
independent delivery, 37, 38
hybrid vectors, 41
promoter-specific expression, 39, 40
replication-selective viruses, 38, 39
selection considerations, 281
VEGF, *see* Vascular endothelial growth
factor promoter
VNP2009, *see Salmonella*

Western blot, nitroreductase, 469

Lightning Source UK Ltd.
Milton Keynes UK
UKOW04f1502310315

248862UK00001B/1/P